CLINICAL MANAGEMENT AND EVOLVING NOVEL THERAPEUTIC STRATEGIES FOR PATIENTS WITH BRAIN TUMORS

Edited by **Terry Lichtor**

Clinical Management and Evolving Novel Therapeutic Strategies for Patients with Brain Tumors
http://dx.doi.org/10.5772/45956
Edited by Terry Lichtor

Contributors

Kost Elisevich, Ryuya Yamanaka, Mihail - Lucian Pascu, Pinar Atukeren, M.Ramazan Yigitoglu, Zamzuri Idris, Jafri Malin Abdullah, Rahman I Ghani, Muzaimi Mustapha, Badrisyah Idris, W M Nazaruddin W Hassan, Maysa Al-Hussaini, Kalkanis, Sanjay Patra, Jiro Akimoto, Hala Mostafa Goma, Amr Abo Ela, Jarosław Paluch, Jarosław Markowski, Agnieszka Piotrowska - Seweryn, Joanna Lewin-Kowalik, Włodzimierz Dziubdziela, Maciej Kajor, Czesław Zralek, Robert Kwiatkowski, Jan Pilch, Yasushi Shibata, Domenico La Torre, Adrianna Ranger, Concetta Alafaci, Alfredo Conti, Francesco Tomasello, Milena Cankovic, Kamil Zeleňák, Viera Cisáriková, Hubert Poláček, Takeshi Okuda, Avila, Mitsutoshi Nakada, Edivaldo De Oliveira, Fabio Da Silva, Andrej Pala, Marc-Eric Halatsch, Georg Karpel-Massler, Christian Rainer Wirtz, Mark M. Souweidane, Zhiping Zhou, Rui Reis, Gerardo Caruso, Francesca Granata, Mariella Caffo, Mariano Cutugno, Francesco Maria Salpietro, Shinji Kohsaka, Shinya Tanaka, George Theodore, Lynn Feun

Published by InTech

Janeza Trdine 9, 51000 Rijeka, Croatia

Notice

Publishing Process Manager Iva Simcic
Technical Editor InTech DTP team
Cover InTech Design team

Additional hard copies can be obtained from orders@intechopen.com

Clinical Management and Evolving Novel Therapeutic Strategies for Patients with Brain Tumors, Edited by Terry Lichtor
p. cm.
ISBN 978-953-51-1058-3

For EU product safety concerns:
IN TECH d.o.o., Prolaz Marije Krucifikse Kozulić 3, 51000 Rijeka, Croatia,
info@intechopen.com or visit our website at intechopen.com.

Meet the editor

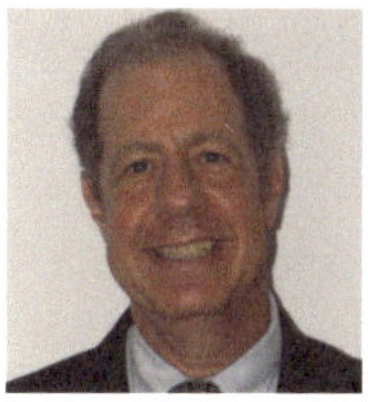

Dr. Lichtor is a practicing neurosurgeon. He has a number of research interests, and his brain tumor work is largely focused on the development of a DNA vaccine for treatment of primary and metastatic intracerebral tumors. In particular Dr. Lichtor has shown that vaccines prepared by transfer of DNA from the tumor into a highly immunogenic cell line can encompass the array of tumor antigens that characterize the patient's neoplasm. Poorly immunogenic tumor antigens, characteristic of malignant cells, can become strongly antigenic if they are expressed by highly immunogenic cells. The introduction of the vaccine directly into the tumor bed of animals with an intracerebral tumor stimulates a systemic cellular anti-tumor immune response associated with a prolongation of survival. It is hopeful that this vaccine strategy will be efficacious in the treatments of patients with brain tumors. Dr. Lichtor is a member of the neurosurgery faculty at Rush University Medical Center in Chicago, Illinois.

Contents

Preface

Although technical advances have resulted in marked improvements in the ability to diagnose and surgically treat primary and metastatic brain tumors, the incidence and mortality rates of these tumors is increasing. Particularly affected are young adults and the elderly. The present standard treatment modalities following surgical resection including cranial irradiation and systemic or local chemotherapy each have limited efficacy and serious adverse side effects. Furthermore the relatively few long-term survivors are inevitably left with cognitive deficits and other disabilities. The difficulties in treating malignant gliomas can be attributed to several factors. Glial tumors are inherently resistant to radiation and standard cytotoxic chemotherapies. The existence of blood-brain and blood-tumor barriers impede drug delivery to the tumor and adjacent brain infiltrated with tumor. In addition the low therapeutic index between tumor sensitivity and toxicity to normal brain severely limits the ability to systemically deliver therapeutic doses of drugs or radiation therapy to the tumor. New treatment strategies for the management of patients with these tumors are urgently needed.

In this book a review of the important features involving the clinical management of patients with these tumors are outlined. In addition advances in radiology both for pre-operative diagnostic purposes along with surgical planning are described. Furthermore a review of newer developments in chemotherapy along with the evolving field of photodynamic therapy both for intra-operative management and subsequent therapy is provided. Hopefully this information coupled with advances in the understanding of the pathology and molecular biology of brain tumors which are also outlined in this book will translate into additional novel therapeutic treatment strategies that should lead to the prolongation of survival without a decline in cognitive functions or other side effects in patients with brain tumors.

Dr. Terry Lichtor
Rush Medical College,
Department of Neurosurgery,
Chicago, United States of America

Section 1

Radiologic Issues Relevant to Brain Tumors

Chapter 1

Navigated Brain Stimulation (NBS) for Pre-Surgical Planning of Brain Lesion in Critical Areas: Basic Principles and Early Experience

Concetta Alafaci, Alfredo Conti and
Francesco Tomasello

Additional information is available at the end of the chapter

http://dx.doi.org/10.5772/53216

1. Introduction

Modern neurosurgery attempts to get the difficult goal of combining an "aggressive" resection of brain tumors with the fundamental purpose of preserving brain functions and best possible quality of life.

One of the most important evolutions of neurosurgical therapies is the opportunity to provide a customized surgical intervention by using modern methods to "map" the eloquent areas of the brain. This allows the identification of brain functional areas to be preserved from possible inadvertent intraoperative damage.

Direct cortical stimulation (DCS) is an intraoperative technique that uses electrodes placed directly on the exposed cortical surface of the brain to stimulate activity of functional areas by simultaneously recording the evoked responses peripherally. DCS is very precise and reliable and can be considered the gold standard in brain mapping and intraoperative functional monitoring. Nevertheless, the neurosurgeon discovers the spatial relationship between the disease and eloquent cortical surfaces only after having completed a craniotomy and dural opening.

A pre-surgical mapping method would give the opportunity to plan the treatment of brain diseases optimizing many aspects of the surgical treatment, including patient positioning, type of anesthesia, size of craniotomy, and extent of resection. Moreover, pre-surgical mapping would allow more precise prediction of the efficacy and risks of treatments that can be discussed with the patient and influence the therapeutic strategy.

New techniques have been proposed in an attempt to provide a reliable method for the functional study that can be, however, exploited pre-operatively. The most recent of these methods of mapping cortical activities is navigated brain stimulation (NBS), which is based on the neurophysiological technique of transcranial magnetic stimulation (TMS) of the cerebral cortex combined with the conventional neuronavigation. Basic principles of NBS will be here discussed together with our preliminary experience using this technique in different neurosurgical diseases.

2. Navigated Brain Stimulation for mapping the motor system

Navigated brain stimulation is a technique for mapping the motor cortex using a transcranial magnetic stimulation (TMS) of brain areas. In NBS, conventional TMS is combined with a sophisticated neuronavigation software that allows the navigation of each single "stimulated" point in the cortex. The electromagnetic stimulus delivered by the TMS coil overcomes the activation threshold of the underlying motor neurons, so that the impulse may propagate to the corticospinal tract determining a muscle contraction. Muscles responses to electric field (motor evoked potential, MEP) are recorded using EMG channels (Figure 1).

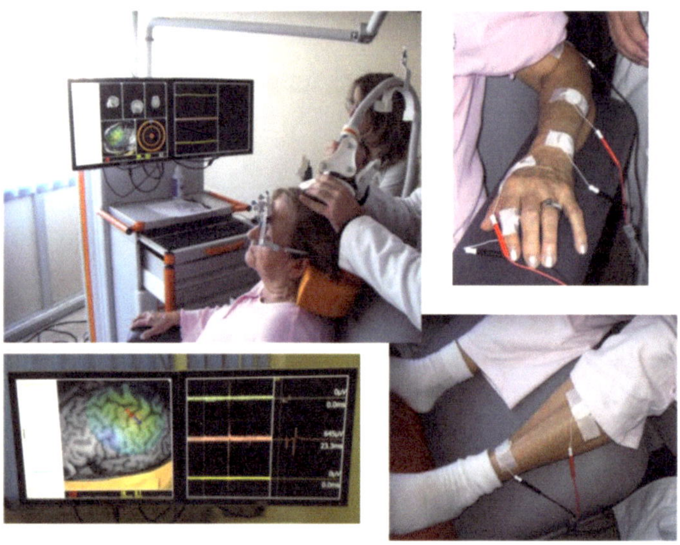

Figure 1. The navigated brain stimulation system Nexstim (Nexstim Ltd., Helsinki, Finland). With NBS, conventional transcranial magnetic stimulation is combined with a neuronavigation system that allows precise identification of each single "stimulated" point in the cortex on three-dimensional imaging study of the patient brain. Muscles responses to electric field (motor evoked potential, MEP) are recorded using EMG channels. The motor map obtained can be used for pre-surgical planning and integrated in the neuronavigation during surgical procedures.

This technique, that has been very recently developed [14], has several exciting clinical and research applications including:

Mapping motor areas for surgical oncology and epilepsy

Checking the integrity of post-stroke motor system

Mapping the motor response in post-traumatic spinal cord injury

Mapping of the areas that control language

Guiding the implantation of stimulating electrodes in the motor cortex

Stimulating the brain plasticity

Treating pain, tinnitus, depression

The first studies on NBS confirmed the safety and tolerability of this technique with no adverse events including pain and seizures, despite the majority of patients in the series had a history of epilepsy. Few patients may have a slight discomfort, and even fewer, a transient headache [14-16].

2.1. Transcranial Magnetic Stimulation

Transcranial magnetic stimulation is a noninvasive technique that allows a focal cortical stimulation. TMS uses electromagnetic induction to produce weak electric currents using a rapidly changing magnetic field. A plastic-enclosed coil of wire is held next to the skull and when activated, it produces a magnetic field oriented orthogonally to the plane of the coil. The magnetic field passes unimpeded through the skin and skull, inducing an oppositely directed current in the brain that activates nearby nerve cells in much the same way as currents applied directly to the cortical surface. The magnetic cortical stimulation is, therefore, a tool to drive in the brain an electrical stimulus generated outside of the head.

The method has, however, an inherent limitation: using a single coil the stimulus that results is not particularly focal and the magnetic field does not penetrate very deeply into the brain. This limitation has been solved through the use of "figure eight " or "butterfly" coils that make the area of overlap of the stimulus significantly more focal and increase the depth of the effect. A single stimulus generated by means of TMS lasts less than 1 ms; despite its brevity it has sufficient power to trigger the activation of many neurons below the coil and a consequent physiological complex chain reaction in the brain tissue that lasts for 50 - 100 ms. In fact, if initially only the neurons immediately below the coil reach the action potential, then it propagates through the synapses also to the adjacent neurons so that the neural response results amplified. This activation of neurons can then be followed by an inhibitory postsynaptic potential and by a period of electrical silence [17].

2.2. Electromyography

The NBS system records motor evoked potentials (MEP) produced by TMS through an electromyography system. Cortical representation of each muscle is a function of its level of innervation, being this latter an index of the degree of fineness of the movements that each muscle can accomplish. The muscles of the face, hand and leg have an extensive somatotopic cortical representation, and recording EMG activity of these muscles allow an almost complete map of the primary motor cortex. It is possible to simultaneously map up to 6 muscles using the 6 EMG channels available in the NBS system.

Muscles of the thenar eminence are usually chosen in the group of muscles of the hand for their wide cortical representation (Figure 1). The mental muscle, being simple to relax for the patient, is frequently used for the group of facial muscles. The tibialis muscle is commonly used for leg function mapping [6].

It is possible to characterize the motor cortex on the basis of the amplitude of the MEP of each stimulated point. A map of colored dots, built on the basis of EMG recordings, provides the accurate localization of the motor cortex at end of the procedure (Figure 2).

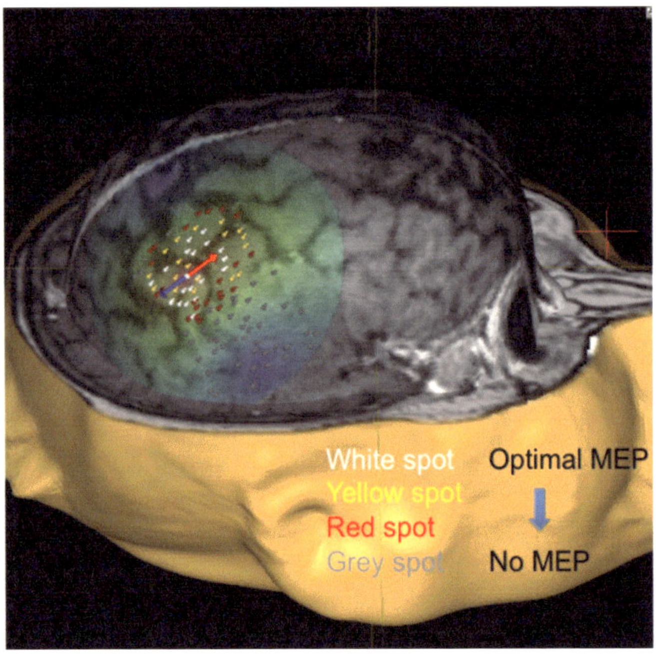

Figure 2. The NBS System uniquely determines the actual location of the stimulating electric field (E-field) in the cortex. Moving the transcranial magnetic stimulation coil over the patient's head, it is always possible to see, in real-time, the stimulation location, strength and direction in the 3-D intracranial rendering. During the mapping, the areas in the cortex with maximal EMG responses are automatically highlighted with different colors.

2.3. Neuronavigation

The NBS can accurately display, in a 3D rendering of the individual patient's magnetic resonance image (MRI), the induced electric field generated by TMS (Figure 3). A standard volumetric MRI is uploaded in the NBS System to obtain a detailed 3D rendering of the head and intracranial structures. Visualization of the brain cortex can be obtained by a tool that allow a layer-by-layer peeling of the skin, bone and dura mater to view the 3D rendering of the brain at any desired intracranial depth. Overlay fMRI, DTI or PET data on the 3D rendering is needed can be registered as well.

With the patent wearing a head tracker (eye-frame), a pointer registers 12 scalp points and computer-aided landmark identification ensures accurate alignment to the MRI data (Figure 3).

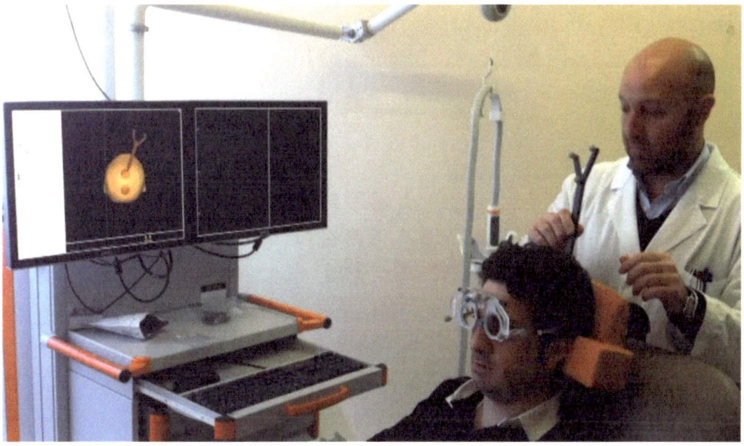

Figure 3. With the patent wearing a head tracker (eyeframe), computer-aided landmark identification ensures accurate alignment of the patient to the MRI data.

Therefore, the NBS system determines the actual location of the stimulating electric field in the cortex, taking into account the size and shape of the individual patient's head, as well as the TMS coil and stimulator parameters. Moving the TMS coil over the patient's head, it is possible to always see, in real-time, the electric field location, strength and direction in the 3-D intracranial rendering. As the session proceeds, a map of the cortical somatotopy, can be created and a post-hoc analysis can be performed offline.

3. Other potential clinical applications of NBS

3.1. Mapping the language

The identification of cortical areas controlling the language can be performed by direct cortical stimulation. The cortical area responsible for the motor function of language can localized by the so-called "speech arrest" caused by its electrical stimulation. Prerequisite of this type of mapping is that the patient must be awake and cooperative. Nevertheless, these conditions cannot be always achieved, especially when patients are children or poorly cooperative adults. In these patients, therefore, it is imperative to find a method of tracking and monitoring the language during a surgery performed under general anesthesia.

In a recent study, navigated TMS was used in combination with video recording of the patient involved in an objects naming task [10]. A repetitive TMS (rTMS) must be used to this purpose. A train of five consecutive TMS pulses was delivered at repetition rate of 5 Hz [4] and with intensity range 80–110% of the motor threshold (MT). The induced electric field ranged between 45 and 80 V/m. To cover speech-related activity and make the possible speech arrest more clear, the train started 300 ms after the presentation of the picture.

Video recording was used for post-hoc review of "errors" caused by repetitive navigated TMS. During stimulation of cortical areas in proximity of the Broadman 44 area, complete anomia and semantic errors have been recorded. In some patients, the stimulation of the right cortex produced similar errors.

Three different cortical areas in the frontal cortex have been identified as responsible for the arrest of speech: primary motor areas negative (NMA), opercular portion of Broca's area (Brodmann area 44) and area of primary motor cortex (M1). M1 cortex is responsible for controlling muscle movements necessary for vocalization, whereas the pars opercularis of Broca's area is responsible for phonological tasks. The responses of the laryngeal muscles can be clearly distinguished by their different latencies to stimulation: stimulation of the M1 produces a short latency response (SLR), whereas stimulation of the part opercularis of the Broca's area produces a long latency response (LLR) [3].

3.2. Therapeutic use of navigated TMS

Repetitive TMS (rTMS) has a potential therapeutic effect in several psychiatric and neurological diseases as well as in stroke and pain. In October 2008, the FDA approved rTMS in the USA for the treatment of major depressive disorders in adults who have failed at least one antidepressant medication.

With rTMS, one challenge is finding the optimal location and dose. In fact, despite multiple successful investigations showing positive effects of rTMS in depression, recent reports have indicated that non-responders may have received rTMS to suboptimal locations [6]. Navigation can help the identification of the optimal brain structure for targeting rTMS, but solving this problem still leaves the question of dose optimization. While specific pulse train parameters have been extensively reviewed in the literature, there is little knowledge of the intracranial strength of applied stimulation and dose-response behavior.

With regard to stroke, MEPs s may have an important role in quantifying the remaining capacity of the motor cortex and the corticospinal tract to generate muscular activity [13]. Navigated TMS may show the development of post-stroke neuronal plasticity with shifting of the primary representation areas. This advances our prognostic evaluation and offers insights for innovative therapeutic strategies [11].

The stimulation of the motor cortex through surgically implanted epidural electrodes is a safe and effective technique to treat chronic neuropathic pain. About ten years ago, it was demonstrated that repetitive TMS of the motor cortex could also produce analgesic effects in patients with neuropathic pain resistant to drugs. Since rTMS is not invasive, the technique is particularly suited to the study of the mechanisms involved in the modulation induced by cortical stimulation. Furthermore, the use of a navigated repetitive TMS may increase accuracy and reliability of the procedure. It exploits the ability to view "hot spots" of cortical stimulation, provided by the maximum amplitude of motor evoked potentials in the muscles of the painful body area, directly on the three-dimensional reconstruction of magnetic resonance imaging of the brain of each individual patient.

There is a critical frequency of stimulation to achieve the analgesic effect of rTMS. Repetitive TMS of the motor cortex has been proven of relieving pain when applied high frequency (> 5Hz), but not at low frequency (<1 Hz). The high frequencies are used to enhance synaptic transmission, without regard to time of stimulation, while the low frequency would be inhibitory. Unlike the frequency, increasing the intensity does not potentiate the analgesic effect of the stimulation. This is because the increased intensity only leads to recruitment of fibers placed in the deepest portion of the cortex, while the pain relief is achieved by activating neural circuitry in the upper layers of the cortex. The peak of analgesic effect of repetitive TMS due to synaptic plasticity, is reported from about 2-3 days after a single session of rTMS and can last for a week. The use in daily sessions of rTMS for several weeks may increase the degree and duration of pain reduction, beyond the time of stimulation. To date, however, the long-term relief, can only be achieved by implanting epidural motor cortex stimulation.

It has also been shown that the analgesic effect of rTMS depends on the precise location of the site of stimulation on the precentral gyrus contralateral to the site of pain. Conventionally, TMS relies solely on the skull anatomy. Using navigated TMS, it is possible to directly visualize the target area. For the hand, the target is located at the knee of the median motor gyrus, which is easily identifiable in 90% of cases, in the front portion of the central sulcus. If the hand knob cannot be accurately identified, the target can be set at the level of the apparent interruption of the central sulcus corresponding to the motor representation of the muscles of the hand. In rare cases where neither the joint nor the apparent interruption of the motor central sulcus can be identified (3% of cases), the target can be identified on the front arm of the central sulcus at the level of the superior frontal sulcus. The effectiveness of repetitive TMS depends also on the orientation of the coil. Analgesia is usually obtained when the coil has an antero-posterior orientation in the precentral gyrus. Repetitive TMS may modulate affective and emotional components of pain, perhaps connected with the effects of stimulation on limbic structures. A positive response to rTMS could be used to identify patients responding to epidural stimulation surgery, even though a negative response is not an exclusion criterion for the implant [1].

4. Materials and methods

All patients admitted to our clinic from November 2011 to May 2012 with lesions (primary brain tumors, brain metastases, vascular malformations) in the motor area underwent preoperative mapping by NBS (Nexstim system 4, Nexstim Ltd., Helsinki, Finland).

Ten patients (5 women and 5 men), aged between 27 and 82 years (mean age = 54 years) underwent NBS. Four patients underwent also preoperative DTI tractography. Seven patients had a lesion of the left cerebral hemisphere.

Neuroimaging was performed using a 1.5-T MRI unit acquiring high-resolution T1 weighted (T1-w) isotropic volumetric data set with a 3D-magnetization prepared rapid gradient echo (3D-MPRAGE) sequence with 1 x 1 x 1 mm voxel size. During the same session DTI was performed. Patients were imaged with parallel imaging technique (IPAT GRAPPA implementation with acceleration factor of 2) and a 4-channel coil with different parameters of the same diffusion-weighted echo-planar sequence with a diffusion-weighted single-shot spin echo, echoplanar sequence with isotropic voxel of 2.3 x 2.3 x 2.3 mm.

Diffusion tensor images were transferred to a personal computer, converted in analyze format and then initially corrected for the effects of eddy-current-induced distortion using FSL modules. After returning them to the DICOM format the images were then processed with the Diffusion Toolkit software (Martinos Center for Biomedical Imaging, Massachusetts General Hospital, Boston, MA, USA) to calculate voxel-based fractional anisotropy maps. Fiber tracking was then performed with the same software using the interpolated streamline propagation algorithm.

The NBS study was performed using a "figure-eight" coil applied perpendicular to the sagittal line of the patient head, with an inclination of 45° and with a posterior-to-anterior flow of direct current.

The procedure was performed according to the following steps:

1. the patient's brain MRI was uploaded in the NBS system so that it can to elaborate a three-dimensional reconstruction; layer–by-layer peeling of superficial cortical structures was performed.

2. the electrodes for recording of electromyographic activity were placed on the surface of the muscles to be activated. Amplitude and latency of evoked potentials engines from 6 EMG channels will be automatically calculated and recorded.

3. The patient wore a special eye-frame for the "head tracking". The operator then tracked the head of the patient with a pointer. The NBS system aligned the points virtually drawn on the patient's head with their corresponding coordinates on the 3D magnetic resonance.

4. The TMS was then performed. Once the brain area for the target muscle was found, the NBS System found the patient’s individual motor threshold (MT). With the stimulator output now set to the optimal mapping intensity, the NBS System automatically and reliably measured MEPs – enabling the high spatial resolution needed for accurate mapping.

5. Before NBS mapping, the resting motor threshold of each individual patient (resting motor threshold = minimal intensity of stimulation that can elicit at least 5 of 10 PEM, with an amplitude of 50 mV) was determined. The cortex of patients was thus activated with a stimulation intensity of 20-30% higher than the resting motor threshold.

http://dx.doi.org/10.5772/53216

6. A cortical somatotopic map was generated by stimulating different parts of the cortex, and identifying those in which the motor response was more intense.

7. The whole data set including the volumetric MRI and a co-registered functional map were exported and uploaded into the operative neuronavigation system.

The motor area has been mapped, on average, twice for each patient: the first mapping was usually carried out one week before surgery. The second determination was obtained the day before surgery.

In one patient, rTMS was performed in order to map language areas. This was done at a frequency of 5 Hz with trains of 7 stimuli (because the area of language is placed in a deepest portion of the cortex than the area motor) and a very low intensity (close to the motor threshold) to minimize the risk of seizures.

Motor evoked potentials of the following muscles were recorded: first interosseous, for the group of muscles of the hand; the tibialis anterior, for the group of muscles of the leg; mental muscle, for the group of muscles of the face.

The software classified the recorded MEP intensities using a chromatic scale of four colors: white, yellow, red, gray. Adjoining white spots (maximum cortical representation of the muscle activated by TMS) with yellow and red spots (MEPs of intermediate intensity, and excluding the grey points (no muscle activation following stimulation of that point = no cortical representation of the muscle at that point), the profile of the motor cortex was so elaborated offline (Figure 4).

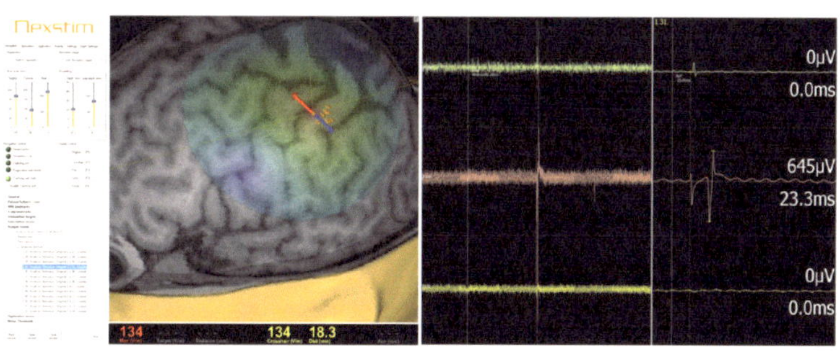

Figure 4. Once the representation area for the target muscle has been found, the NBS System finds thepatient's individual motor threshold (MT). With the stimulator output now set to the optimal mapping intensity, the NBS System automatically and reliably measures MEPs enabling the high spatial resolution needed for accurate mapping.

The data obtained were exported and uploaded on a neuronavigation system Stealthstation 7 (Medtronic, Louisville, CO) and used in the operating room during surgery (Figure 5).

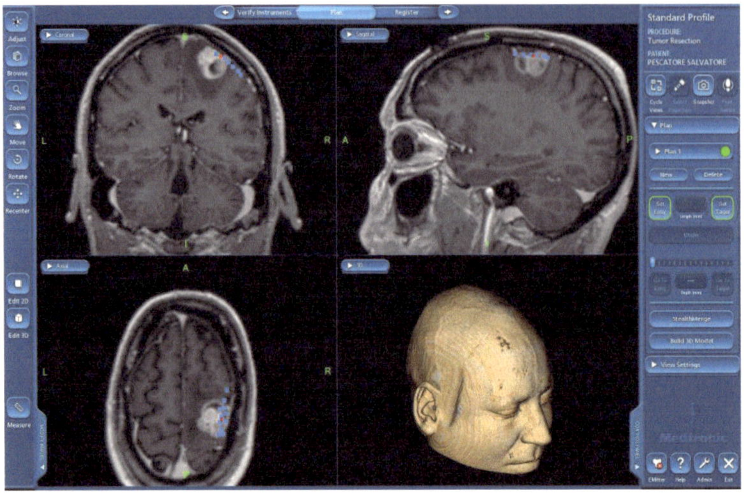

Figure 5. Once the mapping has been completed it is possible exporting images in DICOM format to the neuronavigator. In the operating room, NBS cortical maps may facilitate the optimal placement of direct cortical stimulation electrodes and facilitate surgical guidance.

5. Results and Discussion

All patients underwent gross total resection of tumors or vascular malformations. Post-operatively, only 1 out of 10 patients presented a right facial paresis of the central type associated to motor aphasia; both recovered within 48 hours. In 5 of the patients neurological examination showed no changes as compared to the pre-operative status. Finally, 4 patients had an improvement of neurologic status (Figure 6).

With regard to the tolerability of NBS, we did not record any discomfort for the patients, nor side effects or seizures due to the cortical stimulation, despite the majority of patients had a history of epilepsy (9 of 10 patients).

In this our preliminary experience, albeit the limitation of a small number of cases, NBS met the expectations with successful clinical results. Up to now, functional magnetic resonance imaging (fMRI) was the only non-invasive and readily available method to study brain functions, cognitive activities and potential functional circuitry. fMRI technique uses BOLD (blood oxygenation level dependent) sequences, namely a sequence able to detect increased level of cerebral blood flow and oxygen consumption of brain areas that are activated by appropriate stimulation tests. Although it is less available, positron emission tomography (PET) is the alternative technique that measures the oxygen or glucose consumption of activated brain areas. Both fMRI and PET have a sufficient spatial resolution, but a low temporal resolution. Moreover, the growth of brain tumors may transform local vascularization and cell metabolism, for which a method sensitive to hemodynamic or metabolic changes, may be less accurate.

http://dx.doi.org/10.5772/53216

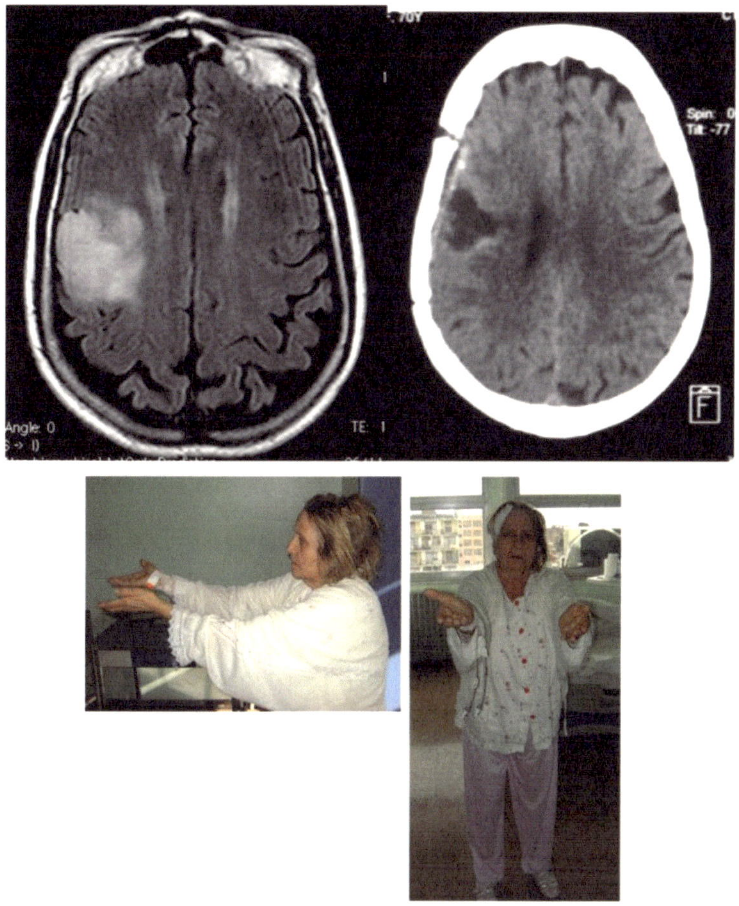

Figure 6. Preoperative MRI (upper left) and post-operative CT (upper right) imaging of a patient with a low grade gliomas of the right pre-rolandic area. The day after surgery the patient present no motor deficits.

Finally, these examinations could be cumbersome, or even not feasible in children and in patients with severe neurological impairments.

Navigated brain stimulation, among the methods of pre-operative brain mapping, has a number of potential advantages. Actually, NBS possesses a very high temporal resolution, since the muscle response to the stimulus electromagnetic is immediate, just as for the DCS. The spatial resolution is extremely high since we can record difference of cortical response within few millimeters. Furthermore, it does not passively record brain activity during voluntary patient movements, but detect an electromyographic response evoked by the TMS.

The identification of the relationships between the lesion and the motor area was possible in all our patients, whereas conventional MRI studies had only provided information on the location of the lesion and its possible relationship with the anatomical structures (e.g. precentral gyrus), but no information on their functional relevance. The peculiarity of the NBS, with respect to the DCS, resides in the possibility of obtaining the cortical mapping preoperatively. Therefore, the surgeon gains the ability to make an accurate surgical plan before the patient arrives in the operating room. This allows a more accurate definition of the craniotomy site and its size, selection of extent of surgical resection prior to surgery, and last but not least, the possibility to predict neurological outcome of treatment and to provide a more accurate information to the patient. In our series, for instance, the indication for surgery was primarily determined on the basis of histology presumed by imaging studies and/or medical history, the location and the size of the lesion, its relation with the cerebral vessels, taking also into account patient age and the risks of comorbidity. Nevertheless, the information obtained with NBS influenced the overall surgical strategy with a planned treatment of extensive resection of noneloquent areas with maximal preservation of the motor area.

NBS functional maps were than "navigated" during surgical resection of the lesion and combined with DCS. The NBS and DCS share similarities, so that the combined use is reliable and can be of great utility. The pre-operative plan, obtained on the basis of NBS, can be applied intraoperatively with the support of DCS. The spatial deviation between DCS and NBS data ranges within the calculated accuracy of the nTMS system, which is 5.73 mm [18]. Such precision has been documented in previous reports on nTMS accuracy, indicating that a spatial resolution of 5 mm is obtainable [2,7,8].

Furthermore, it should be noticed that for lower extremity mapping, nTMS was possible more frequently than DCS, most likely because of the comparatively large stimulated cortical volume, which was calculated to be 1–2 cm^3 for the figure-8 coil used [9].

NBS can also map the cortical areas involved in the control of language. We attempted the use of repetitive transcranial magnetic stimulation (rTMS), with trains of stimuli (between 5 and 10), in that the areas to be mapped are positioned deeper than the area motor of the hand or leg, and the stimulation is made almost at "threshold" level. The use of the repetitive stimulation increases the depth of the stimulus but the low intensity prevents the onset of epileptic seizures. The localization is done by displaying, on the 3D reconstruction of the image of magnetic resonance imaging of the patient, the "hot spot" corresponding to the "speech arrest", i.e. from the errors generated in the naming of objects that are shown, on a screen, to the patient in the course of stimulation. The moments of speech arrest are filmed by a video camera and subsequently analyzed. The method is very promising for the presurgical planning, but also in the neurophysiological study of neuronal networks underlying the function of language. In fact, previous studies have suggesteda revision of the current view, perhaps too simplistic, that Broca's and Wernicke's areas were the only ones involved in the control of language. Already fMRI showed that cortico-cortical connections are much more complex [12]. However, studies in patients with intracranial lesions were found to be more reliable when performed by nTMS; this method, in fact, does not possess the "limit" of relying on cerebral blood flow or metabolism, which could be altered in the presence of brain pathologies. Moreover, fMRI shows the entire cortical network underlying a specific activity, such as aspects of language. The combination with NBS may identify the hierarchy that exists between the different functional areas.

http://dx.doi.org/10.5772/53216

A further opportunity of NBS is the possibility to be integrated in the treatment planning of stereotactic radiosurgery. Radiosurgery is an ablative procedure, but it lacks the possibility of intraoperative brain function mapping and monitoring. NBS is a very good candidate.

Author details

Concetta Alafaci*, Alfredo Conti and Francesco Tomasello

*Address all correspondence to: calafaci@unime.it

Department of Neurosurgery, University of Messina, Messina, Italy

References

[1] Ahdab, R., & Lefaucheur, J. P. (2010). Repetitive transcranial magnetic stimulation and implanted cortical stimulation in the treatment of neuropathic pain. *Proceedings 2nd International Workshop on Navigated Brain Stimulation in Neurosurgery, Berlin, Germany, October 08-09.*

[2] Brasil-Neto, J. P., Cohen, L. G., Panizza, M., Nilsson, J., Roth, B. J., & Hallett, M. (1992). Optimal focal transcranial magnetic activation of the human motor cortex: effects of coil orientation, shape of the induced current pulse, and stimulus intensity. *J Clin Neurophysiol*, 9, 132-136.

[3] Deletis, V., & Rogić, M. (2010). Neurophysiologic markers generated by motor speech-related cortical areas. *Proceedings 2nd International Workshop on Navigated Brain Stimulation in Neurosurgery, Berlin, Germany, October 08-09.*

[4] Epstein, C. M., Lah, J. J., Meador, K., Weissman, JD, Gaitan, L. E., & Dihenia, B. (1996). Optimum stimulus parameters for lateralized suppression of speech with magnetic brain stimulation. *Neurology*, 47, 1590-1593.

[5] Herbsman, T., Avery, D., Ramsey, D., Holtzheimer, P., Wadjik, C., Hardaway, F., et al. (2009). More lateral and anterior prefrontal coil location is associated with better repetitive transcranial magnetic stimulation antidepressant response. *Biol Psychiatry*, 66, 509-515.

[6] Julkunen, P., & Jääskeläinen, J. E. (2010). Transfer of NBS motor mapping data through neuronavigator into optic field of operating microscope. *Proceedings 2nd International Workshop on Navigated Brain Stimulation in Neurosurgery, Berlin, Germany, October 08-09.*

[7] Krieg, S. M., Shiban, E., Buchmann, N., Gempt, J., Foerschler, A., Meyer, B., & Ringel, F. (2012). Utility of presurgical navigated transcranial magnetic brain stimulation for the resection of tumors in eloquent motor areas. *J Neurosurg*, 116(5), 994-1001.

[8] Krings, T., Buchbinder, B. R., Butler, W. E., Chiappa, K. H., Jiang, H. J., Rosen, B. R., et al. (1997). Stereotactic transcranial magnetic stimulation: correlation with direct electrical cortical stimulation. *Neurosurgery*, 41, 1319-1326.

[9] Levy, W. J., Amassian, V. E., Schmid, U. D., & Jungreis, C. (1991). Mapping of motor cortex gyral sites non-invasively by transcranial magnetic stimulation in normal subjects and patients. *Electroencephalogr Clin Neurophysiol*, 43, 51-75.

[10] Lioumis, P., Zhdanov, A., Mäkelä, N., Lehtinen, H., Wilenius, J., Neuvonen, T., Hannula, H., Deletis, V., Picht, T., & Mäkelä, J. P. (2012). A novel approach for documenting naming errors induced by navigated transcranial magnetic stimulation. *J Neurosci Methods*, 204, 349-54.

[11] Mäkelä, J. P., Vitikainen, A. M., Lioumis, P., Paetau, R., Ahtola, E., Kuusela, L., Valanne, L., Blomstedt, G., & Gaily, E. (2012). Functional plasticity of the motor cortical structures demonstrated by navigated TMS in two patients with epilepsy. *Brain Stimul. May 23. [Epub ahead of print]*.

[12] Ojemann, G., & Mateer, C. (1979). Human language cortex: localization of memory, syntax, and sequential motor-phoneme identification systems. *Science*, 205(4413), 1401-1403.

[13] Peurala, S. H., Tarkka, I. M., Juhakoski, M., Könönen, M., Karhu, J., Jäkälä, P., et al. (2008). Restoration of normal cortical excitability and gait ability in acute stroke after intensive rehabilitation. *Cerebrovasc Dis*, 26, 208-209.

[14] Picht, T., Mularski, S., Kuehn, B., Vajkoczy, P., Kombos, T., & Suess, O. (2009). Navigated transcranial magnetic stimulation for preoperative functional diagnostics in brain tumor surgery. *Neurosurgery*, 93-98.

[15] Picht, T., Mularski, S., Kuehn, B., Vajkoczy, P., Kombos, T., & Suess, O. (2009). Navigated transcranial magnetic stimulation for preoperative functional diagnostics in brain tumor surgery. *Neurosurgery*, 65, 93-98.

[16] Picht, T., Schulz, J., Hanna, M., Schmidt, S., Suess, O., & Vajkoczy, P. (2012). Assessment of the influence of navigated transcranial magnetic stimulation on surgical planning for tumors in or near the motor cortex. *Neurosurgery*, 70(5), 1248-1256.

[17] Rothwell, J. (2010). TMS principles. *Proceedings 2nd International Workshop on Navigated Brain Stimulation in Neurosurgery, Berlin, Germany, October 08-09*.

[18] Ruohonen, J., & Karhu, J. (2010). Navigated transcranial magnetic stimulation. *Neurophysiol Clin*, 40, 7-17.

Chapter 2

Functional MRI, Diffusion Tensor Imaging, Magnetic Source Imaging and Intraoperative Neuromonitoring Guided Brain Tumor Resection in Awake and Under General Anaesthesia

Zamzuri Idris, W M Nazaruddin W Hassan,
Muzaimi Mustapha, Badrisyah Idris,
Rahman Izaini Ghani and Jafri Malin Abdullah

Additional information is available at the end of the chapter

http://dx.doi.org/10.5772/52032

1. Introduction

Neuroimaging has evolved from Computed Tomography (CT), CT-Positron Emission Tomography (CT-PET) and Magnetic Resonance Imaging (MRI) scanner in 1970s and 1980s to functional MRI (fMRI), Diffusion Tensor Imaging (DTI) and Magnetic Source Imaging (MSI) or Magnetoencephalography-MRI (MEG-MRI) fusion in 1990s and 2000s. Anatomical and functional neuroimages are currently regarded by most as vital in planning for brain tumors surgery. These anatomical and functional neuroimages can be fused and exported to the neuronavigation system in the operating theatre (Figure 1). Collectively, these images are known as extraoperative neuroimages. On the contrary, intraoperative neuroimages are images that obtained intraoperatively and can be exported regularly to the navigation system. The intraoperative images can be obtained by using either intraoperative CT (iCT), MRI (iMRI) or ultrasound [3D-iUS) [1-3]. Safer and successful brain tumors surgery requires not only neuroimages-guided surgery but also properly defined the eloquent (important and functional) cortices and monitoring of the vital areas of the brain and other organs. Awake surgery with intraoperative brain mapping, and surgery under general anaesthesia with intraoperative monitoring (IOM) which are guided by neuroimages are two operative techniques for brain tumors that are currently regarded by most as gold standard [4-8]. This chapter describes the current functional neuroimaging modalities (fMRI, DTI and MSI), brain mapping, surgery under awake and unconscious states with intraoperative neuromonitorings as adjuncts and techniques to plan and guide the surgeon to resect the brain tumors successfully. We also describe briefly the current treatment modalities for residual brain tumors after the surgery and new concept of brain oscillations and networks as derived from the functional neuroimagings and awake surgery.

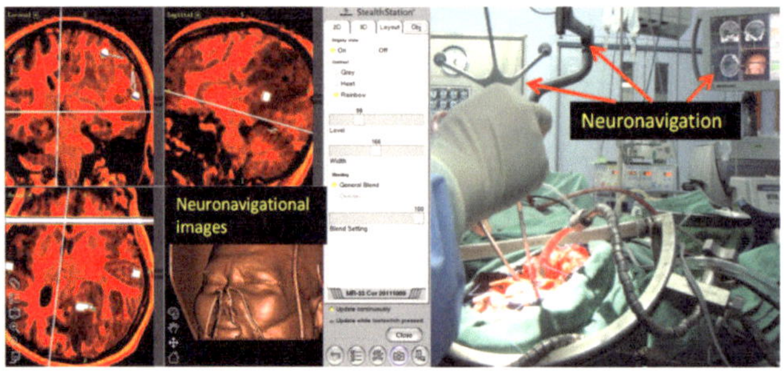

Figure 1. Neuronavigation system in the operating theatre (Medtronic StealthStation TREON™ cranial software; Medtronic Inc., Minneapolis, USA)

2. Neuroimaging

Functional MRI, MSI (MEG-MRI) and transcranial magnetic stimulation (TMS) are three current extraoperative methods that are widely used to locate the eloquent areas of the brain. Functional MRI is based on the increase in cerebral blood flow that accompanies neural activities. The primary form of fMRI uses the blood-oxygen-level-dependent (BOLD) contrast (Figure 2A). In contrast, functional mapping of the brain by using MSI is based on measuring the magnetic fields generated by brain activity (Figure 2B). A basic neural generator of MEG is a magnetometer which consists of a pickup coil paired with a superconducting current detector or better known as superconducting quantum interference device (SQUID). MEG consists of a rigid whole-head helmet containing up to 306 sensors. The sampling rate can reach up to 5 kHz on all channels. The superconducting sensing technology necessary to keep instrumental noise levels at less than a few femtotesla per square root hertz requires cooling at -269°C with liquid helium [9]. A magnetically shielded room made of layers of metal alloys attenuates external perturbations and makes MEG recordings possible (Figure 2C). The equivalent current dipole (ECD) method has been the primary means of analyzing clinical MEG data to identify the location of source activity. Beamforming is a relatively new technique introduced to analyse the brain signals. It is useful to analyse brain activity that may involve multiple active brain regions or networks [10]. Transcranial magnetic stimulation brain mapping is performed by stimulating the cortex with the external figure-of-eight coil (is preferred than circular coil) and single pulse technique, and recording the resulting motor or language responses (note: repetitive pulses or rTMS is preferred than single pulse technique for language mapping) on the navigated anatomical MRI, MSI or fMRI images (see subheading 4.4).

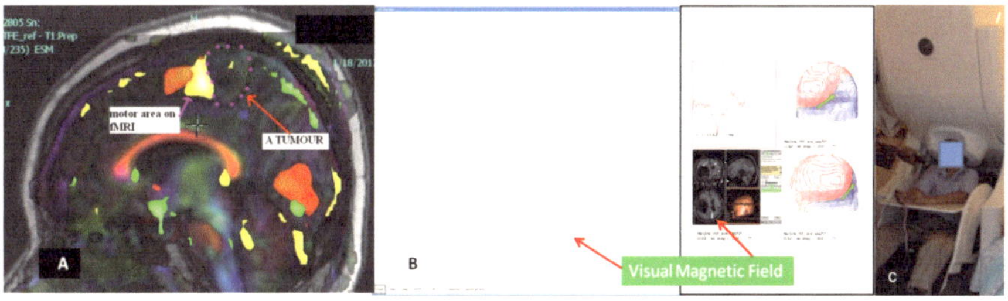

Figure 2. A: Functional MRI depicts the motor hand area lies anterior to the tumor. B: Magnetoencephalography localizes the area for visual evoked magnetic field. C: MEG recording.

Diffusion Tensor Imaging is an anatomical white matter imaging that is useful to elucidate details of the white matter fibres and tracts (Figure 3A). It is an MRI-based technique that can demonstrate white matter anatomy by measuring the directional anisotropy of water (~ non-uniform water flow) [11]. Essentially, in the analysis of the DTI data, a tensor model is used to represent the orientation of the fibers. If there are areas where single fiber population is predominant, the principal diffusion direction is aligned with the white matter fiber tract direction. By following the principal diffusion directions, we can estimate the main directions and reconstruct the fiber tracks, process known as tractography. These reconstructions may then be displayed in 3D, providing a detailed map of the configuration of the tracts and their relationship to other structures [12, 13]. A variety of summary statistics have been proposed to describe the degree to which anisotropy is evident, one of the most common being fractional anisotropy (FA). FA tells the integrity of the fibres and ranged from 0 to 1 (Figure 3B). Nonetheless, one should aware of possible erroneous tractography or erroneous FA values for crossing, kissing, merging or diverging fibres which commonly occurs at subcortical short U fibres and callosal-corona radiata-junctional areas.

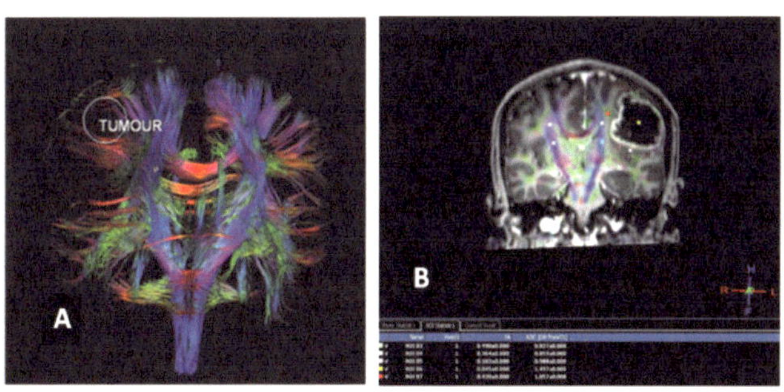

Figure 3. A: Tractography shows various tracts inside the white matter. Blue signifies up-down or down-up fibres, red signifies right-left or left-right fibres and green signifies anterior-posterior or posterior-anterior orientated fibres. B: DTI with FA values.

2.1. Intra- and extraoperative neuroimages and neuronavigation

fMRI, MSI and DTI images are regarded as extraoperative images. They can be fused with anatomical images such as MRI or CT and exported to the neuronavigation. Neuronavigation is a large computer commonly located inside the operating theatre. It helps the surgeon to correlate and localize the eloquent areas of the brain and quickly identify the area of the lesion [14, 15]. Nonetheless, extraoperative images are limited in several ways. They could not give an imaging-update to the operating surgeon with the new images and they may become invalid due to brain shift whenever there is cerebrospinal fluid leak [16]. To solve these problems, an intraoperative imaging modality such as 3D-iUS, iCT (Figure 4) and iMRI can update the operating surgeon with the new and current images. The ultrasound based neuronavigation is interesting and cost a lot less than iCT or iMRI. Combination of these neuroimages with awake brain mapping surgery is regarded by most as a gold standard for brain tumor surgery which lies near the eloquent area of the cortex [17-23].

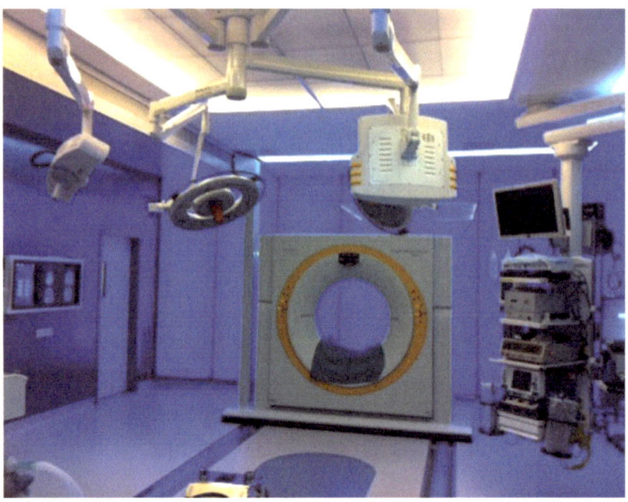

Figure 4. Intraoperative CT with endoscopic and neuronavigational systems.

2.2. Archimedes principle, brain shift and validness of extraoperative neuroimages

The CSF baths the brain and spinal cord, and occupies the ventricular system as well as the subarachnoid spaces or cisterns. The average brain weights 50 g in CSF and 1400 g without CSF [24]. The reduction in brain weight is believed to have resulted from the antigravity effect of CSF buoyancy. In this respect, we motion that there are three ways to overcome gravity: a) acceleration or aerodynamic force b) buoyant force and c) object with no (or negative) mass or time. Speeding rocket or aeroplanes, with their force of accelerations, is the obvious examples of resisting the earth gravity, whilst buoyant force achieves the same effect by reducing the weight of an object within a buoyant setting, say in a fluid or water environment. Archimedes in 212 BC had first coined the buoyant force as "any submerged object is subject to a greater pressure force on its lower surface than on its upper surface, creating a tendency for the object to rise. This tendency is counteracted by the weight of the object, which will sink if it is heavier than the surrounding fluid and will rise if it is lighter. If the object weights the same as an equivalent volume of the fluid, it will be in equilibrium and remains motionless" (Figure 5). Since we know that the average brain's weight is only 50 g in CSF (and the actual weight is 1400 g), buoyant force created by CSF has succeeded to overcome the gravity force. In this context, buoyant force exerts a lifting effect against gravity and creates a "floating brain". The buoyant environment is disturbed once either there is communication between our normal atmosphere with intracranial compartment (gradual obliteration of buoyant environment) or in presence of CSF leak (fast obliteration of buoyant environment)[25, 26]. During craniotomy for brain tumor surgery, brain shift normally happens when there is removal of CSF. Shift in the brain makes the extraoperative images used in neuronavigation fast to be invalid. In conclusion, despite different patient's positioning adopted during imaging and surgery, the extraoperative images incorporated to the neuronavigation system would remain reliable as long as no CSF leak or removal occurs at the actual surgery.

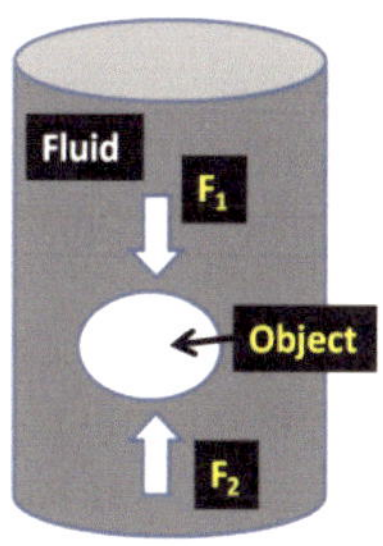

Figure 5. The Archimedes principle: any submerged object is in equilibrium and remains motionless whenever weight of the object (F1) equals to object lower surface fluid pressure (F2).

2.3. Intraoperative neuroimages

The microgravity or buoyant environment created by CSF vanishes once the brain becomes a non-floating organ. At time of actual surgery, opening in CSF cisterns would irrevocably lead to leakage of CSF and hence conversion of buoyant to non-buoyant environment of the brain. Consequently, the localisation onto or into the brain as guided by the extraoperative neuroimages would become imprecise. Thus, surgery that requires precise brain localisation should pay meticulous attention to avoid CSF leak by appropriate positioning of the patient or by using intraoperative neuroimages [27, 28]. Intraoperative neuroimages give updated images to the operating neurosurgeon which can be done on a regular basis. However, note that any extraoperative functional images that are fused with intraoperative images remain inaccurate because of distortion of the brain in the non-buoyant environment and the brain contour itself tends to be different in shape due to the surgery. Therefore, iCT, iMRI or 3D-iUS such as SonoWand system (SonoWand InviteTM Elekta) appears crucially useful to guide the surgeon on the amount and site of the residual (Figure 6), but for a precise functional brain mapping, it is best done under awake state [15, 16, 21].

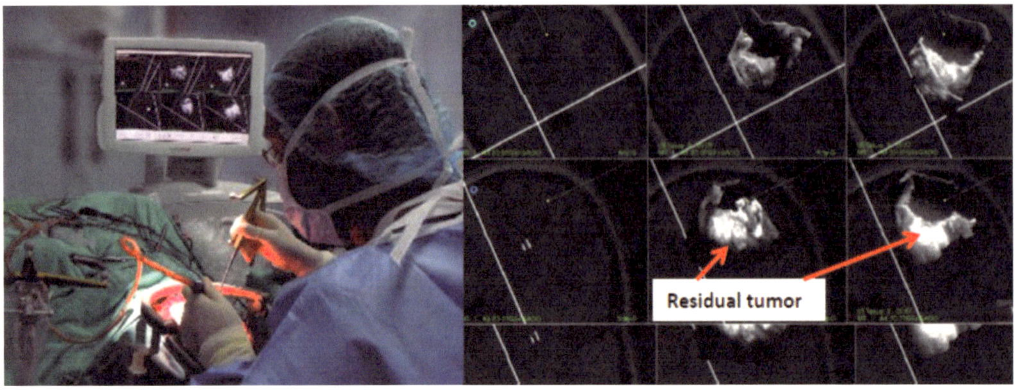

Figure 6. Intraoperative ultrasound using SonoWand system (Elekta) by which the neurosurgeon was informed with the new updated-brain-tumor images.

3. Brain mapping

Mapping the eloquent areas of the brain is vital prior to the definitive tumoral resection. This is especially true for tumors located close to or within the eloquent areas of the brain. Lately, as a result from knowledge gained from intraoperative brain mapping, the previously labeled non-eloquent areas of the brain are no longer considered *silent* brain areas. These areas appeared to be active and and involved in various loops for many brain functions including language, movements and neurocognition. De Benedictis and Duffau in 2011 highlighted the relatively new concept whereby the entire cerebral cortex is involved in execution of functions. The *one-to-one* correspondence between cortical location and function seems inappropriate to explain the complexity of brain processing, especially for higher functions. The brain processing is currently viewed as *many-to-one* or *one-to-many* correlations. Many-to-one concept means multiple brain areas are able to process a single function whilst one-to-many refers to the concept of one region of the brain is capable in eliciting more than one brain functions [30, 31]. Intraoperative brain mapping can be done by using either intraoperative cortical stimulating electrodes such as Ojemann bipolar neurostimulator (Radionics, Inc., Burlington, MA) or grid/strip electrodes, and either done under general anaesthesia or awake state. As a common practice, brain mapping is done under fully awake state using bipolar neurostimulator.

3.1. Technical aspects of brain stimulation

Brain stimulation is currently regarded as important. Brain stimulation is commonly divided into extracranial (or transcranial) and intracranial stimulations. Intracranial stimulation can be further divided into superficial brain stimulation such as cortical-subcortical stimulation and deep brain stimulation. The cortical-subcortical stimulation is commonly used to detect the functional areas of the cortex and subcortical pathways (white matter tracts) prior to and after removal of brain lesions. In contrast to superficial brain stimulation, deep brain stimulation is currently used to treat some neurological or psychiatric diseases. Treating those diseases by giving electrical stimulation works by altering the oscillation rates and amplitudes of the in-

http://dx.doi.org/10.5772/52032

volved networks [32-35]. Transcranial or extracranial stimulation can either be transcranial electrical-digitimer (transcranial electrical stimulation) or magnetic stimulation coil, better known as transcranial magnetic stimulation (TMS) which uses to map the brain motor and language cortices and to treat some neurological or psychiatric diseases [36-38] (see subheading 4.40). Table 1 and figure 7 depict those three common methods of brain stimulation.

Parameters commonly used in electrical brain stimulation (Type of macrostimulation) [note: microstimulation uses glass pipette to penetrate single cell]		
Direct cortical electrical stimulation (source: neurostimulator such as Ojemann neurostimulator)	Deep brain stimulation (DBS) (source: Internal Pulse Generator or IPG)	Transcranial electrical stimulation (TES) [alternative is Trancranial Magnetic Stimulation (TMS).
a) Pulse type can either be monophasic or biphasic pulses.	a) Continuous or reverse pulse type [this differs from mode of stimulation commonly called: unipolar (the case or IPG is positive and a single contact on the lead as cathode. Commonly use because greater current spread typically allows lower stimulation settings) or bipolar mode [2 contacts on the leads as anode and another as cathode – produces narrower field of current spread or more focus effect).	a) Bidirectional square waves (with each cycle, one negative and one positive pulse) or some other pulse type such as brief pulses etc.
b) Frequency: 25 – 60 Hz (low frequency < 30 Hz; intermediately high frequency 30 – 100 Hz: Both normally cause stimulatory effects).	b) Frequency range of 2 - 185 Hz (high frequency > 100 Hz). In DBS, high frequency stimulation or 'hyperstimulation' is used (inhibitory effect on neuronal firing) and mostly at 130 - 185 Hz.	b) Commonly, the frequency ranges from 50 – 130 Hz.
c) Pulse width 0.5 – 1 msec and pulse intervals (length of time between individual impulses; but sometimes it can also mean pulse width) of 1 - 4 msec.	c) Pulse width of 60 – 450 μsec.	c) Single pulse or 2 - 5 train of pulses [0.2 – 0.5 msec pulse width) with 2 - 4 msec interstimulus interval (pulse interval)
d) Intensity of stimulation: microscale [0 – 0.9 mA) to macroscale stimulation [1 – 20 mA).	d) Intensity of stimulation: 0 - 10.5 V (voltage is mostly used) or 0.5 – 2.5 mA (current).	d) Intensity of maximum stimulation is 200 mA [100 to 750 V) (note: for TMS, the stimulus intensity is in the percentage [0-100%], normally at 70 – 90% of magnetic tesla)

Table 1. Comparison among three brain stimulation methods.

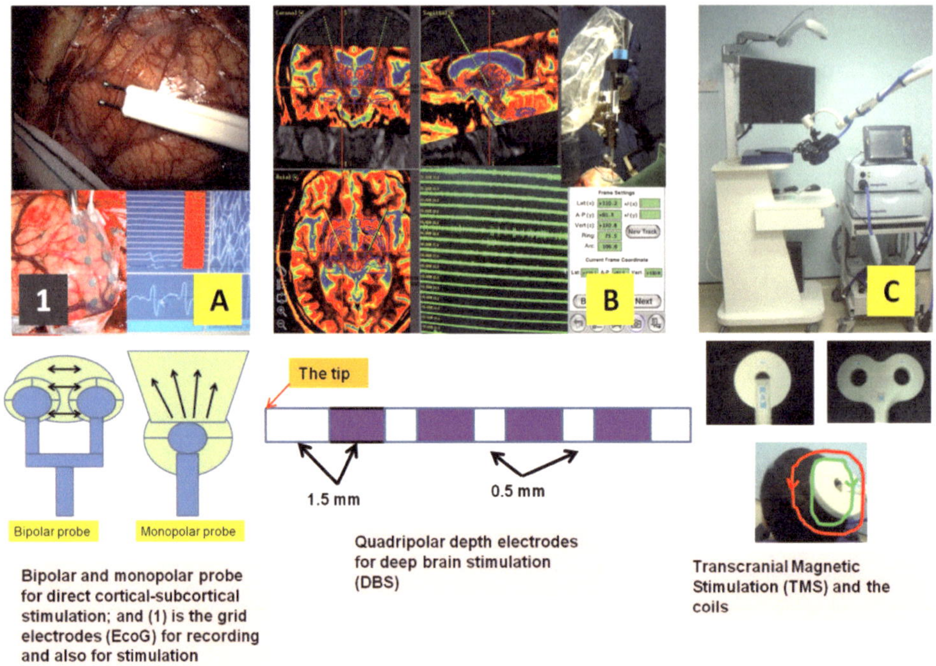

Figure 7. Three methods of brain stimulation. A: Direct cortical stimulation. B: Deep brain area stimulation (in this case, bilateral subthalamic nucleus stimulation or STN-DBS). C: Transcranial Magnetic Stimulation (TMS) using magnetic coils. Note, the induced current in the neural tissues flows in opposite direction to the current generated in the coils and electric energy always coexist with magnetic force (electro-magnetic force).

The most crucial part of brain stimulation is the technical aspects. The elements to this include the stimulator device, the stimulation parameters consisting of pulse type, pulse width (pulse interval), frequency of stimulation, intensity of the stimulation and the stimulation probe. The followings are key points mentioned by Szelenyi et al. that any neurosurgeon who practices direct cortical electrical stimulation need to be familiar with [4]:

i. Stimulator device - Constant-current stimulators are considered safer and more reliable than the constant-voltage stimulators. Unlike the constant-voltage stimulators, constant current stimulators deliver the current independently from the impedance or resistance of the cortical-subcortical surface. Therefore, it is safer and more reliable because constant current is delivered irrespective of possible changes in resistance of brain tissues.

ii. Pulse type – It can be monophasic or biphasic pulse (Figure 8). The first phase of the pulse should be anodal because a lower stimulation intensity is needed to see a stimulation effect. If a monophasic pulse is used, it should be anodal or positive and if biphasic pulse is used, it should be in an anodal/cathodal mode.

iii. Pulse width – The monophasic anodal pulse duration can vary between 0.1 – 2 msec. For biphasic current, the duration of the pulse includes both, the positive and negative phases. Therefore, only half of the pulse duration is anodal and effective for stimulation.

iv. Frequency of stimulation – Transcortical stimulation requires only a low frequency stimulation ranges from 25 – 60 Hz. The most commonly applied frequency is 50-60 Hz.

v. Intensity of the stimulation – For safety reason, the maximum transcortical stimulation intensity should not exceed 40 μC/cm^2/phase and is commonly limited to 16 - 20 mA.

vi. Stimulation probe – Bipolar probe with two ball tips separated by 6 – 10 mm is our probe of choice (Ojemann neurostimulator), the current density appears homogenous and well concentrated at the stimulation site. In contrast, monopolar electrode (single tip) with a frontal reference electrode would cause wider or spacious stimulation effects that leads to the probability of stimulating brain tissues at a more distant site.

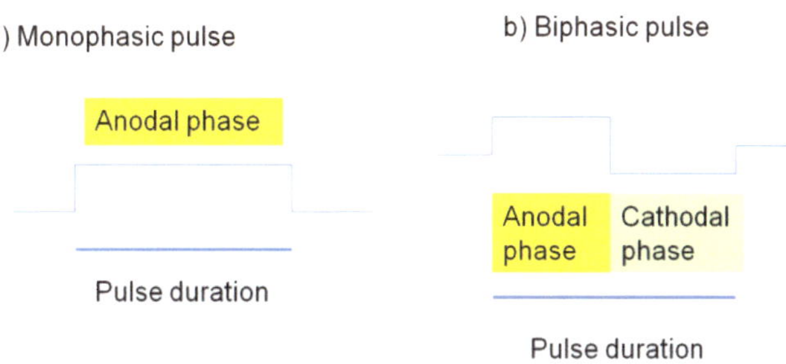

Figure 8. Monophasic and biphasic pulse type.

3.2. Intraoperative brain mapping and awake tumoral surgery

Prior to proper positioning, scalp block is performed at six sites of scalp nerve innervations using mixture of 25 mls ropivacaine 0.75% and adrenaline 5 ug/ml. Additional 20 mls of the same local anaesthetic is infiltrated at the pinning and incision site. Then, the patient is positioned supine with in-situ bladder catheterisation, head fixation in flexed position with the pins and Mayfield head clamp and the thorax is elevated to 40 degrees to ensure comfort to the patient (Figure 9A). Neuronavigation system is arranged such that the monitor is situated at the feet end. Prior to craniotomy, conscious sedation is achieved with dexmedetomidine infusion between 0.2 – 0.5 ug/kg/hr and remifentanil target controlled infusion between 0.25 – 1 ng/ml. Oxygen is only supplied via nasal prong throughout the surgery and the patient is not intubated at all. Needles electromyography (EMG) (or surface EMG electrodes) are inserted into muscles thought to be related to brain mapping (Figure 9B). For the upper limbs, dorsal interrosseus, thenar or hypothenar muscles, brachioradialis, biceps, deltoid and pectoralis major are commonly selected. For the lower limbs, common ones include first dorsal interrosseus, anterior tibialis, gastrocnemius, soleus and anterolateral thigh muscles. For facial muscles, frontalis and orbicularis oris are preferred. In addition to the above mentioned sites for either surface or needle EMG, surface EMG electrode is commonly used for mapping of pharngeal region (anterior neck). Needles EMG are considered important because of their ability to detect muscular response with low amplitudes of stimulation parameters. With that low stimulation parameters, afterdischarges will unlikely occur, intraoperative seizures are prevented and true effect of stimulation is identified. This principle is thought as important for cases with history of focal seizures and tumor is located near the cortical areas which elicit spikes, polyspikes or spike- or sharpwaves on MEG [39, 40]. Registration of neuronavigation system is made after the head is fixed to the Mayfield head clamp. Extraoperative neuroimages are then used to localise the tumor and functional cortical areas. The planned skin incision is marked to cover the tumor and the identified eloquent areas noted on fMRI, DTI and/or MEG. The craniotomy is made large enough to expose brain cortex for mapping purposes. Surgical patties that are soaked with lignocaine are placed onto the dura for few minutes and all sedative medications are stopped. Patient is started to be fully alert on opening the dura layer. Neuronavigation probe is then used to confirm the tumor, eloquent cortex and areas identified on extraoperative neuroimages. CSF leak is kept minimal by proper positioning of the patient's head and no arachnoid opening is made until tumoral resection begun.

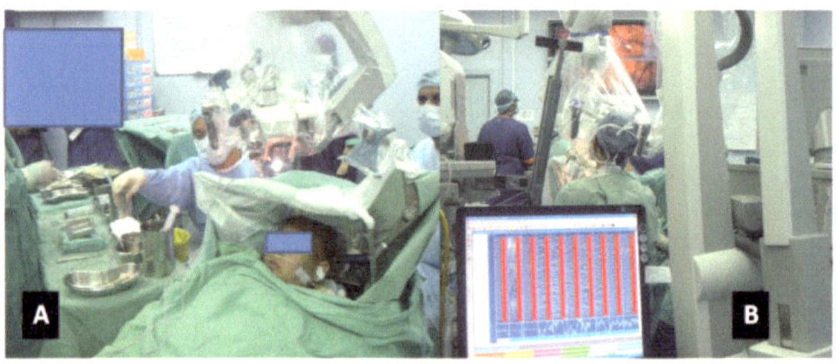

Figure 9. A: Awake craniotomy procedure and B: Intraoperative neuromonitoring with EMGs or motor evoked potentials (MEPs).

Brain mapping is acquired using Ojemann cortical neurostimulator. Stimulating parameters are set normally at anodal biphasic pulse polarity, 50-60 Hz pulse frequency, 0.5-1 milliseconds pulse width/duration (ranges from 0.1 to 2 ms) or pulse intervals and current starting at 1 mA, then increasing gradually until the response is obtained. The sensory response in forms of abnormal sensations is normally noted at 3 – 4 mA stimulus intensity, the motor response is higher at around 3 – 5 mA, manifested as movements or contractions (important to ask the feeling of pharyngeal muscles contraction inside the throat) and EMG responses. If negative motor phenomenon is suspected, especially mapping at the region of association motor cortex, the stimulation induced muscle inhibition can be done by asking the patient to continuously extend and flex the wrist while doing the stimulation (the movement is inhibited by the stimulation). For the language assessment, the longer duration of stimulation is oftenly needed [2 msec pulse width) and every stimulation should start after the patient has said an introductory sentence. The speech or counting arrest is normally noted at 4 – 6 mA. Although no convincing data to support the association between preoperative epilepsy and intraoperative seizures, in the case of a patient known to have seizures or epilepsy, the following precautions are undertaken for cortical stimulation [39, 41]:

i. The antiepileptic drugs must be served prior and on day of surgery (Consider to load the antiepileptic prior to craniotomy in operating theatre if anti-epileptics were missed).

ii. Get the anaesthetist prepared for intravenous diazepam or lorazepam throughout the procedure.

iii. The operating neurosurgeon must ensure the cold isotonic saline or Hartmann's/ Ringer solution is available when needed.

iv. The bipolar stimulating parameters should be started at low values. For patient with history of focal seizure, stimulation is started at low values, example: 20 - 50 Hz pulse frequency, highest micro or lowest macroscale stimulation intensity which subsequently increase to higher values. Needle EMG to detect the responses and nearby grid or strip electrodes to detect afterdischarges are preferred.

v. Short train or train-of-two to five stimulation technique by using monopolar probe or strip electrodes [which commonly used for continuous motor evoked potential (MEP) monitoring] thought to reduce the risk (anodal constant current, or 2-5 pulses, individual pulse width of 0.3 – 0.5 msec and stimulus interval 3 - 4 msec).

vi. Given enough resting time prior to restimulation (or bath the cortex with cold saline prior to restimulation). Never stimulate same cortical area twice successively [stimulate the cortex which is located closed to and far from the lesion alternately].

Cold irrigation of brain surface is made possible by preparing cold isotonic saline or cold Hartmann's/Ringer solution. This is important to treat episode of seizures or afterdischarges during cortical stimulation. Afterdischarges are type of clinical or subclinical seizure recordings which persist despite stopping the stimulation. These can be in the form of polyspike bursts, spike-waves, sequential spikes, rhythmic waves or mixed, usually with more than 10 seconds duration or with clinical seizures. Figure 10 and 11 show the intraoperative brain mapping procedures in our centre and table 2 shows the summary of stimulation effects of various common brain areas as reported by Duffau [42].

The removal of the tumor is made after confirming the functions of identified cortex. Additional knowledge to the operating surgeon regarding the functions of the adjacent cortices would remind him not to injure them during tumoral resection. In addition, knowledge gained from brain mapping can be used to supplement knowledge in neurosciences [43, 44]. For tumor that involves eloquent cortices such as motor cortex, maximal tumoral resection is the aim since most patients already presented with gross neurological deficits secondary to the tumor. If no or minimal deficit is noted prior to definitive surgery, tumoral resection should be made less aggressive by sparing those in the eloquent cortices. Depending upon the intraoperative fresh frozen biopsy results (if no biopsy done prior to excision), this tumoral residual volume

Site of electrical stimulation	Effects
Left Insula	Articulatory disturbances or autonomic disturbances
Left dominant supplementary motor area	Transient speech disorders or mild objective language deficits. Later mild word finding difficulty. Other possibility: agraphia
Left superior longitudinal fascicle (subcoritcal and lateral to the ventricle)	Conduction aphasia (poor repetition), disconnection syndrome
Left inferior frontal gyrus	Reduce capacity for articulate speech/Broca or motor aphasia
Left superior posterior temporal gyrus	Wernicke aphasia/Disturbance in speech comprehension
Left angular gyrus	Alexia with agraphia
Right hemispheric language cortex (language disturbances noted during patient having seizures or on presurgical neuropshychological assessments or language activation in the right hemisphere noted on fMRI)	Crossed aphasia
Temporo-parietal-occipital or optic radiation areas	Transient visual disturbance such as perception of shadow or illusion at certain visual field quadrant
Right angular or temporal gyrus	Complex vestibulo-somatosensory sensations such as out-of-body sensory illusion
Right superior temporal gyrus or supramarginal gyrus or superior longitudinal fascicle	Deficit in visual search (transient spatial neglect)
Left parietal lobe (near left angular gyrus)	Impaired calculation (multiplication and substraction)
Temporo-parietal or frontal areas	Recent memory can be affected (especially, left temporal cortex)
Anterior temporal lobe or dominant frontal premotor area	Famous face recognition affected
Frontal eye field	Ocular deviation or saccade suppression (inattention)
Right posterior perisylvian cortex	Facial emotion recognition
Primary motor cortex	Movements or motor evoked response
Primary sensory cortex	Abnormal sensations

Table 2. The stimulation effects of various common brain areas.

can mostly be treated conservatively with regular clinical assessment and imaging (mostly for low grade tumors) or by precision radiation therapy (for high grade tumors) either using stereotactic radiotherapy (SRT), radiosurgery (SRS) or intraoperative radiotherapy (IORT) and chemotherapy. Sometimes, patient presents with focal seizures and radiologically as well as histologically confirmed benign looking tumor is found at the eloquent area of the cortex, resection of this tumor should be done after thorough investigation to determine if the epileptic focus arises outside the tumoral and eloquent areas. If so, resection of the tumor (simple surgery) is made together with resection of normal looking and non eloquent cortical epileptic

http://dx.doi.org/10.5772/52032

focus (epilepsy surgery). However, if the adjacent normal looking cortical epileptic focus is an eloquent area, multiple subpial transections by using epilepsy knife is a more appropriate choice [45]. The tumoral edge, margin between abnormal and normal looking cortices are stimulated to identify eloquent cortices and important white matter fibres. Information gained from DTI can be used to identify white matter fibres which normally located at the base of the tumor. Therefore, neurostimulation should also be made at the base to identify and confirm those tracts which normally feasible at the end of the surgery. Hemostasis was properly secured prior to closure of the dura. Closure is made in layers after resedation. The patient is normally observed for 24 hours in neurointensive care prior to discharge to a normal ward.

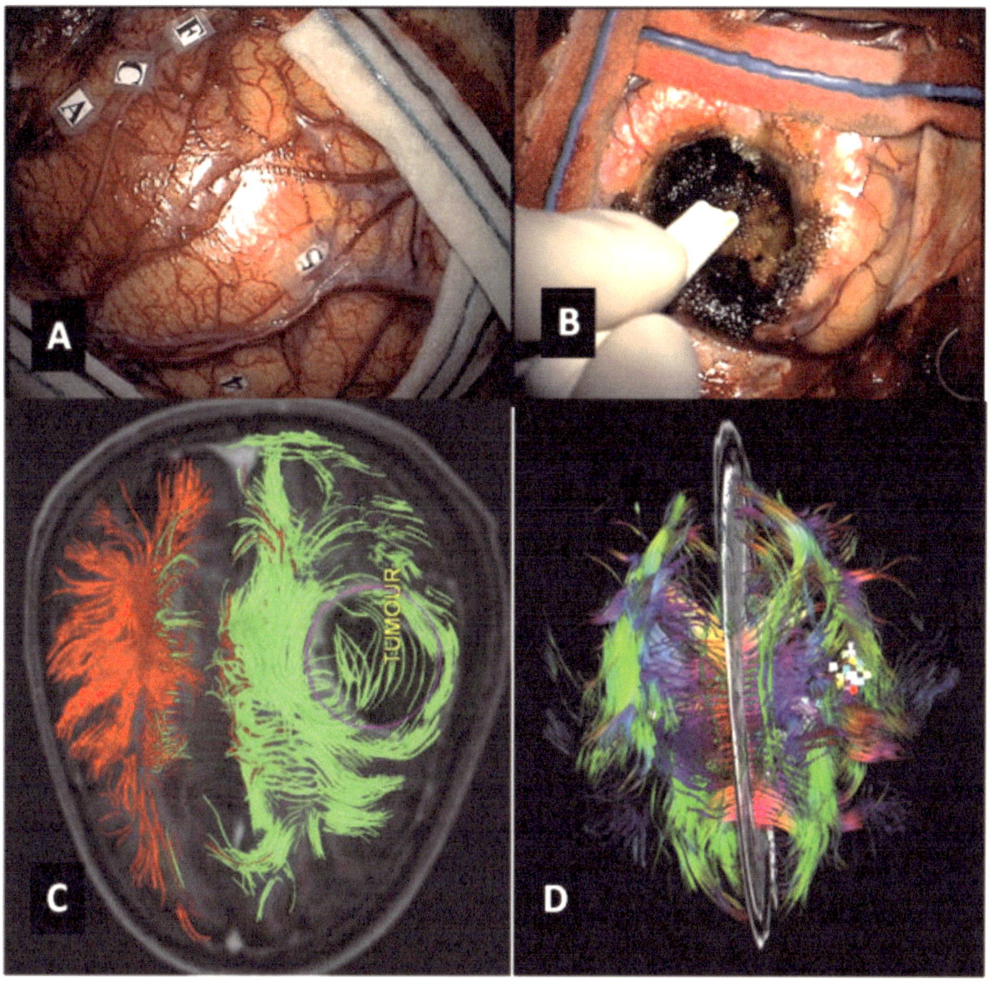

Figure 10. A: Intraoperative brain mapping prior to tumor resection. When areas labeled as A, C, 4 and 5 are stimulated, one would note facial twitching and EMG responses. B: After tumor resection, subcortical stimulation should be done to assess the white matter tracts. C: DTI shows splaying of white matter fibres around the tumor. D: DTI taken months after the surgery revealed more white matter fibres at previous tumor site.

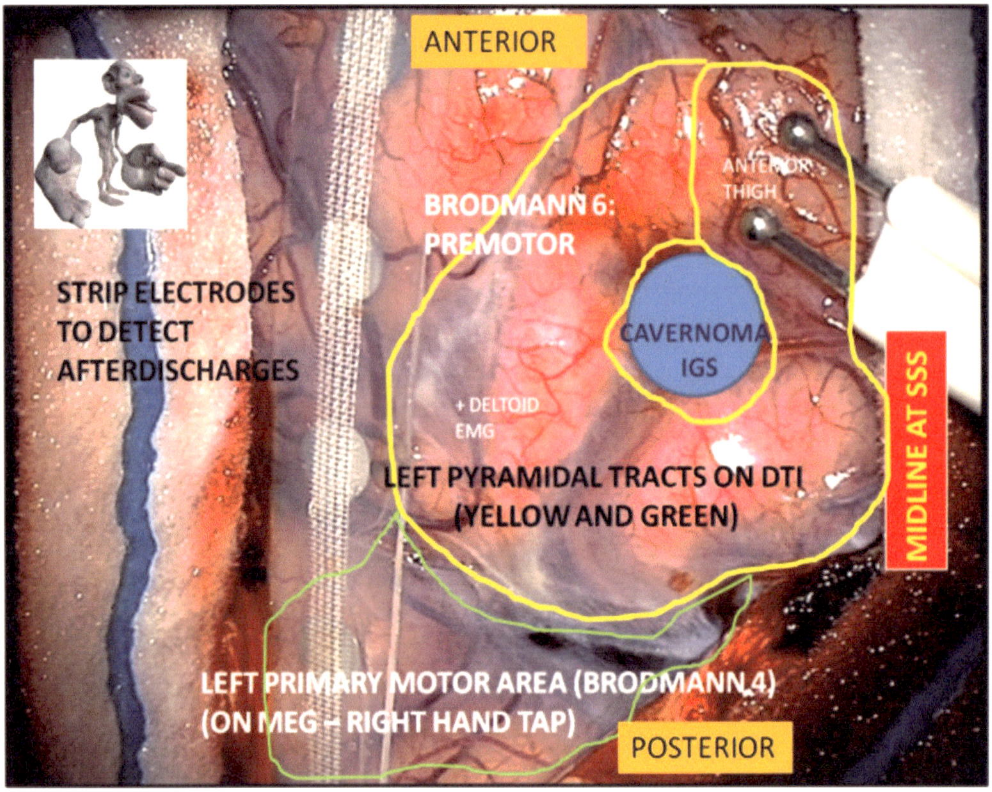

Figure 11. Intraoperative brain mapping under awake state. Cavernoma is identified on image guided system (IGS) or neuronavigation which then resected after complete mapping of adjacent cortical areas.

3.3. Extraoperative brain mapping

Other method of brain mapping is known as extraoperative brain mapping which can be done by using extraoperative neuroimages such as fMRI, MSI, transmagnetic stimulation (TMS) and subdural electrodes (Figure 12A). Subdural grid or strip electrodes (*electrocorticography [EcoG] or intracranial EEG [iEEG]*) are commonly used to record the epileptic discharges and hence identify the epileptic focus prior to resection (mapping the epileptogenic zones) [46]. They can also be used to stimulate the cortex to identify the functional areas of the cortex and to detect afterdischarges during cortical stimulation (functional brain mapping). Brain mapping using grid or strip electrodes are commonly used to identify the language functional areas in cases where the tumor lies closed to language cortices [47]. The electrodes are implanted and secured adequately, clear intraoperative surgical images captured and a thorough language assessment is completed outside the operating theatre. This method is preferred because: a) calmer and appropriate environment outside the operating theatre, b) absence of any residual sedative effects from the drugs used during craniotomy and c) ample time to assess various language functions optimally.

Combined extra- and intraoperative brain mapping is used in our institution. Our findings in comparing extra- with intraoperative brain mapping are in agreement with others, yielding MSI or MEG-MRI signals correlated better with intraoperative cortical stimulation for motor cortices (Figure 12B)[48]. The maximum intraoperative motor response is noted at area which corresponds with area of maximum magnetic signal or vector for motor evoked task. Nonetheless, the information obtained from fMRI should not be regarded as totally unreliable, this is because multiple areas or networks have been shown to be involved in cognitive or motor tasks at different scales [31, 49]. Our experience in awake surgery did show similar findings whereby multiple areas at opposite hemisphere recorded using scalp EEG had shown multiple evoked responses to the electrical stimulation. This finding is further elaborated under the heading of brain waves, oscillations and networks.

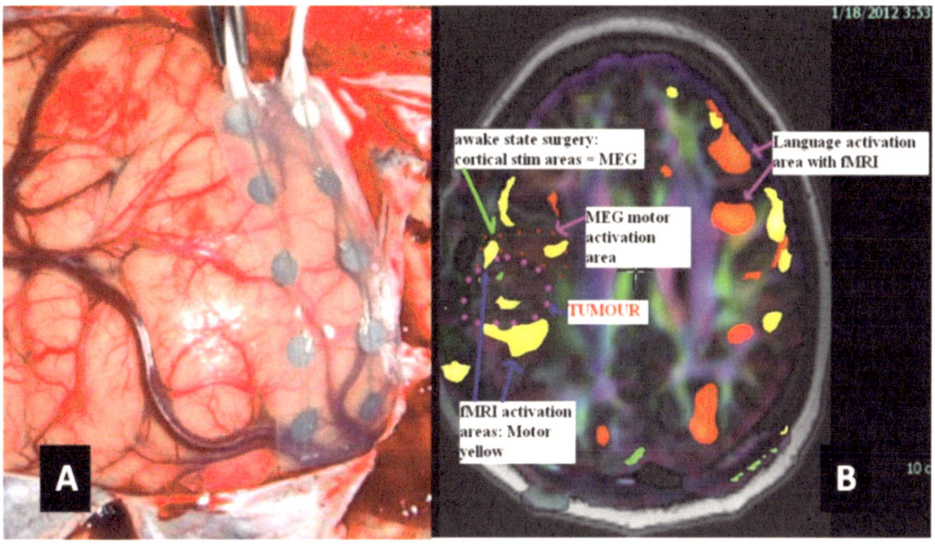

Figure 12. A: Grid electrodes are commonly used to map, stimulate the cortex and to detect afterdischarges. B: Combined extra- and intraoperative information gained from various modalities.

The drawback of brain mapping using fMRI, MSI, TMS is anatomical inaccuracy due to brain shift during surgery and technologically speaking, they lack reliability at an individual scale [42]. Likewise, extraoperative brain mapping with subdural electrodes is limited in terms of inability to stimulate or map the subcortical areas (Figure 12A). Therefore, intraoperative brain mapping of cortical-subcortical brain areas using bipolar probe neurostimulation is regarded as more valid and adaptable than extraoperative brain mapping methods [50]. Nonetheless, not all patients with brain tumors can be operated in awake state. The exclusion criteria include: a) deep seated tumor, b) very young (< 14 years old) or elderly patient (> 65 years old), c) non-educated or non-motivated patients, d) agitative or fretful patients, e) demented patients, and f) presence of other co-morbidity. In such cases, surgery under general anaesthesia is frequently undertaken and therefore new methods in ensuring safety to the patients are required. In that respect, intraoperative monitoring (IOM) seems as an ideal option where it can monitor the functions of the neurons and nerve tracts of the nervous system during state of unconsciousness [6, 7, 51].

4. Intraoperative neuromonitoring for brain tumor surgery

Intraoperative monitoring or neuromonitoring (IOM) is an electrophysiological technique to monitor the functions of neurons and/or nerve tracts during surgery which provides information regarding functional integrity of nervous system in a patient who is anaesthetized and otherwise could not be examined neurologically. IOM consists of somatosensory evoked potential (SSEP), motor evoked potential (MEP), brainstem auditory evoked potential (BAEP), visual evoked potential (VEP), electromyography (EMG) and electroencephalography (EEG).

IOM records spontaneous activity for averaged EEG and non averaged EMG, and evoked response resulted from external stimulation for averaged values of VEP, BAEP, SSEP and MEP. The recorded spontaneous activities are affected by factors such as ischaemia, mechanical injury, blood pressure, body temperature, anaesthetic regime, electrocardiography, electrical interference and muscle activity. During monitoring, ones should be watchful of: a) drop in the amplitude of the response, b) increase in the latency of the response and c) change in the waveform. The goals of IOM are therefore to identify impaired function along the monitored pathways, to alert the surgeon to any impending complications and to reduce risk of postoperative neurological sequelae.

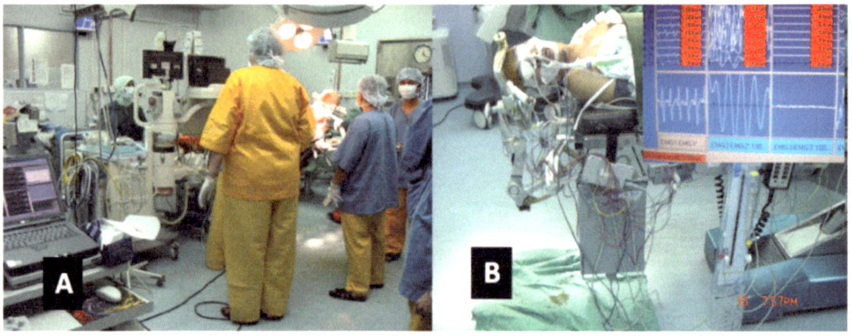

Figure 13. A: Intraoperative neuromonitoring set-up in our operating theatre B: Patient was operated under general anaesthesia with various neuromonitorings.

In general, alarms in neuromonitoring include evoked potentials of ≥ 50% reduction in amplitude and/or increment in latency of ≥ 10%; for EMGs, a change in morphology; and for EEGs monitoring as hints for impending ischaemia or mechanical compression, a decrease or loss in high frequency component, an increase in high amplitude of slower component, burst suppression (periods of silence alteration with periods of activity) which occurs typically in more severe ischaemia and finally flat EEG which is the severest form of an insult. Figure 13A and B show typical IOM set-up in our operating theatre.

4.1. Upper and lower limbs SSEP

Somatosensory evoked potentials monitor the status of ascending white matter fibres from upper or lower limbs. The recording electrodes are situated strategically at certain points along the monitored pathways, for instance, the Erb point for upper limb SSEP commonly records the N9 waveform generated at the brachial plexus (N for negativity - the wave is deflected upwards and P for positivity - the wave is deflected downwards, its amplitude or shape is important; values 9 signifies the expected time for electrical wave to reach the recorded point from the stimulation site in 'milliseconds' or better known as *latency*. *Velocity* is therefore value of measured distance with a tape from the stimulus site to the recorded site and divided with its latency). Table 3 summarises the stimulation parameters, stimulation and recording sites and examples of surgeries that require these types of monitoring.

Upper limb SSEP (ULSSEP)		
Stimulation parameters	**Stimulation and Recording Sites**	**Surgeries requiring ULSSEP and tips**
Stimulus duration: 250 usec. Stimulus intensity: 20 - 30 mA Stimulus rate: 4 - 5 Hz. (note: distal stimulation and recording proximally in the direction in which physiological sensory conduction occurs is known as *orthodromic*. Antidromic study or method is the reverse)	Stimulation site: Median nerve has the most sensory connections within the palm of the hand therefore optimal choice for obtaining ULSSEP. Stimulate the ulnar nerve for cases where T1 nerve root is at risk since median nerve is only innervated by C6 - 7 nerve roots. Recording site: a) Erbs - Generator site is Brachial plexus: waveform N9 b) C2 (cervical level 2) Cervical/medullary: wavefrom N13 c) CP3 - Left somatosensory cortex: wavefrom N20 - P25 d) CP4 - Right somatosensory cortex: waveform N20-P25	Intracranial tumor, chiari malformation, acoustic neuroma, AVM, aneurysm, carotid endarterectomy, spinal decompression, fusion, instrumentation, tethered cord, syringomyelia, intra and extra dural spinal tumors. Damage to the spinal cord or cortex should never result in a loss of the Erbs point. Loss of the Erbs point (N9) indicates a peripheral injury or decrease temperature of the arm. Always be sure of exactly where the lesion is located on the patient you are about to monitor. It helps predicting when and where a change may occur during surgery (*peak monitoring hours*)

Lower limb SSEP (LLSSEP)		
Stimulation parameters	**Stimulation and Recording Sites**	**Surgeries requiring LLSSEP and tips**
Stimulus duration: 250 usec. Stimulus intensity: 20 - 30 mA Stimulus rate: 4 - 5 Hz.	Stimulation site Posterior tibial nerve. Recording site a) C2 (cervical level 2) - Generator site is cervical/medullary: waveform N31 b) CPz - Midline somatosensory cortex: waveform N37-P45 c) CP3 - Left somatosensory cortex: waveform N37-P45 d) CP4 - Right somatosensory cortex: waveform N37-P45	Intracranial tumor, chiari malformation, acoustic neuroma, carotid endaterectomy, AVM, aneurysm, spinal decompression, fusion, instrumentation, tethered cord, syringomyelia, spinal tumor. LLSSEP can be difficult to obtain especially in older patients or those with oedema surrounding the ankles. In this context, do increase the stimulus intensity to 40 - 50 mA [2X) Loss of LLSSEP is not always an indicator of spinal cord or brain injury, decrease in response can be due to peripheral injury. If U/LLSSEP showed partial or total recovery of the responses by the end, often indicates a positive outcome.

Table 3. Summary of stimulation parameters, stimulation and recording sites and examples of surgeries that require SSEP monitorings.

4.2. Brainstem auditory evoked potentials (BAEP)

BAEP monitors the auditory pathways from peripheral to central components. Auditory clicks are delivered directly to the external auditory canal via the foams that are firmly secured and the responses were recorded at A1 and A2 sites (superior to the ears). In BAEP, there are 7 waves generated, each wave or peak has a specific generator site, loss of a particular peak can help you locate where the intraoperative injury has occurred. Figure 14 shows the pattern of BAEP waveforms. The putative generator sites of the major components of the BAEPs are as follows: Peak I - post-synaptic distal cochlear nerve; Peak II - ipsilateral cochlear nucleus in the upper medulla; Peak III - superior olivary complex in the pons (ipsi and contralateral); Peak IV - ascending lateral lemniscus in the pons (ipsi and contralateral); Peak V - inferior colliculus in the midbrain (ipsi and contralateral); Peak VI - medial geniculate in the thalamus and Peak VII - thalamo-cortical auditory radiations or auditory cortex. BAEPs are primarily analyzed for the presence of waves I, III, and V; waves II and IV have been found to be inconsistent even in normal adults, therefore not considered significant for clinical interpretation [52]. Wave V is the most clearly defined because it has the largest amplitude and a characteristic sharp drop immediately after it and the wave that most likely to be present

http://dx.doi.org/10.5772/52032

despite hearing deficits and manipulation of stimulation and recording parameters. Wave V of the BAEP is therefore considered as the most important component of BAEP [52, 53].

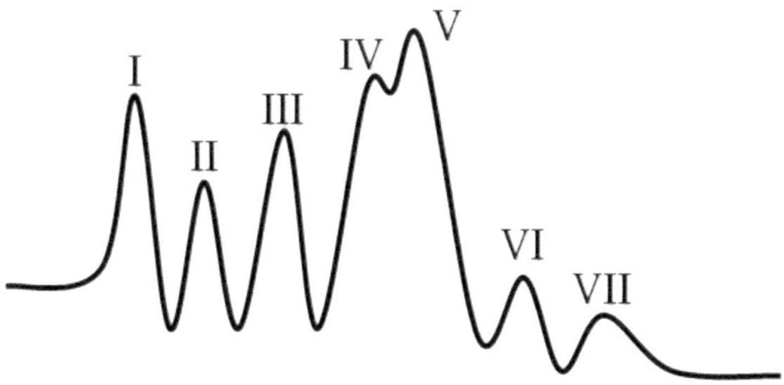

Figure 14. Brainstem auditory evoked potential (BAEP) waveforms.

Interpreting BAEP (also SSEP/MEP) requires baselines waveforms. Baselines are ideally obtained *just prior* to surgical manipulation and after positioning in the operating theatre as a mean of comparison to subsequent averages throughout the case in order to detect any changes. BAEPs that are reliably recorded intraoperatively provide good indication of good neurological outcome. Transient changes are often associated with good prognosis, examples: retraction, manipulation, or compression of the auditory nerve, cerebellum, or brainstem tend to produce transient and reversible changes. Note that these changes usually manifest as increases in latency but with persistence of the insult, loss of BAEP components may occur that could lead to signficant neurological deficits. Specifically, criteria for evaluation of BAEP changes are based on two variables:

i. Latency (timing) - Absolute latency for waves I, III, and V and interpeak latency for waves I-III, III-V, and I-V

ii. Amplitude - Amplitude of waves I and V and amplitude ratio of wave V/I

Generally accepted standard of significant change is a latency increase of peak V exceeding 1.5 ms and a decrease of 50% or more in amplitude [52, 53]. Good *communication* between the surgeon and neurophysiologist is vital to detect early any significant changes which can urge fast intervention by the surgeon and a subsequent change in the surgical procedure and outcomes. Table 4 summarises the stimulation parameters, stimulation and recording sites and recommended types of surgery for BAEP.

Brainstem auditory evoked potentials (BAEP)		
Stimulation parameters	**Stimulation and Recording Sites**	**Surgeries requiring BAEP**
Stimulus duration: 100 usec. Stimulus intensity: 100 – 120 peSPL. Stimulus rate: 11 to 30 Hz.	Stimulation site Auditory clicks delivered directly to the external auditory canal. Recording site a) A1 - Left auditory pathway and brainstem b) A2 - Right auditory pathway and brainstem	Skullbase tumor, posterior fossa tumor, acoustic neuroma, CPA tumor, microvascular decompression, basilar aneurysm, post fossa AVM and EC-IC bypass.

Table 4. Summary of stimulation parameters, stimulation and recording sites and recommended types of surgery for BAEP.

4.3. Electromyography (EMG) and F-wave

Any electrical or magnetic stimulation along the motor pathways will generate involved muscles compound evoked or action potentials, better known as CMAP [compound muscles evoked/action potential – a type of motor evoked potential (MEP) and/or EMG (muscle activity). IOM that uses EMG does monitor wave as well as its sound. On some occasions, muscles twitching, contraction or movement can be noted during the monitoring. It is used during resection of tumor that is located close to motor nerves, for instances, cerebellopontine angle (CPA) tumoral surgery whereby muscles innervated by the facial nerve (orbicularis oris, oculi and nasalis) are monitored using EMGs. The most important factor affecting EMG monitoring is the depth of muscle paralysis. This can be determined by delivering a train of four electrical pulses at approximately 25 mA to usually median or facial nerve, and observing resulting number of twitches: four twitches suggesting no paralysis whereas zero twitches suggesting complete paralysis. For monitoring purposes, ones should have at least 3 twitches in order to detect EMG activity. Interpretation criteria for significant EMG activity are:

i. Sustained firing of a high frequency train lasting for tens of seconds

ii. Large bursts of EMG activity of complex morphology

iii. Sudden bursts of high amplitude spikes

These patterns of activity are usually indicative of nerve irritation but also confirm that the pathway to the specific muscles are intact. Other tips during monitoring are always helpful to turn the volume up high on EMG monitoring machine so that one can hear the EMG activity. If a nerve root can not be electrically stimulated after repeated trials, it may be safe to conclude that the nerve is no longer functionally intact. Figure 15 illustrates the muscle responses that you might get from stimulating the motor cortex, motor pathway, root or nerve.

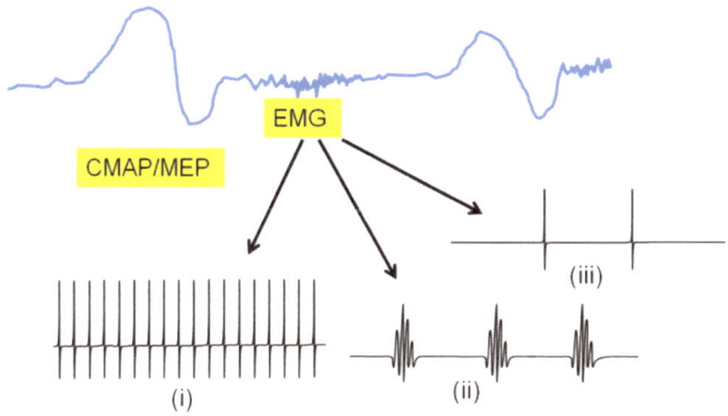

Figure 15. Muscle recording from motor cortical stimulation produces CMAP (which is a type of MEP) or 3 subtypes EMG responses (note: the MEP and EMG monitorings normally display on two different monitors).

F waves (F for foot where they were first described) are a type of late motor response. When a motor nerve axon is electrically stimulated at any point, an action potential is propagated in both directions away from the initial stimulation site. The distally propagated impulse gives rise to the CMAP or M response. However, an impulse also conducts proximally to the anterior horn cell, depolarising the axon hillock and causing the axon to backfire which leads to a small additional muscle depolarisation (F wave) at a longer latency (Figure 16). Because of the long pathway, normal values have to be related to limb length or body height. F waves allow testing of proximal segments of the nerves or roots that would otherwise be inaccessible to routine studies.

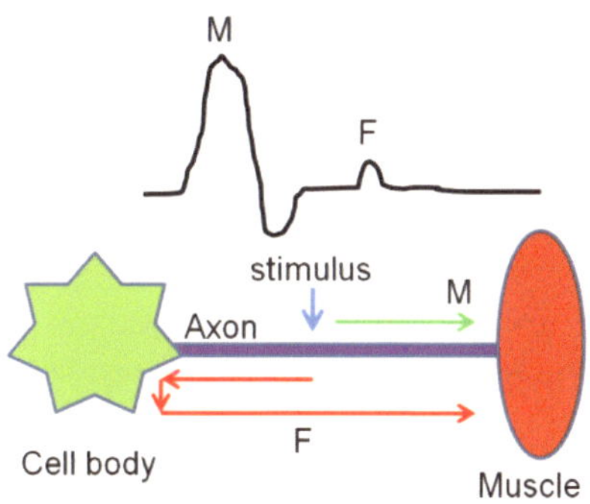

Figure 16. Schematic representation of M and F waves.

4.4. Transcranial electrical and magnetic stimulation and transcortical stimulation

Transcranial electrical stimulation (TES) can be done by using electrical-digitimer stimulation which normally sets at stimulus intensity of 100 to 750 V (max 200 mA), stimulus duration of 0.3-0.5 msec and train of 2 - 5 pulses with 2-4 msec interstimulus interval. On the contrary, the transcranial magnetic stimulation (TMS) uses magnetic stimulation coil to generate electrical current in the brain tissue [54, 55]. The stimulus intensity can be adjusted from 0 to 100% of the magnetic tesla (normally for single pulse motor mapping, 80-90 % stimulus intensity is needed). The stimulation sites can be determined by image guided system (preferred) or based on the scalp EEG 10-20 system electrodes: the left and right motor cortex correspond to C3 and C4 electrode regions (sometimes use C1 and C2 electrode areas). Recordings are made at the spinal cord or nerve level in forms of motor evoked potentials *(MEP:wave forms/neurogenic potentials – repetitive or train of pulses are needed to produce MEPs for continuous monitoring of the waveforms/pathway, therefore transcortical method, strip or grid electrodes are preferred to create persistent stimulation)*, or on the surface (surface electrode) or inside (needle – well tolerated) the muscles in forms of either MEP *[note: when MEP is recorded in or on the surface of the muscle, it is commonly called as CMAP. This can be either at rest - resting MEP or with grip – facilitated MEP]* or EMG responses *(EMG:muscle activity/myogenic potentials)* [56, 57]. Examples of recorded muscles are dorsal interrosseus, abductor pollicis brevis, brachioradialis, biceps, deltoid, thenar or hypothenar muscles or extensor digitorum longus for upper limb and first dorsal interrosseous, extensor hallucis longus, tibialis anterior, gastrocnemius, soleus, anterolateral thigh groups of muscles for the lower limb and for the face; frontalis and orbicularis oris in awake state and orbicularis oculi, oris or nasalis in unconscious state. Examples of Surgeries requiring MEP are for tumors located along the pyramidal-descending pathways *(transcranial stimulation is better since craniotomy is not desired just for the purpose to only stimulate the motor cortex)* or those near or embedded within the motor strip and cortex *(transcortical stimulation is better because craniotomy for tumor resection can also incorporate the motor strips)*. Eventhough transcranial magnetic stimulation is less painful, transcranial electrical stimulation is the optimal choice for obtaining MEPs because it is capable of delivering a more stable stimulus. Total intravenous anaesthesia (TIVA) should be requested before the case begins, since inhalational anaesthetics will reduce the MEPs amplitude. It is helpful to be in constant communication with anaesthesiologist in order to know level of paralysis as an aid in interpretation.

Transcranial Magnetic Stimulation (TMS) is a method to non-invasively probe and reversibly alter neural processing in the human brain. TMS relies on the Faraday principles of electromagnetic induction to generate electrical currents in neural tissue [58]. The direct impact of a TMS is limited to a patch of cortex of a few square centimetres and the induced field falls off exponentially with distance. The effective penetration depth of TMS is estimated to be ~ 2 cm [59]. The intensity of the stimuli can be controlled by changing the current intensity flowing in the coil, thus changing the magnitude of the induced magnetic field and of the secondarily induced electrical field. The focus of the magnetic field depends on the shape of the stimulation coil: figure-of-eight shaped coil (preferred for mapping) or circular coil. The former provides a more focal stimulation, allowing proper mapping of the cortex and the latter induces a more widely distributed electric field allowing for bihemispheric stimulation [60]. The operator can also control the frequency of the delivered stimuli which will determine the effects of TMS on the targetted region of the brain. Frameless stereotactic system helps to precisely localise the brain region during the procedure (Figure 17). Technique for TMS can be either single pulse TMS (spTMS) which can be used to study motor evoked potentials and map the brain cortex, paired-pulse TMS (ppTMS) to study the inhibitory and facilitatory interactions in the cortex and repetitive TMS (rTMS) whereby a train of TMS pulses of the same intensity applied to a single brain area at a given frequency that can range from 1 – 20 Hz. Lower frequencies of rTMS in the 1 Hz range, can suppress excitability of motor cortex, while 20 Hz stimulation can cause temporary increase in cortical excitability [61, 62]. rTMS is mainly used to study the brain-behaviour relationship and mapping the language cortex. Important to note that in a child of less than 10 years old, it may not yield localising response due to relative inexcitibility of child cortex [63]. The contraindication to brain stimulation is presence of pacemaker; and relative contraindication for transcranial stimulation is presence of holes or fracture of skull.

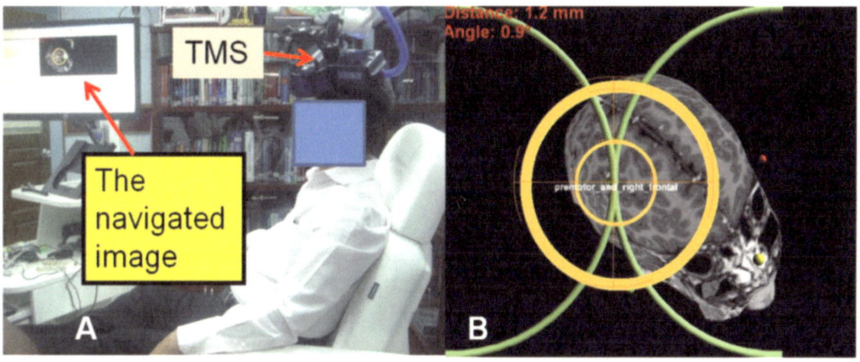

Figure 17. A: The navigated transcranial magnetic stimulation. B: The site of the stimulation is identified on the navigation image.

Transcortical stimulation has been discussed in details at earlier headings and commonly applied in awake surgery. It is a direct method for cortical stimulation which commonly uses neurostimulator *(more precised to elicit EMGs: for brain mapping – tumor within or closed to eloquent cortices)* or strip/grid electrodes for repetitive firing of stimuli to elicit MEP-waves for continuous motor tract monitoring *(example: use for insular region tumor where the surgical approach is at the inferior part relative to the strip/grid electrodes-continuous-stimulation site)* rather than coils *(non-focal and need larger craniotomy than usual).* In general, it requires craniotomy and commonly applies for tumour at region of motor cortex, subcortical motor areas or adjacent to the descending motor pathways. The Penfield technique using neurostimulator is used for transcortical brain mapping: 50-60 pulses per second (frequency 50 – 60 Hz) on motor cortex or subcortically via continuous cortical stimulation over few seconds, with initial current of 1 mA, if no movement or contraction elicited, increase by 1 mA till 16 mA [64]. If no response, then consider non-functional *(Rules of maximum stimulation: < 20 mA for direct (transcortical) and < 200 mA for transcranial/indirect stimulation).*

4.5. Visual evoked potential (VEP)

Goggles containing light emiting diode stimulates retina by light produces evoked responses of occipital cortex at O1 and O2 electrodes or better known as visual evoked potentials (VEPs). P100 of positive polarity and has 100 msec latency is usually used for IOM. Because of high percentage of false positivity associated with VEP, It is mainly used in chiasmatic, optic nerve or sellar region tumour surgery and requires very conservative interpretation (note: patient can close the eyelids during VEP monitoring).

4.6. Tips on anaesthesia

Our IOM anaesthetic protocol encourages use of propofol infusion, opiod infusion (alfentanil etc), with or without inhalational N_2O of less than 50% and intravenous infusion of muscle relaxant with limited dosage, during EMG and/or MEP procedures. Bispectral EEGs (BIS) is good to monitor level of anaesthesia during IOM. Table 5 lists out the anaesthetic tips for IOM procedure.

Intraoperative monitoring (IOM)	Tips for anaesthesia
SSEP	Both techniques of anaesthesia, either inhalational anaesthesia or total intravenous anaesthesia (TIVA) can be used. TIVA can be done with combination of propofol infusion and opioid infusion (remifentanil, sufentanil, alfentanil or fentanyl). Propofol and remifentanil combination is preferable TIVA technique because it can be delivered using target-controlled infusion (TCI) technique. TCI is a technique to deliver certain drugs using special infusion pump incorporated with a software that contains a pharmacokinetic profile of the drugs. If only SSEP is monitored, muscle relaxant can be used if necessary.
EMG	Both techniques of anaesthesia, either inhalational anaesthesia or TIVA can be used. The only important thing is to avoid muscle relaxant during the testing. If muscle relaxant is initially used, it needs to be stopped earlier or reversed when necessary during EMG monitoring
MEP	TIVA is the main anaesthesia technique. Inhalational agents are better totally avoided except desflurane supplement just limited between 0.2- 0.3 minimum alveolar concentration (MAC) is reported to be acceptable in combination with TIVA. Muscle relaxant is better avoided. If indicated to be used, paralysis should be minimal or limited: 1 - 2 twitches per 4 train. Bite block may be used to avoid tongue injury.

Table 5. The anaesthetic tips during IOM procedures.

4.7. Brain tumor surgery under general anaesthesia and neuromonitoring

Intraoperative neuromonitoring is commonly utilised to monitor the status of important neurostructures or tracts whenever surgical removal is planned for tumor that lies close to them. This seems important whenever surgery is planned under general anaesthesia (GA). Under non-awake state, monitoring neurological status of the patient is impossible, therefore many surgeons rely on alternative techniques of IOM to safeguard those neural

http://dx.doi.org/10.5772/52032

structures. The first example is an elderly lady with right frontal high grade tumor presented with left upper limb weakness. The surgery was done under GA with neuronavigation guided surgery and motor cortex stimulation with EMG monitoring. The MEG-MRI (MSI) extraoperative images were uploaded to the neuronavigation system (Medtronic StealthStation TREON™, Minneapolis, USA) and were used to localise the tumor and left leg motor area (Figure 18A). Prior to removal of the tumor, the transcortical motor stimulation was made to localise the hand and facial areas (Figure 18B). Tumor removal was uneventful and immediately after, she received adjuvant intraoperative radiation therapy (IORT) to the periphery and chemotherapy (Figure 18C).

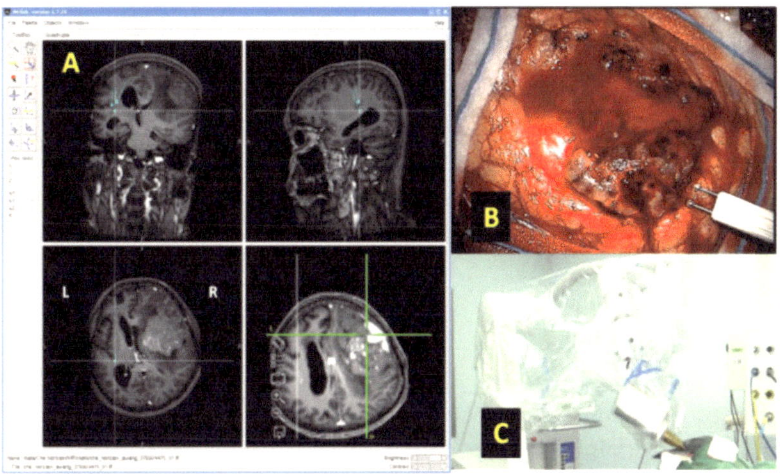

Figure 18. A: MSI was used to localize the eloquent cortices. B: Limited motor cortex stimulation can still be done under general anesthesia as long as no muscle relaxant was given and EMG recordings were made at specific muscles. C: Adjuvant intraoperative radiation therapy (IORT) for residual tumor.

The second case illustration was the ventral brainstem tumor arisen years after radiation therapy to the neck and parotid region for extracranial meningiomas (Figure 19A). The surgery was done under GA and endoscopic true endonasal transphenoidal transclival approach was used to debulk the tumor (Figure 19B). SSEP, BAEP and multiple lower cranial nerve EMGs *(V – Masseter, VI – lateral rectus, VII – nasalis, orbicularis oris and oculi, IX and X – endotracheal tube with adhesive EMG sensors [note: surface EMG electrode at anterior neck is valid for purpose of cortical brain mapping], XI - upper sternomastoid and XII – tongue muscles)* were used to safeguard the important neural structures (Figure 19C). Extraoperative neuroimages were used to localise the tumor and important white matter tracts in the brainstem (Figure 19D). Tumor debulking was completed without causing new neurological deficits (Figure 19E).

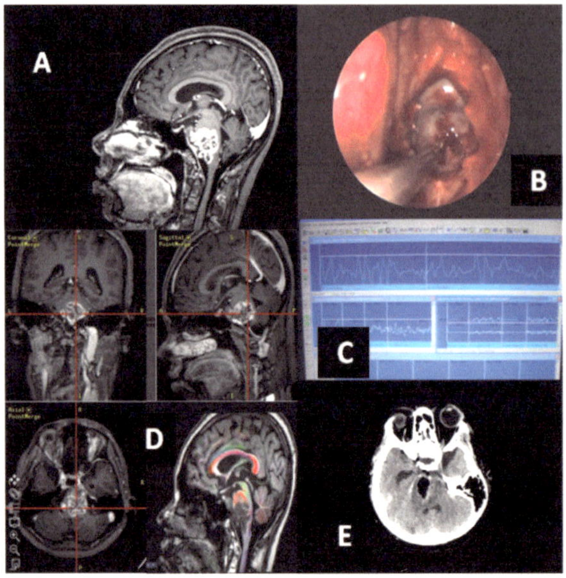

Figure 19. A: Ventral brainstem tumor. B: Endoscopic view during resection. C: Intraoperative neuromonitoring recordings during surgery. D: Neuronavigational images during resection. E: Postoperative image.

5. Brain tumor and adjuvant precision radiation therapy

Several factors known to influence the prognosis of high grade tumors include tumor resection without causing deterioration in patient's neurological functions, adjuvant radiotherapy and chemotherapy [65, 66]. Since high grade tumors tend to be infiltrative in nature, precision radiation therapy should target both the tumor and its infiltrative margin. Hochberg and Pruitt performed series of autopsy studies in patients with high grade brain tumors, where the microscopic margin of tumour was within 2 cm of the enhanced region [67]. This rule of 2 - 3 cm margin from the tumour in radiation therapy seems practical with precision radiation therapy.

Stereotactic radiosurgery (SRS) is an external irradiation technique in which multiple collimated beams of radiation are stereotactically aimed at a radiographically discrete target volume to deliver a single, high dose of radiation to a small volume of tissue (commonly ≤ 3 cm in diameter) (Figure 20A). Stereotactic radiotherapy (SRT) is a technique whereby high precision techniques of SRS with potential radiobiological benefits of fractionation are combined. Therefore SRT involves multiple irradiation sessions and generally used for brain tumors that are irregular in shape and larger than 3 cm in diameter (Figure 20B). Intraoperative or intrabeam radiation therapy (IORT) is a type of intraoperative brachytherapy in which the therapeutic irradiation is administered immeditaley after surgical debulking of brain tumors (Figure 21B). These three techniques of precision radiation therapy are commonly used in our centre to treat high grade tumors after surgical debulking.

http://dx.doi.org/10.5772/52032

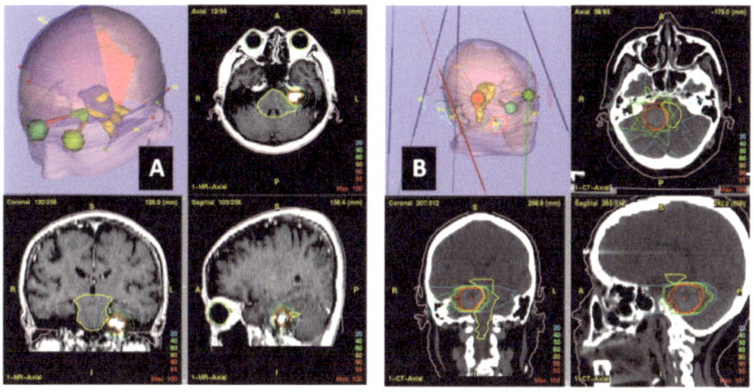

Figure 20. A: Stereotactic radiosurgery (SRS) planning for brain tumor. B: Brain tumor planning for stereotactic radiotherapy (SRT).

In many instances, surgical resection of the tumour is required to reduce the tumor bulk to suit adjuvant therapy, but radiating the *empty* tumoral bed with SRS seems inappropriate. Besides, size of the tumor is also a limiting factor for SRS. As for the time-consuming SRT technique, it is potentially inaccurate because of the different timing of radiation with non-fixed referral points. Thus, such limitations of the two techniques made IORT our most favourable option [66]. The key advantages of IORT are: a) radiation to the tumoral bed can be administered directly after surgical resection; b) radiation can be given circumferentially from the centre of the empty tumoral bed whereby the plan tumour volume is better defined and irradiated; and c) size of the tumor is not a hindrance for high dose irradiation therapy.

At our centre, the IORT procedure had been performed under general anaesthesia immediately after completing the tumoral resection or few days after the surgery. Patient's head was fixed with Mayfield head clamped and rotated adequately so that the tumoral bed localises at the uppermost part. The tumoural bed was measured in all three dimensions and filled up with wet tissue-equivalent cotton strips. Beam directions measured by means of a specially constructed device called the BDI (beam direction indicator). The beam direction was selected according to the shape and depth of the resection cavity and the region presumed at risk of recurrence. The intended beam direction was maintained by using BDI. The BDI consists of a mobile arm with several joints which can be mounted at the edge of the operating table and prepared for the placement of radiation source or better known as Intrabeam Miniature X-ray Source (xRS). The applicator or probe was then fixed to the radiation source. A complete set of spherical applicators or probes from 1.5 to 5.0 cm in diameter are available to enable accurate placement into the tumoral bed, ensuring contact with all surfaces of the treatment area, and uniform dose delivery. The spherical applicator or probe was selected according to the diameter of the resection cavity including a safety margin of at least 1-2 cm. The electron energy was chosen according to the depth of the resection cavity including a margin of at least 1 cm. Dosage of focal irradiation therapy was calculated in Gy and administered intraoperatively (Figure 21A and B).

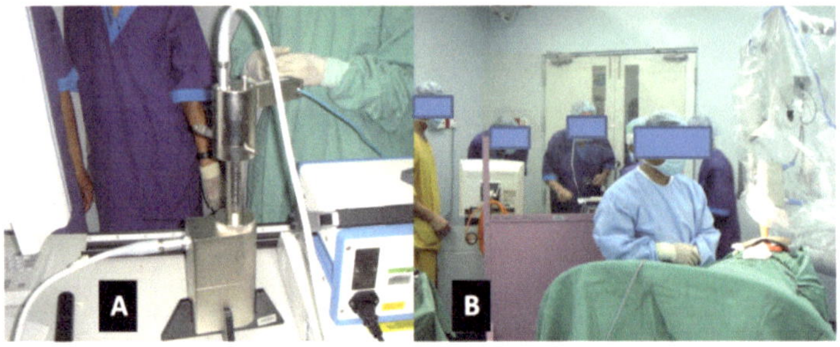

Figure 21. A: Dosage processing prior to irradiation for intrabeam Miniature X-ray Source (xRS). B: Intraoperative radiation therapy procedure, the histologically confirmed tumor bed was irradiated immediately after the surgery.

After completion of the procedure, absolute hemostasis was achieved, dura was closed primarily and the wound was closed in layers. After an interval of 3 – 4 weeks, standard external beam irradiation was started in patients receiving IORT. Besides intracavitary technique of IORT (using spherical applicator as explained above), interstitial IORT is an alternative and commonly used for deep seated high grade brain tumor, such as thalamic gliomas. Initially, tumoral biopsy was made using stereotactic frame (CRW) and once the intraoperative fresh frozen biopsy results confirmed a high grade tumor, the irradiation source was mounted onto the stereotactic frame and the radiation tip was localized into the central part of the tumor for proper irradiation (Figure 22A and B).

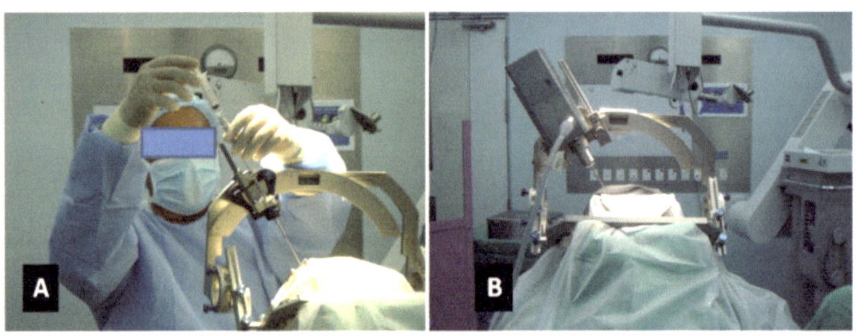

Figure 22. A: Tumoral biopsy procedure completed prior to interstitial IORT. B: An accurate irradiation was administered by using CRW stereotactic frame after knowing the fresh frozen biopsy results.

6. New concept – Brain waves, oscillations and networks

Oscillation with synchronisation does exist inside (~ small universe) and outside (large universe) our brain. Neural oscillation can be stratified into microscale-oscillation (activity of a single neuron), mesoscale-oscillation (activity of local group of neurons or vertices) and macroscale-oscillation (neural activity of different brain regions/networks). Neurons can generate action potentials or spike trains (multiple action potentials in sequence) at microscale oscillation and can be studied using intracellular single-unit recordings. When a group of neurons firing action potentials, synaptic interactions play major role to synchronise the input to other brain regions. Synchronised firing patterns give rise to large-amplitude mesoscale oscillations of local field potentials which can be detected by using EEG or MEG. Neural oscillations which arise from interactions between or among brain regions are known as macroscale-oscillation. It forms various network loops with edges and vertices inside our brain and it is also best detected by using EEG or MEG [31, 68-72]. Neuronal property of creating oscillation inside our brain is important for normal brain functioning. Neural oscillation contributes to neural coding, brain rhythms with different types or frequency of oscillatory activity *[5 type of brain waves: gamma (above 30 Hz), beta [13 – 30 Hz), alpha (8 – 13 Hz), theta [4 – 8 Hz) and delta [0.5 – 4 Hz); sleep spindles; Mu waves; thalamocortical oscillations; epileptic seizures and bursting]* and fast information processing and transfer. Interestingly, neural oscillations also play an important role in many neurological disorders such as excessive synchronisation during seizure in epilepsy or tremors in movement disorders [69]. Lately, it is also being used in controlling the external devices in brain-computer interface [73-74]. Its principle has a potential basis to invent new devise which can restore the functions of the paretic limbs by implanting the devices and get connected to the residual survived-brain networks *(an example: a case with middle-cerebral-artery infarct with hemiparesis, infarctectomy is performed prior to rewiring using advanced DTI and the procedure is completed with implantation of cortical-subcortical stimulatory device)* and subsequently programming the oscillatory outputs (rhythms and amplitudes) via wireless external computers.

Apart from intrinsic properties of neurons, network properties are also an important source of oscillatory activity. The introduction of modern network theory of small-world or scale-free networks appears plausible to describe the real complex brain networks [49, 69]. Small-world network has high clustering coefficient (many vertices/brain areas/rhythms-generating-brain areas) and short path length (connections or edges between vertices/white matter tracts on DTI), and is therefore regarded as the best and economical network model to explain our extremely efficient brain networks or loops. Oscillations produced by the networks are synchronised-large-scale oscillations which can be recorded by using EEG or MEG and studied for:

i. Evoked and event related potentials (ERPs). Evoked or event activity is the brain responses that are directly related to stimulus-related activity. Evoked potentials are commonly used for sensory or motor stimulus, and ERPs are mainly for cognitive tasks. They are obtained by stimulus-locked averaging (averaging different trials at fixed latencies around the presentation of a stimulus). In this analysis, the spontaneous brain activity is regarded as noise and one only focuses on evoked or event related responses

ii. Resting-state activity or spontaneous activity. Oscillatory activities do exist when subjects do not engage in any activity. It is used to study brain maturiy in different ages or pathology, seizure focus, level of consciousness and many else

iii. Complex analysis for brain networks, using neurodynamics-mathematical models or formula of statistical-physics such as spectral analysis (for large-scale data)

From the experiences at our centre, we presented three clinical examples that display features of brain oscillation which were detected by the aforementioned three main studied methods.

Case 1: This is an example of an *evoked response* to display brain oscillation (Figure 23). A 51-year-old man presented with mild left upper limb and facial weakness without history of focal seizures. The brain MRI disclosed a tumoral lesion at right motor cortex. DTI revealed the lesion was surrounded by important pyramidal tracts. He underwent awake tumoral surgery and the tumor was successfully removed. Prior to tumor removal, cortical stimulation was made at right hand motor cortex [60 Hz, 2 ms pulse interval, at 3 – 4 mA) which was confirmed by EMGs responses in the left hand's muscles. Interestingly, there were also obvious evoked potentials responses detected by the opposite side scalp EEGs. Since there is falx structure at the midline, the transfer of the electrical waves from right to left cerebral hemisphere must have gone through appropriate anatomical pathways or loops (corpus callosum or thalamo-cortical loops). This case example proves that inside our brain, there are networks or loops that play significant role in exhibiting their functions.

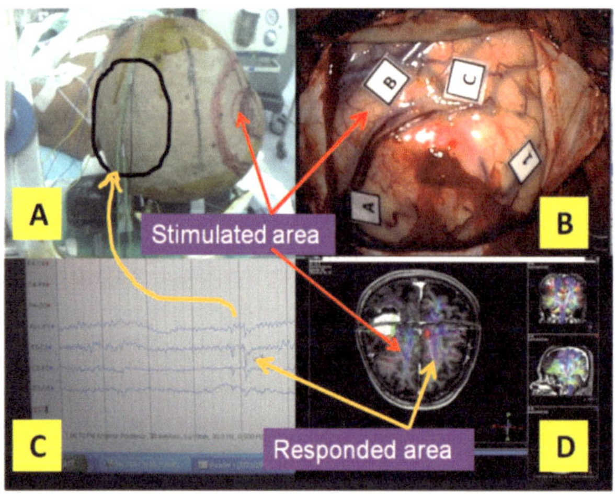

Figure 23. A: Craniotomy for tumor resection was on the right and scalp electrodes were inserted on the left. B: Intra-operative image shows functional brain areas labeled A-C and 1. When area labeled B was stimulated, evoked responses were noted mainly at F3-C3 and C3-P3 at opposite hemisphere (C). D: The stimulated and responded areas seen on DTI.

Case 2: This is an example of resting state or *spontaneous activity* to display brain oscillation (Figure 24). A 41-year-old man who had posterior limb of right internal capsule haemorrhage secondary to cerebral arteriovenous malformation (AVM). He has weakness and dystonia of his left hand. The spontaneous MEG recordings before radiosurgical treatment revealed marked slowings of brain waves at both, right and left motor cortices. This case illustrates lesioning at one point in the network or loop would cause bilateral spontaneous brain waves abnormality. Comparatively similar to above conclusion, it suggests that brain networks or loops do exist in our brain, and they contribute significantly to brain functions.

http://dx.doi.org/10.5772/52032

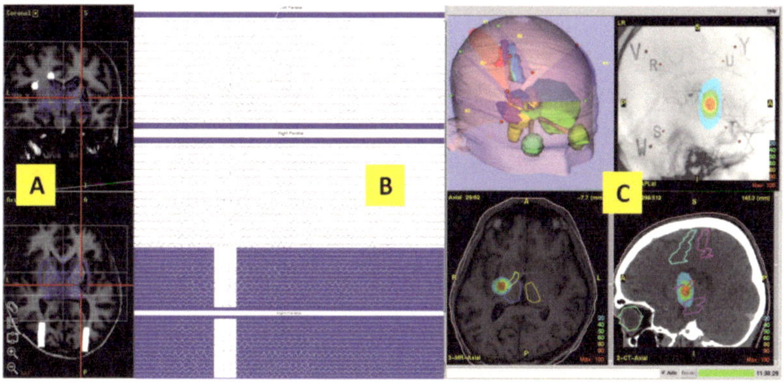

Figure 24. A: The AVM anatomical area was fused with Schaltenbrand-Wahren atlas. B: Spontaneous MEG recordings prior to SRS, shows slowing at bilateral motor cortices. C: Radiosurgical planning for that AVM.

Case 3: This is our third example to display brain oscillation through *complex mathematical model analysis*. Figure 25 disclosed MEG fast-fourier-transformation (fft) analysis for spontaneous brain waves, recorded before and after brain tumor removal in both hemisphere. The tumor was located at frontotemporoparietal brain region. The detail analysis revealed marked changes in brain waves patterns after tumor removal not only in the hemisphere which harbors the tumor, but also in the opposite hemisphere. More activities or less slowing waves patterns were recorded in both hemispheres after tumor resection. This corresponds to marked improvement in patient clinical status. This proves that brain networks or loops do exist in our brain and work via brain waves oscillation.

TUMOURAL HEMISPHERE SIDE		OPPOSITE HEMISPHERE SIDE	
Preoperation	Postoperation	Preoperation	Postoperation
Right frontal	Right frontal	Left frontal	Left frontal
Beta power: 0.14×10^{-24} T/cm	0.18×10^{-24} T/cm	Beta power: 0.39×10^{-24} T/cm	0.15×10^{-24} T/cm
Alpha power: 0.56×10^{-24} T/cm	0.28×10^{-24} T/cm	Alpha power: 0.87×10^{-24} T/cm	0.29×10^{-24} T/cm
Theta power: 0.29×10^{-24} T/cm	0.88×10^{-24} T/cm	Theta power: 0.76×10^{-24} T/cm	0.26×10^{-24} T/cm
Delta power: 7.2×10^{-27} T/cm	6.11×10^{-27} T/cm (less slowing)	Delta power: 5.63×10^{-27} T/cm	1.83×10^{-27} T/cm (less slowing)
Right temporal	Right temporal	Left temporal	Left temporal
Beta power: 0.99×10^{-24} T/cm	0.88×10^{-24} T/cm	Beta power: 1.66×10^{-24} T/cm	0.88×10^{-24} T/cm
Alpha power: 1.94×10^{-24} T/cm	2.08×10^{-24} T/cm	Alpha power: 4.53×10^{-24} T/cm	2.98×10^{-24} T/cm
Theta power: 1.69×10^{-24} T/cm	0.01×10^{-21} T/cm (more)	Theta power: 3.51×10^{-24} T/cm	0.46×10^{-24} T/cm (less ; Oscillate with opposite hemisphere which has more activity???)
Delta power: 0.03×10^{-24} T/cm	0.07×10^{-24} T/cm	Delta power: 0.06×10^{-24} T/cm	0.02×10^{-24} T/cm (less)
Right Parietal	Right Parietal	Left Parietal	Left Parietal
Beta power: 0.53×10^{-24} T/cm	0.23×10^{-24} T/cm	Beta power: 0.31×10^{-24} T/cm	0.22×10^{-24} T/cm
Alpha power: 0.80×10^{-24} T/cm	0.48×10^{-24} T/cm	Alpha power: 1.07×10^{-24} T/cm	0.69×10^{-24} T/cm
Theta power: 0.01×10^{-24} T/cm	0.83×10^{-24} T/cm (more)	Theta power: 0.35×10^{-24} T/cm	0.64×10^{-24} T/cm (more)
Delta power: 0.27×10^{-24} T/cm	4.76×10^{-27} T/cm (less DELTA or slowing waves; more activity after surgery)	Delta power: 0.01×10^{-24} T/cm	6.92×10^{-27} T/cm (less slowing/more activity in opposite parietal lobe too!!!!!)

Figure 25. MEG fast-fourier-transformation analysis for brain tumor patient, before and after the surgery for both hemispheres. Analysis revealed enhanced activities in both hemispheres after the surgery.

7. Conclusion

Intraoperative use of anatomical and functional neuroimages plays crucial roles to quickly identify the tumor and to better define the eloquent areas of the brain. This extraoperative-neuroimages guided brain mapping approach commonly combines either with intraoperative brain mapping technique when patients with brain tumors undergo awake craniotomy surgery or with intraoperative neuromonitoring technique when surgery was done under general anaethesia. Both techniques appear to be useful to the neurosurgeons and acceptable to the patients whilst ensuring a safer removal of brain tumors. Besides, information gained from awake surgery, neuromonitoring and functional neuroimagings expands further insights and potential novel understanding in the field of fundamental and cognitive neurosciences.

Acknowledgements

We would like to thanks Mr Azmi Kass Rosman, Dr Saiful Azli Mat Nayan and Dr Gee Teak Sheng from Department of Neurosurgery, Sungai Buloh Hospital, Kuala Lumpur for providing us iCT photo which was depicted in figure 4 in this chapter.

Author details

Zamzuri Idris[1], W M Nazaruddin W Hassan[2], Muzaimi Mustapha[1], Badrisyah Idris[1], Rahman Izaini Ghani[1] and Jafri Malin Abdullah[1]

1 Department of Neurosciences, Universiti Sains Malaysia, Malaysia

2 Department of Anaesthesiology, Universiti Sains Malaysia, Malaysia

References

[1] Lee CC, Lee ST, Chang CN, Pai PC, Chen YL, Hsieh TC, et al. Volumetric measurement for comparison of the accuracy between intraoperative CT and postoperative MR imaging in pituitary adenoma surgery. AJNR Am J Neuroradiol. 2011;32(8): 1539-44.

[2] Shah MN, Leonard JR, Inder G, Gao F, Geske M, Haydon DH, et al. Intraoperative magnetic resonance imaging to reduce the rate of early reoperation for lesion resection in pediatric neurosurgery. J Neurosurg Pediatr 2012;9(3):259-64.

[3] Lindner D, Trantakis C, Renner C, Arnold S, Schmitgen A, Schneider J, et al. Application of intraoperative 3D ultrasound during navigated tumor resection. Minim Invasive Neurosurg. 2006;49(4):197-202.

[4] Szelenyi A, Bello L, Duffau H, Fava E, Feigl GC, Galanda M, et al. Intraoperative electrical stimulation in awake craniotomy: methodological aspects of current practice. Neurosurg Focus. 2010;28(2):E7.

[5] Yordanova YN, Moritz-Gasser S, Duffau H. Awake surgery for WHO Grade II gliomas within "noneloquent" areas in the left dominant hemisphere: toward a "supratotal" resection. Clinical article. J Neurosurg. 2011;115(2):232-9.

[6] Ritzl EK. Intraoperative neuromonitoring during glioma surgery: bring in the expert neurophysiologists! J Clin Neurophysiol. 2012;29(2):151-3.

[7] Weinzierl MR, Reinacher P, Gilsbach JM, Rohde V. Combined motor and somatosensory evoked potentials for intraoperative monitoring: intra- and postoperative data in a series of 69 operations. Neurosurg Rev. 2007;30(2):109-16;discussion 16.

[8] Duffau H. New concepts in surgery of WHO grade II gliomas: functional brain mapping, connectionism and plasticity-a review. J Neurooncol. 2006;79(1):77-115.

[9] Sylvain B. Magnetoencephalography. In: Duffau H. (ed.) Brain Mapping: from neural basis of cognition to surgical applications. 1st ed: Springer-Verlag; 2011.p77-89.

[10] Herdman AT, Cheyne D. A practical guide for MEG and beamforming. In: Handy TC. (ed.) Brain Signal Analysis: advances in neuroelectric and neuromagnetic methods. 1st ed. Cambridge: MIT Press; 2009.p99-140.

[11] Assaf Y, Pasternak O. Diffusion tensor imaging (DTI)-based white matter mapping in brain research: a review. J Mol Neurosci. 2008;34(1):51-61.

[12] Beaulieu C. The basis of anisotropic water diffusion in the nervous system - a technical review. NMR Biomed. 2002;15(7-8):435-55.

[13] Nucifora PG, Verma R, Lee SK, Melhem ER. Diffusion-tensor MR imaging and tractography: exploring brain microstructure and connectivity. Radiology. 2007;245(2): 367-84.

[14] Bello L, Castellano A, Fava E, Casaceli G, Riva M, Scotti G, et al. Intraoperative use of diffusion tensor imaging fiber tractography and subcortical mapping for resection of gliomas: technical considerations. Neurosurg Focus. 2010;28(2):E6.

[15] Gonzalez-Darder JM, Gonzalez-Lopez P, Talamantes F, Quilis V, Cortes V, Garcia-March G, et al. Multimodal navigation in the functional microsurgical resection of intrinsic brain tumors located in eloquent motor areas: role of tractography. Neurosurg Focus. 2010;28(2):E5.

[16] Kuhnt D, Bauer MH, Nimsky C. Brain Shift Compensation and Neurosurgical Image Fusion Using Intraoperative MRI: Current Status and Future Challenges. Crit Rev Biomed Eng. 2012;40(3):175-85.

[17] Rasmussen IA, Jr., Lindseth F, Rygh OM, Berntsen EM, Selbekk T, Xu J, et al. Functional neuronavigation combined with intra-operative 3D ultrasound: initial experiences during surgical resections close to eloquent brain areas and future directions in automatic brain shift compensation of preoperative data. Acta Neurochir (Wien). 2007;149(4):365-78.

[18] Schulder M, Maldjian JA, Liu WC, Holodny AI, Kalnin AT, Mun IK, et al. Functional image-guided surgery of intracranial tumors located in or near the sensorimotor cortex. J Neurosurg. 1998;89(3):412-8.

[19] Prabhu SS, Gasco J, Tummala S, Weinberg JS, Rao G. Intraoperative magnetic resonance imaging-guided tractography with integrated monopolar subcortical functional mapping for resection of brain tumors. J Neurosurg. 2011;114(3):719-26. .

[20] Nossek E, Korn A, Shahar T, Kanner AA, Yaffe H, Marcovici D, et al. Intraoperative mapping and monitoring of the corticospinal tracts with neurophysiological assessment and 3-dimensional ultrasonography-based navigation. . J Neurosurg. 2011;114(3):738-46.

[21] Parney IF, Goerss SJ, McGee K, Huston J, 3rd, Perkins WJ, Meyer FB. Awake craniotomy, electrophysiologic mapping, and tumor resection with high-field intraoperative MRI. World Neurosurg. 2010;73(5):547-51.

[22] Benzagmout M, Gatignol P, Duffau H. Resection of World Health Organization Grade II gliomas involving Broca's area: methodological and functional considerations. Neurosurgery. 2007;61(4): 741-52;discussion 52-3.

[23] Duffau H, Capelle L, Denvil D, Sichez N, Gatignol P, Lopes M, et al. Functional recovery after surgical resection of low grade gliomas in eloquent brain: hypothesis of brain compensation. J Neurol Neurosurg Psychiatry. 2003;74(7):901-7.

[24] Hartmann P, Ramseier A, Gudat F, Mihatsch MJ, Polasek W. Normal weight of the brain in adults in relation to age, sex, body height and weight. Pathologe. 1994;15(3): 165-70.

[25] Isago T, Nozaki M, Kikuchi Y, Honda T, Nakazawa H. Sinking skin flap syndrome: a case of improved cerebral blood flow after cranioplasty. Ann Plast Surg. 2004;53(3): 288-92.

[26] Coenen VA, Abdel-Rahman A, McMaster J, Bogod N, Honey CR. Minimizing brain shift during functional neurosurgical procedures - a simple burr hole technique that can decrease CSF loss and intracranial air. Cent Eur Neurosurg. 1055;72(4):181-5.

[27] Coenen VA, Abdel-Rahman A, McMaster J, Bogod N, Honey CR. Minimizing brain shift during functional neurosurgical procedures - a simple burr hole technique that can decrease CSF loss and intracranial air. Cent Eur Neurosurg. 2011;72(4):181-5.

[28] Huston OO, Watson RE, Bernstein MA, McGee KP, Stead SM, Gorman DA, et al. Intraoperative magnetic resonance imaging findings during deep brain stimulation surgery. J Neurosurg. 2012;115(4): 852-7.

[29] Vitaz TW, Inkabi KE, Carrubba CJ. Intraoperative MRI for transphenoidal procedures: short-term outcome for 100 consecutive cases. Clin Neurol Neurosurg. 2011;113(9):731-5. .

[30] De Benedictis A, Duffau H. Brain hodotopy: from esoteric concept to practical surgical applications. Neurosurgery. 2011;68(6):1709-23.

[31] Sporns O, Tononi G, Edelman GM. Theoretical neuroanatomy: relating anatomical and functional connectivity in graphs and cortical connection matrices. Cereb Cortex. 2000;10(2):127-41.

[32] Zaidel A, Spivak A, Grieb B, Bergman H, Israel Z. Subthalamic span of beta oscillations predicts deep brain stimulation efficacy for patients with Parkinson's disease. Brain. 2007;133(Pt 7):2007-21.

[33] Cohen MX, Axmacher N, Lenartz D, Elger CE, Sturm V, Schlaepfer TE. Good vibrations: cross-frequency coupling in the human nucleus accumbens during reward processing. J Cogn Neurosci. 2009;21(5):875-89.

[34] Tsang EW, Hamani C, Moro E, Mazzella F, Saha U, Lozano AM, et al. Subthalamic deep brain stimulation at individualized frequencies for Parkinson disease. Neurology. 2012;78(24):1930-8.

[35] Liu X, Wang S, Yianni J, Nandi D, Bain PG, Gregory R, et al. The sensory and motor representation of synchronized oscillations in the globus pallidus in patients with primary dystonia. Brain. 2008;131(Pt 6):1562-73.

[36] Pallanti S, Cantisani A, Grassi G, Antonini S, Cecchelli C, Burian J, et al. rTMS age-dependent response in treatment-resistant depressed subjects: a mini-review. CNS Spect. 2012;17(1):24-30.

[37] Prikryl R, Mikl M, Prikrylova Kucerova H, Ustohal L, Kasparek T, Marecek R, et al. Does repetitive transcranial magnetic stimulation have a positive effect on working memory and neuronal activation in treatment of negative symptoms of schizophrenia? Neuro Endocrinol Lett. 2012;33(1):90-7.

[38] Lefaucheur JP, Drouot X, Von Raison F, Menard-Lefaucheur I, Cesaro P, Nguyen JP. Improvement of motor performance and modulation of cortical excitability by repetitive transcranial magnetic stimulation of the motor cortex in Parkinson's disease. Clin Neurophysiol. 2004;115(11):2530-41.

[39] Niesen AD, Jacob AK, Aho LE, Botten EJ, Nase KE, Nelson JM, et al. Perioperative seizures in patients with a history of a seizure disorder. Anesth Analg. 2010;111(3): 729-35.

[40] Stefan H, Scheler G, Hummel C, Walter J, Romstock J, Buchfelder M, et al. Magnetoencephalography (MEG) predicts focal epileptogenicity in cavernomas. J Neurol Neurosurg Psychiatry. 2004;75(9):1309-13.

[41] Szelenyi A, Joksimovic B, Seifert V. Intraoperative risk of seizures associated with transient direct cortical stimulation in patients with symptomatic epilepsy. J Clin Neurophysiol. 2007;24(1):39-43.

[42] Duffau H. Indications of awake mapping and selection of intraoperative tasks. In: Duffau H. (ed.) Brain Mapping: from neural basis of cognition to surgical applications. 1st ed: Springer-Verlag; 2011.p321-334.

[43] Crone NE, Sinai A, Korzeniewska A. High-frequency gamma oscillations and human brain mapping with electrocorticography. Prog Brain Res. 2006;159:275-95.

[44] Jerbi K, Ossandon T, Hamame CM, Senova S, Dalal SS, Jung J, et al. Task-related gamma-band dynamics from an intracerebral perspective: review and implications for surface EEG and MEG. Hum Brain Mapp. 2009;30(6):1758-71.

[45] Behdad A, Limbrick DD, Jr., Bertrand ME, Smyth MD. Epilepsy surgery in children with seizures arising from the rolandic cortex. Epilepsia. 2009;50(6):1450-61.

[46] Maehara T. Intraoperative Monitoring of epileptic foci: usefulness of multimodality image-guided epilepsy surgery performed in combination with electrocorticography. Brain Nerve. 2011;63(4):321-9.

[47] Crone NE, Hao L, Hart J, Jr., Boatman D, Lesser RP, Irizarry R, et al. Electrocorticographic gamma activity during word production in spoken and sign language. Neurology. 2001;57(11):2045-53.

[48] Korvenoja A, Kirveskari E, Aronen HJ, Avikainen S, Brander A, Huttunen J, et al. Sensorimotor cortex localization: comparison of magnetoencephalography, functional MR imaging, and intraoperative cortical mapping. Radiology. 2006;241(1):213-22.

[49] Sporns O, Tononi G, Edelman GM. Theoretical neuroanatomy and the connectivity of the cerebral cortex. Behav Brain Res. 2002;135(1-2):69-74.

[50] Duffau H. Contribution of cortical and subcortical electrostimulation in brain glioma surgery: methodological and functional considerations. Neurophysiol Clin. 2007;37(6):373-82.

[51] Krammer MJ, Wolf S, Schul DB, Gerstner W, Lumenta CB. Significance of intraoperative motor function monitoring using transcranial electrical motor evoked potentials (MEP) in patients with spinal and cranial lesions near the motor pathways. Br J Neurosurg. 2009;23(1):48-55.

[52] Markand ON. Brainstem auditory evoked potentials. J Clin Neurophysiol. 1994;11(3): 319-42.

[53] Legatt AD. Mechanisms of intraoperative brainstem auditory evoked potential changes. J Clin Neurophysiol. 2002;19(5):396-408.

[54] Lorenzano C, Gilio F, Inghilleri M, Conte A, Fofi L, Manfredi M, et al. Spread of electrical activity at cortical level after repetitive magnetic stimulation in normal subjects. Exp Brain Res. 2002;147(2):186-92.

[55] Levy WJ, York DH, McCaffrey M, Tanzer F. Motor evoked potentials from transcranial stimulation of the motor cortex in humans. Neurosurgery. 1984;15(3):287-302.

[56] Woodforth IJ, Hicks RG, Crawford MR, Stephen JP, Burke DJ. Variability of motor-evoked potentials recorded during nitrous oxide anesthesia from the tibialis anterior muscle after transcranial electrical stimulation. Anesth Analg. 1996;82(4):744-9.

[57] Mallik A, Weir AI. Nerve conduction studies: essentials and pitfalls in practice. J Neurol Neurosurg Psychiatry. 2005;76(Suppl 2):ii23-31.

[58] Nollet H, Van Ham L, Deprez P, Vanderstraeten G. Transcranial magnetic stimulation: review of the technique, basic principles and applications. Vet J. 2003;166(1): 28-42.

[59] Reithler J, Peters JC, Sack AT. Multimodal transcranial magnetic stimulation: using concurrent neuroimaging to reveal the neural network dynamics of noninvasive brain stimulation. Prog Neurobiol. 2011;94(2):149-65.

[60] Kobayashi M, Pascual-Leone A. Transcranial magnetic stimulation in neurology. Lancet Neurol. 2003;2(3):145-56.

[61] Chen R, Classen J, Gerloff C, Celnik P, Wassermann EM, Hallett M, et al. Depression of motor cortex excitability by low-frequency transcranial magnetic stimulation. Neurology. 1997;48(5):1398-403.

[62] Maeda F, Keenan JP, Tormos JM, Topka H, Pascual-Leone A. Interindividual variability of the modulatory effects of repetitive transcranial magnetic stimulation on cortical excitability. Exp Brain Res. 2000;133(4):425-30.

[63] Nezu A, Kimura S, Uehara S, Kobayashi T, Tanaka M, Saito K. Magnetic stimulation of motor cortex in children: maturity of corticospinal pathway and problem of clinical application. Brain Dev. 1997;19(3):176-80.

[64] Penfield W, Boldrey E. Somatic motor and sensory representation in the cerebral cortex of man as studied by electric stimulation. Brain. 1937;60:389-443.

[65] Simpson JR, Horton J, Scott C, Curran WJ, Rubin P, Fischbach J, et al. Influence of location and extent of surgical resection on survival of patients with glioblastoma multiforme: results of three consecutive Radiation Therapy Oncology Group (RTOG) clinical trials. Int J Radiat Oncol Biol Phys. 1993;26(2):239-44.

[66] Zamzuri I, Rahman GI, Muzaimi M, Jafri AM, Nik Ruzman NI, Lutfi YA, et al. Polymodal therapy for high grade gliomas: a case report of favourable outcomes following intraoperative radiation therapy. Med J Malaysia. 2012;67(1):121-2.

[67] Hochberg FH, Pruitt A. Assumptions in the radiotherapy of glioblastoma. Neurology. 1980;30(9):907-11.

[68] Battaglia D, Witt A, Wolf F, Geisel T. Dynamic effective connectivity of inter-areal brain circuits. PLoS Comput Biol. 2012;8(3):e1002438.

[69] Bullmore E, Sporns O. The economy of brain network organization. Nat Rev Neurosci. 1038;13(5):336-49.

[70] Sporns O, Tononi G, Edelman GM. Connectivity and complexity: the relationship between neuroanatomy and brain dynamics. Neural Netw. 2000;13(8-9):909-22.

[71] Momjian S, Seghier M, Seeck M, Michel CM. Mapping of the neuronal networks of human cortical brain functions. Adv Tech Stand Neurosurg. 2003;28:91-142.

[72] Ahmadlou M, Adeli H, Adeli A. Graph theoretical analysis of organization of functional brain networks in ADHD. Clin EEG Neurosci. 2012;43(1):5-13.

[73] Birbaumer N, Cohen LG. Brain-computer interfaces: communication and restoration of movement in paralysis. J Physiol. 2007;579(Pt 3):621-36.

[74] Prasad G, Herman P, Coyle D, McDonough S, Crosbie J. Applying a brain-computer interface to support motor imagery practice in people with stroke for upper limb recovery: a feasibility study. J Neuroeng Rehabil. 2010;7:60.

Chapter 3

Modern Neuroimaging Techniques in The Diagnosis of Brain Tumours

Concetta Alafaci, Francesca Granata,
Mariano Cutugno, Maria Caffo, Gerardo Caruso and
Francesco Maria Salpietro

Additional information is available at the end of the chapter

http://dx.doi.org/10.5772/53217

1. Introduction

Intracranial tumors represent a significant health problem. The annual incidence of primary and secondary central Nervous system neoplasms ranges from 10 to 17 per 100.000 persons. The main histological types of brain tumors in adults include: high-grade (gliomas, primary cerebral lymphomas, medulloblastomas), low-grade (meningiomas, acoustic neuromas, neurofibromas) and Secondaries (common malignancies spreading to the brain include lung cancer, breast cancer, stomach cancer, prostate cancer, thyroid cancer, colorectal cancer, melanoma and kidney cancer). In recent years, the diagnosis of brain tumors has considerable progressed due to continuous advances in neuroradiology.

Neuroradiology is a part of general radiology dedicated to the diagnostic examination of the brain and spinal cord. The history of neuroradiology, as a whole, reflects the history of radiological development. It is, on one hand, the history of collaboration of radiologists, neurologists and neurosurgeons in the development of clinical methods of Central Nervous System (CNS) radiological examination. On the other hand, it is the history of collaboration of physicists, mathematicians, engineers and radiologists in the design and creation of new devices for brain and diagnostics of spinal cord diseases.

Neuroradiology began in the early 1900s as soon after Roentgen discovered X-rays. He made the first X-ray image - a skull - in December 1895. X-rays promptly became the new tool in physics research and in medicine, providing many opportunities to visualize the internal structures of the human body. This was followed by the development of ventriculography in 1918 while the 1920s was the era of pneumoencephalography development thanks to the work of Walter Dandy, a prominent neurosurgeon at Johns Hopkins Hospital [1]. The 1930s were marked by the introduction of cerebral angiography. From 1935 to 1946, the phenomenon of nuclear magnetic resonance was discovered [2]. The 1950s and 1960s witnessed questions for practical solutions of tomography problems in neuroradiology and subsequent development of electronics and computer techniques. The 1970s and 1980s were the years of wide introduction of Computed Tomography (CT) in the clinical setting. When CT became available, the use of uncomfortable procedures was abruptly stopped because CT could depict the ventricular system and the intracranial suarachnoid spaces directly, without introducing air into the subarachnoid space itself [3]. As regard to the development of cerebral angiography, in the early 1960s, it was performed by means of direct puncture of the common carotid artery and the vertebral artery. In the late 1960s and early 1970s cerebral angiography was predominantly performed by means of selective catheter angiography following puncture of the femoral artery [3]. Progress in neuroradiology continued rapidly with the development of MR imaging in the late 1970s and early 1980s. The advantages of MRI imaging were that it could be performed in any plane and with various pulse sequences, obtaining more details of the cerebral anatomy [4]. By the end of 20th century, Magnetic Resonance Imaging (MRI) had been strongly incorporated into the clinical practice, and in some cases (spinal cord examination) became a method of choice compared to the CT. The high tissue resolution and the wide variety of types of contrast for MR images are typical for MRI. Currently, MRI employs several physical factors defining the brightness of tissue on the image such as: proton density; $T1$ and $T2$ relaxation time of protons in tissue; movement of protons in the large vessels with a blood–cerebrospinal fluid (CSF) flow and passage of protons through a capillary net; random thermal water molecule motion; anisotropy of the diffusion proton motion and magnetic susceptibility of tissues; chemical shift of proton's resonance frequency in molecular complexes. In addition, volumetric CT and super-fast MRI have opened wide diagnostic opportunities of CNS examination not only on a level of anatomic structures (simulation and support of surgery, endoscopy), but also on a level of molecular and gene biology. Neuroradiology has become the quantitative method of brain function examination, able to monitor and predict the results of therapeutic treatment and surgical intervention of many diseases [5].

Further development of neuroradiology is closely linked with the increase of processing speed and improvements in computer technologies, increase of (MRI) magnetic field induction, development of "open" magnets for biopsy, intra-operative control, examination of critical patients.

This chapter focuses on the role of the most commonly used advanced MR imaging techniques – perfusion imaging, diffusion-weighted imaging, and MRI spectroscopy- for the diagnosis of the most common brain tumors in adults.

1.2. Conventional MRI imaging

When dealing with a patient with a brain tumor, standard X-rays and CT scan is initially used in the diagnostic process. However, MRI is generally more useful because it provides detailed informations about tumor type, position and size, tumor anatomy, cellular structure and vascular supply, making it an important tool for the diagnosis, treatment and monitoring of the disease. For this reason, MRI is the study of choice of brain tumors.

Discussion of MRI physic details is beyond the scope of this chapter. The concept that is important to remind is that conventional MRI exploits three physical properties of tissue protons to generate signal imaged as areas of different contrast, which reflect the anatomy and physiology of the organ under investigation. Those protons properties which contribute to MRI signal generation are Proton Density (defined as the number of hydrogen protons per unit of volume of tissue), T1 relaxation time (which is the time requested to recover 63% of the longitudinal magnetization) and T2 relaxation time (which is defined as the time requested to recover 63% of the transverse magnetization to be lost). T1 and T2 relaxation time and proton density are all specific for different type of tissues and increase as the magnet`s field strength increases [6]. In all three types of images, bright areas correspond to tissue with high signal intensity (i.e. areas with large transverse magnetization) and are referred to as hyperintense, whereas dark areas correspond to low signal intensity (i.e. small transverse magnetization) and are referred to as hypointense.

Different types of acquisition of MR imaging give different informations (table 1):

- T1-weighted images give a lot of anatomical informations as well as informations about venous sinus permeability or pathologic blush. CSF is dark and fat is white in T1-weighted sequences. Lesions bright in T1- weighted sequences are: fat (lipoma, dermoid), subacute haemorrhage (metHb), metastatic melanoma (melanotic), protein-containing fluid (colloid cyst) and paramagnetic agents (gadolinium).

- T2-weighted images give informations about oedema, arteries and sinus permeability. Water is white in T2- weighted sequences, fat appears intermediate to dark, and haematomas have a variable signal intensity. Some dark lesions on T2-weighted images are acute haemorrhage (deoxyHb), haemosiderin, iron and mucinous lesions.

- A proton density-weighted image is an image primarily dependent on the density of protons in the imaging volume. The higher the number of protons in a given unit of tissue, the brighter the signal is. Proton density-weighted images have excellent grey matter–white matter contrast, as their brain CSF contrast is much lower. It is useful to study basal nuclei anatomy and differentiate lacunar infarctions from Virchow-Robin spaces, and to evaluate also cerebral gliosis.

Conventional MRI gives morphological informations about brain tumors. Some authors name Conventional MRI as Morphological MRI, to differentiate it from Functional MRI that will be discussed later. Those morphological informations are both macroscopic and microscopic (T2 sequences give useful information in this sense, with a low signal intensity in the presence of calcification, melanin, lipids and haemosiderin). The vascularization of the neoplasm can be seen with the typical vessel aspect characterized by absence of signal in all sequences (the so called "Signal Void").

Most of the tumors are iso-hypointense in T1 and hyperintense in DP and T2. A hyperintensity in T1, however, can only be caused by fat (lipomas) and paramagnetic substances, such as melanin (melanoma metastases) and different degradation products of hemoglobin. Tumors with high cellularity (medulloblastomas, lymphomas) are characterized by a hyperintensity in DP and relatively low signal on T2-weighted images. Meningiomas are usually isointense in all sequences, and- if small - may be disregarded on the basic examination.

The cystic-necrotic areas usually associated with malignant tumor such as glioblastoma multiforme (GBM) are markedly hypointense on T1 and hyperintense on T2. Signal can be differentiated, in most cases, from that of CSF in the proton density, as necrotic areas are slightly hyperintense, while CSF is slightly hypointense. It is important the concentration of proteins within cystic tumors, being the hyperintensity in the T2 sequences directly proportional to the protein concentration. It must be noted, on the other hand, that when the protein concentration in the cystic lesion is too high there can be a paradoxal hyperintensity in T1 and hypointensity in T2 sequences. The hemorrhagic areas cause the typical alterations of signal that follow the steps of degradation of haemoglobin. Calcifications are highlighted as areas of signal void, hypointense in T2 and DP. Perilesional edema is characterized as an area slightly hypointense on T1 and hyperintense in DP and T2. The mass effect can be evaluated in a much more accurate way than CT in studying the behavior of convolutions of the brain. A lesion may be considered intra-axial if it expands the adjacent cerebral convolutions. Anyway an intra-axial lesion may invade the meninges (eg, metastasis, glioblastoma multiforme) and an extra-axial lesions can invade the brain tissue (eg, dural metastases).

Another important sequences in MRI is "Fluid Attenuated Inversion Recovery" (FLAIR) also called the "dark fluid technique". It is used to remove the effects of fluid from the resulting images. Lesions that are normally covered by bright fluid signals on T2-weighted images are visible by FLAIR. Its use is very common in many specific diseases, such as multiple sclerosis. Particularly, the correct evaluation of site and extension of the tumour is an important step to define the possibility of surgical resection. FLAIR sequences, available in 3D form on modern MRI equipment, seem to be mandatory to assess the extension of a glioma, usually with a hyperintense signal. 3D T1 weighted GRE sequences can provide images with high inplane spatial resolution without interslice gaps. This technique can be, therefore, very useful, after gadolinium injection, to obtain volumetric MRI data that can be reconstructed in any desired plane, suitable for presurgical planning or surgical navigation system.

Another important tool in MRI imaging is the use of contrast medium. Gadolinium, a rare earth metal, is frequently used in MRI. The paramagnetic properties of gadolinium affect free protons and hence shorten Tl-weighted signal. Gadolinium is not visualized but its effect on free protons. Increased concentrations of gadolinium will result in high signal, i.e. enhancement, on Tl weighting. It highlights areas of blood-brain barrier breakdown, areas of inflammation and increased vascularity. Marked enhancement is normally visible in the pituitary gland, choroid plexus, nasal mucosa and turbinates, and in slowflowing blood in vessels. Contrast enhancement is frequently used to improve detection and definition of tumors, infections, meningeal diseases, vascular diseases and "post-operative spine". Gadolinium is an extremely safe substance and has been used worldwide with less side-effects compared to iodinated contrast media. Gadolinium is a substance that allows the study of the blood-brain barrier permeability in brain tumors: low-grade tumors, which contain capillaries with a structure similar to the normal nervous tissue with tight junction, are characterized by no enhancement, while high-grade tumors have pathological capillaries with a high enhancement after gadolinium administration, expression of the blood-brain barrier disruption. As regard to extra-axial tumors, they usually have high enhancement because, being extra-axial lesions, they have no blood-brain barrier.

Basically the most important goals of conventional MRI in the diagnosis of brain tumors are:

- discover the lesion and define its nature (blood, ischaemia, tumor).

- localize the lesion (intra- or extra-axial, above or under the tentorium) and define its limits and relations with the surrounding structures, with the use of gadolinium.

- evaluate mass effect (compression, dislocations, cerebral erniation).

- evaluate the characteristics (necrosis, calcifications, surrounding oedema, haemorrhage, rupture of blood-brain barrier).

- give indications about the most probable histological nature and grade of malignancy of the tumor.

- define the vascularization and the relations with the closest cerebral vessels (very important in meningiomas, where it is necessary to evaluate the feeding arteries, in order to consider the possibility of a preoperative endovascular embolization, and the possible infiltration of dural sinus or cerebral vessels).

Substance	**On T1 weighting**	**On T2 weighting**
Water	Black	White
Fat	White	Gray/white
White matter	Gray	Gray/black
Gray matter	Gray/black	Gray/white
Bone		
Cortex	Black	Black
Marrow	White	Gray/white
Calcification	Gray/white	Black
Intervertebral disk	Gray	White
Air	Black	Black
Hematoma	Depends on the phase	Depend on the phase
Most pathology	Gray/black	White

Table 1. Signal intensity on MRI

1.3. Digital Subtraction Angiography (DSA)

Catheter angiography is an invasive technique which has progressively become safer with the introduction of DSA, non-iodate contrast media and improved catheters and guide wires.

The right femoral artery is punctured using the Seldinger technique. The catheter is then advanced up to the aortic arch and then, selectively, into the required artery. The catheters are usually 4F or 5F in size and pre-shaped to facilitate selective catheterization. Once in position in the desired artery, the formal DSA is undertaken with the contrast injection by hand or mechanical pump. Multiple projections are used to demonstrate the vasculature and images are obtained as far as the venous phase in several planes. Commonly, the internal carotid circulation is studied in lateral, posteroanterior 20° and oblique projection, e.g. 30° cranio-caudal, 30° lateral.

The posterior circulation is studied in lateral and Townes' projection (30° fronto-occipital). Numerous supplementary projections can be performed according to which vessel has to be demonstrated. This is particularly Important in the diagnosis of aneurysms where a clear demonstration of the neck of the aneurysm is required, especially if endovascular treatment has to be considered.

Local complications occur in about 5% of cases and range from self-limiting hematoma to fatal retroperitoneal hematoma. Vessel injury can result in pseudo-aneurysm, arteriovenous fistula and distal emboli.

Systemic complications are related to the contrast media or, very occasionally, to local anesthetics and sedation. Contrast media reactions are common to all radiological procedures using iodinated contrast. The risk is increased by history of previous reaction and in asthma sufferers, where the risk of severe reaction is about 0.2%. Neurological complications range from headache to disabling stroke or death. The risks are increased in the older population (over 50 years), particularly if there is atherosclerosis, vasculitis or sickle cell disease.

Cerebral DSA remains the investigation of choice in a number of conditions despite improvements in Doppler ultrasound, MRAand CTA. The most common reason for its use is in the investigation of Subarachnoid hemorrhage (SAH), where DSA remains the gold standard. Other indications for angiography include: assessment of aneurysms (e.g.fusiform, dissecting, mycotic, giant) that have not presented with SAH; assessment of AVMs and other vascular lesions, such as carotido-cavernous fistula or dural fistula; investigation of various cerebrovascular disorders, such as vasculitis and demonstration of tumor vascularity, particularly if pre-operative embolization has been considered. This is particularly true for intracranial meningiomas. Meningiomas are commonly supplied by dural arteries such as middle meningeal artery, accessory meningeal arery, ascending pharyngeal, or occipital transmastoid perforating branches of the external carotid artery. Dural arteries also include the tentorial and infratentorial trunk branches of the internal carotid artery, as well as the posterior meningeal branch of the vertebral artery. Secondary supply to meningiomas may be derived from pial branches (of the anterior, middle and posterior cerebral arteries). Embolization involves the devascularization of the tumor's supply through the placement of an embolic agent via a microcatheter into the feeding arteries. Because meningiomas are usually vascularized, preoperative tumor embolization can easily complete tumor resection by diminishing operative time and intraoperative blood loss [7]. Diagnostic angiography can also identify important informations for the surgeon such as a potential occlusion of a dural sinus adjacent to the tumor and the pattern of collateral venous drainage around such an occlusion.

Angiography in gliomas is not specific. Many gliomas, especially low-grade, are seen as avascular or hypovascular areas surrounded by displaced normal vessels. High-grade gliomas may show intense tumor neovascularization in a disorganized pattern, a prominent tumor blush in the mid-arterial phase, hypovascular areas representing necrosis or cysts and arteriovenous shunting with early draining veins which represent the most angiographically common finding in glioblastoma multiforme. These characteristics do not allow the differentiation of a primary glioblastoma from a secondary lesion. Some authors propose the possibility to use DSA in patients with brain metastases, in order to get a regional chemoinfusion to the arteries feeding the metastatic foci [8].

1.4 . New Functional Methods in Neuroradiology

The increase of the processing speed of CT and MRI scanners, the invention of new data-registration technologies and the algorithms of data-processing transfer neuroradiology allowed great development in neuroradiology. Functional MRI can detect areas of the brain having increased neuronal and metabolic activity, and areas of damage in the brain–blood barrier. It makes a quantitative assessment of microvascular permeability of brain tissue, evaluates the state of receptors on the cell surface as well as hormonal activity, and reveals the presence of certain antigen and protein structures [5]. Thus, CT and MRI perform diagnostics not only on a cellular, but also on a molecular level. Diffusion, perfusion, MR spectroscopy and functional MRI belong to the so-called methods of molecular visualization.

1.4.1. Diffusion Weighted Imaging

Diffusion is the basic physical process occurring during the cell's metabolic reactions. Kinetic energy leads to Brownian motion (random walk) of molecules (thermal motion; the speed is about 10–3 mm2/s). As a whole, the molecular motion of protons in physiological systems is divided into three types:

1. movements with moderate speed in macroscopic vessels (about 10–100 mm/s);
2. slow flow in a capillary net, or perfusion (the speed is about 0.1–10 mm/s); and
3. diffusion motion of molecules (the speed is about 10–3 mm2/s).

Blood flow in large vessels is measured as a volume-in-time unit, perfusion flow (a local blood flow) is measured as the volume of blood passing in and out of a given tissue weight (volume) per unit of time and the diffusion factor is estimated by the average square of the distance made by molecules for a time unit.

The image appearance in "*isotropic*" Diffusion Weighted Imaging (DWI) is based on the principle that molecules in any living tissue routinely undergo random (brownian) motion. Isotropic DW images are typically obtained by measuring loss of signal after a pulse sequence that consists of a series of two sequential gradient pulses added to a 90°–180° spin-echo sequence on either side of the 180° pulse [9]. The degree of MR signal loss after application of the second gradient pulse is related to two factors:

a. the duration and strength of the magnetic field gradients and

b. the diffusion coefficient of the substance.

The apparent diffusion coefficient (ADC) is a value that describes microscopic water diffusibility in the presence of factors that restrict diffusion within tissues (eg, cell membranes, viscosity). The ADC can be derived on a voxel-by-voxel basis and depicted on an ADC map, which allows ADCs in specific regions to be measured by using regions of interest. Measurement of the ADC would be expected to be useful in tumor assessment because variations in water content (and diffusivity), which can be found within tumors for various reasons (eg, necrosis, variations in cellularity) and adjacent to tumors (eg, vasogenic edema), provide information that is not readily available from conventional MR imaging.

The motion of the water molecules in live tissues occurs within the cell limits (the limited diffusion), as well as in intercellular spaces among structures, which restrict the molecules motion but still leaves them some freedom for manoeuvring between obstacles (the complicated diffusion). Water diffusion inside extracellular space is inversely proportional to the density of the intracellular space constituents.

The tendency for water molecules to diffuse in some directions rather than equally in all directions is termed "*anisotropy*." Highly compact white matter fiber tracts exhibit a high degree of anisotropy, and less compact white matter pathways exhibit lesser degrees of anisotropy. All types of white matter typically show greater degrees of anisotropy than are seen in gray matter structures, which have a low degree of anisotropy.

Diffusion Tensor Imaging (DTI) represents a magnetic resonance imaging method that is expression of fractional water anisotrophy (FA) and is available in many modern clinical scanners. DTI is similar to DWI but involves the collection of additional data necessary to define the tensor (vector) which describes the preferential direction and magnitude of water diffusion. FA maps has been used to investigate the microstructure of white matter that can be altereted in many pathologic conditions such as brain tumors. DTI provides a sensitive means to detect alterations in the integrity of white matter structures. In fact, in many settings, white matter abnormalities can be seen on diffusion-tensor images being not evident on routine MR images [2,3]. Diffusion-tensor imaging also provides a means of depicting white matter pathways (tractography). This may be useful in neurosurgical procedures by preoperatively depicting important white matter tracts, helping determine infiltration of white matter tracts by tumor, and providing evidence of degeneration of white matter tracts distal to tumor sites (ie, wallerian degeneration). In the real biological environment, water molecules can encounter natural barriers, such as cellular membranes and large albumin molecules, which can interfere with free motion of protons. Therefore, in practice, the apparent diffusion coefficient is calculated, and its value is lower than diffusion coefficient for pure water at temperature.

All diffusion-weighted examinations are performed without contrast injection. This is important for critically ill and restless patients, and especially for special examinations of brain development in children, beginning with the prenatal period. In the last case, DWI enables to obtain both the additional qualitative (visualization) and quantitative tissue characteristics.

1.4.1.2. Clinical Application of DWI and DTI

Today, DWI is one of the fastest and highly specific methods of early-phase ischaemic stroke diagnostics (within 6 h of onset), during which there is a therapeutic window for restoration of the affected brain tissue. In acute phase of stroke, the affected area on DWI typically has a high MR signal, whereas the surrounding tissues look dark. The ADC maps provide a reverse-in-brightness picture. Diffusion ADC maps are a tool in the diagnosis and monitoring of cerebral ischaemia.

DWI provides invaluable informations for inflammatory lesions of brain and spinal cord (abscesses, empyema). Purulent abscess content has a typical hyperintense MR signal on DWI and can be easily visualised on pretreatment (before draining) and as well on postoperative images. In addition, DWI can be used in the assessment of drainage intervention effectiveness or in the case of verification of the purulent complication in incision wound.

DWI and ADC maps provide great help in the diagnosis of brain tumors, providing additional diagnostic informations for differentiation of neoplasms with similar signs on *T*1 and *T*2 MRI (glioma, tumours with ring-shaped contrast accumulation), peritumoral oedema (vasogenic or cytotoxic) or the presence or absence of intratumoral cysts, only to name a few [10]. At the same time, as some authors demonstrate, DWI data alone do not allow differentiation between benign astrocytoma and anaplastic tumours, or between anaplastic astrocytoma and glioblastoma [5].

In many observations, the peripheral part of a tumor (as a rule in the case of malignant gliomas) is hyperintense on DWI; presumably it is linked to more dense cellular arrangement in the most actively growing tumor area (accordingly, there is a limitation on diffusive proton motion in this area). In fact, it has been demonstrated that the higher the tumor cellularity is the greater is the ADC value . It is demonstrated that value of ADC higher than 100×10^{-3} mm^2/s is typical of high grade tumors while ADC values lower than 100×10^{-3} mm^2/s are related to low grade lesion [11].

A low ADC in an intra-axial neoplasm should raise suspicion for lymphoma or metastatis, depending on the conventional MRI appearance, because the higher cellularity of these tumors generally produces an ADC which is significantly lower than in glioma. However, although most gliomas have a higher ADC (related to their lower cellularity), a number of case reports have demonstrated a low ADC in a small number of glioblastoma. Thus it is important to integrate DWI with other advanced and conventional neuroimaging data for accurate clinical interpretation [12].

In other brain neoplasms—in particular meningiomas and neurinomas— DWI may predict tumour histological type, with high reliability even before surgery. Based on this method data, the epidermoid and arachnoid cysts can be precisely differentiated. In fact DWI has a sensivity and specificy of over 90% for distinguishing epidermoid (low ADC) from aracnoid cyst (high ADC) and distinguishing abscess (low ADC) from necrotic tumor (high ADC). The viscous keratin and cholesterol in epidermoid and the viscous and cellular pus in abscess produce a very low ADC that distinguishes these lesions from increased diffusivity in necrotic tumor and from normal or slightly low diffusivity in demyelinating plaque. Meningiomas, a lower ADC has been demonstrated in atypical and malignant subtypes. It is also demonstrated that the eterogeneity of ADC within tumor reflects heterogeneity of cellularity within it [12].

Recently, DWI and DTI methods have begun to be applied to visualisation of a neural tract lines—tractography. This is a new and promising technique that enables non-invasive viewing of the brain neural tracts [13]. Despite some technical problems, the first results in tractography application to neurosurgery seem promising [5]. It is possible to plan operational access and to estimate the scope of brain hematoma to be removed, taking into account neural tracts and their involvement in the pathological process (dislocation–deformation, invasion, damage), with an aim to maximise the radical tumour resection and to minimise the subsequent complications [14].

In gliomas, the infiltration of the tumor disrupts the organization of the white matter tracts: FA derived from DTI defines of the degree of tumor infiltration. [12]. Some studies also suggest that DTI may distinguish vasogenic edema in brain metastases and meningiomas from non-enhancing tumor infiltration in gliomas. It has to be considered that white matter adjacent to glioma generally contains different proportions of vasogenic edema and tumor infiltration at different distances from the center of the tumor, making more difficult to define an unbiased region of interest for valid data analysis.

1.4.2. Perfusion Weighted Imaging

Perfusion studies are useful to quantify blood movement supplying each element of organ or tissue volume. It is widely known that, unlike the majority of parenchymatous tissue, brain tissue does not accumulate glucose, and brain cells can produce energy via anaerobic glycolysis only for several minutes.

Meanwhile, the brain consumes about 25% of all glucose consumed in the entire body, and for neurons, the uninterrupted and sufficient supply of oxygen and glucose is necessary.

There are complex mechanisms of autoregulation that manage brain perfusion to satisfy the demands of the nervous system for energy (released in a course of metabolic processes).

There are several modern quantitative methods of brain haemodynamic examination: MRI, CT with contrast enhancement, CT with Xe, single-photon emission computed tomography (SPECT) imaging and positron emission tomography (PET). The obvious advantages of CT and MRI are minimally invasive, high sensitivity in tissue microcirculation assessment, high resolution, the short examination time (within the framework of standard protocols), and

http://dx.doi.org/10.5772/53217

last, but not least, the reproducibility of results. The most widespread perfusion examination in neuroradiology is based on intravenous bolus administration (CT and MRI). The dynamic studies of bolus passage demonstrate its distribution in tissue in each given image pixel, depending on time. The following main haemodynamic characteristics are used for quantitative assessment: cerebral blood flow (CBF), cerebral blood volume (CBV) and mean transit time (MTT).

The blood flow characteristics are measured in the ratio to 100 g of brain tissue. Accordingly, the value of CBV is measured in millilitres per 100 g of brain tissue, and CBF is measured in millilitres per 100 g per minute. The local (regional) CBV is defined as percentage of blood volume in a single element of brain tissue volume. MTT is measured in seconds.

Perfusion CT

CT approaches to perfusion imaging were first proposed in the early 1980s. However, clinical uses of perfusion CT were slow to progress because the technique suffered initially from relatively limited imaging volumes and poor temporal resolution. With the advent of multidetector CT, rapid scanning of larger volumes at faster speeds has been possible. Also, because CT uses ionizing radiation while MR imaging does not, MR imaging would seem to offer an advantage. However, CT techniques requiring lower milliampere-second values have been developed, associated to lower radiation dose. The use of iodinated contrast agents, with the associated risks of allergic reaction and nephrotoxicity, remains a drawback in some patients. However, perfusion CT has some clear advantages compared to perfusion MR imaging. CT scanners are generally more widely available, and CT does not suffer from magnetic susceptibility artefacts, which can compromise perfusion MR images when hemorrhage or other causes of magnetic susceptibility effect are present in the area of interest.

Initial analyses of CT data with deconvolution methods used indicator-dilution methods that suffered from the same problems as dynamic susceptibility contrast (DSC) MR approaches. The modern spiral CT scanners present new opportunities in tissue perfusion examination during the first passage of the iodide contrast bolus. This method has high resolution and provides quantitative assessments of tissue perfusion, and currently, it is one of the most perspective methods. Perfusion CT is based on analysis of CT density increase during contrast media passage through brain vascular structures. Contrast bolus (iodine agent with concentration 350–370 mg/ml, speed of administration is 4 ml/s) is administered intravenously. Spiral CT obtains a series of scans with 1-s intervals, within 50–60 s after contrast administration

Perfusion MRI (PWI)

There are MRI methods of haemodynamic perfusion examination, aided by exogenous and endogenous markers. The methods of perfusion assessment during contrast bolus passage are called perfusion-weighted MRI, or PWI. Perfusion-Weighted MRI can be performed by using either a gradient-echo or a spin-echo pulse sequence. Gradient-echo DSC sequences tend to be more sensitive to larger vessels, such as veins, in the imaged region. Spin-echo DSC techniques tend to show greater sensitivity to smaller vessels (and therefore are more representative of capillary density) or tumor-specific vessels.

These examination methods are currently widely used in MR diagnostics, especially in combination with MR angiography and MR spectroscopy. PWI uses changes of *T*1 or *T*2 tissues contrast due to infusion of gadolinium into blood as a contrast agent. Normally, gadolinium does not pass through blood–brain barrier. It can pass into intracellular spaces only in cases of blood–brain barrier disruptions. The CM bolus is administrated quickly (about 2–3 s); the speed of administration is 4–5 ml/s and is higher than in the standard infusion. The bolus passage on consecutive (in time) scans corresponds to the sharp decrease of MR signal intensity. In the process of CM bolus passage through the vascular system, multiple registration of the image from the same location occurs (usually it is 10 different levels).

The scanning takes place for 1–2 min. The graph of intensity decrease during CM bolus passage provides the curve "signal intensity–time" in each pixel of the scan. The form of this curve for arteries and veins provides arterial and venous function data. With these data, the haemodynamic tissue parameters are calculated. The regional CBV (rCBV) is estimated on the basis of area under curve "concentration–time"; the MTT calculation is performed on the basis of centre of gravity in CM distribution position, regional CBF (rCBF) = rCBV/MTT. The perfusion maps are built in "off-line" mode in the specialised workstations. The method of dynamic *T*1 MRI is used in cases of examination of CM distribution in extracellular spaces.

1.4.2.3. Clinical Applications of CT and MRI Perfusion

Currently, perfusion examinations are performed to estimate the haemodynamic of brain tumours, monitor tumour-state after chemo- and radiotherapy, detect the tumour recurrence and radiation necrosis. This procedure gives informations in cases of brain injury and CNS damage like ischaemia, hypoxia, large-arteries stenosis, blood diseases, vasculitis and moyamoya disease. Epilepsy, migraine, vasospasm, various mental diseases (including dementia), autism, and so forth are prospective in terms of perfusion methods application.

CT and MRI perfusion allow building of parametric maps and quantitative characterization of areas of hyper- and hypo-perfusion, which is very important in diagnosis of tumours and cerebrovascular diseases. Perfusion maps provide important additional information about characteristics of normal and pathological tissues (in areas of tumour, oedema, necrosis). In neurosurgery, Perfusion Weighted Imaging (PWI) is used in primary differential diagnosis of tumor grading, in particular gliomas. However, perfusion CT and MRI do not specifically allow differentiating tumours according their histology, nor does it enable estimation of the tumour spreading into brain tissue [5].

The hyperperfusion in the structure of astrocytoma can indicate increase of tumour malignancy because the degree of perfusion is related to the development of abnormal vascular net (angiogenesis). In other words, the tumor perfusion is related to the grade of the tumor itself and the most important value to evaluate it is rCBV (higher rCBV values indicates high grade tumors while rCBV values $< 1,5$ are usually related to tumor with low grade of malignancy) [15]. Maia et al demonstrated that rCBV correlates with the vascular endothelial growth factors (VEGF) which is expression of the angiogenesis in gliomas [16].

If the abnormal vascular net in a tumour can be the evidence of its aggressiveness, on the other hand the decrease of perfusion in a tumour tissue under the influence of chemo- or radiotherapy can be a sign of response to treatment. The use of PWI in target selection for stereotactic intervention is helpful, especially in cases of gliomas characterized by full absence of contrast accumulation with the use of standard CT and MRI. (Fig 1 c)

PWI potential is higher in assessment of histological type and spreading of extra-axial neoplasms than of intra-axial ones. PWI successfully visualizes meningiomas and neurinomas of cerebellopontine angle, according to the high haemodynamic parameters of these tumors. In addition, it has been demonstrated that there is a clear correlation between local blood flow (CBF, CBV) and direct angiography data in patients with meningiomas. The tumours with radiopaque shadows in the early capillary phase of angiography have high perfusion, and such tumours are characterised by high risk of a intraoperational bleeding. CT PWI data are highly specific in demonstrating the blood supply of haemangiomas located in posterior cranial fossa; in this case, early and marked contrasting is combined with high perfusion.

PWI is also successfully used in differential diagnosis of postoperative residual tumour growth and radionecrosis. In both cases, standard CT and MR examinations can show the accumulation of contrast in the lesion and blood–brain barrier disruption. Blood–brain barrier disruptions cause CM extravasation in pathological tissues, with subsequent contrast accumulation. However, the pathophysiological reasons in both cases are different. For tumoral tissues, the perfusion increase or the reaching of normal perfusion level are typical, while in necrotic tissues the blood supply is absent. Blood–brain barrier disruption in tumours is related to the invasive growth of tumour cells and vascular wall damage. In case of radionecrosis, the disruption of blood– brain barrier is an initial step, but the radionecrosis is characterized by a decrease perfusion level (iso- or hypoperfusion). The areas of radionecrosis appear as areas of weak blood filling on CBV maps.

Undoubtedly, ischaemic brain damage takes the first place in the frequency of PWI methods used. Currently, PWI is an integral part of diagnostics in patients in whom cerebral ischaemia is suspected. The first clinical PWI application in brain lesion diagnostic in humans was performed for stroke diagnosis. At present, perfusion MRI is the only method to verify early ischaemia, is capable to show the haemodynamic decrease in certain brain areas (as the main mechanism of ischaemic damage), even in the first minutes after appearance of focal neurogical deficit.

1.4.3. Proton MR Spectroscopy

MR spectroscopy (MRS) is a non-invasive method of brain metabolism assessment. Proton (1H) MRS is based on a "chemical shift" which is the change of proton resonant frequency. This term was developed by N. Ramsey in 1951, for defining a distinction between frequencies of separate spectral peaks. The chemical shift measured unit is in parts per million (ppm). The main metabolites and corresponding values of the chemical shift are: *N*-acetylaspartate (NAA), 2 ppm; choline (Cho), 3.2 ppm; creatine (Cr), 3.03 and 3.94 ppm; *myo*-inositol (mI), 3.56 ppm; glutamate and glutamine (Glx), 2.1–2.5 ppm; lactate (Lac), 1.32 ppm; and a complex of lipids (Lip), 0.8–1.2 ppm.

Multinuclear MRS, based on phosphorus, carbon and other element nuclei, are entering the clinical practice.

Currently in proton MRS, two basic methods are used, single voxel (SV) and multivoxel (MV, or chemical shift imaging). MRS is a single-stage detection of spectra from several brain areas.

MV-MRS simultaneously obtains MR spectra for several voxels, and thus it is possible to compare spectra from different elements in an examination area. Processing of the MV-MRS data enables construction of a parametrical map of brain. The concentration of particular metabolites on this map is marked by colour, and thus it is possible to visualize the metabolite distribution in brain, i.e. to obtain an image weighed on the chemical shift. *NAA* is the most visible peak in the 1H spectrum (at 2 ppm). In the adult brain, NAA plays at least two roles:

1. as a predecessor of brain lipids, and
2. as a participant in coenzyme A interactions.

Some researchers believe that NAA is metabolically inert, and it participates only in maintenance of "deficiency anion" balance in neutral tissues, so it is the indicator of processes with neurotransmitter–neuromodulator participation, and its basic function is to be the form of free storage of aspartate. In an adult brain, the concentration of NAA in the cortex is higher than in the white matter, as the majority of NAA is located in neurons and their branches.

Due to the mainly neuronal and axonal NAA location, the NAA peak decreases in cases of neurodegenerative diseases.

The *choline* contribution is a sum of signals from several choline-containing chemical compounds (phosphoryl choline, glycerophosphoryl choline and free choline), and probably together with choline, which is present in a form of a polar head group in lipid membranes. MRS might not detect the compounds of choline embedded in a membrane; however, in the case of cell membrane destruction caused by the disease, choline is released, accumulated and may be them detected. Choline is a structural component of cellular membranes, especially myelin membranes. The choline peak tends to increase in highly malignant tumours and neurodegenerative diseases. Focal inflammation, which leads to considerable local cellularity and often to significant cellular membranes damages, could also result in increasing of choline peak.

The *creatine* peak at 3.03 ppm is caused by protons of methyl (CH3) group of creatine, phosphocreatine, lysine and glutathione. It appears that phosphocreatine is the basic molecule for maintenance of energy-dependent systems in all brain cells. Its concentration is maximal in cerebellum, followed by grey, and then by white, matter. Usually, it is assumed that the general creatine level is stable in different situations; therefore, the height of creatine peak is often used as reference in comparison with the height of other metabolites peaks.

MI has two peaks at 3.56 and 4.06 ppm, and it is supposed to function as storage of membranous phosphoinositides, which are the second messengers of the hormonal systems and participate in CNS enzyme regulation. It is one of the major growth factors, and it is a predecessor of phosphatidylinositol, which in turn is a part of the lipid layers of cellular membranes. It is primarily located in glial cells and, therefore, could serve as a specific glial marker.

The low combined peak at 3.56 ppm is from glycine and inositol-1-phosphate.

Another important metabolite that can be detected is lactate, which is a marker of anaerobic glycolisis. Lactate is detected by its typical doublet located in 1H MRS spectra around 1.32 ppm. It is believed that lactate, if found in greater quantities, especially in the first hours of life, is an indicator of brain damage. Lactate concentration varies as the brain matures: it is higher in newborns and in less-matured areas of the brain, such as parietal, anterior frontal and temporal. In more mature brains, lactate concentration is higher, for example in the basal ganglia and central gyri. Lactate is also a pathological metabolite in cases of high grade tumours, together with lipids (frequency range 0,8-1,3 ppm) that represent a marker of myelin disruption and necrosis.

Currently, the following areas of proton MRS clinical application are: injury, metabolic and mitochondrial damages, as well as inflammatory and volumetric disorders.

1.4.3.1. Proton MR Spectroscopy and Brain Tumours

MRS is now widely used to estimate various volumetric brain formations [17]. The most important goals of H-MRS are:

- *differentiate neoplastic from non-neoplastic lesion.* MRS accuracy is 95% to 100% in distinguishing neoplastic from non-neoplastic lesions. Cho is considered the most specific marker of intracranial neoplasm and increase in Cho levels and Cho/Cr and Cho/NAA ratio is very suggestive of neoplasm.

- *differentiate primary neoplasm versus metastases.* Absent or practically absent NAA and Cr levels are suggestive of a metastatic lesion. If the spectral analysis of the peritumoral region shows an increase in Cho level, it is probably an infiltration related to primary neoplasm. If there's no increase in Cho level it is probably vasogenic edema associated with metastasis.

- *indicate tumor grade and extension.* Sensitivity, specificity and accuracy of proton MRS are 100%, 86% and 96% respectively, in discriminating between high and low grade neoplasm. The most important metabolites to estimate tumour grade are Cho (higher Cho levels are related to cell density and correlate with the grade of the tumors), Lactate (there's a correct correlation between lactate levels and tumor grade), lipids (they are tipically found in high grade tumors), NAA and Cr (they usually decrease in high grade tumors), Mi (In low grade tumors Mi/Cr ratio is typically greater than in high grade tumors).

- *assess the ideal site for biopsy:* if performed in the site where the Cho/NAA ratio is maximum the biopsy will show high tumor infiltration.

- *demonstrate tumour extension*: intracranial neoplasm often extend beyond enhancement demonstrated in gadolinium-enhanced MRI. The high signal area on T2 surrounding the neoplasm may represent vasogenic edema, tumor infiltration, and or abnormalities induced by radiotherapy and chemiotherapy.

- *demonstrate tumour progression*: Cho and lactate levels are considered prognostic factors in patients with intracranial neuroepithelial tumors. An increase in Cho levels > 140% in the lesion is related to high risk of tumor progression.Tumor progression is characterized by an increase in Cho levels greater than 45%, while in tumors that do not progress Cho levels decrease, maintain or rise less than 35%.

- *demonstrate therapeutic response:* Proton MRS is very useful in follow therapeutic response, identify residual or recurrent tumor earlier than conventional MRI and, above all, differentiate residual or recurrent tumor from post-treatment abnormalities. Evidence of radiation necrosis is typically observed within 6 months and is characterized by reduced Cho and increased lipid and lactate levels or by a normal spectral pattern. Postradiation and postchemotherapy necrotic areas are usually characterized by absent or decreased brain metabolites (NAA, Cr, Cho, Mi), elevated lipid and lactate levels, large peak between 0 and 2 ppm indicating cell necrosis products.

Definitively, even if it is impossible to predict with sufficient confidence the neoplasm histological type, nevertheless, the majority of researchers agree that tumoural processes as a whole are characterised by a low NAA–Cr ratio, increase in Cho–Cr ration, and in some cases, by the lactate peak.

In the majority of performed MRS examinations, proton spectroscopy is used in differential diagnostics of astrocytoma, ependymoma and primitive neuroepithelial tumors (PNET). Typical signs of astrocytoma and ependymoma are the decrease in the NAA–Cho ratio and increase in the ratio of Lac–Cho peaks in relation to those in a healthy hemisphere. Although the typical pattern of glioma spectra is well defined with high choline and low or absent NAA peaks, with lipid and lactate peaks often seen in GBM, studies of MRS for prediction of tumor histology have not shown sufficient specificity to make MRS a clinically useful adjunct in most cases.

MRS of extra-axial tumors that do not arise from glial precursors, such as meningiomas, generally reveals very high choline and no NAA, because the tumors contain no neurons. Although the presence of a very high alanine peak in rare meningioma's subtype can be useful to suggest the diagnosis, a recent well-controlled study suggests that the presence of low levels of alanine detected in up to 80% of meningioma is not useful because it is detected in similar frequency in metastases and schwannoma [12].

In comparison to these tumours, PNET are characterized by an increase in the NAA–Cho ratio and a lower Lac– Cho ratio, which is related to a higher level of Cho in patients with PNET, as with malignant neoplasm. For astrocytoma, in general, the increase of the Cho peak, the change of mI peak (depends on the malignancy level), the significant reduction of the NAA peak and the appearance of a Lac peak are typical.

For low grade astrocytoma, the reduction of NAA peak is typical, and the increase of Cho peak is observed. The height of the mI peak can remain unchanged, or it can not rise significantly in comparison with contralateral tissues not affected by tumours. The Lac peak is characterised by small elevation, and in rare cases, it cannot be detected at all. The Cho and Lak peak rises, while the mI peak falls with the increase of malignancy level—in particular, in cases of anaplastic astrocytoma. The NAA peak is reduced in comparison with its height in the spectrum of benign astrocytoma.

The marked or full reduction of NAA and mI peaks, and the sharp increase of the Lac peak, are observed in spectrum of glioblastoma, which is characterised by the presence of necrotic areas. At the same time, the Lip peak appears and overlaps the Lac peak and these peaks look like single complex. Generally, the height of Cho peak is sharply increased.

It is important to use MRS during postoperatory period for diagnostics of the continued neoplasm growth, tumour relapse or radiation necrosis. As a rule, treatment of brain tumours is a combination of surgery with chemo- and radiotherapy. However, current methods and doses of radiotherapy could cause death of tumour cells and also of normal cells, especially in cases of lowered sensitivity threshold for radiotherapy. First, vessels endothelium cells suffer, then brain oedema appears, and as a result, a zone of radiation necrosis could appear. According to statistics, in more than 5% of all patients who undergo radiotherapy because of a tumor, brain damage is diagnosed by the end of the first year near the tumour as well as in other areas.

The diagnosis of lymphomas is an important neuroradiology problem. Differential diagnosis of these tumours based on only routine CT and MRI is complicated, and combined chemo- and radiotherapy treatment is more preferable than surgical removal [5]. Therefore, the correct diagnosis influences the tactic choice in the treatment and prognosis of the disease. In the majority of cases, it is necessary to differentiate lymphomas with glial tumours and metastases. The common trend of changes in peaks of Cho, Lac and NAA is observed in lymphoma spectrum as well as in that of astrocytoma. However, these changes are different. With the lymphoma spectrum, the changes of peak heights are not so expressed. The Cho peak moderately increases, and the increased of peak of the Lac–Lip complex is substantial, whereas the decrease in the NAA peak is not significant.

1.4.4. Functional MRI

Brain activity mapping enables to reveal the areas of neuronal activation in response to tests, motor, sensor, and other stimuli. Until recently, similar mapping was performed with the help of radionuclide methods: PET and SPECT imaging. Functional MRI (fMRI) is based on increase of brain haemodynamics in response to cortical neuronal activity due to a certain stimulus [18; 19]. BOLD (*Blood Oxygenation Level Dependent contrast*) EPI-GRE registers hyperintense MR signal from active areas of the brain cortex. The registration time of one MR image is about 100 ms. fMRI signal intensity, registered by physiological load, is compared with the intensity, registered in the event of its lack. During MRI examination, the stimulation periods (duration of 30 s) alternate with control periods (without stimulation) of the same duration. The areas of statistically significant MR signal increasing during activation, revealed in the course of subsequent mathematical processing of images, correspond to areas of neuronal activity. They are marked with colour— in this way the neuronal activity maps are built and these maps are imposed on *T*1 MRI sequences. Map construction methods (for instance, brain wave algorithms) subtract images obtained during neuron stimulation from control images obtained in the absence of stimulation. The subtracted image is imposed on a control scan according to its location, and areas of increased neuronal activity are marked with colour. The revealed functionally significant areas could be "imposed" on a *T*1 MRI sequence of the same section or on a three-dimensional (3D) brain model, and thus it is possible to estimate the ratio between the affected area (tumour) and functionally active brain areas, for example, motor, sensory or visual cortex.

1.4.4.1. Clinical Application of fMRI

Neuronal activity mapping enables planning the surgical approach and studying the pathophysiological processes in brain. This method is used in neurosurgery to study cognitive functions. Its perspective is in revealing the epileptic foci. Currently, fMRI is an integral part of MRI protocol in patients with brain tumours located close to functional critical brain areas. In the majority of cases, the examination results adequately reflect the location of sensomotor, speech and acoustical areas of brain cortex. However, according to the literature, 8–30% of all observation are not informative due to motion artefacts, lack of precise tests execution by the patients and damage to the above-mentioned cortical centres by tumours. In cases in which fMRI can localize active cortical areas, in 87% of cases there is a correspondence with the results of intraoperational electrophysiological methods, within 1-cm limits, and in 13% of cases, within 2 cm. This is evidence of the high accuracy of the fMRI technique [20]. Performing fMRI (currently it is conducted for somatosensory and visual cortices) and tractography with mapping of the functionally active cortical areas, pyramidal or optic tracts is becoming a standard in patient suffering from lesions located in eloquent areas. Imposition of these maps over 3D brain images is promising within the framework of one MRI examination for patients with brain tumours who are going to be operated. Based on these data, neurosurgeons plan the interventional approach and estimate the volume of neoplasm resection, and radiologists assess the areas of radiation and its distribution in tumour.

Conclusions

Advances in imaging technology have led to a better understanding of brain tumors and have advanced neuro-imaging from a purely anatomical to functional assessment of the nervous system.

MRI is the preferred imaging study for brain tumors diagnosis, providing detailed informations on lesion type, size and location. Although gadolinium-enhanced T1-weighted images and T2-weighted images are the MRI modalities of choice for the initial assessment, their usefulness in identifying tumor types, distinguishing tumors from nontumoral lesions, and assessing treatment effects is limited. For this reason, these sequences are used in combination with other MRI technicques, including Diffusion Weighted Imagin (DWI), Diffusion-Tensor-Imaging (DTI), Perfusion MRI, and Magnetic Resonance Spectroscopy (MRS). The most important application of MRI is intraoperative MRI (iMRI). Used with or without cortical stimulation, iMRI can maximize tumor resection while minimizing damage to healthy tissue, reducing the risk of neurological deficits and improving patient survival [21].

Advanced brain tumor MRI evaluation can now routinely produce an impressive array of in vivo data reflecting tumor cellularity, metabolism, invasiveness, neocapillary density and permeability. Ongoing technical improvements and additional metrics, currently reported in the literature in a preliminary way, promise to bring to the clinic further dramatic increases in the quantity and quality of imaging data over the next years [12]. The greatest current challenge in advanced tumor imaging is the need for a new tumor classification method that can allow better integration of advanced imaging data into brain tumors research and clinical decision making. In essence, what is needed is a significant revision of brain tumor nosology. It is conceivable that a new tumor classification, advanced-MRI metrics in addition to nucleoside positrone emission tomography data and cellular and molecular microarray data could define novel pathophysiologically relevant subtypes that would better predict brain tumor patient prognoses and responses to targeted chemotherapeutic agents, than our current histopathologic grading system. A number of recent reports have been published evaluating imaging markers by direct comparison with molecular genotype [16] and phenotype and patient outcomes [22]. This approach seems likely to become the dominant paradigm in the future [12].

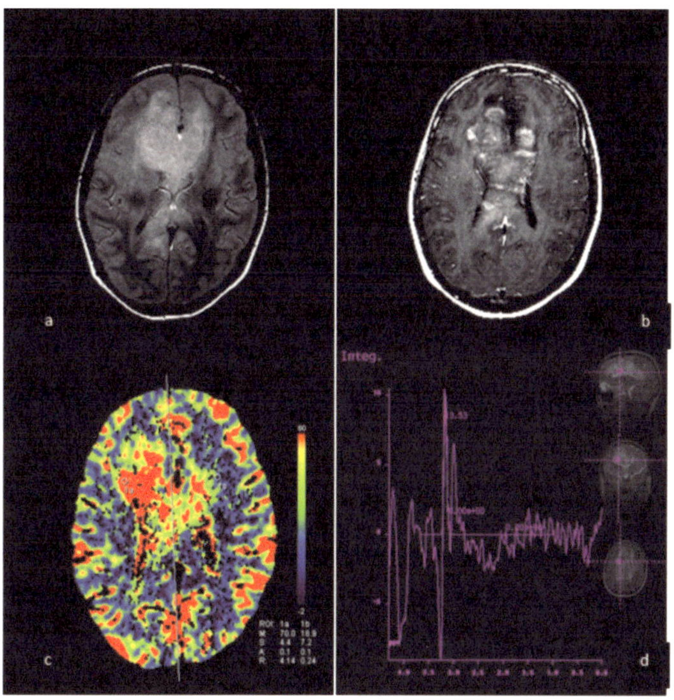

Figure 1. a) MRI Flair sequences demonstrate a frontal lesion with homogenous hyperintensity. b) T1 weighted MRI with gadolinium administration demonstrating no enhancement of the lesion. c) Perfusion CT scan showing a circular area of the tumor with higher r-CBV, expression of hypervascularization of that part of the tumor. d) MRI Spectroscopy showing an increased choline/NAA ratio. The neuroradiological findings suggested the diagnosis of low grade glioma with an area within it of higher grade (the area with hypervascularization). Definitive histological results was positive for anaplastic oligodendroglioma.

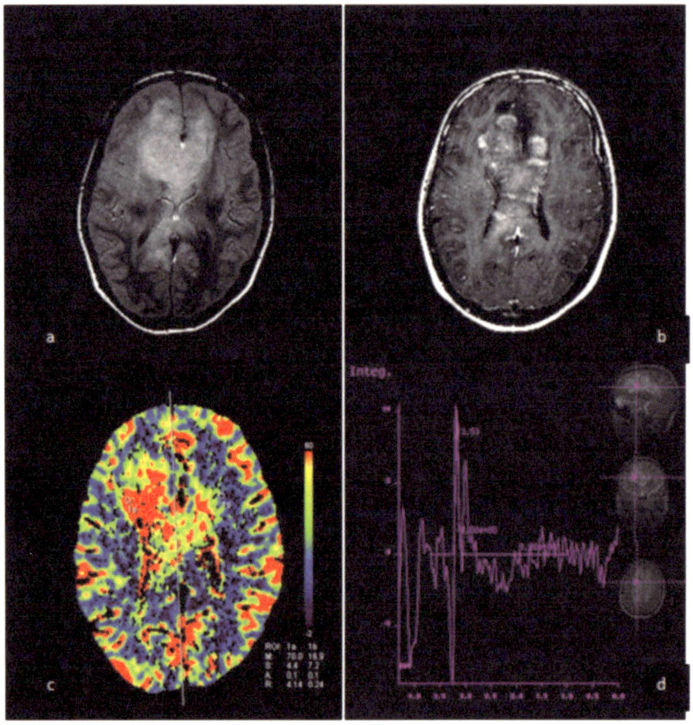

Figure 2. a) MRI Flair sequences demonstrate a frontal lesion with involvement of corpus callosum and bilateral extrinsecation (butterfly glioma). b) T1 weighted MRI with gadolinium administration demonstrating disomogenous enhancement of the lesion.. c): Perfusion CT scan showing a high vascularization of the tumor with high r-CBV. d) MRI Spectroscopy showing an increased choline/NAA ratio (higher than in case 1). The neuroradiological findings suggested the diagnosis of high grade glioma. Definitive histological results were positive for glioblastoma multiformis.

Author details

Concetta Alafaci[1*], Francesca Granata[2], Mariano Cutugno[1], Maria Caffo[1], Gerardo Caruso[1] and Francesco Maria Salpietro[3]

*Address all correspondence to: calafaci@unime.it

1 Dept of Neurosurgery, University of Messina, Italy

2 Dept of Neuroradiology University of Messina, Italy

3 Dept of Neurosurgery, Papardo Hospital, University of Messina, Italy

References

[1] Dandy, W. E. (1919). Roentgenography of the brain after the injection of air into the spinal canal. *Ann Surg*, 70, 397.

[2] Zavoisky, E.K. (1945). Spin-magnetic resonance in paramagnetics. *J Phys Acad Sci USSR*, 9, 211-245.

[3] Leeds, N. E., et al. (2000). Evolution of diagnostic neuroradiology from 1904 to 1999. *Radiology*, 217, 309-318.

[4] Leeds, N. E., et al. (1999). Neuroimaging of brain tumors. *In: Evans RW, eds. Diagnostic testing in neurology.Philadelphia, PA: Sauders*, 169-199.

[5] Kornienko, V.N, & Pronin, I.N. (1999). Neuroradiology: History and New Research Technologies. *In Springer-Verlag Berlin Heidelberg eds. Diagnostic Neuroradiology*, 1-28.

[6] Westbrook, C., et al. (2005). MRI in Practice. *3rd ed. Oxford, United Kingdom: Wiley Blackwell.*

[7] Dowd, C.F, et al. (2003). Meningiomas: the role of preoperative angiography and embolization. *Neurosurg Focus*, 15(1), Article 10, 1-4.

[8] Meshechkin, A. V., et al. (2011). Regional chemoinfusion and radiation therapy to patients with breast cancer metastase to the brain: preliminary report. *Vestn Khir Im I Grek*, 170(3), 17-19.

[9] James, M., et al. (2006). Diffusion-weighted and Perfusion MR Imaging for Brain Tumor Characterization and Assessment of Treatment Response. *Radiology*, 239, 632-649.

[10] Mulkern, R. V., et al. (1999). Multi-component apparent diffusion coefficients in human brain. *NMR Biomed*, Feb, 12(1), 51-62.

[11] Bulakbasi, N., et al. Combination of single voxel proton MR spectroscopy and apparent diffusion coefficient calculation in the evaluation of common brain tumors. *AJNR*, Feb, 24(2), 225-33.

[12] Geoffrey, S., & Young, . (2007). Advanced MRI of adult brain tumors. *Neurol Clin*, 25-947.

[13] Patel, M. D., et al. (2010). Distribution and fibre field similarity mapping of the human anterior commissure fibres by diffusion tensor imaging. *Magma*, Dec, 23(5-6), 399-408.

[14] Merhof, D., et al. (2007). Correction of susceptibility artifacts in diffusion tensor data using non-linear registration. *Med Image Anal*, Dec, 11(6), 588-603.

[15] Lev, M. H., et al. (2004). Glial tumor grading and outcome prediction using dynamic spin-echo MR susceptibility mapping compared with conventional contrast-en-

hanced MR: confounding effect of elevated rCBV of oligodendrogliomas. *AJNR*, Feb, 25(2), 214-21.

[16] Maia, , et al. (2005). Mr cerebral blood volume maps correlated with vascular endhotelial growth factor expression and tumor grade in non-enhancing gliomas. *AJNR Am J Neuroradiol*, Apr, 26(4), 777-83.

[17] Hourani, R., et al. (2006). Proton magnetic resonance spectroscopic imaging to differentiate between nonneoplastic lesions and brain tumors in children. *J Magn Reson Imaging*, Feb, 23(2), 99-107.

[18] Ramsey, N. F., et al. (2002). Functional MRI experiments: acquisition, analysis and interpretation of data. *Eur Neuropsychopharmacol*, Dec, 12(6), 517-26.

[19] Sunaert, S. (2006). Presurgical planning for tumor resectioning. *J Magn Reson Imaging*, Jun Review, 23(6), 887-905.

[20] Blatow, M., et al. (2007). fMRI reflects functional connectivity of human somatosensory cortex. *Neuroimage*, Sep 1, 37(3), 927-36.

[21] Tonnarelli, L. Magretic resonance imaging of brain tumor. *CEwebsource.com*.

[22] Chackis, C., Stadnik, T., Michotte, A., et al. (2006). Prognostic value of perfusion-weighted imaging in brain glioma : a prospective study. *Acta Neurochir*, (Wien), 148(3), 277-85.

Chapter 4

Radiology Imaging Techniques of Brain Tumours

Kamil Zeleňák, Cisáriková Viera and Poláček Hubert

Additional information is available at the end of the chapter

http://dx.doi.org/10.5772/53470

1. Introduction

The development of radiological imaging techniques for the evaluation of brain tumours has progressed significantly in recent years. Two modalities that play a crucial role in the evaluation of brain tumours in preoperative time to detach are computed tomography (CT) and magnetic resonance imaging (MRI).

Despite the new digital radiological techniques, which are used widely in clinical practice, imaging methods such as CT and MRI eliminate x-ray from the examination algorithm of brain tumours. An x-ray of the skull may detect changes that can lead to suspicion of a tumour in the intracranial space and subsequent examination using CT or MRI.

It is important to distinguish tumoural from non-tumoural lesions, and to determine their spatial location. New, advanced imaging CT and MRI techniques provide more detailed characteristics of brain tumours, and thus, more choices of appropriate therapeutic management of the patient. These techniques also play a significant role in monitoring the effect of the therapy.

Diagnosis of tumours has improved considerably due to the introduction of new imaging CT and MRI techniques. These techniques, and the contrast medium in particular, provide anatomical and structural information about brain tumours, and information about the physiology, metabolism, and haemodynamics of individual tumours. The importance of radiology imaging techniques, and their role, in the diagnosis of brain tumours are listed in Tables 1 and 2.

Radiology Imaging Techniques of Brain Tumours	
MODALITY	**IMPORTANCE**
CT	screening method
MRI	method of choice
DSA	mostly used for determination of blood supply and embolization of hypervascular tumours
US	intraoperative navigation
X – ray	limited
Conventional invasive X – ray methods	obsolete

Table 1. Importance of radiology imaging techniques in the diagnosis of brain tumours.

Role of Radiology Imaging Techniques		
Preoperatively	Detection	
	Characterization	localization
		size
		margins
		extension
		midline shift
		compression
		contrast enhancement
		vascularity
		supplying vessels
		perifocal oedema
	Differentiation	benign vs malignant
	Staging	
	tumour embolization	
	surgical planing	
Intraoperative	surgical navigation	
Postoperatively	monitoring the effect of treatment	
	exclude recurrence	
	distinguishing recurrent tumour from radiation necrosis	

Table 2. Role of radiology imaging techniques in brain tumours

http://dx.doi.org/10.5772/53470

2. Conventional imaging methods

For decades, diagnostic imaging dominated conventional non-invasive and invasive methods, and later invasive contrast x-ray techniques. During the second half of the twentieth century, a number of different projection x-ray radiographs of the head and their modifications, as well as complex invasive contrast imaging techniques, such as pneumoencephalography, ventriculography, and myelography, were improved [1]. Another imaging method is ultrasonography, which can be used for neuronavigation during operation of brain tumours.

2.1. Conventional non-invasive X-ray methods

In the past, conventional non-invasive x-ray examination (radiography of the head) was the basic diagnostic method in neuroradiology. The baseline projections are posteroanterior (PA) and lateral x-ray projections of the skull. A PA projection is centred by orbitomeatal lines and provides anatomical information about the skull and frontal structures. A lateral projection shows the configuration of the skull and the skull base.

Modification of a PA projection by Caldwell with an x-ray beam inclination of 15°–23°, caudal to the orbitomeatal line, provides a clearer view of the *os petrosum*. With an x-ray beam inclination of 37°, caudal to the orbitomeatal line, we obtain a semiaxial Waters projection, which shows paranasal cavities and structures of the zygomaticomaxillar complex. An x-ray beam inclination of 30°, caudal to the orbitomeatal line, in the anteroposterior (AP) direction provides the Towne's projection, which is appropriate for imaging the *os spheoidale*, foramen magnum, and pyramids, and their dorsal edges in particular.

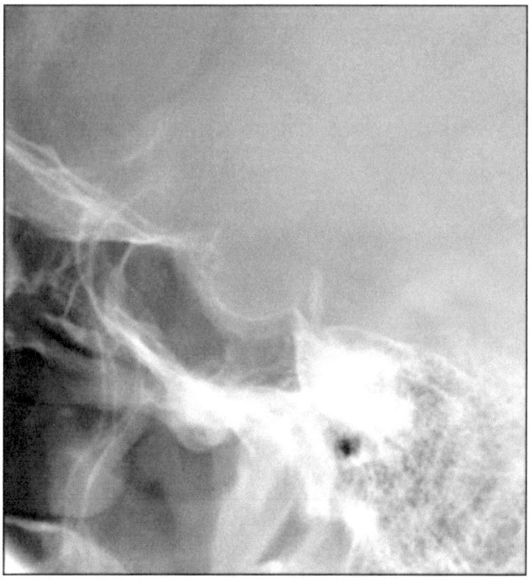

Figure 1. Sella turcica (lateral projection): destruction by tumour

A submentovertical projection is an axial projection of the skull with the x-ray beam passing approximately perpendicular to the orbitomeatal line, and is suitable for imaging the *os sphenoidale* and the base middle *fossa foramina*. The Stenvers projection with a 45° rotation of the head from the PA line, and with a caudal x-ray beam inclination of 10°–15°, is the most common projection for imaging the *os petrosum*, providing a good display of the tip of the pyramid, the structures of the inner ear, and the *meatus acusticus internus*. The Schüller projection is a lateral projection with a caudal x-ray beam inclination of 30° and is employed for enhanced imaging and evaluation of the *processus mastoideus* pneumatization. A modification of these projections is a lateral projection by Runström I, with an x-ray beam inclination of 15° and a projection by Runström II with a caudal x-ray beam inclination of 45° [1]. Other special projections focus on the *sella turcica* (Figure 1.), *canalis opticus.*

2.2. Conventional invasive X-ray methods

Pneumoencephalography is an imaging method in which the lumbar or suboccipital approach is used to instill air into the cerebral ventricles and the subarachnoid spaces after removing approximately 10–30 mL of cerebrospinal fluid [2].

Ventriculography is an imaging method in which, through a trepanation hole, air is introduced into each lateral brain ventricle after the collection of cerebrospinal fluid [3].

These imaging x-ray methods are currently not used in clinical practice.

Before the era of CT and MRI, panangiography was the essential imaging technique of neuroradiology in the diagnosis of brain tumours. A brain tumour manifests itself in angiographic images by indirect signs, such as dislocation of intracranial arteries, depending on tumour size and location; tumoural vessels filling with the contrast medium, tumour vascularization; or vascular occlusion and stenosis [2].

With the onset of CT and MRI, the position of angiography has gradually changed. Currently, due to a new generation of digital radiological technology and rapid development of intracranial catheterization techniques and instrumentation, digital subtraction angiography is a highly specialized imaging method in interventional radiology, with many therapeutic implications.

2.3. Ultrasound

Ultrasound is a widely available, non-invasive diagnostic method without negative biological effects. Principally, it is applied, in the primary examination of the brain in prenatal and postnatal diagnoses, and in the examination of cerebral arteries. Currently, ultrasonography, used in planning operational strategy and choice of neurosurgery access, has been replaced by new, and more accurate, neuronavigation systems using MRI data. Ultrasound with a high-frequency transducer can be used to monitor changes during brain tumour operations in real time [1] (Figure 2.).

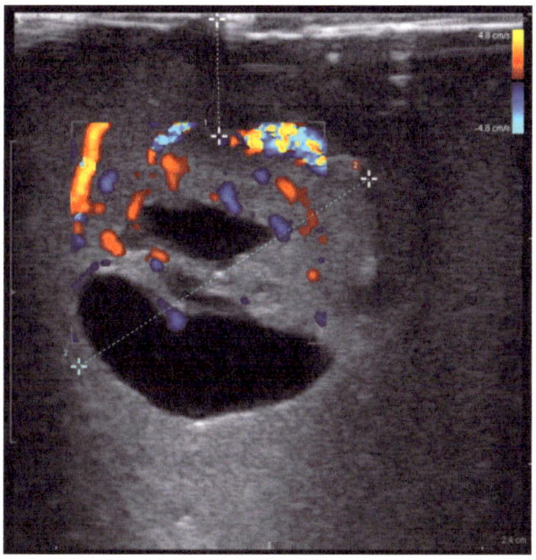

Figure 2. Intraoperative ultrasound navigation with colour flow mapping, showing peripheral vascularization of a brain tumour with solid and cystic parts

3. Computed Tomography – CT

From its first test scan on a mouse, in 1967, to current medical practice, the CT scanner has become a core imaging tool. Initially financed by money from Beatles' record sales, the first patient scan was performed in 1971. Only 8 years later, a Nobel Prize in Physics and Medicine was awarded to Gofrey Newbold Hounsfield and Allan McLeod Cormack for their discovery [4]. The prototype (EMI Ltd.) was installed at Atkinson Morley's Hospital in South London where the first patient, a middle aged lady with a suspected frontal lobe tumour, was scanned on 1st October 1971 [5].

The rapid development of CT scanners, a new generation of CT devices, and advanced post-processing technologies in recent years has enabled the creation of progressive, advanced CT protocols for the diagnosis of individual anatomical regions with respect to the pathological processes that can be diagnosed. Technological improvements and new CT applications in neuroradiology are mainly related to CT angiography and CT perfusion with a dynamic contrast agent bolus [1].

The basic CT examination of brain tumours involves standard non-contrast enhanced and contrast enhanced imaging (Figure 3.). Compared to MR, CT is superior in the detection of calcification and bone abnormalities, and it is also less time consuming.

In CT diagnosis, depending on the type of examination, iodinated contrast agents are administered, in different quantities and by different modes. Iodinated contrast agents are divided into ionic, high-osmolar contrast agents and non-ionic, low-osmolar or iso-osmolar contrast agents. Intravenous administration of contrast agents may cause various negative allergic reactions, which are divided into early (within 20 min) and late effects. In practice, non-ionic contrast media are generally preferred as, due to their low osmolarity, they result in significantly fewer negative effects [6].

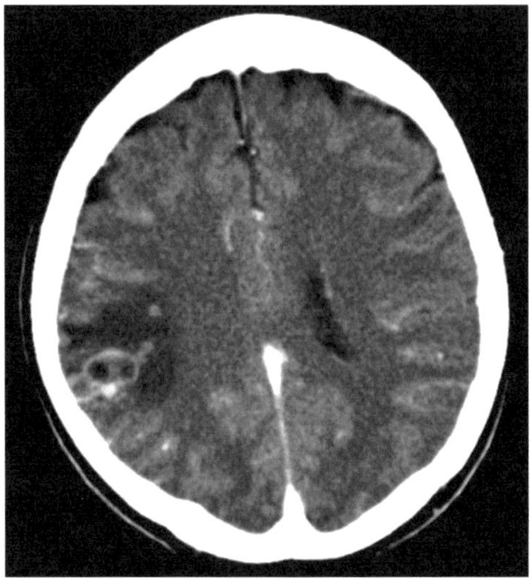

Figure 3. Contrast enhanced CT of brain tumour: irregular peripheral enhancement of glioblastoma (the image displayed is of the same patient as displayed in Figure 2)

Examination of blood vessels using CT angiography is a non-invasive imaging method which is conducted in various ways: imaging individual sections, maximum-intensity projection (MIP), shaded surface display (SSD), the volume-rendering technique (VRT), multiplanar reconstruction (MPR), and virtual angiography. Improvement in the quality of CT angiography, and the new generation of CT equipment gives rise to the possibility of longer scans, faster scan times with display of the arterial phase of contrast filling with the lowest venous infiltration, and better resolution with improved vascular details.

CT perfusion (Figure 4.) in the diagnosis of brain tumours allows assessment of tumours on the microvascular level through a dynamic scanning sequence during an intravenous bolus injection of a contrast agent. This is a relatively new technique that is used in neuroimaging for quantitative and qualitative assessment of cerebral perfusion by the parameters of cerebral blood flow (CBF), cerebral blood volume (CBV), mean transit time (MTT), and time to peak (TTP). Maps with colour-coded flow rates can be obtained by using postprocessing software. Due to this technique, it is possible to assess the state of vascularization and haemodynamics of brain tumours and their differentiation [7 - 9].

4. Magnetic resonance imaging – MRI

Historically, many scientists have contributed to the study of NMR (MRI), which led to construction of reliable MR scanners for clinical practice. Isidor Isaac Rabi in 1930 began by studying the magnetic properties of atomic nuclei (Nobel Prize in Physics in 1944) [10]. The first successful nuclear magnetic resonance experiment with NMR precision measurements was made independently in 1946 by Felix Bloch and Edward Mills Purcell (they jointly received the Nobel Prize in Physics in 1952). In 1971, Raymond Vahan Damadian, measured T1 and T2 relaxation times of excised normal and cancerous rat tissue and stated that tumour tissue had longer relaxation times than normal tissue. He is the inventor of the first MR Scanning Machine (1977) [11]. In March 1973 Paul C. Lauterbur published the first 2D NMR images of two 1 mm capillaries filled with water [10] and in 1974 the image of thoracic cavity of mouse. He called his imaging method zeugmatography. This term was later replaced by NMR imaging [12]. Peter Mansfield with Grannel described the use of magnetic field gradients to acquire spatial information in NMR. P.C. Lauterbur and Sir Peter Mansfield received the Nobel Prize in 1952. The first commercial MR scanner (Picker Ltd.) in Europe was installed in 1983 in Manchester Medical School.

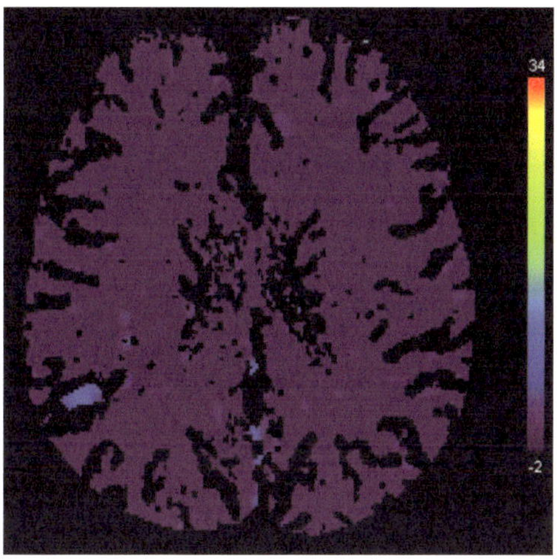

Figure 4. CT perfusion of a brain tumour across the solid part of the tumour (the image displayed is of the same patient as displayed in Figure 2).

The main advantages of MRI are the possibilities of imaging individual anatomical regions in vivo with high tissue contrast, imaging in arbitrary planes, non-invasivity, and the absence of demonstrable detrimental effects on human health. Qualitative evaluation of tissues allows for four basic physical attributes: T1 and T2 relaxation, proton density, motion, and flow.

4.1. Conventional MRI techniques

Conventional MRI techniques provide information about the anatomical conditions of brain tissue, the tumour itself, and its relationship with its surroundings. In contrast to CT, conventional MRI techniques are significantly more sensitive, but as they are nonspecific, they often provide limited information about tumour physiology.

The conventional MRI protocol in the diagnosis of brain tumours includes standard T1-weighted imaging (spin echo [SE], turbo spin echo [TSE], gradient echo, three-dimensional [3D] sequences, and dynamic studies), T2-weighted imaging (SE, fast spin echo [FSE] or TSE, and 3D sequences), "dark fluid" T2-weighted imaging (proton density [PD] and fluid-attenuated inversion recovery [FLAIR]), gradient echo (GRE T2, T2 * GRE, and GRE 3D T1), inversion recovery (IR) (FLAIR, T1 IR, and short-time inversion recovery [STIR]), and fat suppression (FS) (STIR and T1 FS) [13] (Figure 5.).

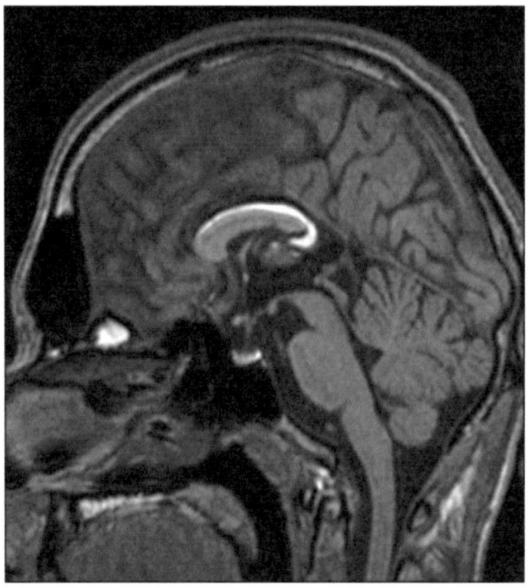

Figure 5. Sagittal non-contrast enhanced T1W image: hyperintense signal of pericallosal lipoma.

Brain tumours show variable pathomorphological manifestations in MRI, which depend on the structure of different types of tumours. They may have a homogeneous or an inhomogeneous structure, and depending on whether they are focal lesions or infiltrative and growing, they are sharply contoured or diffuse [14].

In general, brain tumours in T1-weighted imaging are hypo- or isointense and in T2-weighted imaging are hyper- or isointense. The tumour's signal is modified by the intralesional proportion of individual components. Tumours may contain solid, cystic, necrotic, or haemorrhagic components, fatty tissue, or an increased proportion of protein in intracystic components. Not all tumours cause oedema of the brain tissue, which may have a different range [13, 15].

In some cases, visualization of brain tumours in non-contrast imaging can be difficult; therefore administration of a paramagnetic contrast agent is necessary. Contrast enhancement of brain tumours is variable and dependent on tumour neovascularization.

MRI shows intracranial arteries, veins, and venous sinuses at high-quality. Magnetic resonance angiography (MRA) can be implemented using several techniques: phase-contrast MRA (PC MRA), time-of-flight MRA (TOF MRA), and contrast-enhanced MRA (CE MRA) [16].

http://dx.doi.org/10.5772/53470

Tumour angiogenesis can be dynamically monitored in vivo by 3D-CTA and 4D-CE-MRA. Of the two methods, 3D-CTA has better spatial resolution, but 4D-CE-MRA allows temporal resolution of tumour angiogenesis [17].

MRA allows detailed evaluation of intracranial vascular structures, not only because of purely pathological changes of vascular origin, but also in relation to brain tumours.

4.1.1. Contrast agents

In addition to non-contrast enhanced imaging, magnetic resonance examination is realized with contrast agents, which improves visualization and demarcation of the tumour. Contrast agents used in MRI are paramagnetic substances containing gadolinium chelates; they cause shortening of the T1 and T2 relaxation times, resulting in a stronger T1 and a lower T2 signal, and they also increase the contrast between two tissues with different quantities of the contrast agent. Increase of T1 signal is more significant, compared with the degree of weakness of the T2 signal; therefore T1-weighted sequences are used after contrast administration (Figures 6-8.).

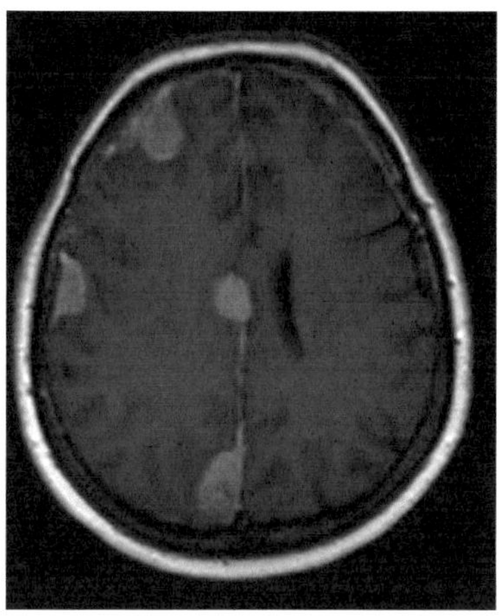

Figure 6. Axial contrast enhanced T1W image: homogeneous enhancement of multiple meningiomas right supratentorial in patient with neurofibromatosis type 2.

Contrast agents for MRI can be divided into several categories: intravenous contrast agents, which include the majority of non-specific and specific contrast agents; oral contrast agents for display purposes of the gastrointestinal tract; and interstitial contrast agents. According to the space distribution of contrast agents, they are classified into extracellular organ-non-specific and intracellular organ-specific contrast agents. In the diagnosis of brain tumours intravenous extracellular organ-non-specific contrast agents are used, which have the ability to pass through the blood–brain barrier [18].

Different types of contrast enhancement and common types of brain tumour are listed in Table 3.

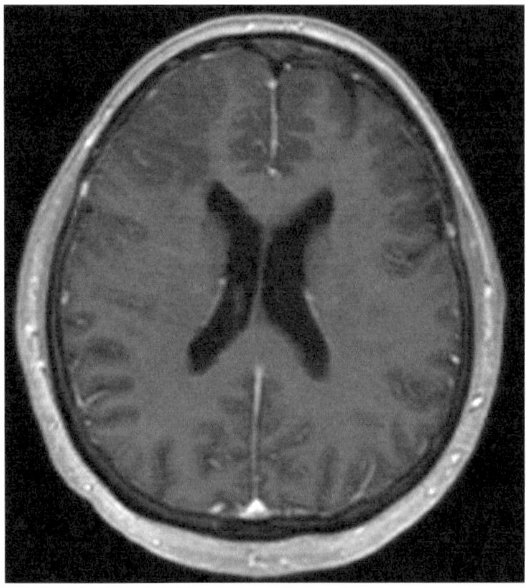

Figure 7. First patient examination. Axial contrast enhanced T1W image displays almost no contrast enhancement in the right frontal

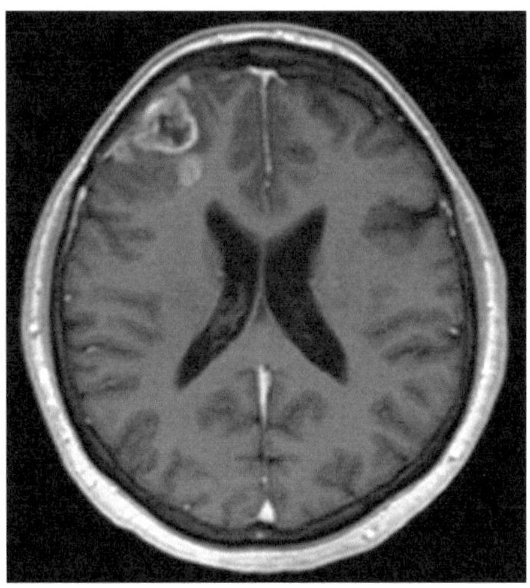

Figure 8. Second patient examination. Axial contrast enhanced T1W image displays irregular peripheral enhancement of right frontal tumour (the image displayed is of the same patient as displayed in Figure 7, 3 months later; glioblastoma was confirmed by histology).

Different types of contrast enhancement	
no enhancement	Low grade astrocytoma
diffuse homogeneous	Meningioma
diffuse inhomogeneous	Pleomorphic xanthoastrocytoma
ring enhancement	Metastasis
irregular peripheral enhancement	Glioblastoma
mural nodule enhancement	Haemangioblastoma

Table 3. Different types of contrast enhancement of brain tumours and common types of brain tumour.

4.2. Advanced MRI techniques

Early and accurate diagnosis is the first precondition of the successful treatment of brain tumours. The basic method of determining species diagnosis and grading is the histopathological examination. Biopsy is an invasive method with the risk of possible complications. At the time of the development and practical use of modern, advanced diagnostic techniques, the role of radiodiagnostic imaging modalities was not limited to the assessment of pathological-anatomical conditions [9].

Advanced magnetic resonance techniques in neuroradiology evaluate changes at the microvascular, haemodynamic, and cellular levels of brain tumours, and in addition to structural changes, evaluate changes at the metabolic and biochemical levels [19].

Incorporation of new diagnostic techniques, such as diffusion-weighted imaging (DWI), diffusion tensor imaging (DTI), tractography, perfusion-weighted imaging (PWI), magnetic resonance spectroscopy (MRS), and functional MRI (fMRI), into the diagnostic protocol allows us to obtain detailed information about tumour lesions. This presents the best possibility of accurate grading of brain tumours in the preoperative time, allowing us to select the most appropriate therapeutic management for the patients [20].

New techniques lead to better quality monitoring of the effects of therapy.

4.2.1. Diffusion-weighted imaging (DWI)

The theory of diffusion is based on constant, disordered, random motion of water molecules in all directions (Brownian motion). Biological tissues in which diffusion is the same in all directions is isotropic; if diffusion is restricted in one direction, tissues are anisotropic. The most common barrier to diffusion is the cell wall. Cerebrospinal fluid is the isotropic field; diffusion in gray matter in all directions compared to the liquor is limited but also isotropic. White matter is the anisotropic region because here diffusion progresses with greater intensity in the direction within axons [21].

DWI is echo-planar imaging that measures the random motion of water molecules (i.e. diffusion in biological tissue). The diffusion capacity of water protons is tissue-specific and creates a specific contrast on DWI. On diffusion sequences, the motion of water protons in biological tissue causes changes in the signal. These signal changes are quantified by calculating the apparent diffusion coefficient map (ADC) [22] (Figure 9.).

DWI, which is currently a routine part of imaging protocols, plays an important role in the assessment of the cellularity of biological tissue. In the diagnosis of brain tumours, DWI is applicable in differential diagnosis of cystic lesions, abscesses, necrosis, and metastases. In addition, DWI has a fundamental role in the evaluation of the age of brain ischemia, in imaging of traumatic changes, and in evaluation activities of demyelinating lesions [23].

Possibilities of using the ADC in differential diagnosis of intracranial tumours, and differentiating peritumoural oedema and infiltration, have been studied since the beginning of the 21st century. Most studies have concluded that the ADC is useful for distinguishing peritumoural infiltration only and cannot provide information on the degree of differentiation of glial tumours. However, they found that in tumour tissue with high cellularity, ADC values were reduced compared to tumours with low cellularity; thus the probability of higher grading is reduced for solid tumours with high values of the ADC. For tumours with a cystic component, such as glioblastoma multiforme, the relationship between the ADC and the grading is below the level of statistical significance [24].

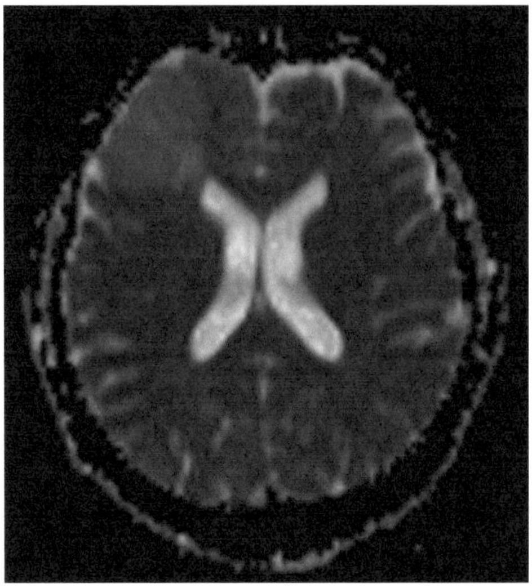

Figure 9. Axial ADC map showing the right frontal hyperintensity of a tumour (the image displayed is of the same patient as displayed in Figure 7).

4.2.2. Diffusion tensor imaging (DTI)

DTI is an advanced magnetic resonance technique that allows visualization of white matter tracts, and describes the movement of water molecules by using two parameters, mean diffusivity (MD) and fractional anisotropy (FA), which represent the directionality of water diffusion [25].

The postprocessing of DTI data using software generates maps of FA and ADC using DWI images. Reduction of FA surrounding white matter of the tumour indicates the suspicion of peritumoural white matter infiltration by tumoural elements [26]. Using 3D software applications, 3D image tracts are created, allowing imaging of the spatial configuration of white matter structures, such as the corticospinal tract, and configuration of the *corpus callosum* [27]. DTI is able to demonstrate structural changes of white matter tracts related to brain tumours, such as the detection of alterations, integrity, or dislocation of individual tracts (Figure 10.).

Thus, DTI provides other important information that can help distinguish infiltrative growing tumours from bounded tumours and, together with assessment of the ADC and conventional MRI with a contrast agent, the grading of tumours can be better specified [28 - 30].

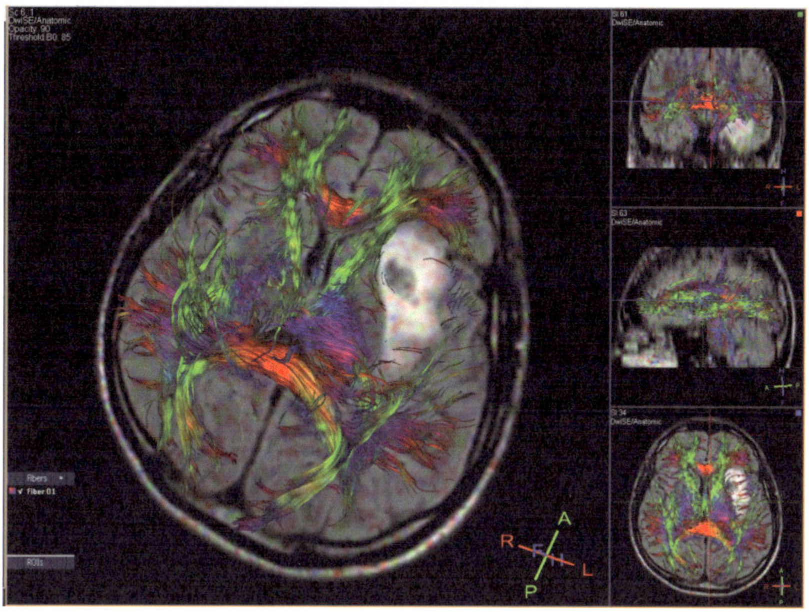

Figure 10. DTI: destruction and deviation of white matter tracts by anaplastic astrocytoma.

4.2.3. *Perfusion-weighted imaging (PWI)*

The rapid growth of cells is a result of the increased metabolic demands of a tumour. Cellular hypoglycaemia and hypoxia result in the production of cytokines of angiogenesis (vasoactive endothelial growth factor) followed by tumour neovascularization, which leads to a higher volume of blood flow through tumour tissue. Tumour neovascularization and haemodynamic changes are the basic principles of perfusion MRI, which evaluate the blood supply to brain tissue by four parameters: CBV (the quantity of blood in a given volume in mL/100mg), CBF (the blood flow in brain tissue in mL/100g/min), MTT (the average time for arteriovenous passage of blood in a given volume in seconds), and TTP (the average time to maximum density in the scanning area in seconds) [31, 32].

PWI uses fast, dynamic, epiplanar imaging sequences with a bolus of a paramagnetic contrast agent, 0.2 mmol/kg body weight, at an injection rate of 5 mL/s, approximately 5-10 seconds after the start of imaging sequences, followed by an injection of 20-30 mL of saline. The passage of the contrast agent through vascularized parts of the tumour leads to a reduction in signal intensity. Converting the values of individual parameters by postprocessing to the colour range creates maps with different blood flows. Regional cerebral, and tumour, vascularity is correlated with the CBV.

With PWI it is possible to determine tumour grading non-invasively. In general, high-grade tumours have higher CBV values than low-grade tumours. PWI is also used for localization of the parts of a tumour with a high degree of vascularity for the purpose of stereotactic biopsy. PWI helps to define the edge of a tumour, which is important in planning surgical treatment radiotherapy. PWI is also used to monitor the effect of treatment on patients. In the field of radiation changes, using conventional magnetic resonance techniques, it is difficult to differentiate the eventual recurrence of a tumour. Postirradiation changes have lower CBV values, and through PWI, it is possible to detect areas with increased perfusion, which correspond to tumour recurrence. Increasing specificity in these cases allows the combination of PWI with MRS [33].

4.2.4. Magnetic resonance spectroscopy (MRS)

Based on recent achievements in the field of MRS, the diagnostic proportion of proton MRS has significantly increased, in the past decade progressing from basic and clinical research to routine clinical practice. MRS is a non-invasive method and currently is part of the advanced diagnostic protocol in neuroradiology. MRS can determine pathological changes in brain tissue long before conventional techniques [34].

MRS provides biochemical and metabolic information about brain tumours and their surrounding tissues. Thus MRS, contributes significantly to the distinguishing of tumour from non-tumour lesions, the type of diagnosis and tumour grading in preoperative time, oedema from infiltrative growing tumours, the monitoring of tumour response to treatment and distinguishing postirradiation necrosis from tumour recurrence [35].

MRS by non-invasive and non-destructive methods detects, in vivo in brain tissue, diagnostically important compounds such as those containing choline (Cho – a key marker of cell membrane stability), creatine (Cr – an indicator of the energy status, often used as a reference value), *N*-acetylaspartate (NAA – the main indicator of the structure and function of neurons), lactate (Lac – in normal tissue its concentration is on the edge of detectability and is increased in anaerobic metabolism), and lipids. The magnetic resonance spectrum of human brain metabolites is relatively constant [36].

Changes in biochemical processes at the cellular level precede macroscopic changes; therefore, MRS is able to detect the development of pathological processes in brain tissue before conventional MRI techniques. MRS and MRI use magnetic characteristics of the atomic nucleus; in obtaining the signal, they work on the same physical principle, but the data processing and interpretation for each are different. MRI provides detailed information about the pathological-anatomical state of brain tissue [37].

Whereas, MRS detects metabolic signals and results in a spectrum in which the position of the signal of a specific metabolite is expressed on the horizontal axis in chemical shifts specified in parts per million (ppm), and the vertical axis reflects the intensity of the signal. The chemical shift and shape of the signal is characteristic for each metabolite [38] (Figure 11.).

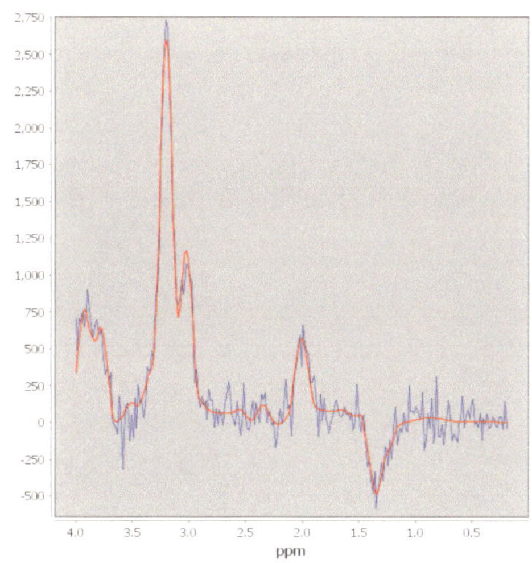

Figure 11. MRS: a typical sample 1H MR spectrum in the lesion. Cre2, Cho, Cre, NAA, lac (the image displayed is of the same patient as displayed in Figure 10).

In practice, there are two basic techniques of MRS, single voxel spectroscopy (SVS) and chemical shift imaging (CSI). The result of SVS is one spectrum, which shows the overall distribution of individual metabolites in a limited volume of tissue (voxel) in a volume of 2-8 mL. CSI measures the concentration of metabolites in a selected volume of brain tissue divided into many small voxels. The result is an individual spectrum for each voxel, and the imaging of the distribution of the concentration of individual metabolites in the examined area is produced as a spectroscopic map (Figure 12.).

In clinical practice, MRS is realized through the anatomical imaging of brain tissue using conventional MRI. The spectra are displayed together with conventional MRI images, which characterize the anatomical location of the measured area selected for spectroscopy [38].

The results of the spectra are evaluated by the relative intensity of the signals and the ratios of observed metabolites are typically set to creatine or choline (for example, NAA/Cr, NAA/Cho, or NAA/Cr + Cho). Different types of tumours are manifested by a characteristic spectroscopic profile. Primary tumours are characterized by reducing the concentrations of NAA and *N*-acetylaspartylglutamate, Cr, and creatinephosphate, and increasing the concentrations of Cho and (in astrocytoma) inositol (Ins). Increased concentrations of Lac and lipids (Lip) are characteristic of necrosis. Peritumoural oedema is characterized by low concentrations of all metabolites. The interpretation of results may not be accurate using ratios in the evaluation of the spectra; therefore, different quantification programs using standard reference values are currently being tested and used [35 - 36].

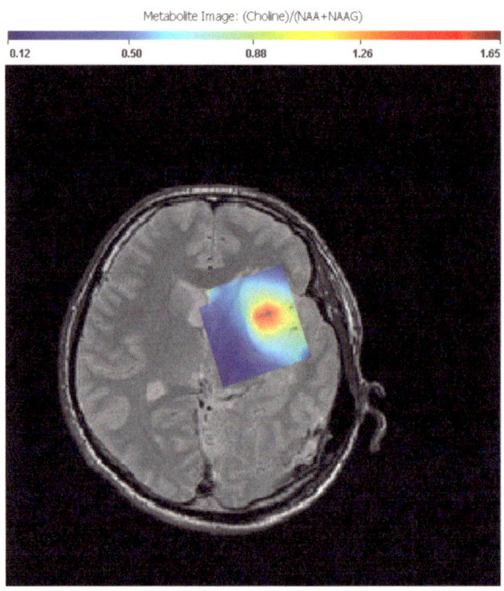

Figure 12. MRS: Coloured metabolic map of the metabolic ratio of total cholines to the signal of the total NAA signal (not resolved to its components), tCho:tNAA (the imaged displayed is of the same patient as displayed in Figure 10).

4.2.5. *Functional magnetic resonance imaging (fMRI)*

Functional magnetic resonance imaging (fMRI) is an MRI procedure that indirectly measures the brain activity by means of deoxyhaemoglobin concentration or blood perfusion changes.

The 1st technique, known as BOLD (blood oxygenation level dependent), is the most popular and frequently used [39]; a relative decrease in deoxyhaemoglobin concentration in the active brain tissue, due to an excessive increase of regional blood flow, and corresponding increase of oxyhaemoglobin. Oxyhaemoglobin is, however, less effectively deoxygenated by active brain tissue compared to inactive brain tissue in physiological conditions. Relative changes of diamagnetic oxyhaemoglobin and paramagnetic deoxyhaemoglobin can be easi-

http://dx.doi.org/10.5772/53470

ly measured by fast T2-weighted echo-planar (EPI) acquisitions. Their temporal resolution, approximately 100 ms per image slice, is good enough to compare several brain images in rest and active (performing sensory, motor or cognitive task) conditions. The statistical maps that result from this, coregistered with structural MRI (Figure 13.), can provide precise information (in the order of millimetres) about the position and the size of brain regions involved in the processing of each respective task, and, sometimes the dynamics of such processing.

The 2nd group of techniques can evaluate the changes of blood flow in brain tissue using special exogenous diffusible tracers like fluorinated halocarbons, deuterated water, ^{17}O -water and ^{13}C-hydrocarbons, or magnetically labelled endogenous blood water (arterial spin labelled perfusion, ASL). The latter technique is non-invasive and very promising for future clinical applications. It can substitute some nuclear medicine diagnostic methods while providing images with better spatial and temporal resolution. Compared to BOLD techniques, ASL can provide not only relative differential maps, but it also provides quantifiable information about absolute blood flow values (in ml/g/min) in selected brain regions [40]. Thus, it can show the regions activated by some tasks, and also pathological tissue with increased or decreased perfusion compared to normal brain tissue [41]. However, the intrinsic signal-to-noise ratio of ASL is lower compared to BOLD measurements, and currently the majority of scanners are not equipped with the respective product sequences to perform routine clinical ASL procedures.

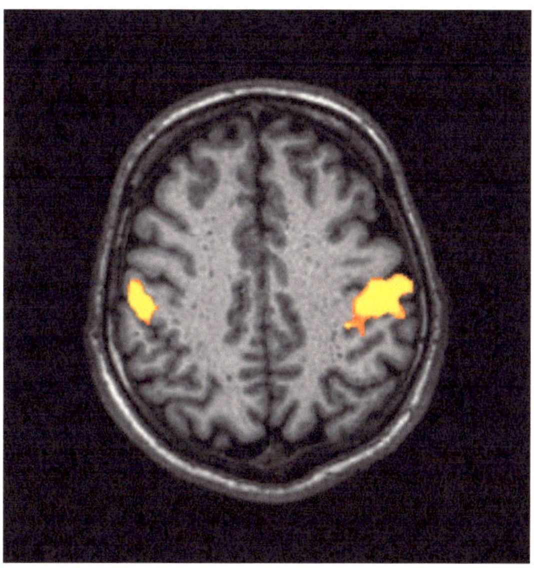

Figure 13. fMRI: activation of motor cortex during physical stimulation.

Presently, in tumour imaging, fMRI is used predominantly for the preoperative localization of eloquent cortical regions that may have been displaced, distorted or compressed by the tumour [42]. FMRI can provide an alternative to invasive mapping techniques (IMTs), with many benefits, particularly in those patients that are unable to undergo awake craniotomy or other stereotactic diagnostic procedures. FMRI data can be very helpful in neuronavigation, especially if the eloquent region is hidden in the depth of sulci and/or cannot be stimulated during the surgery [43].

The sensitivity of fMRI recordings can be increased by the use of stronger magnetic fields. A shorter scanning procedure, higher signal-to-noise-ratio, and increased spatial resolution of the resultant images favour the usage of 3T and are stronger compared to conventional 1,5T scanners [44].

However, the limitations of fMRI are not a result of poor engineering or the low power of the scanners; the main pitfalls are due to complicated functional brain organization and inappropriate diagnostic protocols that ignore this organization [45]. There are always several brain regions involved in the processing of every sensory/motor/cognitive task. It is upon the examiner to choose the best one, to adjust the statistical thresholds of the fMRI map (which determines the number and the size of activated brain regions), and to recognize which regions are eloquent.

A coregistration of the data provided by several different functional and/or structural MRI techniques (e.g. BOLD, ASL, diffusion tensor imaging, MR spectroscopy, ^{23}Na-MRI) is suitable for future improvements of functional MRI diagnostics.

4.2.6. Neuronavigation and intraoperative imaging modalities

Introduction of CT, MRI, and microsurgical operating techniques into clinical practice have resulted in progress in the neurosurgical therapy of brain tumours. The application of new MRI techniques and microsurgery allows for the resection of tumours in functionally important brain regions.

Neuronavigation is a common method of preoperative localization of brain tumours. It uses imaging materials of preoperative MRI examinations, 3D sequences and DTI and fMRI data, that are transferred to a computer database of a neuronavigation device; which, after data processing and registering of the patient's head position, allows for planning of an optimal trajectory for operating on the brain tumour [46].

According to the virtual reality planning, neurosurgeons could obtain more anatomic information and choose the best approach for tumour resection, which would result in a better prognosis for patients [47].

The disadvantage of current navigation systems is that it is impossible to update data during the neurosurgical procedure. A shift in brain structures and tracts of white matter as a result of the evacuation of cerebrospinal fluid, tumour resection, or gravity makes navigation inaccurate. These disadvantages deal intraoperative using of imaging methods – intraoperative ultrasonography and MRI [48].

http://dx.doi.org/10.5772/53470

Intraoperative MRI displays actual dynamic changes in deformable brain tissue during surgery, and helps in early detection of potential tumour residue. Data transfer from intraoperative MRI to the neuronavigation system is possible, and data for neuronavigation can be updated repeatedly. For this purpose, different types of magnetic resonance devices are used. The presence of a magnetic field requires the use of compatible surgical instruments.

Intraoperative ultrasonography with new devices and high resolution is a cheaper alternative to MRI, with the advantage of imaging in real time; it provides actual images of the tumour, surrounding structures, and major blood vessels during surgery [1].

5. Digital subtraction angiography - DSA

Digital subtraction angiography (DSA) is a computer-assisted x-ray technique that subtracts images of bone and soft tissue to permit viewing of the cardiovascular system [49].

At the beginning of the process of subtraction, an image (the mask) is obtained before arrival of contrast material at the area of interest, and the mask image is placed into one of two digital memories. Then, one or more subsequent images are obtained after the arrival of a contrast bolus and placed into a second digital memory. The mask image is digitally subtracted from the succeeding contrast image, resulting in contrast-filled structures that are rendered visible free of background detail. Subtraction is performed in real time [50].

Iodine contrast media are used for the visualization of vessels, however cerebral angiography using gadolinium as an alternative contrast medium in a patient with severe allergy to iodinated contrast medium may be performed [51].

Radiation, today known as X-rays, was discovered by the German physicist Wilhelm Röntgen (March 27, 1845–February 10, 1923) on November 8, 1895 [52]. Discovery of X-rays is ranked as one of the best discoveries in medicine. X-rays are electromagnetic waves. The range of wavelengths corresponding to diagnostic imaging span from about 0.1 nm (at 12.4 keV) to 0.01 nm (at 124 keV) [53]. This type of radiation is ionizing.

In a vacuum X-ray tube, the electrons that make up the beam are emitted by a heated cathode filament. The electrons are then focused and accelerated towards the focal spot by a high voltage that is applied between the cathode filament and the anode. A generator is used to supply the X-ray tube with a controlled high voltage between the cathode and anode, and a controlled current to the cathode. The electron beam strikes the rotating anode "target" and part of its kinetic energy (less than 1%) is converted into X-ray photons, while the rest is converted into heat, which heats up the anode. The X-ray beam leaves the tube through the tube window and passes onto the patient. Some of the X-rays pass through the patient, while some are absorbed. The resulting radiation pattern is detected by a flat panel digital X-ray detector (FPD).

FPD system is superior to the image intensifier as it visualizes small intracranial vessels combined with a significant reduction of radiation dose, and is able to create high-quality 3D DSA images on which high spatial resolution allows precise visualization of small vessels, such as perforating vessels [54]. DSA images are then displayed on the LCD monitor with high resolution and different screen layouts, which can be connected to several image sources.

The first carotid angiography was performed by Portuguese Egas Moniz (1874-1955) in 1927; he is considered as a pioneer of cerebral angiography. He reported the first case of cerebral angiography at the Societe de Neurologie in Paris on July 7, 1927 [55]. Surprisingly, most angiograms were performed to visualize the intracranial portion of the carotids in cases of tumours, to look for abnormal displacement of arterial branches, with little interest in the vascular disease itself [56].

The technique, how to obtain safe access to blood vessels was published by Sven-Ivar Seldinger (1921-1998) in 1953 [57]. DSA is an invasive technique, performed using a catheter; the most commonly used approach is the transfemoral approach. At the end of angiography, the puncture site can be safely closed by a closure device [58].

DSA is used to detect the blood vessels supplying the brain tumours, and also to control the hypervascular tumour embolization (meningiomas, paragangliomas, haemangiopericytomas, juvenile nasopharyngeal angiofibromas and intraaxially located tumours: haemangioblastomas (Figure 14.), hypervascularized metastases and ependymomas). Presurgical or palliative embolization of a tumour can be performed by either an intraarterial catheterization approach or direct puncture of the tumour artery [59].

DSA may also be used for a balloon occlusion test [60]. Although 4D-CE-MRA may be useful for evaluating tumour stain in hypervascular brain, head and neck tumours, it is not able to replace DSA in planning interventional procedures [61].

Modern biplane DSA devices are very useful for neurovascular interventions, which also allows: 2D and 3D navigation for advanced embolization guidance; overlay of a DSA reference image over the matching live fluoro for guidance with less contrast media and less dose; cross-sectional imaging to view anatomical structures of tumours in combination with the feeding vessels of the tumour; single-colour vascular flow visualization from a 2D DSA image series to visualize tumour perfusion tumour vascularization, tumour blush and demonstrate postembolization result; to fuse the dataset with a preprocedural CT, MR or PET image to show tumour activity; synchronize the 3D image to the gantry position; PACS connectivity; the reporting of patient exposure following an intervention.

Modern systems update dynamically to movements of the C-arm, table, zoom and source-to-image distance to facilitate efficient workflow during interventional procedures. By providing more effective and faster guidance, this potentially reduces the use of contrast agents and radiation dose. Pulse frequencies can be adapted to clinical needs according to the ALARA principle (As Low as Reasonably Achievable).

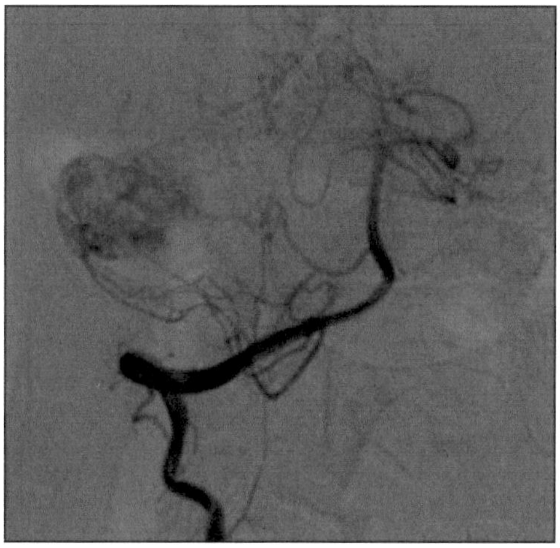

Figure 14. DSA (right vertebral angiogram): intra-axial hypervascularized haemangioblastoma supplied mainly by right anterior inferior cerebellar artery.

6. Conclusion

Radiology has an important role in the diagnosis of brain tumours. A significant factor for success in the treatment of brain tumours is the determination of the extent of the tumour and infiltration of important structures using the CT and MRI imaging methods. Currently, conventional CT protocols, and particularly MRI protocols, have been expanded by sophisticated new techniques that are used in practice. They have significantly contributed to the more detailed species diagnosis of tumours, and to a more accurate estimate of their malignant potential and relationship to the surrounding tissue. With the new techniques, we can evaluate not only detailed tumour morphology, but also the character of the tumour at the microvascular, haemodynamic and cellular level, and the metabolic and biochemical level. With new methods of imaging, exact operational planning approaches on brain tissue can be achieved. Postoperative monitoring of the effect of therapy is highly refined, with more accurate detection of tumour recurrence, and differentiation from postoperative and postradiation changes. Some characteristics of selected brain tumours are presented in Tables 4 and 5.

Hybrid systems have presented new possibilities in brain tumour imaging. The hybrid brain PET/MR allows for molecular, anatomical and functional imaging with uncompromised MR image quality and a high accordance of PET results between PET/MR and PET/CT [62].

Characteristics of selected intracranial tumours

AGE		LOCALIZATION	TYPE		CHARACTERISTIC	TYPICAL CT / MR FINDINGS
Children	Intra-axial tumours	Supratentorial tumours	Astrocytoma		infiltrative / non-infiltrative types	No contrast enhancement in low-grade astrocytomas
			Meduloblastoma		highly malignant	variable contrast enhancement
		Infratentorial tumours	Posterior fossa astrocytoma	Pilocytic astrocytoma	most common (85% of cerebellar astrocytomas); solid/cystic focal lesion	well-demarcated cysts with a contrast enhancing mural nodule
				Brainstem astrocytoma	95% of brainstem neoplasms	variable MR appearance (may be totally or partly solid with a cystic, necrotic, or haemorrhagic component)
			Meduloblastoma		highly malignant, frequently disseminate into the leptomeninges; cystic components may be present in up to 80%; hydrocephalus is often observed	variable contrast enhancement
			Ependymoma		arise from the ependyma of the fourth ventricle	foci of high intensity (necrotic areas and cysts) and low intensity (calcifications or haemorrhage) on T2-WI
			Haemangioblastoma		Uncommon except in patients with von Hippel Lindau disease	small contrast-enhancing nodule with or without cyst
			Teratoma		in infants, second most commoon type of germ cell tumours, occurs more common in males, may contains calcification, cysts; fatty components can cause a chemical meningitis	variable signal on T1-WI and T2-WI
	Extra-axial tumours	Supratentorial tumours	rare			
		Sella region	Craniopharyngioma		may contain cysts, lipid components, and calcification	variable signal on T1-WI and T2-WI
		Infratentorial tumours	rare			

Table 4. Characteristics of selected intracranial tumours in children

Characteristics of selected intracranial tumours

AGE	LOCALIZATION		TYPE	CHARACTERISTIC	TYPICAL CT / MR FINDINGS
Adults	Intra-axial tumours (located in the brain or brainstem)	Supratentorial tumours	MTS (metastases)	approximately 33% of intracranial tumours	circumscribed sphenoid peripheral to nodular enhancing lesion, often multiple, axonal oedema
			Glioblastoma	most common primary CNS tumour, highly malignant, can cross corpus callosum	irregularly marginated tumour with necrosis and peripheral oedema
			Astrocytoma	infiltrative / non-infiltrative types	No contrast enhancement in low-grade astrocytomas
			Lipoma	benign fatty lesion commonly affecting corpus callosum	density of fat, high T1-WI signal, signal suppression on FS (fat suppression) or STIR method
			Oligodendroglioma	uncommon slow-growing gliomas	clump-like calcification
		Infratentorial tumours	Cerebellar metastases	especially lung and breast cancer, also melanoma, thyroid malignancies, and renal cell cancer; can present with obstructive hydrocephalus	melanoma MTS – high T1-WI signal
			Haemangioblastoma	typically multiple in patients with von Hippel-Lindau disease	small contrast-enhancing nodule with or without cyst
			Lymphoma	primary CNS lymphoma – more common than secondary (can involve the leptomeninges), B cell lymphoma more common; in immunocompromised patients	diffuse leptomeningeal enhancement
			Choroid plexus papilloma	Choroid plexus papilloma of fourth ventricle, rare neoplasm, usually prominent contrast enhancement, calcifications may be associated, hydrocephalus	MR features of choroid plexus carcinoma and papilloma overlap
	Extra-axial tumours	Supratentorial tumours	Meningioma	most common extraaxial tumour, usually benign, multiple in neurofibromatosis type 2	dural-based lesions (the dural tail sign), prominent enhancement, calcifications may be associated
		Sella region	Pituitary adenoma	common benign slow-growing, endocrine abnormalities	microadenomas typically enhance less than normal pituitary tissue – early phase of dynamic imaging
		Infratentorial tumours	Acoustic schwanoma	90% of intracranial schwannomas 75% of lesions in the cerebellopontine angle cisterns	prominent contrast enhancement; can be heterogeneous in large lesions

Characteristics of selected intracranial tumours				
AGE	LOCALIZATION	TYPE	CHARACTERISTIC	TYPICAL CT / MR FINDINGS
	(arise from the skull, meniges, or tissues other than brain)		multiple seen with neurofibromatosis type 2	
		Meningioma	can result in compression of dural venous sinuses; rarely invasive – malignant type	same as supratentorial
		Paraganglioma	lesions, also referred to as chemodectomas, arise from paraganglia	prominent contrast enhancement; tubular zones of flow voids; often erosive bone changes

Table 5. Characteristics of selected intracranial tumours in adults

Tables 4 and 5 are modified according to [13 – 14, 63 - 64].

Author details

Kamil Zeleňák, Cisáriková Viera and Poláček Hubert

Department of Radiology, University Hospital Martin, Slovakia

References

[1] Černoch Z, Eliáš P, Krajina A, Ryška J, Šercl M, Žiška J. Neuroradiologie. Hradec Králové: Nucleus HK; 2000.

[2] Leeds NE, Kieffer SA. Evolution of Diagnostic Neuroradiology from 1904 to 1999. Radiology 2000; 217(2) 309-318.

[3] Adson AW, Ott WO, Crawford AS. A study of ventriculography. Radiology 1924;2(2) 65-73.

[4] Goodman LR. The Beatles, the Nobel Prize, and CT scanning of the chest. Radiol Clin North Am 2010;48(1) 1-7.

[5] Beckmann EC. CT scanning the early days. Br J Radiol 2006;79(937) 5-8.

[6] Prokop M, Galanski M. Spinal and Multislice Computed Tomography of the Body. Stuttgart: Thieme; 2003.

[7] Hoeffner EG, Case I, Jain R,Gujar SK, Shah GV, Deveikis JP, Carlos RC, Thompson BG. Cerebral perfusion CT: Technique and clinical applications. Radiology 2004;231(3) 632-644.

[8] Ellika SK, Jain R, Patel SC, Scarpace L, Schultz LR, Rock JP, Mikkelsen T. Role of Perfusion CT in Glioma Grading and Comparison with Conventional MR Imaging Features. American Journal of Neuroradiology 2007;28(10) 1981-1987.

[9] Wintermark M, Dillon WP. Advanced CT and MR Imaging Techniques: An Academic Whim or Clinical Standard in the making. American Journal of Neuroradiology 2006;27(6) 1257.

[10] Geva T. Magnetic Resonance Imaging: Historical Perpective. J Cardiovasc Magn Reson 2006;8(4) 573-580.

[11] Timeline of MRI. http://www.fonar.com/timeline_print.htm (accessed 3 July 2012).

[12] Lauterbur PC. Progres in n.m.r. zeugmatography imaging. Philos Tans R Soc London B Biol Sci 1980;289(1037) 483-487.

[13] Reimer P, Parizel PM, Stinoth FA. Clinical MR Imaging. Berlin: Springer; 2003.

[14] Burgener FA, Meyers SP, Tan RK, Zaunbauer W. Differential diagnosis in Magnetic Resonance Imaging. Stuttgart-New York: Thieme; 2002.

[15] Osborn AG, Blaser S, Salzman K, Katzman GL, Provenzale J, Castillo M, Hedlund GL, Illner A, Harnsberger HR, Cooper JA, Jones BV, Hamilton BE. Diagnostic Imaging Brain. Salt Lake City: Amirsys; 2004.

[16] Prince MR, Grist TM, Debatin JF. 3D contrast MR angiography. Berlin: Springer; 2003.

[17] Wang H, Zheng LF, Feng Y, Xie XQ, Zhao JL, Wang XF, Zhang GX. A comparison of 3D-CTA and 4D-CE-MRA for the dynamic monitoring of angiogenesis in a rabbit VX2 tumor. Eur J Radiol 2012;81(1) 104-10.

[18] Kalva SP, Blake MA, Sahani DV. MR contrast agents. Applied Radiology 2006;35(1) 18-27.

[19] Al-Okaili RN, Krejza J, Wang S, Woo JH, Melhem ER. Advanced MR Imaging Techniques in the Diagnosis of Intraaxial Brain Tumors in Adults. Radiographic 2006;26(Suppll) S173-189.

[20] Karimi S, Petrovich NM, Peck KK, Hou BL, Holodny AI. Advanced MR techniques in brain tumor imaging. Applied Ragiology 2006;35(5) 9-18.

[21] Moritani T, Ekholm S, Westesson PL. Diffusion-Weighted MR Imaging of the Brain. Berlin Heidelberg: Springer; 2009.

[22] Bammer R. Basic principles of diffusion-weighted imaging. European Journal of Radiology 2003;45(3) 169-184.

[23] Timothy PL, Rowley HA. Diffusion weighted magnetic resonance imaging in stroke. European Journal of Radiology 2003;45(3) 185-194.

[24] Herneth AM, Guccione S, Bednarski M. Apparent Diffusion Coefficient: a quantitative parameter for in vivo tumor characterization. European Journal of Radiology 2003;45(3) 208-213.

[25] Romano A, Fasoli F, Ferrante M, Ferrante L, Fantozzi LM, Bozzao A. Fiber density index, fractional anisotropy, ADC and clinical motor findings in the white mater of patients with glioblastoma. European Radiology 2008;18(2) 331-336.

[26] Sinha S, Bastin ME, Whittle IR, Wardlaw JM. Diffusion tensor MR imaging of high-grade cerebral gliomas. American Journal of Neuroradiology 2002;23(4) 520-507.

[27] Bammer R, Burak A, Moseley ME. In vivo MR tractography using diffusion imaging. European Journal of Radiology 2003;45(3) 223-234.

[28] Mori S, Crain BJ, Chacko VP, Van Zijl PC. Three-dimensional tracking of axonal projections in the brain by magnetic resonance imaging. Annals of neurology 1999; 45(2) 265-269.

[29] Kono K, Inoue Y, Nakayama K, Shakudo M, Morino M, Ohata K, Wakasa K, Yamada R. The role of diffusion-weighted imaging in patients with brain tumors. American Journal of Neuroradiology 2001;22(6) 1081-1088.

[30] Kleiser R, Staempfli P, Valavanis A, Boesiger P, Kollias S. Impact of fMRI-guided advanced DTI fiber tracking techniques on their clinical applications in patients with brain tumors. Neuroradiology 2010;52(1) 37-46.

[31] Petrella JR, Provenzale JM. MR Perfusion Imaging of the Brain Techniques and Applications. American Journal of roentgenology 2000;175(1) 207-219.

[32] Pollock JM, Tan H, Kraft RA, Whitlow CHT, Burdette JH, Maldjan JA. Arterial Spin Labeled MRI Perfusion Imaging: Clinical Applications Magnetic resosnance imaging clinics of North America 2009;17(2) 315-338.

[33] Forsting M, Weber J. MR perfusion imaging: a tool for more than stroke. European Radiology 2004;14(Suppl5) M2-M7.

[34] Majós C, Aguilera C, Cos M, Camins A, Candiota AP, Delgado-Goni T, Samitier A, Castaner S, Sánchez JJ, Mato D, Acebes JJ, Arús C. In vivo proton magnetic resonance spectroscopy of intraventricular tumors of the brain. European Radiology 2009;19(8) 2049-2059.

[35] Schlemmer HP, Bachert P, Henze H, Buslei R, Herfarth KK, Debus J, vanKaick G. Differentiation of radiation necrosis from tumor progression using proton magnetic resonance spectroscopy. Neuroradiology 2002;44(3) 216-222.

[36] Howe FA, Barton SJ, Cudlip SA, Stubbs M, Saunders DE, Murphy M, Wilokins P, Opstad KS, Doyle VL, McLean M, Beel BA, Griffiths JR. Metabolic profiles of human

brain tumors using quantitative in vivo 1H magnetic resonance spectroscopy. Magnetic resonance in medicine: official journal of the Society of Magnetic Resononance in Medicine / Society of Magnetic Resonance in Medicine 2003;49(2) 223-232.

[37] Law M, Cha S, Knopp EA, Johnson G, Arnett J, Litt AW. High-grade gliomas and solitary metastases: differentiation by using perfusion and proton spectroscopic MR imaging. Radiology 2002;222(3) 715-721.

[38] Burtscher IM, Holtas S. Proton MR spectroscopy in clinical routine. Journal of Magnetic Resonance Imaging 2001;13(4) 560-567.

[39] Huettel SA, Song AW, McCarthy G. Functional Magnetic Resonance Imaging (2 ed.). Massachusetts: Sinauer Associates; 2009.

[40] Detre JA, Wang J, Wang Z, Rao H. Arterial spin-labeled perfusion MRI in basic and clinical neuroscience. Current Opinion in Neurology 2009;22(4) 348-355.

[41] Weber MA, Kroll A, Günther M, Delorme S, Debus J, Giesel FL, Essig M, Kauczor HU, Schad LR. Nichtinvasive Messung des relativen zerebralen Blutflusses mit der MR-Blutbolusmarkierungstechnik (arterial-spin-labeling): Physikalische Grundlagen und klinische Anwendungen. Der Radiologe 2004; 44(2) 164-173.

[42] Vlieger EJ, Majoie CB, Leenstra S, Den Heeten GJ. Functional Magnetic Resonance Imaging for Neurosurgical Planning in Neurooncology. European Radiology 2004;14(7) 1143-1153.

[43] Salvan CV, Ulmer JL, Mueller WM, Krouwer HG, Prost RW, Stroe GO. Presurgical and intraoperative mapping of the motor system in congenital truncation of the precentral gyrus. American Journal of Neuroradiology 2006;27(3) 493-497.

[44] Duchin Y, Abosch A, Yacoub E, Sapiro G, Harel N. Feasibility of using ultra-high field (7 T) MRI for clinical surgical targeting. PLoS One 2012;7(5) e37328.

[45] Logothetis NK. What we can do and what we cannot do with fMRI. Nature 2008;453(7197) 869-878.

[46] Ganslandt O, Behari S, Gralla J, et al., Neuronavigation: concept, techniques and applications. Neurol India 2002;50(3) 244-255.

[47] Tang HL, Sun HP, Gong Y, Mao Y, Wu JS, Zhang XL, Xie Q, Xie LQ, Zheng MZ, Wang DJ, Zhu HD, Tang WJ, Feng XY, Chen XC, Zhou LF. Preoperative surgical planning for intracranial meningioma resection by virtual reality. Chin Med J (Engl) 2012;125(11) 2057-61.

[48] Rasmussen Jr. IA, Lindseth F, Rygh OM, Berntsen EM, Selbekk T, Xu J, Nagelhus Hernes TA, Harg E, Haberg A, Unsgaard G. Functional neuronavigation combined with intra-operative 3D ultrasound: Initial experiences during surgical resections close to eloquent brain areas and future directions in automatic brain shift compenzation af preoperative data. Acta neurochirurgica 2007;149(4) 365-378.

[49] Digital subtraction angiography. Dictionary.com. The American Heritage® Stedman's Medical Dictionary. Houghton Mifflin Company. http://dictionary.reference.com/browse/digital subtraction angiography (accessed: 20 July, 2012).

[50] Harrington DP, Boxt LM, Murray PD. Digital subtraction angiography: overview of technical principles. American Journal of Roentgenology 1982;139(4) 781-6.

[51] Sakamoto S, Eguchi K, Shibukawa M, Kiura Y, Yamasaki F, Kajiwara Y, Matsushige T, Kurisu K. Cerebral angiography using gadolinium as an alternative contrast medium in a patient with severe allergy to iodinated contrast medium. Hiroshima J Med Sci 2010;59(1): 15-6.

[52] Stanton A [translator]. On a new kind of rays. By W.C. Rontgen. Translated by Arthur Stanton from the Sitzungsberichte der Würzburger Physic-medic. Gesellschaft, 1895. Nature, January 23, 1896. Radiography 1970;36(428) 185-8.

[53] Beutel J, Kundel HL, Van Metter RL. Handbook of Medical Imaging, Vol. 1. Bellingham: SPIE Press; 2000.

[54] Hatakeyama Y, Kakeda S, Korogi Y, Ohnari N, Moriya J, Oda N, Nishino K, Miyamoto W. Intracranial 2D and 3D DSA with flat panel detector of the direct conversion type: initial experience. Eur Radiol 2006;16(11) 2594-602.

[55] Moniz E. L'encephalographie arterielle, son importance dans la localisation des tumeurs cerebrales. Reviews Neurology 1927;(2) 72-90.

[56] Estol CJ. Dr C. Miller Fisher and the history of carotid artery disease. Stroke; a journal of cerebral circulation 1996;27(3) 559-66.

[57] Seldinger SI. Catheter replacement of the needle in percutaneous arteriography; a new technique. Acta radiologica 1953;39(5) 368-76.

[58] Reekers JA, Müller-Hülsbeck S, Libicher M, Atar E, Trentmann J, Goffette P, Borggrefe J, Zeleňák K, Hooijboer P, Belli AM. CIRSE vascular closure device registry. Cardiovascular Interventional Radiology 2011;34(1) 50-3.

[59] Krajina A, Cesak T, Zelenak K, Rehak S. Therapeutic Embolization of Cranial Tumors. In: Diagnostic Techniques and Surgical Management of Brain Tumors. Rijeka: InTech Europe; 2011.

[60] Hertel A, Görling S, Schwager K, Hofmann E. Angiography and cerebral perfusion scintigraphy in balloon test occlusion of carotid artery in head and neck tumors. Rofo 2012;184(3) 214-9.

[61] Nishimura S, Hirai T, Shigematsu Y, Kitajima M, Morioka M, Kai Y, Minoda R, Uetani H, Murakami R, Yamashita Y. Evaluation of brain and head and neck tumors with 4D contrast-enhanced MR angiography at 3T. AJNR Am J Neuroradiol 2012;33(3) 445-8.

[62] Schwenzer NF, Stegger L, Bisdas S, Schraml C, Kolb A, Boss A, Müller M, Reimold M, Ernemann U, Claussen CD, Pfannenberg C, Schmidt H. Simultaneous PET/MR

imaging in a human brain PET/MR system in 50 patients-Current state of image quality. Eur J Radiol 2012 Jan 17. [Epub ahead of print]

[63] Gaillard F, et al. Posterior fossa tumours. http://radiopaedia.org/articles/posterior-fossa-tumours (accessed: 18 July, 2012).

[64] Louis DN, Ohgaki H, Wiestler OD, Cavenee WK, Burger PC, Jouvet A, Scheithauer BW, Kleihues P. The 2007 WHO classification of tumours of the central nervous system. Acta Neuropathol 2007;114(2) 97-109.

Chapter 5

Recent Developments of Single Photon Emission Computed Tomography for the Diagnosis of Brain Tumors

Yasushi Shibata

Additional information is available at the end of the chapter

http://dx.doi.org/10.5772/52352

1. Introduction

1.1. Diagnostic ability of ^{201}thallium SPECT and ^{99m}technetium methoxyisobutylisonitrile SPECT for patients with initial glioma

Single photon emission computed tomography (SPECT) is a valuable diagnostic modality for the evaluation of brain tumor malignancy and activity. Thallium-201 (Tl) SPECT and Technetium-99m methoxyisobutylisonitrile (Tc-MIBI) SPECT were clinically used to evaluate brain tumor malignancy and activity. In addition, both early and delayed images were taken depending on the preference of each institute. The results of SPECT examinations always include some false positive or false negative findings. The diagnostic value of brain tumor SPECT has been evaluated using sensitivities and specificities with arbitrary cut off values [1-8]. These arbitrary cut off values depend on the measurement methods used by each institute, as a result, studies using these arbitrary cut off values are not useful for evaluating tumor malignancy at other institutes.

A receiver operating characteristic (ROC) analysis is useful for evaluating the diagnostic ability of different examinations that include some errors [9, 10]. In order to investigate the ability of each SPECT modality to evaluate tumor malignancy, each SPECT modality was directly compared for the patients with an initial glioma using an ROC analysis. The hypothesis is that the one SPECT modality is superior to any other modalities for grading glioma.

1.2. Methods

The study population included 59 patients with glioma who were admitted to Tsukuba University hospital between 1999 and 2005 and who underwent SPECT imaging. None of the patients had received any previous radiation therapy to the brain and recurrent cases were excluded. Tl and Tc-MIBI SPECT images were taken before surgery, radiation or chemotherapy in most patients. The SPECT images were taken after surgery but before radiation or chemotherapy in one patient. All pathological diagnoses were confirmed after the surgical removal of the tumor. The benign group included low grade astrocytomas (n=23) and a central neurocytoma (n=1) while the malignant group included anaplastic astrocytomas (n=10) and glioblastomas (n=25). The benign group included 13 men and 11 women, ranging from 3 to 59 years of age and the median age was 32 years old. The malignant group included 17 men and 18 women, ranging from 7 to 79 years of age and the median age was 55 years old.

Tl SPECT and Tc-MIBI SPECT images were obtained 15 min (early) and 3 hr (delayed) after the intravenous injection of 74 MBq of Tl chloride or 740 MBq of Tc-MIBI using a multi-detector SPECT machine (E.CAM, Siemens Medical, Malvern, PA) and a high resolution collimator (LEHR, Siemens Medical, Malvern, PA). The Butterworth pre-correction filter and the Chang method were used for pre and post attenuation corrections. The Ramp filter was used for reconstruction. The image matrixes for Tl and MIBI SPECT were 64x64 and 128x128. The pixel sizes for Tl and MIBI SPECT were 6.61mm and 3.31mm. The slice thickness both of Tl and MIBI SPECT was 6.61mm.

The Regions of Interest (ROI) were set on tumor and contra-lateral normal white matter in reconstructed SPECT images. The ROIs were customized for each patient. In the cases with a hot tracer uptake into the tumor, the ROIs were placed at homogeneously high uptake areas. In cases with no tracer uptake, the ROIs were placed at suspected tumor areas using the MRI findings as references. All ROIs were selected by independent radiology technologists. Tumor/Normal (T/N) ratios were calculated as the ratios of radioactivity in the ROIs. The diagnostic abilities of the T/N ratios for malignancy were analyzed by an ROC analysis using the ROCKIT1.1B2 Beta and PlotROC.xls software programs (University of Chicago). The area z-score (Az) values were calculated from the areas under the ROC curves and the diagnostic accuracy was compared between each imaging modality. Any differences in the Az values were analyzed using the bivariate x2 test.

1.3. Results

Figure 1 shows the ROC curves. The vertical axis is the true positive fraction (TPF) that means sensitivity and the horizontal axis is the false positive fraction (FPF) that is same value of 1-specificity. The ROC curve of the early MIBI shifted to upper right and the sensitivity was better than the other in the high FPF area, however the sensitivity was low in the low FPF area. The ROC curve of the delayed MIBI shifted to the upper left and showed well balanced high sensitivity and specificity. The ROC curves of the early and delayed Tl were almost same and showed lower sensitivity and specificity than that of the delayed MIBI in most areas.

http://dx.doi.org/10.5772/52352

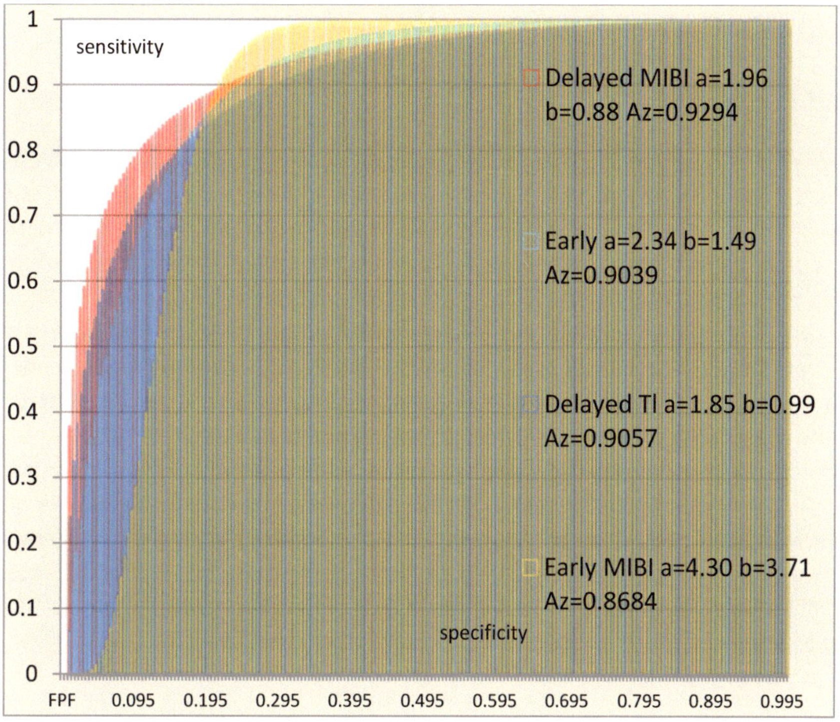

Figure 1. Receiver operating characteristic (ROC) curves

1.4. Discussion

1.4.1. Tl SPECT

Tl SPECT is useful for identifying the presence of a tumor [11], tumor malignancy [1, 6, 12] and for making a differential diagnosis to distinguish tumor recurrence from radiation necrosis [6, 12, 13]. The Tl index, the ratio of radioactivity of ROI at the lesion and normal brain, was used to differentiate low and high grade glioma [1], recurrence and radiation necrosis [2, 3]. The dynamic Tl SPECT is reported to be useful to evaluate tumor vascularity, histology and malignancy [14, 15]. However there are some false positive and false negative cases reported [6, 7, 12, 16, 17]. Inflammation after surgery or radiation is a major cause of false positive Tl uptake. The causes of false negative findings may include small tumor size, histological heterogeneity, cystic or necrotic components, or a low threshold of the detector or imaging [18, 19]. Both of central neurocytoma and ganglioglioma are benign glioma. High Tl uptake in a central neurocytoma and ganglioglioma were reported [20] [21]. High cell density and high metabolic rate are thought to explain the high Tl uptake in these low proliferative tumors. In the present series, one patient with a central neurocytoma showed high Tl uptake and no MIBI uptake. In this case, MIBI SPECT was more accurate than Tl SPECT to evaluate tumor malignancy, because central neurocytoma is a benign tumor. Pilocytic astrocytoma is one of the most benign gliomas and the Tl SPECT findings of a pilocytic astrocytoma are reported to show a variable uptake [8].

1.4.2. Tc-MIBI SPECT

Tc-MIBI SPECT is reported to be useful to diagnose brain tumor recurrence [22, 23], high S-phase fraction and aneuploidy [24], tumor volume and survival [25, 26], and, differential diagnosis of radiation necrosis [27]. The Tc-MIBI index, the ratio of radioactivity of the ROI at the lesion and normal brain, was used to differentiate low and high grade gliomas [28], recurrence and radiation necrosis [22] and the estimation of the prognosis [25, 26]. However there are some false positive and false negative cases reported [23]. Tc-MIBI is concentrated in the mitochondria as the result of active diffusion due to increased metabolic needs [22]. Tc-MIBI uptake is determined by tumor malignancy, viability, density, oxygenation, vascular supply, and blood brain barrier (BBB) disruption [29]. These factors are not linearly correlated, because glioblastoma, the most malignant form of glioma, is pathologically heterogeneous including internal necrosis. False negative MIBI SPECT may occur due to the lack of contrast uptake on MRI and masked by other normal tissue uptake. This was seen in temporal and periventricular tumors [23], because Tc-MIBI is physiologically taken into the orbita, naso-pharyngeal tissues, pituitary, scalp and choroid plexus [30]. Some of the false positive results were due to recent radiation induced local disruption of the BBB [23].

The pixel size of MIBI SPECT was smaller than that of Tl SPECT in this study. Therefore, MIBI SPECT has a higher spatial resolution than Tl SPECT. This study investigated the diagnostic ability of SPECT for glioma malignancy. Higher spatial resolution might influence the diagnostic ability with small or heterogeneous tumors. However, all of the gliomas in this study were larger than the pixel size. In addition, most of the malignant tumors in this study were highly heterogeneous in both of MRI and SPECT. Only the higher spatial resolution of MIBI SPECT could not explain the slightly higher diagnostic ability of MIBI SPECT than that of Tl SPECT. Some authors have reported that Tc-MIBI SPECT has higher sensitivity and specificity than that of Tl SPECT for adult and childhood brain tumors and differential diagnosis of recurrence and radiation necrosis [26, 27, 31]. However, other authors did not [32]. This discrepancy may be caused by small and heterogeneous patient populations and arbitrary selected cut off values. In Tl SPECT there is some normal brain uptake, this makes T/N ratio low. Tc-MIBI has high photon energy level and higher tumor/background ratio in comparison with Tl SPECT and yields clear SPECT images and high sensitivity for malignant brain tumor [22, 27, 31].

P-glycoprotein is one of the drug efflux pumps in the cell membrane and it acts to remove Tc-MIBI from tumor cells [33, 34]. Other studies have suggested that p-glycoprotein expression in malignant glioma is the cause of false negative with Tc-MIBI SPECT [35-37]. The effect of p-glycoprotein expression on clinical Tc-MIBI SPECT images has been investigated, and this effect was negligible in the diagnosis of brain tumor malignancy [38]. Henze also reported that p-glycoprotein efflux does not contribute to false negative MIBI SPECT, since MIBI washout did not occur between the early and late SPECT scans [39].

1.4.3. ROC analysis

Many facilities use a cut off value to evaluate tumor malignancy in Tl or Tc-MIBI SPECT [1, 4-8]. Serizawa reported that simple inter-institutional comparisons of Tl indices are not possible because measurement methods are different in each institute [7].

Most diagnostic tests have some errors and the results are influenced by arbitrary selected cut off values. ROC analysis is useful to evaluate the diagnostic values of each examination that yield some false positive or false negative results [9, 10]. Henze reported that ROC analysis comparing I-123-iodo-α-methyl-L-tyrosine (IMT), Tc-MIBI SPECT and F-18-fluorodeoxyglucose positron emission computed tomography (FDG PET) for detection of tumor progression in irradiated low-grade astrocytoma demonstrated that IMT yielded best diagnostic accuracy [29]. ROC analysis has better diagnostic power than the arbitrary cut off method and independent disease prevalence and decision-making threshold [29]. ROC analysis also provides adequate cut off value with appropriate sensitivity and specificity. Because SPECT image accuracy is dependent on SPECT machine quality, acquisition algorithm, and injected isotope dose, each facility should determine its own cut off value to provide an adequate diagnosis from an ROC analysis of own data.

Some facilities omitted the acquisition of delayed images due to their limited examination time. However, the current results demonstrated the superior diagnostic value of delayed images in both of Tl and Tc-MIBI SPECT. These results revealed both Tl and Tc-MIBI SPECT are useful for the diagnosis of gliomas. However, the SPECT study is not perfect, there are still some false positive and false negative findings. Multi-modality imaging studies may therefore help to diagnose brain tumors more correctly. If it is necessary to limit SPECT examinations due to medical economical issues related to the health insurance policy, then Tc-MIBI SPECT with a delayed acquisition is therefore considered to be the most reasonable choice.

1.5. Conclusion

Both of Tl and Tc-MIBI SPECT are useful imaging modalities for the evaluation of glioma malignancies. Although there was no statistically significant difference, delayed Tc-MIBI SPECT demonstrated the best diagnostic value in our patients with glioma based on an ROC analysis.

2. Coregistration of functional SPECT images and high resolution anatomical MRI

2.1. Introduction

201Thallium Single Photon Emission Computed Tomography (Tl SPECT) is a useful functional imaging modality for the diagnosis of malignancy and activity of brain tumors. One of the drawbacks of Tl SPECT is its low spatial resolution. The coregistration of functional SPECT images and high resolution anatomical magnetic resonance imaging (MRI) is considered to be a reasonable method to improve the low spatial resolution of SPECT.

Some methods developed for the coregistration of multiple images have been reported. One is a prospective method using external markers[40-42]. Another is the retrospective methods based on imaging data[43-46]. Prospective methods need prospective external fiducial marker placement and only the image with the marker can be coregistered. Retrospective methods do not need external markers, and therefore they are more flexible. Variable images can be retrospectively coregistered using software programs.

A newly developed software Brain Easy Analysis Tool for 201Tl-SPECT (BEAT-Tl, Fuji Film RI Pharma. Tokyo, Japan) was used for the coregistration of Tl SPECT and MRI in patients with brain tumors. The feasibility and reliability of BEAT-Tl was evaluated for patients with brain tumors.

2.2. Materials and methods

The patient population included 98 patients (47 men and 51 women). The age range was from 4 to 84 years of age and the median age was 54. All patients had been admitted to Tsukuba University Hospital between 2004 and 2007. The brain MRI and Tl SPECT images were taken within a 1 week interval. No anti-tumor therapy was administered between the examinations. The sets of MRI and Tl SPECT examinations were taken for 120 times (59 times for men and 61 times for women). MRI showed mass lesions in all of the patients. The final diagnoses included glioma, lymphoma, neurocytoma, metastasis, meningioma, radiation necrosis, encephalitis and multiple sclerosis. Most patients underwent tumor removal surgery and the pathological diagnoses were determined.

MRI was performed using the 1.5 Tesla clinical MRI scanner (Gyroscan NT Intera, Philips, Netherlands). T1 weighted images with or without Gd-DTPA enhancement, T2 weighted images and Fluid attenuated inversion recovery images (FLAIR) were routinely acquired. Tl SPECT images were acquired 15 minutes (early image) and 3 hours (delayed image) after the intravenous injection of 74 MBq of Thallium Chloride (Fuji Film RI Pharma. Tokyo, Japan) using a multi-detector SPECT machine (E.CAM, Siemens Medical, Erlangen, Germany) and a high resolution collimator (LEHR, Siemens Medical, Erlangen, Germany). The Butterworth pre-correction filter and the Chang method were used for pre and post attenuation corrections. The Ramp filter was used for reconstruction. The image matrixes for Tl SPECT were 64 x 64. Both the pixel sizes and the slice thickness for Tl SPECT were 6.61mm.

The MRI and SPECT data were saved as Digital Imaging and Communications in Medicine (DICOM) formats. The DICOM data were converted to the analyze format using File Converter Ver. 2.5 (Fuji Film RI Pharma. Tokyo, Japan). Both the MRI and SPECT data in analyze format were transferred to the co-registration software program BEAT-Tl and then coregistered images were created. The BEAT-Tl program is based on Statistical Parametric Mapping (SPM) and it can be used on personal computers with the Windows operating system. The imaging quality, clinical usefulness and the artifacts of the coregistered images were evaluated by visual inspection.

http://dx.doi.org/10.5772/52352

2.3. Results

The coregistered images were easily and promptly created within one minute. The image quality was sufficient. There were no large displacements of the MRI and SPECT images and no major artifacts. The coregistration was fully automatic and no manual coregistration procedure was required.

The small hot uptake in Tl SPECT always coincided with enhanced tumors in MRI. For large tumors, Gd enhanced T1 weighted MRI showed relatively homogeneous enhancement. However, Tl SPECT showed focal uptake of Tl in the homogeneously enhanced tumor. Therefore, the coregistered images demonstrated metabolic heterogeneity on Tl SPECT. In most patients, Tl hot uptake was in the Gd enhanced tumor. In some patients, Tl uptake was observed outside of the Gd enhanced tumor.

2.4. Illustrative cases

Case 1:A 64-year-old female with an anaplastic oligodendroglioma

Tl uptakes were different between 2 fusion images of Gd enhanced T1 weighted MRI and early Tl SPECT (Fig. 2, Lt) or delayed Tl SPECT (Fig.2,Rt). Tl uptakes were heterogeneous even though the Gd enhanced tumor was homogenous. Most Tl uptakes were within the Gd enhanced tumor. However the part of the delayed Tl uptake was out of the Gd enhanced area, and therefore this region seemed to demonstrate tumor invasion into normal brain tissue.

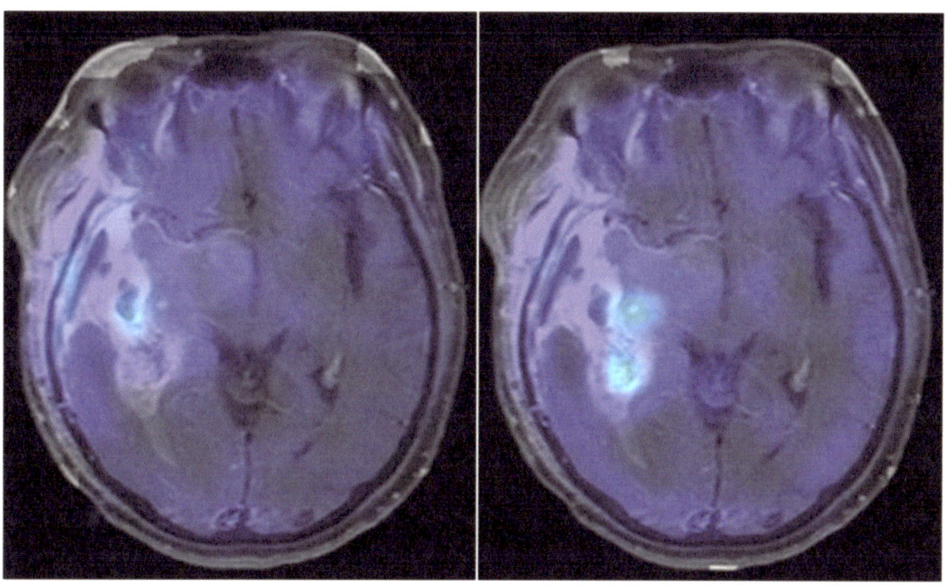

Figure 2. Fusion images of Gd enhanced T1 weighted MRI and early Tl SPECT (Lt) or delayed Tl SPECT (Rt) of Case 1.

Case 2: A 34-year-old male with a frontal glioblastoma.

A fusion image of the preoperative Gd enhanced MRI and delayed Tl SPECT (Fig 3, Lt) showed Rt medial Tl uptake although the Gd enhanced tumor was located in the corpus callosum. Because there was a tumor without Gd enhancement in the left frontal lobe, the left frontal lobe and the tumor at the corpus callosum was removed. After radiation therapy of 60Gy, 2 months after the surgery, tumor recurrence was seen mainly in the Rt medial frontal lobe where the hot Tl uptake was seen in Gd enhanced T1 weighted MRI (Fig 3, Rt).

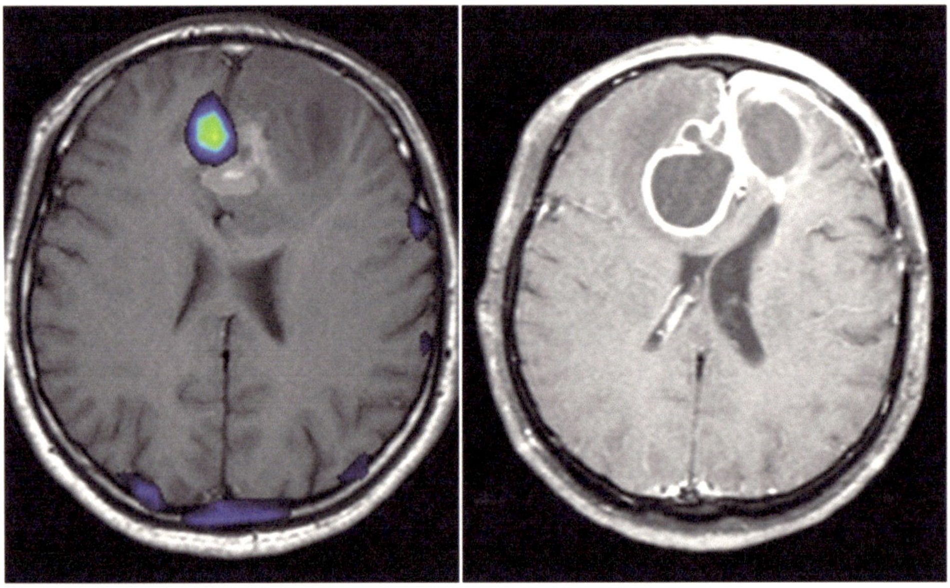

Figure 3. Fusion image of preoperative Gd enhanced MRI and delayed Tl SPECT (Lt) and Gd enhanced T1 weighted MRI (Rt) 2 months after the surgery.

2.5. Discussion

2.5.1. Usefulness of coregistration

The one of the major disadvantages of SPECT is the low spatial resolution caused by scattering radiation. Because no anatomical landmarks are seen in Tl SPECT images, it is sometimes difficult to precisely determine the locations of lesions and the relationships with normal structures based on only Tl SPECT images. The coregistration of Tl SPECT and MRI has thus completely solved these problems.

Even when tumors were found to be homogeneous in MRI, Tl SPECT showed metabolic heterogeneity. These detailed analyses thus become possible by studying coregistration images. Further pathological and clinical studies are expected to reveal the clinical significance of these imaging modalities.

2.5.2. *Method of coregistration*

Other methods for the coregistration of SPECT and MRI has been reported [45-47]. These methods required meticulous and cumbersome procedures and long calculation time. In some cases sufficient coregistration could not be achieved by automatic calculations and thus required manual procedures.

The Brain easy analysis tool (BEAT, Fuji film RI Pharma, Tokyo, Japan) is the coregistration program for cerebral blood flow (CBF) SPECT and MRI. BEAT uses automated image registration (AIR http://bishopw.loni.ucla.edu/) as the coregistration algorithm and ratio image uniformity (RIU) as the cost function. In CBF SPECT image, tracer uptake into normal brain tissue is seen, so the contour of the brain tissue is clear. However, in the brain tumor SPECT image, the tracer uptake into the normal brain tissue is negligible, so the contour of the normal brain tissue is not seen. Because of these factors, the coregistration of brain tumor SPECT and MRI has not been achieved using the same algorithm used for the coregistration of CBF SPECT image and MRI.

BEAT-Tl uses statistical parametric mapping (SPM) 2 (http://www.fil.ion.ucl.ac.uk/spm/) as the voxel based coregistration software and normalized mutual information (NMI) as the cost function to evaluate coregistration accuracy. These algorithms allow automatic coregistration of brain tumor SPECT and MRI with satisfactory accuracy.

The BEAT-Tl program runs on a normal personal computer without any problems. The usual calculation time is within a minute, so it is simple for operators. The results could be fed back to a busy daily clinical practice, so the clinical impact and efficacy are significant. In the current study, the accuracy of the coregistration was satisfactory. There were no major errors or artifacts.

SPECT/computed tomography (CT) or positron emission CT (PET)/CT are thus considered to be alternative methods to create coregistration images. These hardware based coregistrations must be more accurate than the software based coregistrations. Currently, however, these machines are expensive and not available in most clinical settings. As the results, the coregistration software program is both a convenient and sufficiently accurate method to create coregistration images in most clinical facilities.

2.5.3. *Study limitation*

The current study population was relatively small and this study did not evaluate every patient admitted to this hospital. In the future, a prospective study will reveal the exact usefulness and the limitations of the coregistration images of Tl SPECT and MRI.

The uptake of Tl into a lesion is affected by multiple factors, including tumor malignancy, tumor metabolism, cell density, blood brain barrier breakdown, blood flow, blood volume and capillary density [1, 5]. Therefore, the interpretation of Tl SPECT should be done cautiously. The fusion of Tl SPECT and MRI could be helpful to evaluate the mechanisms of Tl uptake into lesions. Although no large displacements of the coregistration were seen in the images created by BEAT-Tl, the coregistration error was not measured in this study. In order to investigate the coregistration error, stereotactic or image guided surgery will be done in a future study. One of the problems of image study for malignant brain tumors is the heterogeneity. Glioblastoma multiforme is pathologically, metabolically, and radiologically heterogeneous. Pathological radiological correlations could reveal the meaning of each finding. Neurosurgeons could remove the tumor; however, the registration of the removed tissue at exact locations on each image is not easy. Image guided surgery using coregistration image should facilitate these studies. The application of fusion images for navigation guided neurosurgery will be developed.

2.6. Conclusion

BEAT-Tl is a useful coregistration software program that is used to evaluate brain tumors. It improves the spatial correlation of SPECT images and such coregistration images demonstrate a metabolic heterogeneity in tumors that is not revealed in MRI.

3. Evaluation of glioma surgical extent using fusion image of Tl SPECT and anatomical MRI

3.1. Introduction

In glioma surgery, removal extent has been evaluated using morphological image, such as MRI or X-ray CT. These morphological images could not completely evaluated surgical removal extent, because glioma is invasive tumor. The contribution of glioma surgery for the improvement of the prognosis is controversial [48, 49]. One of the causes of this discrepancy may be the method of evaluation of glioma surgical extent. We evaluated the glioma surgical extent using fusion image of metabolic Tl SPECT and anatomical MRI. Our hypothesis is these fusion images could more precisely predict the prognosis of the patient received glioma removal surgery.

3.2. Methods

From 2006 to 2008, 146 patients examined both of Tl SPECT and MRI at the same time under the diagnosis of brain tumor. And 58 patients received tumor removal surgery after the examinations. Only 36 patients who were examined MRI within 3 days after the surgery were included because surgical modification of MRI increase after postoperative 4 days [50]. Finally 30 patients who have Gd-DTPA enhanced tumor in MRI and hot tumor uptake in Tl SPECT were included in this study, in order to make image evaluation easy. Final patient population included 17 male and 13 female, age range from 34 to 80 year-old. World Health Organization (WHO) pathological grade are 10 grade 3 and 20 grade 4. Oligodendroglioma component was recognized in 7 grade 3 tumors. All patients received adjuvant standard radiation and chemotherapy.

http://dx.doi.org/10.5772/52352

3.3. Results

Partial removal group were frequently seen in Grade 4. The removal rates with MRI and SPECT were concordant for 24 cases. The removal rates with MRI were higher than those with SPECT in 6 cases. So SPECT more efficiently revealed residual tumor than MRI did (Figure 4,5). The time to progression was short in partial removal group with MRI and SPECT (Figure 6). The removal rates, pathology and oligodendroglioma components were all related with the prognosis in multivariate analysis.

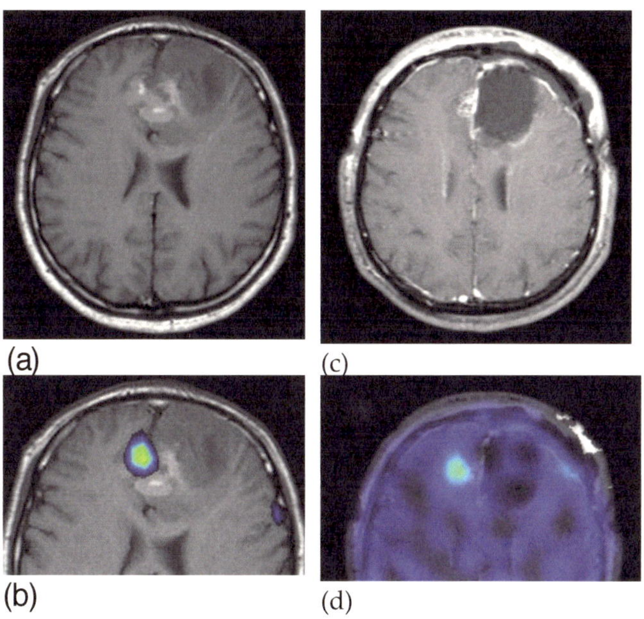

(a): preoperative Gd-enhanced MRI showed left frontal non-enhanced low intensity tumor and Gd-enhanced tumor. Enhanced tumor located at left medial frontal lobe and invaded into right medial frontal lobe.

(b): The fusion image of preoperative Tl-SPECT and MRI showed hot Tl uptake only at right medial frontal lobe.

(c): Postoperative Gd-enhanced MRI showed small residual enhanced tumor at right medial frontal lobe.

(d): The fusion image with Tl-SPECT demonstrated residual tumor at right medial frontal lobe. Surgical extents were evaluated as subtotal removal by MRI, partial removal with Tl-SPECT.

(e): After radiation and chemotherapy, tumor recurrence occurred from right medial frontal residual tumor.

(Reproduced from Y Shibata, CI research 32:19-24, 2010 with permission.)

Figure 4. Case 1, 34 year-old man with glioblastoma. (same case as Fig 2-2)

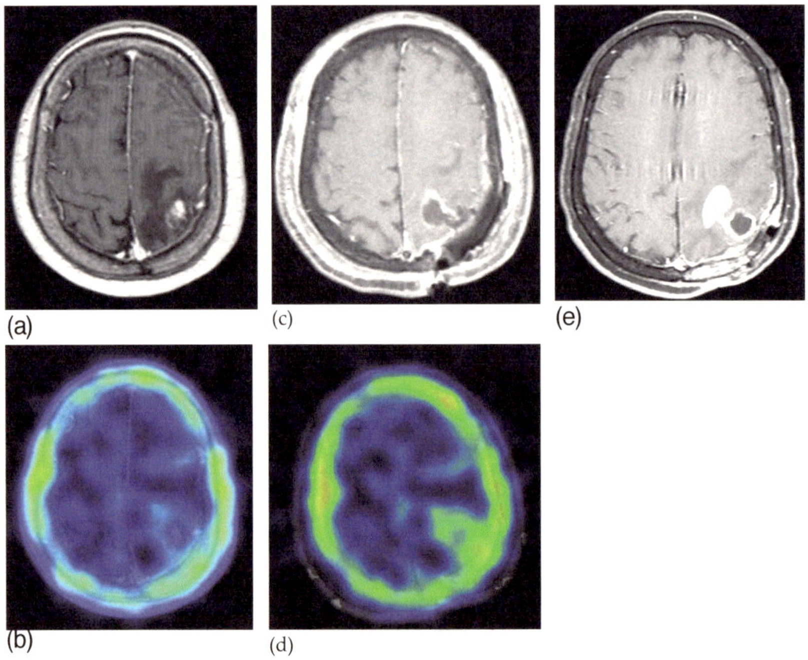

(a): Preoperative Gd-enhanced MRI showed right parietal ring enhanced tumor and perifocal edema.
(b): The fusion image of preoperative Gd-enhanced MRI and Tl SPECT
(c): Postoperative Gd-enhanced MRI showed small residual enhanced tumor at right parietal lobe.
(d): The fusion image of preoperative Tl SPECT and MRI showed hot Tl uptake at right residual parietal lobe.
(e): After radiation and chemotherapy, tumor recurrence occurred from hot Tl uptake area.
(Reproduced from Y Shibata, CI research 32:19-24, 2010 with permission.)

Figure 5. Case 2, 57 year-old woman with glioblastoma.

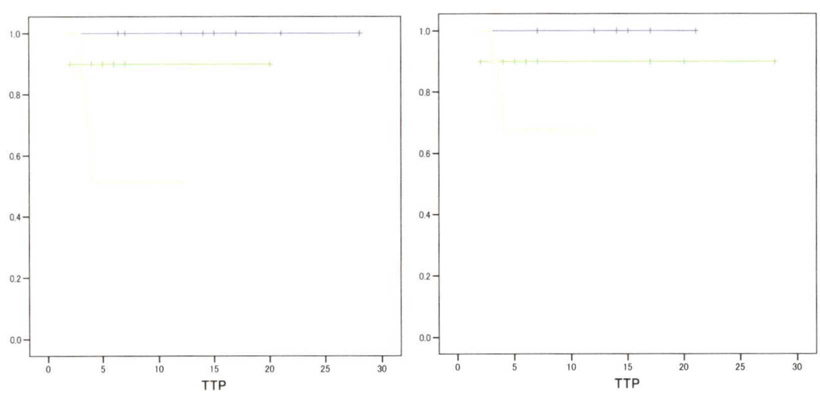

Figure 6. Kaplan-Meier curves of Time to Progression evaluated by removal rate in MRI (Left) and SPECT (Right). Partial removal groups (brown curves) showed significantly early recurrences than both of total (blue curves) and sub-total removal groups (blue curves).

3.4. Conclusion

The fusion image of preoperative Tl SPECT and postoperative MRI is more useful to evaluate glioma removal extent than MRI only. Partial removal groups have poor prognosis, so maximum surgical removal should be aimed using multimodal images including MRI and Tl SPECT. The total removal of Tl SPECT positive lesion improves the prognosis and especially prevents early recurrence.

Acknowledgements

I appreciate my mentors, collaborators and the patients.

Author details

Yasushi Shibata

Department of Neurosurgery, Mito Medical Center, University of Tsukuba, Ibaraki, Japan

I declare that I have no conflict of interest.

References

[1] Black KL, Hawkins RA, Kim KT, Becker DP, Lerner C, Marciano D. Use of thallium-201 SPECT to quantitate malignancy grade of gliomas. J Neurosurg. 1989;71:342-6.

[2] Kosuda S, Shioyama Y, Kamata N, Suzuki K, Tanaka Y, Nakamura O, et al. [Differential diagnosis between recurrence of brain tumor and radiation necrosis by 201Tl SPECT]. Nippon Igaku Hoshasen Gakkai Zasshi. 1991;51:415-21. (In Japaese)

[3] Kosuda S, Fujii H, Aoki S, Suzuki K, Tanaka Y, Nakamura O, et al. Reassessment of quantitative thallium-201 brain SPECT for miscellaneous brain tumors. Ann Nucl Med. 1993;7:257-63.

[4] Kahn D, Follett KA, Bushnell DL, Nathan MA, Piper JG, Madsen M, et al. Diagnosis of recurrent brain tumor: value of 201Tl SPECT vs 18F- fluorodeoxyglucose PET. Am J Roentgenol. 1994;163:1459-65.

[5] Burkard R, Kaiser KP, Wieler H, Klawki P, Linkamp A, Mittelbach L, et al. Contribution of thallium-201-SPECT to the grading of tumorous alterations of the brain. Neurosurg Rev. 1992;15:265-73.

[6] Staffen W, Hondl N, Trinka E, Iglseder B, Unterrainer J, Ladurner G. Clinical relevance of 201Tl-chloride SPET in the differential diagnosis of brain tumours. Nucl Med Commun. 1998;19:335-40.

[7] Serizawa T, Saeki N, Higuchi Y, Ono J, Matsuda S, Sato M, et al. Diagnostic value of thallium-201 chloride single-photon emission computerized tomography in differentiating tumor recurrence from radiation injury after gamma knife surgery for metastatic brain tumors. J Neurosurg. 2005;102 Suppl:266-71.

[8] Comte F, Bauchet L, Rigau V, Hauet JR, Fabbro M, Coubes P, et al. Correlation of preoperative thallium SPECT with histological grading and overall survival in adult gliomas. Nucl Med Commun. 2006;27:137-42.

[9] Metz CE. ROC methodology in radiologic imaging. Invest Radiol. 1986;21:720-33.

[10] Metz CE, A. HB, Jong-Her S. Maximum likelihood estimation of receiver operating characteristic (ROC) curves from continuously-distributed data. Statistics in Medicine. 1998;17:1033-53.

[11] O'Tuama LA, Janicek MJ, Barnes PD, Scott RM, Black PM, Sallan SE, et al. 201Tl/99mTc-HMPAO SPECT imaging of treated childhood brain tumors. Pediatr Neurol. 1991;7:249-57.

[12] Yoshii Y, Satou M, Yamamoto T, Yamada Y, Hyodo A, Nose T, et al. The role of thallium-201 single photon emission tomography in the investigation and characterisation of brain tumours in man and their response to treatment. Eur J Nucl Med. 1993;20:39-45.

[13] Schwartz RB, Carvalho PA, Alexander E, 3rd, Loeffler JS, Folkerth R, Holman BL. Radiation necrosis vs high-grade recurrent glioma: differentiation by using dual-isotope SPECT with 201TI and 99mTc-HMPAO. AJNR Am J Neuroradiol. 1991;12:1187-92.

[14] Ueda T, Kaji Y, Wakisaka S, Watanabe K, Hoshi H, Jinnouchi S, et al. Time sequential single photon emission computed tomography studies in brain tumour using thallium-201. Eur J Nucl Med. 1993;20:138-45.

[15] Sugo N, Yokota K, Kondo K, Harada N, Aoki Y, Miyazaki C, et al. Early dynamic 201Tl SPECT in the evaluation of brain tumours. Nucl Med Commun. 2006;27:143-9.

[16] Buchpiguel CA, Alavi JB, Alavi A, Kenyon LC. PET versus SPECT in distinguishing radiation necrosis from tumor recurrence in the brain. J Nucl Med. 1995;36:159-64.

[17] Rollins NK, Lowry PA, Shapiro KN. Comparison of gadolinium-enhanced MR and thallium-201 single photon emission computed tomography in pediatric brain tumors. Pediatr Neurosurg. 1995;22:8-14.

[18] Kallen K, Burtscher IM, Holtas S, Ryding E, Rosen I. 201Thallium SPECT and 1H-MRS compared with MRI in chemotherapy monitoring of high-grade malignant astrocytomas. J Neurooncol. 2000;46:173-85.

[19] Young RJ, Ghesani MV, Kagetsu NJ, Derogatis AJ. Lesion size determines accuracy of thallium-201 brain single-photon emission tomography in differentiating between intracranial malignancy and infection in AIDS patients. AJNR Am J Neuroradiol. 2005;26:1973-9.

[20] Kumabe T, Shimizu H, Sonoda Y, Shirane R. Thallium-201 single-photon emission computed tomographic and proton magnetic resonance spectroscopic characteristics of intracranial ganglioglioma: three technical case reports. Neurosurgery. 1999;45:183-7.

[21] Kanamori M, Kumabe T, Shimizu H, Yoshimoto T. (201)Tl-SPECT, (1)H-MRS, and MIB-1 labeling index of central neurocytomas: three case reports. Acta Neurochir (Wien). 2002;144:157-63.

[22] Soler C, Beauchesne P, Maatougui K, Schmitt T, Barral FG, Michel D, et al. Technetium-99m sestamibi brain single-photon emission tomography for detection of recurrent gliomas after radiation therapy. Eur J Nucl Med. 1998;25:1649-57.

[23] Le Jeune FP, Dubois F, Blond S, Steinling M. Sestamibi technetium-99m brain single-photon emission computed tomography to identify recurrent glioma in adults: 201 studies. J Neurooncol. 2006;77:177-83.

[24] Ak I, Gulbas Z, Altinel F, Vardareli E. Tc-99m MIBI uptake and its relation to the proliferative potential of brain tumors. Clin Nucl Med. 2003;28:29-33.

[25] Beauchesne P, Soler C. Correlation of 99mTc-MIBI brain spect (functional index ratios) and survival after treatment failure in malignant glioma patients. Anticancer Res. 2002;22:3081-5.

[26] Beauchesne P, Pedeux R, Boniol M, Soler C. 99mTc-sestamibi brain SPECT after chemoradiotherapy is prognostic of survival in patients with high-grade glioma. J Nucl Med. 2004;45:409-13.

[27] Yamamoto Y, Nishiyama Y, Toyama Y, Kunishio K, Satoh K, Ohkawa M. 99mTc-MIBI and 201Tl SPET in the detection of recurrent brain tumours after radiation therapy. Nucl Med Commun. 2002;23:1183-90.

[28] Baillet G, Albuquerque L, Chen Q, Poisson M, Delattre JY. Evaluation of single-photon emission tomography imaging of supratentorial brain gliomas with technetium-99m sestamibi. Eur J Nucl Med. 1994;21:1061-6.

[29] Henze M, Mohammed A, Schlemmer HP, Herfarth KK, Hoffner S, Haufe S, et al. PET and SPECT for Detection of Tumor Progression in Irradiated Low-Grade Astrocytoma: A Receiver-Operating-Characteristic Analysis. J Nucl Med. 2004;45:579-86.

[30] Kirton A, Kloiber R, Rigel J, Wolff J. Evaluation of pediatric CNS malignancies with (99m)Tc-methoxyisobutylisonitrile SPECT. J Nucl Med. 2002;43:1438-43.

[31] O'Tuama LA, Treves ST, Larar JN, Packard AB, Kwan AJ, Barnes PD, et al. Thallium-201 versus technetium-99m-MIBI SPECT in evaluation of childhood brain tumors: a within-subject comparison. J Nucl Med. 1993;34:1045-51.

[32] Nishiyama Y, Yamamoto Y, Fukunaga K, Satoh K, Kunishio K, Ohkawa M. Comparison of 99Tcm-MIBI with 201Tl chloride SPET in patients with malignant brain tumours. Nucl Med Commun. 2001;22:631-9.

[33] Feun LG, Savaraj N, Landy HJ. Drug resistance in brain tumors. J Neurooncol. 1994;20(2):165-76.

[34] Lehnert M. Multidrug resistance in human cancer. J Neurooncol. 1994;22(3):239-43.

[35] Andrews DW, Das R, Kim S, Zhang J, Curtis M. Technetium-MIBI as a glioma imaging agent for the assessment of multi-drug resistance. Neurosurgery. 1997;40(6): 1323-32.

[36] Ballinger JR, Sheldon KM, Boxen I, Erlichman C, Ling V. Differences between accumulation of 99mTc-MIBI and 201Tl-thallous chloride in tumour cells: role of P-glycoprotein. Q J Nucl Med. 1995;39(2):122-8.

[37] Piwnica-Worms D, Chiu ML, Budding M, Kronauge JF, Kramer RA, Croop JM. Functional imaging of multidrug-resistant P-glycoprotein with an organotechnetium complex. Cancer Res. 1993;53(5):977-84.

[38] Shibata Y, Matsumura A, Nose T. Effect of expression of P-glycoprotein on technetium-99m methoxyisobutylisonitrile single photon emission computed tomography of brain tumors. Neurol Med Chir (Tokyo). 2002;42:325-30.

[39] Henze M, Mohammed A, Schlemmer H, Herfarth KK, Mier W, Eisenhut M, et al. Detection of tumour progression in the follow-up of irradiated low-grade astrocytomas: comparison of 3-(123I)iodo-alpha-methyl- L-tyrosine and 99mTc-MIBI SPET. Eur J Nucl Med Mol Imaging. 2002;29:1455-61.

[40] Yamamoto Y, Nishiyama Y, Monden T, Matsumura Y, Satoh K, Ohkawa M. Clinical Usefulness of Fusion of 131I SPECT and CT Images in Patients with Differentiated Thyroid Carcinoma. J Nucl Med. 2003;44:1905-10.

[41] Chajari M, Lacroix J, Peny AM, Chesnay E, Batalla A, Henry-Amar M, et al. Gallium-67 scintigraphy in lymphoma: is there a benefit of image fusion with computed tomography? Eur J Nucl Med Mol Imaging. 2002;29:380-7.

[42] Aqueveque AC, Gonzalez EP, Gutierrez BD, Jaimovich FR, Diaz PJ, Csendes GP, et al. (Fusion of SPECT with computed tomography or magnetic resonance for the interpretation of abnormal tracer uptake.). Rev Med Chil. 2007 (In Spanish);135:725-34.

[43] Pietrzyk U, Herholz K, Fink G, Jacobs A, Mielke R, Slansky I, et al. An interactive technique for three-dimensional image registration: validation for PET, SPECT, MRI and CT brain studies. J Nucl Med. 1994;35:2011-8.

[44] Pietrzyk U, Herholz K, Schuster A, Stockhausen H-Mv, Lucht H, Heiss W-D. Clinical applications of registration and fusion of multimodality brain images from PET, SPECT, CT, and MRI. European Journal of Radiology. 1996;21:174-82.

[45] Sabbah P, Foehrenbach H, Dutertre G, Nioche C, DeDreuille O, Bellegou N, et al. Multimodal anatomic, functional, and metabolic brain imaging for tumor resection. Clin Imaging. 2002;26:6-12.

[46] Komori T, Kanamoto T, Ogura Y, Utsunomiya K, Adachi I, Narabayashi I. The evaluation of thallium-201 SPECT/MRI image fusion in brain tumor. Rinsho Hoshasen. 2004;49:285-90. (In Japanese)

[47] Holman BL, Zimmerman RE, Johnson KA, Carvalho PA, Schwartz RB, Loeffler JS, et al. Computer-assisted superimposition of magnetic resonance and high-resolution technetium-99m-HMPAO and thallium-201 SPECT images of the brain. J Nucl Med. 1991;32:1478-84.

[48] Mitchell P, Ellison DW, Mendelow AD. Surgery for malignant gliomas: mechanistic reasoning and slippery statistics. Lancet Neurol. 2005;4:413-22.

[49] Sanai N, Berger MS. Glioma extent of resection and its impact on patient outcome. Neurosurgery. 2008;62:753-64; discussion 264-6.

[50] Albert FK, Forsting M, Sartor K, Adams HP, Kunze S. Early postoperative magnetic resonance imaging after resection of malignant glioma: objective evaluation of residual tumor and its influence on regrowth and prognosis. Neurosurgery. 1994;34:45-60; discussion -1.

Section 2

Pathology of Brain Tumors

Chapter 6

Pilocytic Astrocytoma: Anatomic, Pathological and Molecular Aspects

Aline Paixao Becker, Cristovam Scapulatempo-Neto, Luciano Neder, Leila Chimelli and Rui M. Reis

Additional information is available at the end of the chapter

http://dx.doi.org/10.5772/53956

1. Introduction

1.1. Epidemiology

Brain tumors are rare neoplasms, however, they represent the second commonest cancer in childhood (the first being hemato-lymphoid neoplasms) and correspond to the main solid tumor in the pediatric context (ages 0-19 years) [1]. In this setting, gliomas, and particularly astrocytomas are the leading group. Pilocytic astrocytoma (PA) is the commonest brain tumor in the ages 5-14 years and the second in the age ranges 0-4 years and 15-19 years, although it represents about only 6% of all gliomas, according to the last Central Brain Tumors Registry (CBTRUS) Report [1]. PA affects males and females equally, and the main affected ages are 6 to 13 years-old, with 75% of cases occurring at this ages [2; 3].

PAs present a good prognosis in general, with 10-year survival >90% [4]. However, about 10-20% of patients suffer with recurrence of completely excised lesions or growing of residual lesions [4]. Besides, 2-3% of the cases may disseminate through the spinal cord [2; 4]. These aggressive tumors are particularly more frequent in adults and older patients, which explains the difference in the 10-year survival [5].Overall, the prognosis between children and adults is significantly different [5]. While in children and young adults the 5-year survival is >90%, in the group of 60+ years patients, this value is about 52% [5]. Likewise, the mortality rates related to PAs are higher in adults than in children. Despite this could be explained by differences in the location of these tumors in adults many evidences suggest that PA is in fact a more aggressive neoplasm in older age groups [5].

2. Anatomical location and neurorradiological features

The main location of PA is the cerebellum, with more than 60% of the cases occurring in cerebellar hemispheres, however, it can arise all through the neuraxis, including hypothalamic region, the optic-chiasmatic tract and spinal cord, with some cases involving the whole spinal cord ("holocord pilocytic astrocytoma") [2; 3; 6]- [9]. This wide distribution in the central nervous system (CNS) may, in part, explain the differences in the prognosis of PA, since GTR of a lesion located near or in eloquent areas of the CNS may be unachievable. In addition, some locations present special features or are related to specific conditions. For example, multiple tumors and tumors located in the optic-chiasmatic region are far more common in patients with neurofibromatosis 1 (NF1), while supratentorial and spinal cord PAs are more frequent in adults than in children [2; 5].

At neurorradiological exams, the typical finding is, generally, a non-infiltrative, well delimited biphasic lesion, with a cystic, hipointense, area associated with a mural nodule, which can be contrast-enhanced at magnetic resonance image (MRI) and computed tomography (CT), however, diverse patterns as solid nodule or complete cystic lesions can be seen [2; 10] (Figure 1). In any case, perilesional edema is not commonly observed, as it is in high-grades primary brain tumors [11]. Anecdotally, PA can be manifested as cerebral hemorrhage [12].

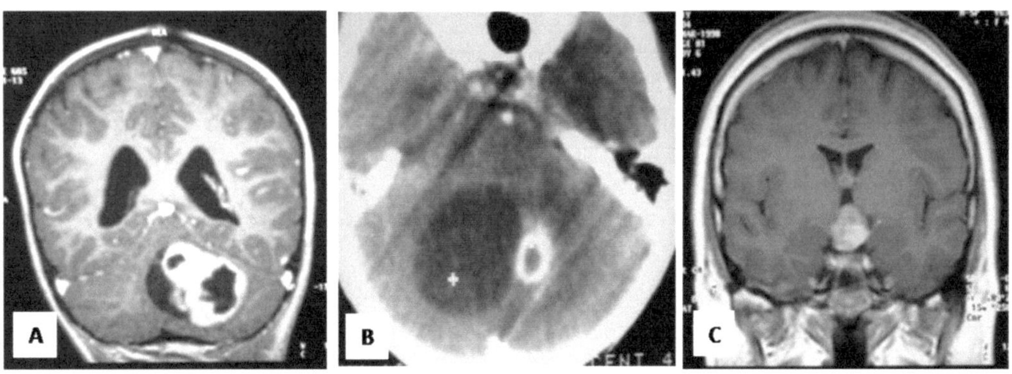

Figure 1. Neurorradiological features of Pilocytic Astrocytomas, after endovenous contrast injection. Note the absence of perilesional edema, even in voluminous lesions. A- Cerebellar lesion – solid with cystic areas. This is the commonest pattern of PA (MRI, coronal view). B- Cerebellar lesion, predominantly cystic with a mural nodule (CT, axial view). C- solid, suprasselar lesion (MRI, coronal view).

3. Clinical signs and symptoms

Due to its highly variable location in the neuraxis, the signs and symptoms of PA depend on the affected area. As the most common location is the cerebellum, headache and neck pain, vomiting, gait disturbance and visual abnormalities are usually referred [2; 3; 6; 13]. In supratentorial tumors, the occurrence of seizures may be seen and is related to cortical involvement [6]. In the hypothalamic area, PA may present with hormonal dysfunctions, for example, diabetes insipidus, obesity [3; 11] and the diencephalic syndrome – emaciation, hiperkinesis, irritability and accelerated growth [11]. The involvement of the optical pathway is related to visual loss or visual-field deficits [6; 11]; proptosis presents only in large, intraorbital tumors [6].

Clinical signs of intracranial hypertension, as hydrocephalus, papilledema, nistagmus, nausea and vomiting are common in virtually all locations, because of the mass effect impinged by the neoplasm [2; 3; 11]. On the other hand, smaller lesions may remain asymptomatic by some variable time [11].

4. Histopathological aspects

Some histopathological features of PA are well-established, for instance, biphasic pattern, with high- and low-cellularity areas; elongated (piloid) and rounded, oligodendroglial-like, cells mixed in various proportions; microcystic areas; Rosenthal fibers, and eosinophilic granular bodies are the commonest findings [2; 6] (Figure 2). In general, these findings support a diagnosis of a low-grade astrocytoma (grade I), according to the World Health Organization (WHO) criteria. However, features like microvascular proliferation, necrosis and degenerative nuclear atypia, more commonly present in infiltrative, high-grade gliomas, may be seen (Figure 3B, C). Diverse from infiltrative tumors, though, these features shall not be interpreted as malignancy signs, unless they are associated to high mitotic activity [2; 3; 10]. Leptomeningeal dissemination is quite common, and apparently is not related to aggressive behavior [14]. Calcification, hemorrhage and perivascular lymphocytic infiltration are less common (Figure 3A, D), but may be seen in some cases [10; 14]. Eventually, neuronal cells can be observed, intermingled in the tumor, but they lack neoplastic features, and can be interpreted as entrapped neurons [6; 10; 14].

Because of the great variation in histopathological appearance, the diagnosis of PA is usually challenging, especially in minute biopsies, and greatly dependent upon correlation with neurorradiological aspects [2; 3]. This can be such a dilemma, that some authors refer huge discordance between pathologists, with half of PAs misdiagnosed as higher-grade tumors at primary diagnosis [15].

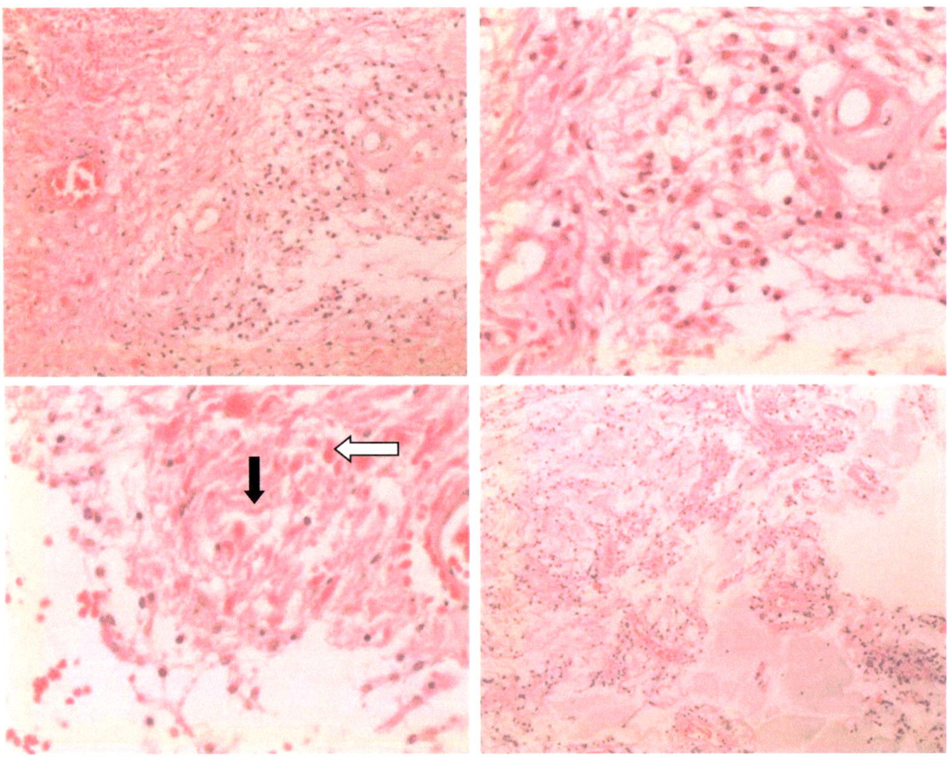

Figure 2. Histopathological aspects of Pilocytic Astrocytoma. All microphotographs represent H&E stain. A- Biphasic pattern – high cellularity at left and lower cellularity at bottom right (100x). B- Round and piloid cells constitute this tumor. Note the vasculature, with typical endothelia (200x). C- Rosenthal fibers (black arrow) and eosinophilic granular body (white arrow) can be seen in higher cellular areas (200x). D- At bottom, a microcystic area is seen (40x).

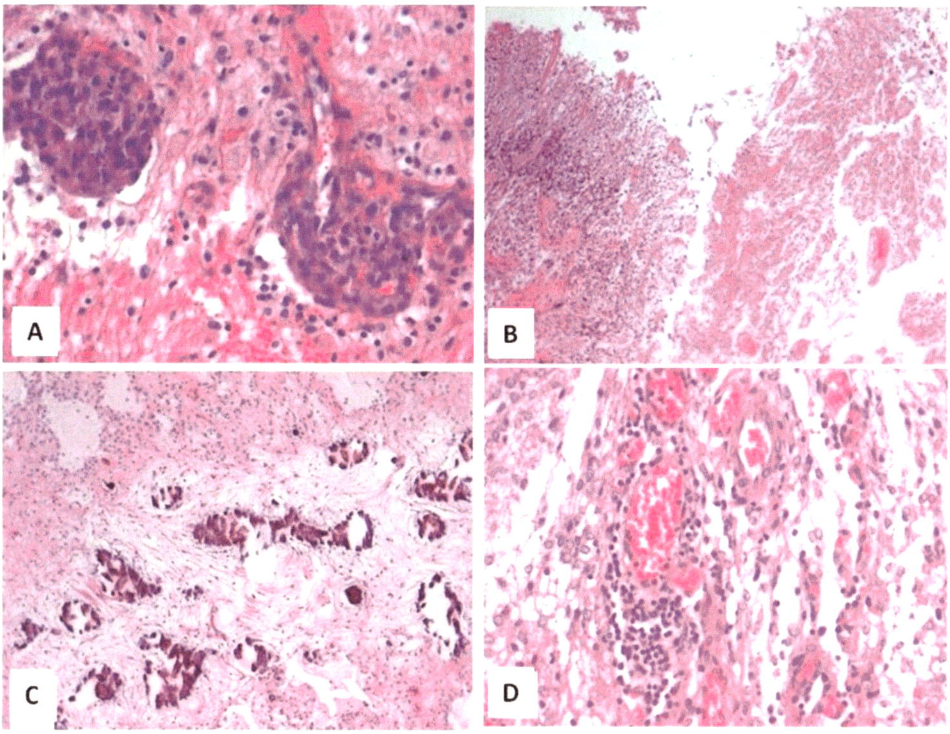

Figure 3. Some other histopathological aspects of Pilocytic Astrocytoma at the H&E stain. A- Microvascular proliferation (200x) B- Areas of necrosis may be seen in some tumors – in this case, the necrosis is at right (40x). C- Calcification foci near a microcystic area of tumor (40x). D- Lymphocytic cuffs may be present (200x).

4.1. Differential diagnosis

Differential diagnoses of PA include low- and high-grade gliomas and the identification of different entities has great importance in the treatment choice and prognosis of patients.

Among low-grade tumors, the most important differential diagnoses include ganglioglioma; pleomorphic xantoastrocytoma (PXA); grade II oligodendroglioma; and diffuse astrocitoma. In these cases, tumor location, neurorradiological and immunohistochemical features can help in the definition, and this will be better discussed later in next sections. Moreover, hypothalamic lesions, especially in infants, must also be distinguished from pilomixoid astrocytoma, a recently described tumor, stated as grade II variant of PA in the last WHO classification [2; 3].

On the other hand, anaplastic astrocytoma and anaplastic oligodendroglioma (WHO grade III) are some of the high grade lesions that can be confounded with PA [2; 3] when there are degenerative atypia and/or oligodendroglial-like areas in the tumor. Finally, glioblastoma (GBM – WHO grade IV), the commonest and most aggressive astrocytoma, share various histological and neurorradiological features with PA, which makes the diagnosis problematic in some cases [16]- [18]. In these cases, clinical correlation and immunohistochemical markers can be used for better defining the diagnosis.

5. Immunohistochemistry in the diagnosis of pylocitic astrocytoma

In order to reduce misdiagnoses, some immunohistochemical markers can be used to elucidate complicated cases. There are no specific markers for PA, but differences between expressions of standard antibodies can help in the task. Some of the main immunohistochemical markers are described herein:

5.1. Glial Fibrillary Acidic Protein (GFAP)

GFAP is a cytoplasmatic intermediate filament, component of the cytoskeleton of normal and neoplastic astrocytes [3]. Like in all astrocytomas, GFAP is persistently, diffusely expressed in PAs, which does not permit the delineation between PA and diffuse astrocytomas. However, it may be a useful tool to differentiate PA from other gliomas, such as ependymomas and oligodendrogliomas.

As described earlier, some PAs may present perivascular lymphocytic cuffs and neuronal cells entrapped among the neoplastic astrocytes. These characteristics are also seen in gangliogliomas [6]. To rule out this possibility, GFAP may help, as stated since 1970s by Eng and Rubinstein [19], since the neoplastic neuronal cells in this tumor are negative and may be highlighted in contrast to the strongly positive neoplastic astrocytes with this marker – this pattern corroborates the mixed nature of ganglioglioma. There are other immunohistochemical markers that help in this differential diagnosis, in addition to GFAP, for example, CD34 (positive in gangliogliomas and negative in PAs) and Neu N (neuronal marker, useful in the identification of neoplastic and entrapped neurons).

Secondly, since PAs may present oligodendroglial-like areas and calcifications, another utility for the use of GFAP is to differentiate these areas (in a small sample, for example) from oligodendrogliomas. Oligodendroglial tumors are mostly negative, however, a peculiar pattern of perinuclear immunoreactivity was recognized after the description of the protoplasmatic oligodendrocytes, present in almost 80% of oligodendrogliomas [17; 20]. Even in those positive cases, the pattern contrasts to the cytoplasmatic, diffuse positivity seen in the PAs. Other immunohistochemical markers can be used in a panel in order to refine this diagnosis, for instance, OLIG-2, a transcription factor involved in oligodendroglial differentiation [21]. Although some weak immunnopositivity may be seen in astrocytomas (low and high grades) and more than 70% of PAs may be immunoreactive for OLIG-2 [22], according to some authors, OLIG-2 can significantly distinguish oligodendroglial and astrocytic tumors [20; 21]. As these both markers (GFAP and OLIG-2) can be simultaneously expressed by PAs and oligodendrogliomas, the interpretation of these immunohistochemical tests must take in account other histopathological findings and even neurorradiological features.

Finally, although GBM is a also a tumor of astrocytic lineage, it may present a different pattern of GFAP immunopositivity. Opposed to the diffuse positivity in PA, GBM is heterogeneously immunoreactive, predominant at the periphery of the tumor or only focal. This happens because the immunoexpression of GFAP tends to decrease with the malignant progression of astrocytomas [16; 17; 23].

http://dx.doi.org/10.5772/53956

In summary, GFAP is an important marker of astrocytic differentiation and can help to distinguish PA from other low- and high grade gliomas, both through the presence or absence of its immunoexpression and the different patterns (subcellular location and distribution over the tumor areas) of immunopositivity.

5.2. Ki67

The non-histone nuclear protein ki67 is a protein codified by genes present in the chromosome 10 [24; 25]. It is expressed in the nuclei of cells in all but G0 and early G1 phases of the cellular cycle [26], which allows a faithful estimative of the proliferative index of a neoplasm. As PA is a grade I astrocytoma, low proliferative index is the rule in these tumors [2; 3] (Figure 4A) with medium values about 2% [14; 27], however medium values as high as 4,4% have been related [10; 28].

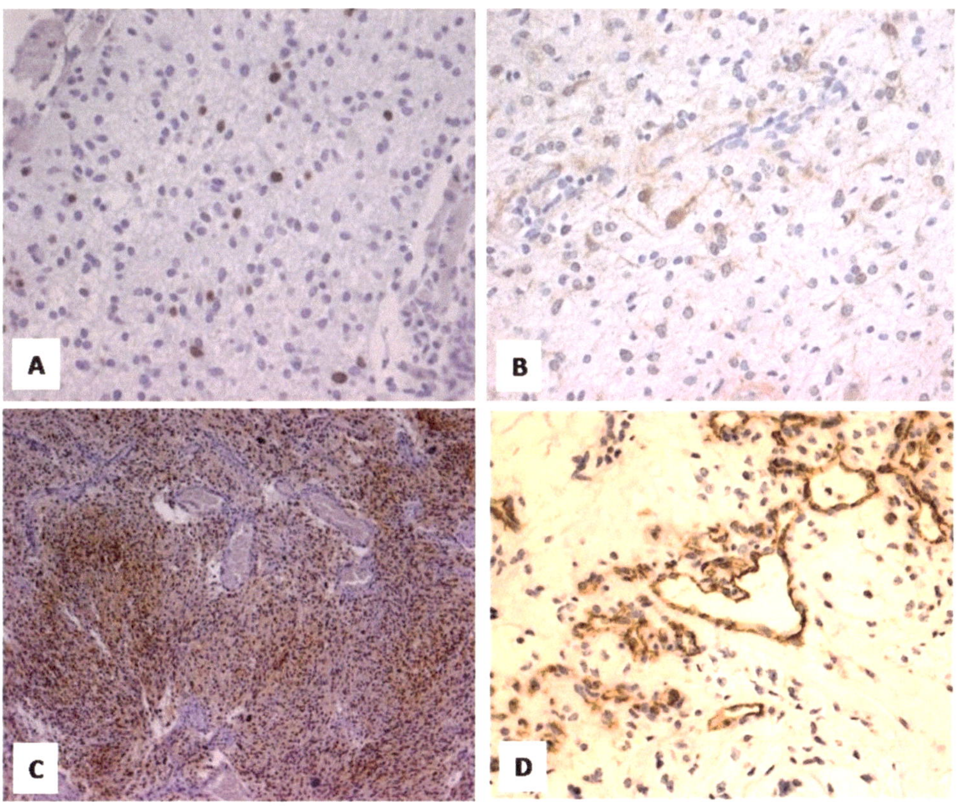

Figure 4. Immunnohistochemical aspects, with avidin-biotin-peroxidade technique. A- Ki67 – nuclear positivity in about 2% of neoplastic cells(100x). B- Galectin-3 – this case showed weak, diffuse immunopositivity and predominant cytoplasmatic location (100x). C- Galectin-3 strong, diffuse positivity and the vascular endothelium showed no reaction (100x). D- CD31 reaction in the endothelia – delicate vessels in the tumor (200x).

Proliferative index by ki67 expression is a well established prognostic factor in diffuse astrocytomas [29], yet, its role in the prognosis of PA is controversial. In 2002, Roessler et al did not show significant differences between cerebellar PA when comparing groups according to the proliferative index with a cut-off value of 5% [28] and this result was further corroborated by other study with even lower cut-off value of 3% [10]. Shortly after, Bowers et al (2003) described a subset of PA with worse prognosis, when the proliferative index determined by Ki67 was >2% [27]. More recently higher medium values (>10%) were described in recurrent and more aggressive PAs [10], and this exceptionally high value is similar to the medium value of proliferative index for GBM (12,28%) described earlier by the same group [29].

Although the proliferative index is still a questionable independent prognostic factor of PAs, it is well accepted that a strict follow up is needed in the cases with high proliferative activity [10; 27].

5.3. Galectin-3

Galectin-3 (gal-3) is a carbohydrate-binding protein that binds specifically to β-galactosides sugars. This protein is involved in various biological processes, such as cellular proliferation, apoptosis, transcriptional regulation, intracellular signalization, adhesion and migration [30; 31]. The expression of gal-3 may be seen in both cytoplasm and nuclei of neoplastic cells (particularly carcinomas) from various organs, such as thyroid, pancreas and prostate [32], but the relation between hyper- or loss of expression and biologic behavior of the tumor varies among the different organs [32].

In APs, gal-3 is expressed in the nuclei and cytoplasm of neoplastic cells in all cases of PA described by various authors [2; 10; 32; 33], but lacks the expression in the vascular endothelia(Figure 4B, C), contrary to what it is seen in non-neoplastic brain parenchyma [10; 33] and in astrocytomas grades II and III and oligodendroglial tumors, which permits a faithful delineation from PA when facing tough cases [17; 31].

Gal-3 is not specific of PA, since other low-grade tumors, such as ependymomas and PXA also present diffuse expression of gal-3 [10; 32; 33]. Interestingly, focal (heterogenous) expression of gal-3 is also seen in GBM [2; 18; 32], and although the vast differences between the biological behavior and molecular pathways of these tumors, this expression may be related to microvascular proliferation and breaking of hematological barrier (and contrast-enhancement at neuroimage) seen in these both entities [10; 18].

Although various studies have tried to relate the intensity and extension of gal-3 expression to the clinical behavior of PA, no prognostic significance was proved until now. Still, as gal-3 expression is a conspicuous finding in PAs, in a pattern that can be differentiated from other grades of astrocytoma, this marker may be very useful in the tumor diagnosis [10; 18; 32; 33]. Besides, recently a group of authors described a close relationship between expression of gal-3 and activation of the RAF-MEK-ERK pathway in pancreatic cancer [34] and, as we shall see later in this chapter, that is an important molecular pathway in the genesis of PA, so gal-3 may be soon proved as a potential target for future treatments.

6. Molecular biology of pilocytic astrocytomas

Since no prognostic factors have been identified to differentiate regular from the more aggressive Pas [5; 10; 14], the genetic characteristics of the PAs have recently been investigated to better understand and try to predict the behavior of this tumor. Among these alterations, chromossomal abnormalities (structural or numerical, as the aneuploidies), single-gene mutations and epigenetic damage are mechanisms that could launch the molecular pathway of oncogenesis.

The molecular pathways of oncogenesis differ in PAs and diffuse astrocytomas. For example, two growth factor receptors, EGFR and PDGFR, related to invasion and malignant progression, which are frequently hyperexpressed in infiltrative diffuse astrocytomas had a lower expression in PAs observed by different groups [35; 36]. Besides, other genes characteristically altered in diffuse gliomas, as *TP53* and *PTEN* are normally expressed in Pas [2; 35; 37].

No cytogenetic abnormalities were detected in PA at first, and the majority of PAs presented normal karyotype, similar to fetal astrocytes [37], and the majority of the altered tumors were from female and adult patients [2]. Since then, a lot of genes have been investigated. We shall see the most studied genes in PAs in the subsequent sessions.

6.1. *NF1* gene

The first genetic studies tried to establish some differences between sporadic PAs and NF1-PA, which present a more aggressive behaviour. It was known that NF1-PAs present germline mutations of *NF1* (in contrast to somatic mutations in GBM of this gene) and this results in a loss of expression of the gene and, at protein level, results in a defective protein, neurofibromin [3], which lastly permits a constitutive activation of the RAS-RAF-MERK-ERK molecular pathway [4], or the mTOR/AKT pathway, activated in more aggressive Pas [4].

The detection of *NF1* mutations can be achieved by molecular methods, by verifying the expression of the gene or even at IHC, through the expression (or loss of expression) of neurofibromin. [2; 3]

6.2. The RAS-RAF-MEK-ERK signaling pathway

The studies of *NF1* gene were "the initial indication that *Mitogen-activated protein kinase* (MAPK) signaling might play a role in the development of PAs", as stated by Jones et al (2011) [4]. Since then, various groups have investigated the participant proteins of these pathways.

The MAPK pathways regulate fundamental biologic processes. In mammalian, there are 4 well-described MAPK pathways [38; 39] (Figure 5) and the most studied is the *extracellular signal-regulated kinase* (ERK)1/2 [39]. Alterations of this pathway are described in both low and high-grade astrocytomas [4], but molecular mechanisms differ between them.

In summary, the ERK1/2 pathway is triggered by the binding of soluble peptides to a Tyrosin-kinase receptor (TKR) at the cell surface, and initiates a cascade of events that terminates in the appropriated cellular response [40]. This pathway is related to various

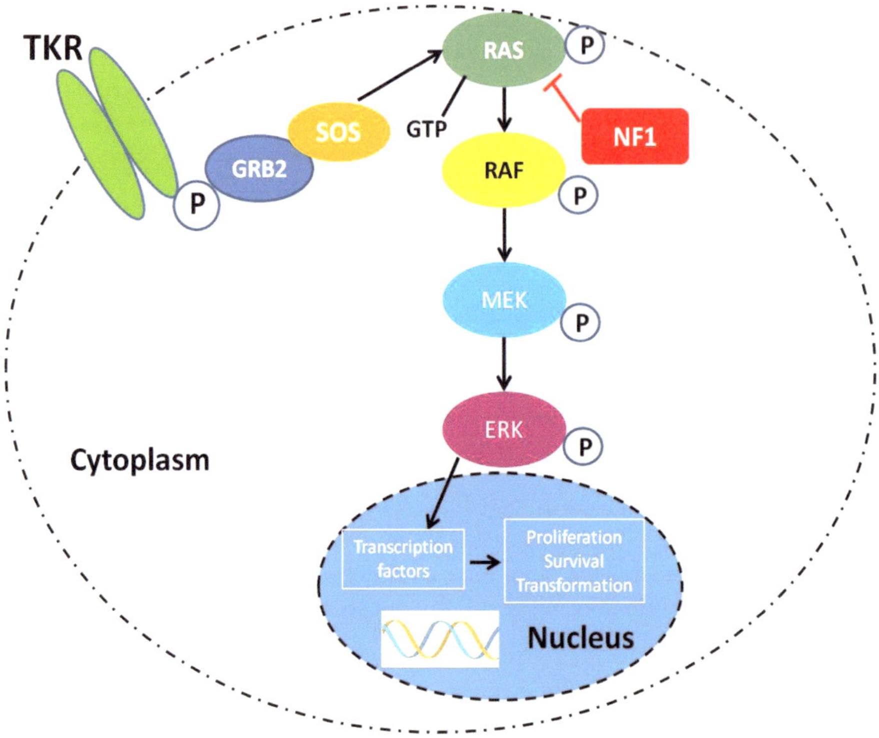

Figure 5. Integration of the MAPK pathways in the cellular response to various environmental stimuli. The sequential phosphorilation of RAS-RAF-MEK ERK, after dimerization of TKR, and the role of negative regulation of NF1.

fundamental cellular processes, such as proliferation, cellular differentiation, survival, migration, and angiogenesis [41; 42].

The ERK cascade is constituted by RAS, Raf, MEK and ERK proteins [39], which are subsequently activated during the process. After the binding of the extracellular peptide with the TKR and its dimerization, it activates the RAS protein, which then activates the Raf family, MEK and, finally, ERK protein [40; 43], that is present in the nuclei, to effectuate the response to the.initiator sign [43]. The RAS-Raf league is considered the regulatory center of the ERK cascade and mutations of any of this genes result in ERK pathway misregulation. It is important to note that the mutations of these proteins are mutually exclusive [39].

The proteins of Raf family are the main effectors of RAS and their action is in phosphorylating MEK 1 and MEK2 [44]. This family is a cytoplasmatic group of proteins, constituted by A-Raf, B-Raf and C-Raf [43], proteins that present similar structure and biological features [44], although they show different tissue distribution and capacity of activating the MEK proteins [45].

6.2.1. Oncogene BRAF

In humans, the most studied Raf protein is the B-Raf (BRAF), which is mutated in about 8% of all human neoplasms [44], and in melanomas this rate can be as high as 60% of the cases, with the commonest mutation being point mutation V600E [46; 47].In the setting of PA, mutations with constitutive activation of BRAF were demonstrated in up to 80% of cases, while they are very rare in diffuse astrocytomas [48]. The mechanisms that explain a constitutive activation of the BRAF are: i) point mutation V600E [44; 49; 50]; ii) duplication of a region in chromosome 7q [51; 52]; and iii) fusion between oncogenes *BRAF* and *KIAA1549*.

The point mutation V600E refers to a single glutamic acid for valin substitution at codon 600 of *BRAF* gene [44], which is the commonest BRAF missense mutation in human cancer [44; 46]. This mutation is not specific for PA and can be detected in various brain tumors, including PXAs, gangliogliomas, and in up to 6% of GBMs [49; 50] and other tumors, such as thyroid cancers and melanomas [44].

The BRAF duplications are due to a somatic rearrangement of the gene in sporadic PAs. It was the first described genetic alteration of PAs [51; 52]. They are more frequent in gliomas in non-cerebellar [52] location, including that of the optical pathways [53], both in NF1-related tumors and in those sporadic ones. Nevertheless, other authors did not identify BRAF duplications in NF1-related tumors, and suggested the activation of a different pathway (mTOR) in the genesis of these frequently more aggressive tumors [54]

Finally, the fusion *BRAF-KIAA1549* is present in 50-100% of the patients with PA [4; 55; 56]. This alteration is highly specific for PAs, and there is a growing tendency for using this marker as a powerful tool of molecular diagnosis in surgical pathology routine [57]. Although this fusion has recently been described in some other low-grade tumors, such as pilomixoid astrocytoma, glioneuronal tumors and unclassifiable low grade gliomas [57; 58], clinical and pathological correlation permit the diagnosis of PA in cases where diffuse component is predominant at histology [57]. Also, this fusion is significantly more frequent in infratentorial and optical pathways-located tumors [57].

The importance of studying the genetic mutations in PAs has grown, since many target therapies against the MAPKs pathway components are recently being developed. For example, concerning tumors with the V600E mutation, in 2012 two groups described the use of Vemurafenib, a BRAF inhibitor, in melanoma [59] and in lung cancer [60], with good results. In addition, other proteins of the ERK cascade can be targeted by novel drugs, as Trametinib, a specific MEK inhibitor, that has also been used successfully in patients with melanomas that present V600E mutation [61]. It is still unknown whether tumors harboring the fusion *BRAF-KIAA1549* are responsive to Vemurafenib and Trametinib. Concerning the former, the distinct studies showed the lack of patient's response in the wildtype BRAF [62]

At last, it is important to note that the resultant protein of the fusion *BRAF-KIAA1549* is cancer-specific and it is potentially a target for future treatments. The most representative example of this possibility is the identification of the fusion *BCR-ABL* in chronic myeloid leukemia (CML), in a similar molecular mechanism. The knowledge of this fusion permitted the development of a target-drug, Imatinib, in the middle 2000's [63].This drug has changed the treatment and prognosis of the CML patients by controlling the disease, with excellent tolerability.

The molecular pathways of PAs are beginning to be faithfully recognized and some of the molecules of these pathways have already some kind of target drug available for inhibition, with efficacy proved in other kinds of tumors. As there are no studies with these novel drugs in PAs, this can become a good direction for future clinical research.

7. Conclusion

Pilocytic astrocytoma is usually a tumor with good prognosis; however some eloquent locations do not permit the total resection of lesions. In these cases and in the ones that can recur even after gross total resection, the patients can suffer with physical limitations and even death. The study of the molecular pathways of PA´s oncogenesis may represent a hope for longer and better quality life for these patients. There is a wide field for research in order to better understand this intriguing tumor, since the understanding of these mechanisms can turn a potentially fatal in a controllable disease.

Acknowledgements

The authors appreciatively thank Dr. Ricardo Santos de Oliveira, M.D., PhD and Dr. Hélio Rubens Machado, M.D., PhD (Department of Neurosurgery- FMRP-USP) for the neurorradiological exams photographs and the Surgical Pathology Department of FMRP-USP (SERPAT) for the microphotographs of the cases.

Author details

Aline Paixao Becker[1,2], Cristovam Scapulatempo-Neto[1,3], Luciano Neder[4], Leila Chimelli[5] and Rui M. Reis[1,6]

1 Molecular Oncology Research Center, Barretos Cancer Hospital, Barretos, São Paulo, Brazil

2 School of Medicine, University of Ribeirão Preto (UNAERP), Brazil

3 Department of Pathology, Barretos Cancer Hospital, Barretos, São Paulo, Brazil

4 Ribeirão Preto School of Medicine, University of São Paulo (FMRP-USP), Brazil

5 Division of Pathology National Institute of Cancer, Brazil

6 Life and Health Sciences Research Institute (ICVS), Health Sciences School, University of Minho, Braga, Portugal

References

[1] CBTRUS Statistical Report: Primary Brain and Central Nervous System Tumors Diagnosed in the United States in (2012). Ref Type: Report

[2] Scheithauer, B. W, Hawkins, C, & Tihan, T. VandenBerg SR, Burger PC. Pilocytic astrocytoma. In: David N.Louis, Hiroko Ohgaki, Otmar D.Wiestler, eds. *WHO Classification of tumours of the central nervous system.* Lyon: IARC, (2007). , 2007, 14-21.

[3] Louis, D. N, Reifenberger, G, Brat, D. J, & Ellison, D. W. Tumours: introduction and neuroepithelial tumours. In: Seth Love, David N.Louis, David W.Ellison, eds. *Greenfield´s Neuropathology.* London: Hodder Arnold, (2008). , 2008, 1855-60.

[4] Jones, D. T, Gronych, J, Lichter, P, Witt, O, & Pfister, S. M. MAPK pathway activation in pilocytic astrocytoma. *Cell Mol Life Sci* (2011).

[5] Johnson, D. R, Brown, P. D, Galanis, E, & Hammack, J. E. Pilocytic astrocytoma survival in adults: analysis of the Surveillance, Epidemiology, and End Results Program of the National Cancer Institute. *J Neurooncol* (2012). , 187-93.

[6] Burger, P. C, & Scheithauer, B. W. Pilocytic astrocytoma. In: Burger PC, Scheithauer BW, eds. *Tumors of Central Nervous System.* Washington: The Armed Forces Institute of Pathology, (1994). , 1994, 77-94.

[7] Sandalcioglu, I. E, Gasser, T, Wiedemayer, H, Horsch, S, & Stolke, D. Favourable outcome after biopsy and decompression of a holocord intramedullary spinal cord astrocytoma in a newborn. *Eur J Paediatr Neurol* (2002). , 6, 179-82.

[8] Tobias, M. E, Mcgirt, M. J, Chaichana, K. L, et al. Surgical management of long intramedullary spinal cord tumors. *Childs Nerv Syst* (2008). , 24, 219-23.

[9] Burger, P. C, & Scheithauer, B. W. Tumors of neuroglia and choroid plexus epithelium- Glioblastoma multiforme. In: P.C.Burger, B.W.Scheithauer, eds. *Tumors of the central nervous system.* Washington: Armed Forces Institute of Pathology., (1994). , 1994, 25-161.

[10] Paixao, B. A, De Oliveira, R. S, Saggioro, F. P, Neder, L, Chimelli, L. M, & Machado, H. R. In pursuit of prognostic factors in children with pilocytic astrocytomas. *Childs Nerv Syst* (2010). , 26, 19-28.

[11] Koeller, K. K, & Rushing, E. J. From the archives of the AFIP: pilocytic astrocytoma: radiologic-pathologic correlation. *Radiographics* (2004). , 24, 1693-708.

[12] Matsumoto, K, Akagi, K, Abekura, M, et al. Hypothalamic Pilocytic Astrocytoma Presenting with Intratumoral and Subarachnoid Hemorrhage- Case Report. *Neurol Med Chir (Tokyo)* (1997). , 849-52.

[13] Abdollahzadeh, M, Hoffman, H. J, Blazer, S. I, et al. Benign cerebellar astrocytoma in childhood: experience at the Hospital for Sick Children 1980-1992. *Childs Nerv Syst* (1994). , 10, 380-3.

[14] Fernandez, C, Figarella-branger, D, Girard, N, et al. Pilocytic astrocytomas in children: prognostic factors--a retrospective study of 80 cases. *Neurosurgery* (2003). , 53, 544-53.

[15] Aldape, K, Simmons, M. L, & Davis, R. L. Discrepancies in diagnoses of neuroepithelial neoplasms: The San Francisco Bay Area Adult Glioma Study. *Cancer* (2000). , 2342-9.

[16] Kleihues, P, Burger, P. C, & Aldape, K. D. et al. Glioblastoma. In: David N.Louis, Hiroko Ohgaki, Otmar D.Wiestler, Webster K.Cavenee, eds. *WHO Classification of tumors of the Central Nervous System.* Lyon: International Agency for Research on Cancer (IARC), (2007). , 2007, 33-49.

[17] Louis, D. N, Reifenberger, G, Brat, D. J, & Ellison, D. W. Tumors: introduction and neuroepithelial tumors- Glioblastoma. In: Seth Love, David N.Louis, David W.Ellison, eds. *Greenfield´s Neuropathology.* London: Edward Arnold Publishers, (2008). , 2008, 1821-2000.

[18] Neder, L, Marie, S. K, Carlotti, C. G, et al. Galectin-3 as an immunohistochemical tool to distinguish pilocytic astrocytomas from diffuse astrocytomas, and glioblastomas from anaplastic oligodendrogliomas. *Brain Pathol* (2004). , 14, 399-405.

[19] Eng, L. F, & Rubinstein, L. J. Contribution of immunohistochemistry to diagnostic problems of human cerebral tumors. *J Histochem Cytochem* (1978). , 26, 513-22.

[20] Ikota, H, Kinjo, S, Yokoo, H, & Nakazato, Y. Systematic immunohistochemical profiling of 378 brain tumors with 37 antibodies using tissue microarray technology. *Acta Neuropathol* (2006). , 111, 475-82.

[21] Mokhtari, K, Paris, S, Aguirre-cruz, L, et al. Olig2 expression, GFAP, and 1p loss analysis contribute to glioma subclassification. *Neuropathol Appl Neurobiol* (2005). , 53.

[22] Takei, H, Yogeswaren, S. T, Wong, K. K, et al. Expression of oligodendroglial differentiation markers in pilocytic astrocytomas identifies two clinical subsets and shows a significant correlation with proliferation index and progression free survival. *J Neurooncol* (2008). , 86, 183-90.

[23] Becker, A. P, Caravina, G, Clara, C, & Reis, R. M. The Role of Immunohistochemistry in Diagnosis and Prognosis of Glioblastoma Patients. Nova Publishers, (2012).

[24] Schonk, D. M, Kuijpers, H. J, Van Drunen, E, et al. Assignment of the gene(s) involved in the expression of the proliferation-related Ki-67 antigen to human chromosome 10. *Hum Genet* (1989). , 83, 297-9.

[25] Gerdes, J, Li, L, Schlueter, C, et al. Immunobiochemical and molecular biologic characterization of the cell proliferation-associated nuclear antigen that is defined by monoclonal antibody Ki-67. *Am J Pathol* (1991). , 138, 867-73.

[26] Burger, P. C, Shibata, T, & Kleihues, P. The use of the monoclonal antibody Ki-67 in the identification of proliferating cells: application to surgical neuropathology. *Am J Surg Pathol* (1986). , 10, 611-7.

[27] Bowers, D. C, Gargan, L, Kapur, P, et al. Study of the MIB-1 labeling index as a predictor of tumor progression in pilocytic astrocytomas in children and adolescents. *Clin Oncol* (2003). , 2968-73.

[28] Roessler, K, Bertalanffy, A, Jezan, H, et al. Proliferative activity as measured by MIB-1 labeling index and long-term outcome of cerebellar juvenile pilocytic astrocytomas. *J Neurooncol* (2002). , 141-56.

[29] Neder, L, Colli, B. O, Machado, H. R, & Carlotti, C. G. Jr., Santos AC, Chimelli L. MIB-1 labeling index in astrocytic tumors--a clinicopathologic study. *Clin Neuropathol* (2004). , 23, 262-70.

[30] Perillo, N. L, Marcus, M. E, & Baum, L. G. Galectins: versatile modulators of cell adhesion, cell proliferation, and cell death. *J Mol Med (Berl)* (1998). , 76, 402-12.

[31] Stillman, B. N, Mischel, P. S, & Baum, L. G. New roles for galectins in brain tumors--from prognostic markers to therapeutic targets. *Brain Pathol* (2005). , 15, 124-32.

[32] Park, S. H, Min, H. S, Kim, B, Myung, J, & Paek, S. H. Galectin-3: a useful biomarker for differential diagnosis of brain tumors. *Neuropathology* (2008). , 28, 497-506.

[33] Borges, C. B, Bernardes, E. S, Latorraca, E. F, et al. Galectin-3 expression: a useful tool in the differential diagnosis of posterior fossa tumors in children. *Childs Nerv Syst* (2011). , 27, 253-7.

[34] Shumei SongBaoan Ji, Vijaya Ramachandran et al. Overexpressed Galectin-3 in Pancreatic Cancer Induces Cell Proliferation and Invasion by Binding Ras and Activating Ras Signaling. *PLoS ONE* (2012). , 7, 1-11.

[35] Huang, H, Hara, A, Homma, T, Yonekawa, Y, & Ohgaki, H. Altered expression of immune defense genes in pilocytic astrocytomas. *J Neuropathol Exp Neurol* (2005). , 64, 891-901.

[36] Rorive, S, Maris, C, Debeir, O, et al. Exploring the distinctive biological characteristics of pilocytic and low-grade diffuse astrocytomas using microarray gene expression profiles. *J Neuropathol Exp Neurol* (2006). , 65, 794-807.

[37] Beatriz, M, Lopes, S, & Scott, R. VandenBerg. Tumors of the central nervous system. In: Christopher D.M.Fletcher, ed. *Diagnostic Histopathology of Tumors.* Philadelphia: Elsevier, (2007). , 2007, 1653-732.

[38] Roberts, P. J. Der CJ. Targeting the Raf-MEK-ERK mitogen-activated protein kinase cascade for the treatment of cancer. *Oncogene* (2007). , 26, 3291-310.

[39] Dhillon, A. S, Hagan, S, Rath, O, & Kolch, W. MAP kinase signalling pathways in cancer. *Oncogene* (2007). , 26, 3279-90.

[40] Marshall, C. J. Ras effectors. *Curr Opin Cell Biol* (1996). , 8, 197-204.

[41] Dunn, K. L, Espino, P. S, Drobic, B, He, S, & Davie, J. R. The Ras-MAPK signal transduction pathway, cancer and chromatin remodeling. *Biochem Cell Biol* (2005). , 83, 1-14.

[42] Yoon, S, & Seger, R. The extracellular signal-regulated kinase: multiple substrates regulate diverse cellular functions. *Growth Factors* (2006). , 24, 21-44.

[43] Mckay, M. M, & Morrison, D. K. Integrating signals from RTKs to ERK/MAPK. *Oncogene* (2007). , 26, 3113-21.

[44] Vakiani, E, & Solit, D. B. KRAS and BRAF: drug targets and predictive biomarkers. *J Pathol* (2011). , 223, 219-29.

[45] Wellbrock, C, Karasarides, M, & Marais, R. The RAF proteins take centre stage. *Nat Rev Mol Cell Biol* (2004). , 5, 875-85.

[46] Davies, H, Bignell, G. R, Cox, C, et al. Mutations of the BRAF gene in human cancer. *Nature* (2002). , 417, 949-54.

[47] Fisher, R, & Larkin, J. Vemurafenib: a new treatment for BRAF-mutated advanced melanoma. *Cancer Manag Res* (2012). , 600

[48] Riemenschneider, M. J, Jeuken, J. W, Wesseling, P, & Reifenberger, G. Molecular diagnostics of gliomas: state of the art. *Acta Neuropathol* (2010). , 120, 567-84.

[49] Basto, D, Trovisco, V, Lopes, J. M, et al. Mutation analysis of B-RAF gene in human gliomas. *Acta Neuropathol* (2005). , 109, 207-10.

[50] Schindler, G, Capper, D, Meyer, J, et al. Analysis of BRAF mutation in 1,320 nervous system tumors reveals high mutation frequencies in pleomorphic xanthoastrocytoma, ganglioglioma and extra-cerebellar pilocytic astrocytoma. *Acta Neuropathol* (2011). , 600E

[51] Bar, E. E, Lin, A, Tihan, T, Burger, P. C, & Eberhart, C. G. Frequent gains at chromosome 7q34 involving BRAF in pilocytic astrocytoma. *J Neuropathol Exp Neurol* (2008). , 67, 878-87.

[52] Pfister, S, Janzarik, W. G, Remke, M, et al. BRAF gene duplication constitutes a mechanism of MAPK pathway activation in low-grade astrocytomas. *J Clin Invest* (2008). , 118, 1739-49.

[53] Rodriguez, F. J, Ligon, A. H, Horkayne-szakaly, I, et al. BRAF Duplications and MAPK Pathway Activation Are Frequent in Gliomas of the Optic Nerve Proper. *J Neuropathol Exp Neurol* (2012). , 71, 789-94.

[54] Jentoft, M, Giannini, C, Cen, L, et al. Phenotypic variations in NF1-associated low grade astrocytomas: possible role for increased mTOR activation in a subset. *Int J Clin Exp Pathol* (2010). , 4, 43-57.

[55] Tian, Y, Rich, B. E, Vena, N, et al. Detection of KIAA1549-BRAF fusion transcripts in formalin-fixed paraffin-embedded pediatric low-grade gliomas. *J Mol Diagn* (2011). , 13, 669-77.

[56] Jones, D. T, Kocialkowski, S, Liu, L, Pearson, D. M, Ichimura, K, & Collins, V. P. Oncogenic RAF1 rearrangement and a novel BRAF mutation as alternatives to KIAA1549:BRAF fusion in activating the MAPK pathway in pilocytic astrocytoma. *Oncogene* (2009). , 28, 2119-23.

[57] Ida, C. M, Lambert, S. R, Rodriguez, F. J, et al. BRAF alterations are frequent in cerebellar low-grade astrocytomas with diffuse growth pattern. *J Neuropathol Exp Neurol* (2012). , 71, 631-9.

[58] Lin, A, Rodriguez, F. J, Karajannis, M. A, et al. BRAF alterations in primary glial and glioneuronal neoplasms of the central nervous system with identification of 2 novel KIAA1549:BRAF fusion variants. *J Neuropathol Exp Neurol* (2012). , 71, 66-72.

[59] Yadav, V, Zhang, X, Liu, J, Estrem, S, Li, S, Gong, X-Q, Buchanan, S, Henry, J. R, Starling, J. J, & Peng, S-B. Reactivation of Mitogen-Activated Protein Kinase (MAPK) Pathway by FGF Receptor 3 (FGFR3)/Ras Mediates Resistance to Vemurafenib in Human B-RAF Mutant Melanoma. Journal of Biological chemistry, 1-20. (2012). Ref Type: In Press, 600E

[60] Gautschi, O, Pauli, C, Strobel, K, Hirschmann, A, Printzen, G, Aebi, S, & Diebold, J. A patient with BRAF lung adenocarcinoma responding to Vemurafenib. Journal of Thoracic Oncology 28. (2012). Ref Type: In Press, 600E

[61] Flaherty, K. T, Robert, C, Hersey, P, et al. Improved Survival with MEK Inhibition in BRAF-Mutated Melanoma. *The New England Journal of Medicine* (2012). , 367, 107-14.

[62] Flaherty, K. T, Puzanov, I, Kim, K. B, et al. Inhibition of mutated, activated BRAF in metastatic melanoma. *N Engl J Med* (2010). , 363, 809-19.

[63] Druker, B. J, Guilhot, F, & Brien, O. SG et al. Five-year follow-up of patients receiving imatinib for chronic myeloid leukemia. *N Engl J Med* (2006). , 355, 2408-17.

Chapter 7

Histology of Primary Brain Tumors

Maysa Al-Hussaini

Additional information is available at the end of the chapter

http://dx.doi.org/10.5772/52356

1. Introduction

Pathological classification of brain tumors is the corner stone upon which the management plan and treatment strategy depends. It is the pathologist who defines the "target" at which the rest of the clinical team members aim their "weapons". Despite of the great advancement of the ancillary studies, the simple H&E stained slide remains an invaluable mean in the diagnosis, classification and stratification of primary brain tumors. Slides should be interpreted in correlation with patient's age and clinical presentation. Radiological findings substitute the macroscopic/gross description in other organs and assessment of the location (supratentorial, infratentorial, intra-ventricular), growth pattern (circumscribed versus infiltrative, solid versus cystic), enhancement pattern (non-enhancing versus enhancing), and the presence or absence of edema, necrosis, calcification should all be consolidated with the microscopic findings in formulating the final diagnosis. The need for an expert neuropathologist is becoming crucial in reviewing the cases before commencing on treatment [1-3]. The importance of multidisciplinary clinics/teams cannot be overemphasized and neuropathologist plays a central role in these clinics [4, 5]. In less developed countries, telemedicine and twinning programs as well as affiliation with recognized international experts may offer an accessible and relatively affordable tool which can help narrowing the knowledge and practice gaps, thus providing patients in these countries with better standards of care [6, 7].

This chapter aims at providing a concise yet comprehensive description of the histology of the most common neuroepithelial primary central nervous system tumors, based on the most recent pathological classification of tumors of the CNS; 2007 WHO Classification of Tumours of the CNS [8]. The morphological features as well as the most useful immunohistochemical stains that can be used to support the diagnosis will be provided. In primary brain tumor there is a considerable overlap in diagnostic features and morphological criteria that are used to grade the tumor, which although is not the primary intention of this chapter, will be alluded to briefly for sake of completeness.

Primary brain tumors are divided into 2 major groups, neuroepithelial and non-neuroepithelial tumors. Table-1.

I: Tumors of Neuroepithelial Tissue		**II: Tumors of non-Neuroepithelial Tissue**
A: Glioma	**C: Neuronal and mixed neuronal-glial tumors**	**A: Tumors of the meninges**
1. Astrocytic tumors	Ganglioglioma and gangliocytoma	**1. Meningiomas**
Pilocytic astrocytoma	Desmoplastic infantile ganglioglioma/astrocytoma	Benign Meningioma variants
Pilomyxoid astrocytoma	Dysembryoplastic neuroectodermal tumor	Atypical
Pleomorphic astrocytoma	Central neurocytoma	Clear cell
Sub-ependymal giant cell astrocytoma	Extra-ventricular neurocytoma	Chordoid
Fibrillary astrocytoma	Cerebellar liponeurocytoma	Anaplastic
Anaplastic astrocytoma	Papillary glio-neuronal tumor	Papillary
Glioblastoma	Rosette forming tumor of the 4th ventricle	Rhabdoid
Gliomatosis Cerebri	**D: Choroid plexus tumors**	**2. Primary Melanocytic lesions**
2. Oligodendroglioma	Choroid plexus papilloma	**3. Other Neoplasms related to meninges**
3. Mixed oligo-astrocytoma	Atypical choroid plexus papilloma	Hemangioblastoma
4. Ependymoma	Choroid plexus carcinoma	**B: Cranial and paraspinal nerve tumors**
Myxo-papillary ependymoma	**E: Tumors of the pineal region**	**C: Germ cell tumors**
Sub-ependymoma	Pineocytoma	**D: Tumors of the sellar region**
Cellular ependymoma	Pineal parenchymal tumor of intermediate differentiation	**E: Hematopoietic cell tumors**
Clear cell ependymoma	Pineoblastoma	
Tanycytic ependymoma	Papillary tumor of the pineal region	
B: Embryonal tumors	**F: Other neuroepithelial tumors**	
Medulloblastoma	Angiocentric glioma	
CNS- primitive neuroectodermal tumor	Chordoid glioma of the 3rd ventricle	
Atypical teratoid rhabdoid tumor	Astroblastoma	

Cribriform Neuroepithelial Tumor (CRINET); This tumor is a recently described neuroepithail tumor and is not part of the WHO classification of primary brain tumors.

Table 1. WHO classification of tumors of the nervous system (2007) [8]

http://dx.doi.org/10.5772/52356

2. Neuroepithelial group of tumors

2.1. Glial tumors

This is by far the most common group of central nervous system tumors, both in adults and pediatrics. They are thought to originate from the brain framework cells; the glial cells. This group is divided into several tumor families which are further divided into entities, patterns and variants based on the presumed cell of origin and the growth pattern.

2.1.1. Astrocytic tumors

Circumscribed astrocytomas

a. Pilocytic astrocytoma (PA)/pilomyxoid astrocytoma(PMA)

Pilocytic astrocytoma (PA) is assumed to arise from reactive astrocytes [9], this tumor predominates in children in the first decade of life and is the prototype of circumscribed tumors. It typically involves midline structures most commonly the cerebellum followed by optic pathway, hypothalamus, basal ganglion and thalamus but can occasionally arise elsewhere. The morphological features are at large similar regardless of the site of origin with one exception; the optic pathway glioma. Typically this is a biphasic tumor with compact and microcystic areas, the proportion of which may vary from one tumor to the other. Proliferation of bipolar spindle "piloid" cells with long fibrillary processes is seen mostly within the compact areas "Figure 1".

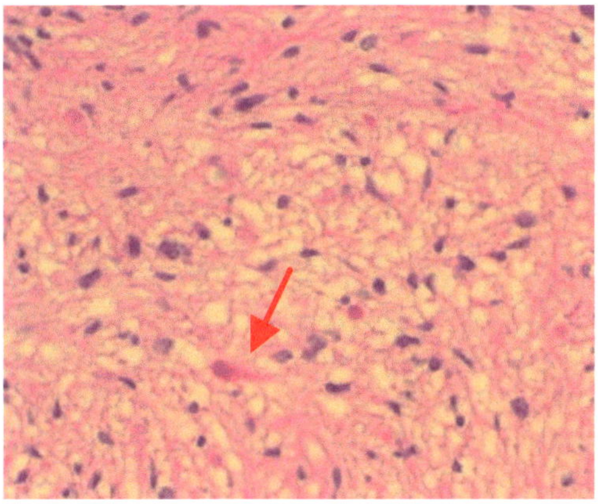

Figure 1. There is proliferation of piloid cells with elongated cytoplasmic processes. Rosenthal fibers are acidophilic processes seen in these areas (arrow).

The microcystic areas, on the other hand show protoplasmic-like astrocytes with multi-polar short cytoplasmic processes and small cell body with round to oval bland nuclei "Figure 2".

Areas with oligodendroglial like proliferation can be encountered, especially in the posterior fossa tumors. Various forms of vascular proliferation can be seen including reactive vascular

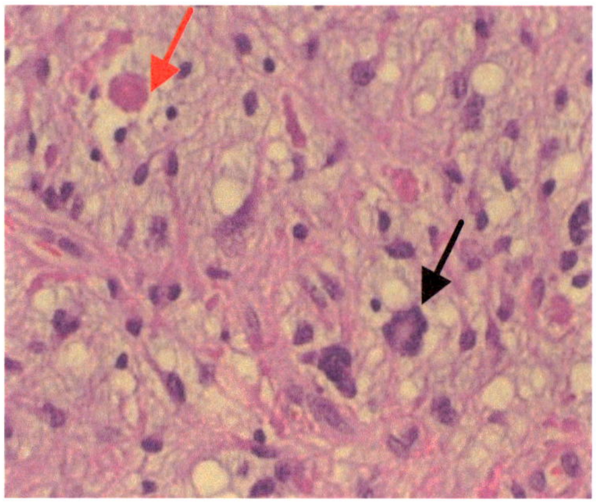

Figure 2. The microsystic areas are composed of proliferation of protoplasmic astrocytes. Eosinophilic granular bodies are seen in these areas (red arrow). Multinucleated giant cells are somtimes seen in pilocytic astrocytoma (black arrow).

proliferation, vessels with hyalinized walls and granulation tissue like vessels, none of which carries a prognostic significance. Conspicuous pleomorphic cells, some of which appear multinucleated can be seen focally within tumor and are not associated with unfavorable outcome. Rosenthal fibers which correspond to thick, tortuous bright acidophilic cytoplasmic processes of variable length are seen mostly in the compact areas, while eosinophilic granular bodies predominate in the microcystic foci, both of which representing products of degeneration [9]. Calcifications with psammoma like spherules, perivascular inflammatory infiltrate and hemosiderin-laden macrophages are detected in few tumors. Scattered mitotic figures and foci of infarction-type necrosis can be identified in anotherwise typical pilocytic astrocytoma. However; unlike fibrillary astrocytoma neither of these features warrant a higher grade diagnosis [10]. Areas with diffusely infiltrative growth pattern with entrapment of normal ganglion producing the "trapped neuron" appearance, can be seen in some tumors. In addition; infiltration into the overlying leptomeninges can sometimes be encountered [9].

Cases that exhibited anaplastic features and persued a more malignant behavior are reported in the literature, especially but not exclusively following radiotherapy [11]. The presence of increased mitotic activity per high power field, hypercellularity, endothelial proliferation and/or palisading necrosis should alert the pathologist to such a possibility. The diagnosis of "anaplastic pilocytic astrocytoma" is the term proposed by the WHO book for such tumors [8, 9]. Atypical pilocytic astrocytoma is, on the other hand assigned to few tumors that display few mitotic figures in conjunction with hypercellularity and marked nuclear atypia [8, 11].

Tumor cells are typically reactive with glial fibrillary acidic protein (GFAP) and vimentin. Reactivity for synaptphysin but not other neuronal markers is seen in some cases [10]. Neurofilament protein (NFP) highlights occasional axons in the background or can be totally negative thus is helpful in confirming the circumscribed nature of the tumor. Rosenthal fibers are reactive for GFAP but not NFP in support of their origin from astrocytic processes. This typically takes the form of positivity at the periphery of the fiber, with negative central core.

In Masson Trichrome special stain they appear bright red. Eosinophilic granular bodies (EGBs) on the other hand are positive for PAS diastase, which highlights their variably-sized granular appearance. Pilocytic astrocytomas are typically negative for P53 and EGFR, an important differentiating point from low and high grade diffuse astrocytoma; respectively [10, 12]. MIB-1 labeling index is variable and can range from 1-8% [10, 13], and this does not seem to be associated with prognosis [14]. BRAF immunostain has been recently described in some cases. However; this is not helpful in determining BRAF duplication [10], the genetic signature of pilocytic astrocytoma.

Pilomyxoid astrocytoma (PMA) is a distinctive tumor that occurs mostly in infants in the hypothalamic/ supra-sellar region. As the name implies this tumor manifests prominent myxoid stroma that can be highlighted with alcian blue stain and a monomorphic piloid astrocytes that arrange themselves in a distinct perivascular growth pattern with sun-ray like orientation "Figure 3".

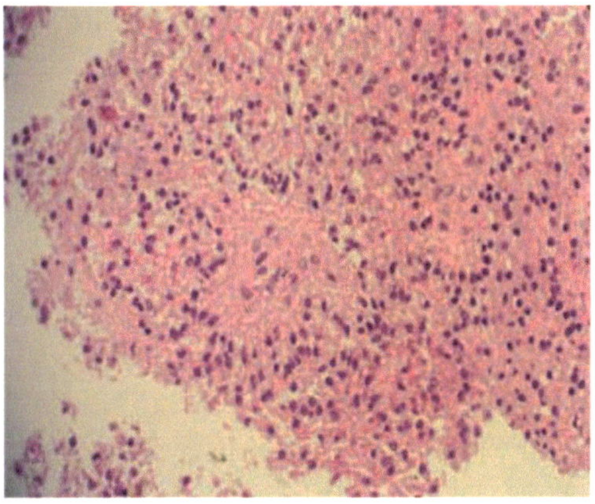

Figure 3. Distinct perivascular pseudorosette is seen in this case of pilomyxoid astrocytoma.

Few mitotic figures can be detected. Unlike pilocytic astrocytoma, there is no biphasic growth pattern, Rosenthal fibers or eosinophilic granular bodies and infiltration into adjacent brain parenchyma is more prominent [15]. Interestingly; some PMA cases have matured into pilocytic astrocytoma following several recurrences [16], suggesting a close relation between both tumors. The tumor cells demonstrate strong and diffuse positivity for GFAP and vimentin and focal positivity for synaptophysin. Neurofilament protein highlights the limited infiltration into adjacent parenchyma [17]. MIB-1 labeling index is around 5%, although higher figures would still be compatible with the diagnosis.

b. Pleomorphic xantho-astrocytoma (PXA)

PXA is a superficially located tumor with close relation to the meninges that predominates in the temporal lobe. It occurs in children and young adults with history of epilepsy [18]. Morphologically it is a composite tumor with a variegated appearance in which spindle cells closely intermingle with small and large mononuclear and multinucleated bizarre tumor giant cells with acidophilic cytoplasm "Figure 4". Intra-nuclear cytoplasmic pseudo-inclusions are frequently seen in the giant cells. Cytoplasmic lipidization in the form of intra-cytoplasmic droplets that occupy much of the cytoplasm and displace the organelles and glial filaments to the periphery is seen in tumor cells scattered through the tumor, hence the "xantho" prefix.

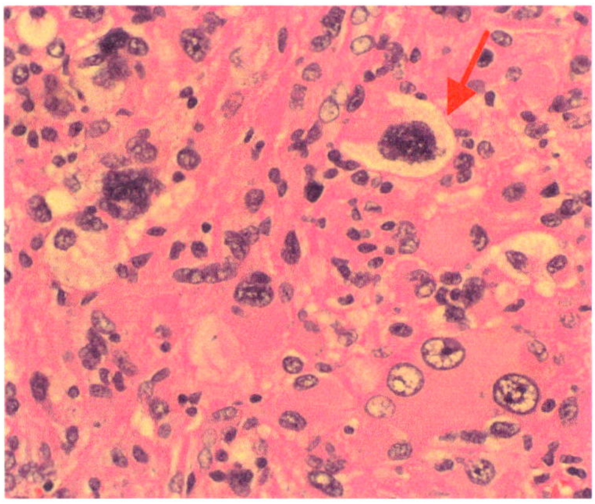

Figure 4. Multinucleated tumor giant cells are seen (right lower) admixed with cells with intracytplasmic fine lipid droplets (arrow).

These lipidized cells can be prominent or alternatively can only be scattered through out the tumor substance. Oil-red O confirms the intra-cytoplasmic lipid content on fresh material. An infiltrating astrocytoma pattern is seen at the deeper aspect of the tumor and this does not affect the outcome [19]. Invasion of the overlying meninges can be encountered in some tumors, creating resemblance with meningioma. Striking positivity for reticulin stain with fibers surrounding groups of cells or individual cells is seen in many tumors; probably representing a reaction to infiltration of the meninges. The blood vessels show peri-vascular lymphoplasmacytic infiltration. Eosinophilic granular bodies, but not Rosenthal fibers can be seen scattered within the tumor substance. Despite of this alarming appearance mitotic figures are not seen and necrosis is at best focal; important discriminating features from giant cell glioblastoma [20]. GFAP labels the tumor cells including the giant cells, and is displaced to the periphery in lipidized cells. Positivity for synaptophysin, NFP and CD34 in tumor cells has been noted in some cases, rendering separation from ganglioglioma difficult [18, 20]. PXA with anaplasia is reserved for tumors showing no or rare degeneration, increased mitoses ≥5 MF/10HPFs and atypical mitoses [14]. MIB-1 and P53 are not helpful in predicting more aggressive tumors, i.e. PXA with anaplasia [21].

c. Sub-ependymal giant cell astrocytoma (SEGA)

This intra-ventricular tumor is typically associated with tuberous sclerosis complex. It exhibits proliferation of three cell types; large gemistocytes -like cells with perivascular pseudorosette pattern, long spindle fibrillary astrocytes arranged in broad fascicles and giant cells, some with ganglioid appearance "Figure 5".

Calcification is noted in some cases and can be prominent in long standing ones [22]. Various combinations of glial and neuronal markers are reported in different cell population. Co-expression of GFAP, neuron-specific enolase (NSE) and synaptophysin is noted in tumor cells, including the spindle cells, while NFP is usually positive in ganglioid cells only. Mitosis, vascular proliferation and necrosis do not seem to affect the prognosis [23, 24].

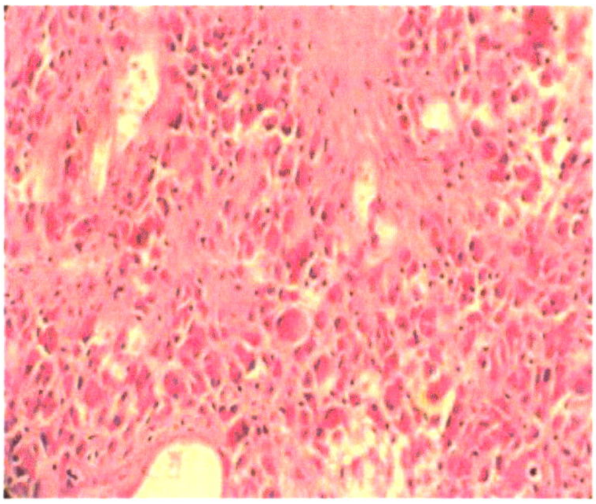

Figure 5. This intraventricular tumor shows admixture of large gemistocytic-like cells, ganglioid cells and spindle cells in a fibrillary background.

Diffuse astrocytoma

This group of tumors is composed of proliferation of astrocytes that diffusely infiltrate pre-existing brain parenchyma, thus precluding successful attempts at complete excision and cure. In addition; there is a natural tendency for progression and transformation from lower into high grades. On a rising scale of malignacy these tumors are divided into the following entities:

a. Fibrillary astrocytoma (FA,

FA is at the lower end of the malignancy scale, and can raise diagnostic difficulties with reactive gliosis on one hand and circumscribed low grade astrocytoma on the other. Morphologically there is proliferation of "well-differentiated" fibrillary astrocytes with elongated, irregular and hyperchromatic nuclei exhbiting angulated contours with many coma-shaped forms that lack nucleoli "Figure 6".

Thin cytoplasmic process originate from the cytoplasm and form the mesh-like fibrillary background. Morphological variation include the proliferation of gemistocytic and protoplasmic astrocytes. Gemistocytes contain a globular acidophilic cytoplasm with distinct membranous accentuation, eccentric irregular nuclei and thick cytoplasmic processes. Protoplasmic astrocytes on the other hand show multi-polar cytoplasmic processes and grow in a myxoid background, forming microcysts [25]. Features of anaplasia are lacking and mitoses are generally not detected [25, 26]. GFAP positivity is seen both as haphazardly crossing processes in which "naked" tumor nuclei are enmeshed, and as dense cytoplasmic rim positivity surrouding the nuclei. Gemistocytes demonstrate diffuse cytoplasmic GFAP positivity with

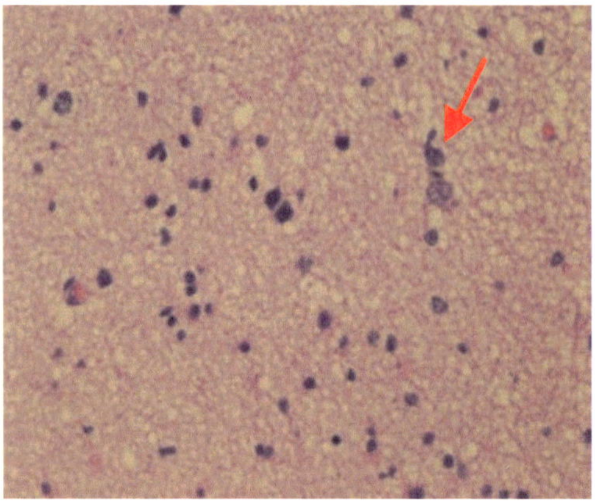

Figure 6. Fibrillary astrocytoma with mild increase in cellularity with scattered dark, elongated and minimally irregular nuclei (arrow).

membranous accentuation; an important discriminating point from mini-gemistocytes seen in oligodendroglioma (see below). To support the infiltrating astrocytoma diagnosis NFP, P53 and IDH1 can be used. Neurofilament protein is useful to highlight the the infiltrative growth pattern "Figure 7".

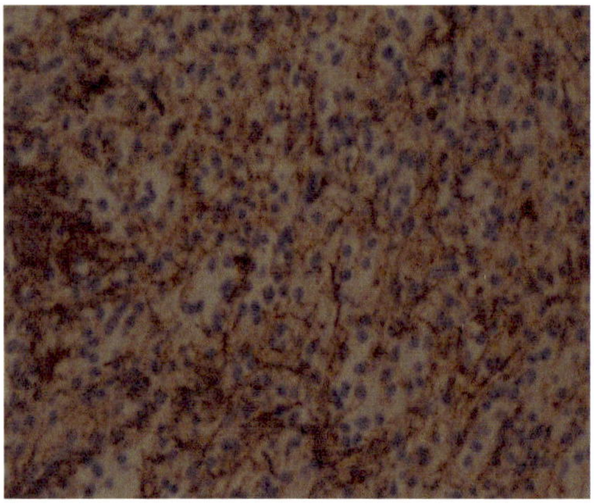

Figure 7. Neurofilament protein immunostain highlights the neuronal processes, with negative tumor cells in between confirming the infiltrative nature of the tumor.

P53 may be strongly positive in tumor cell nuclei versus the negative/ minimal staining in gliosis. [27]. Recently; IDH1 antibody is reported to be positive in all infiltrating gliomas (astrocytoma, oligodendroglioma and mixed oligo-astrocytoma) with granular cytoplasmic reactivity pattern [20, 28].MIB-1 labeling index is low, although the cut-off value is not exactly determined (see below) [29].

A recently described morphological pattern is the "glioneuronal tumor with neuropil-like islands", in which nodules of well differentiated neurocytic cells are embedded within and surround acellular synaptophysin-positive neuropil islands. These are seen focally in what is an otherwise typical infiltrating astrocytoma of either fibrillary or anaplastic types [15]. There is a relative abrupt transition between both components [30]. In these islands the cells are positive for synaptophysin and NeuN, while the neuropil in the background displays granular positivity for synaptophysin [17].

b. Anaplastic astrocytoma (AA)

AA occupies an intermediate position between fibrillary astrocytoma and glioblastoma. Features of anaplasia include higher cellularity, greater degree of pleomorphism and increased proliferation. The exact number of mitotic figures needed to separate this from FA is still debatable and this feature should be evaluated in relation to the amount of tissue sample examined. While the presence of a single mitotic figure in a small stereotactic biopsy justifies assigning grade III to a tumor, the presence of a single mitotic figure in an ample biopsy after careful searching and deeper sections might not be as relevant. In one study; >3MF/10HPFs was the cut-off value proposed [27]. Ancillary studies might help in defining the proliferative activity of a tumor and can be used to support the diagnosis of AA. Although cut-off values are variable an elevated MIB-1 labeling index (>9%) and proliferative activity as measured by PHH3 mitotic index (>4per 1000 cells) were found to be supportive of AA diagnosis over FA, in which MIB-1 and PHH3 labeling indices were low (≤ 9% and ≤4 per 1000 cells) [27]. In addition; MIB-1 labeling index prognostic value independent from histologic grade was reported [14], which might be indicative of an early anaplastic transformation [31], even in the absence of detectable mitoses.

c. Glioblastoma (GBM)

This is the most malignant and unfortunately the single most common primary brain tumor. The essential features for the diagnosis of GBM are microvascular proliferation (MVP) and/or necrosis whether palisading or not. Microvascular proliferation is loosely defined to include endothelial hypertrophy, endothelial hyperplasia and glomeruloid vessels, in which multi-layered tufts of proliferating endothelium are accompanied by smooth muscles and peri-cytes"Figure 8" [32].

As the original name implies glioblastoma "multiforme" is characterized by heterogeneous cell population with proliferation of fibrillary, gemistocytic and scattered tumor giant cells "Figure 9".

On the basis of their origin GBM is divided into primary (type II) and secondary (type I) types. Primary GBM is a tumor of elderly patients, is characterized by short presenting history and it arises de-novo with no detectable pre-existing lower grade tumor. Secondary GBM on the other hand affects younger patients with prolonged history and is typically preceded by a lower grade astrocytoma. Prognosis seems to be better for the secondary tumors. Whether a tumor is primary or secondary GBM cannot be predicted on basis of morphologic features. However; the presence of large vessel thrombosis with large areas of infarction-like necrosis seems to be more prevalent in primary GBM. Immunohistochemically; reactivity for P53,

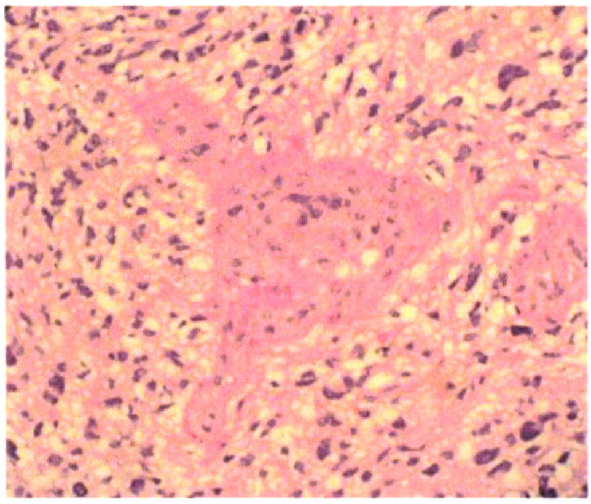

Figure 8. Microvascular proliferation with glomeruloid growth pattern.

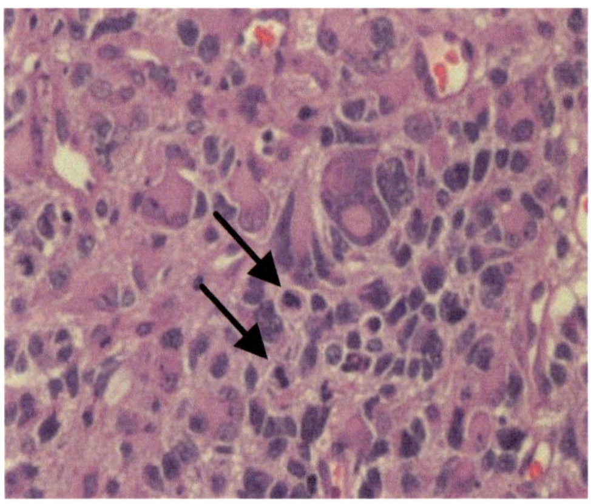

Figure 9. A case of GBM with large cells with abundant acidophilic cytoplasm at the upper left corner, and with intra-nuclear inclusion seen in a single giant tumor cell. The lower right filed is composed of smaller cells. Note multiple mitoses (arrows).

MGMT and IDH1 is more frequent in secondary GBM, while positivity for EGFR is more common in primary GBM [32].

Several GBM variants and patterns are described some of which might be prognostically relevant, Table-2.

Giant cell glioblastoma (GCG)

GCG accounts approximately for 1.5- 5% of GMB cases [32]. This is characterized by the predominance of bizarre markedly enlarged, often multinucleated tumor giant cells that tend to grow in cohesive pattern with rich reticulin-positive stroma, accounting for the deceptively circumscribed nature of the tumor seen radiologically. GFAP tends to be strongly positive in many of the tumor cells. Up to 90% of these tumors are positive for P53 [20]. Recently; it was shown that CD34 can be positive in giant cell glioblastoma, thus losing its discriminating power from pleomorphic xanthoastrocytoma; its main differential diagnosis [33]. Giant cell glioblastoma is claimed to carry a slightly better prognosis than classical GBM [20].

Gliosarcoma (GS)

This is a well-circumscribed, biphasic tumor that brings morphological remembrance to "carcinosarcoma" in other sites. There is a near mutually exclusive staining for GFAP and reticulin in the glial and mesenchymal components; respectively [34]. In the glial component a clear GFAP-positive, reticulin-free usually fibrillary and sometimes gemistocytic astrocytes proliferation is seen with necrosis and vascular proliferation. The sarcoma component, on the other hand is typically GFAP-negative, and reticulin-rich. This component may be fibroblastic with proliferation of long bundles of malignant spindle cells, or can show heterologous component including smooth muscle, adipose tissue, cartilage and osteoid formation [32].

Glioblastoma with oligodendroglial component (GMB-O)

This is thought to represent a variant of glioblastoma with a probable better prognosis [35]. Its relation to the mixed oligo-astrocytic tumors is discussed below. The essential component for establishing this diagnosis is the presence of an oligodendroglial component in addition to the astrocytic component in association with necrosis [15]. In 15-20% of tumors 1p/19q co-deletion is detected.

Small cell glioblastoma (SCG)

This is characterized by proliferation of deceptively bland, uniform, small, round to slightly elongated cells with minimal atypia, but with brisk mitoses. Of note is the rarity of microvascular proliferation and necrosis in most cases [20]. GFAP is at best focally positive in thin cytoplasmic processes. Resemblance to anaplastic oligodendroglioma is further accentuated by the presence of tumor cell satellitosis, chicken-wire vascular proliferation and microcalcifications [15, 20]. The disconnection between the bland cytology and the brisk mitosis should act as a clue in this differential diagnosis. Furthermore; immunreactivity for EGFRvIII supports the diagnosis of small cell GBM [20].

Glioblastoma with primitive neuroectodermal tumor (PNET)-like component

In this variant proliferation of a clone of primitive cells reminiscent of PNET/medulloblastoma is seen, sometimes forming discrete nodule. The cells have high nuclear cytoplasmic ratio and exhibit frequent neuroblastic and Homer-Wright rosettes. Features of anaplasia with cell-cell wrapping, increased cell size with prominent nucleoli are seen in a subset of cases; thus bringing resemblance to anaplastic/large cell medulloblastoma (see below). Mitotic activity is brisk. Immunohistochemistry shows diffuse staining for neural markers including synaptophysin and NeuN and in many cases P53. GFAP is positive only in occasional cells. MIB-1 labeling index shows a nearly diffuse positivity (almost 100%) [31, 36].

Adenoid glioblastoma

This is an extremely rare variant that brings metastatic carcinoma into the differential diagnosis. There is glandular-metaplastic component that intermingles with the better defined glial component. Reactivity for a variety of cytokeratins including CK7 can add further to the confusion [32, 37].

Granular cell glioblastoma (GCA)

This is a deceptively bland tumor with proliferation of astrocytes showing abundant granular PAS-positive cytoplasm and regular nuclei, so they can be confused with macrophages. Reactivity with GFAP is the rule with few cases displaying EMA but not cytokeratin positivity. P53 can be positive in few cases [32].

Table 2 summarizes the clinicopathological features of GBM variants (From Miller et al with modification) [32]

	Tumor								
Features	**1ry**	**2ry**	**Fib**	**Gem**	**GCA**	**GC**	**GS**	**SCA**	**GBM-O**
Peak age (decade)	6-7	5-6	6-7	6-7	6-7	5-6	6-7	6-7	5-6
Circumscription	…	…	-	-	+/-	+	+	-	-
Nuclear irregularity	…	…	++	+	+/-	+++	++	+/-	+
Perinuclear haloes	…	…	-	-	-	-	-	-	++
Cytoplasmic granules	…	…	-	-	+	-	-	-	-
Multinucleated cells	…	…	+/-	+/-	+/-	+++	+/-	+/-	+/-
Reticulin meshwork	…	…	-	-	+/-	+/-	+++	-	-
PVI	…	…	+/-	++	+/-	+	+/-	+/-	+/-
Mucin-filled microcysts	…	…	+/-	-	-	-	-	-	+++

1ry, primary; 2ry, secondary; Fib, fibrillary; Gem, gemistocytic; GCA, granular cell astrocytoma; GC, giant cell; GS, gliosarcoma; SCA, small cell astrocytoma; GBM-O, GBM with oligodendroglial features; …, no data available; -, absent; +/-, infrequent; + to +++, increasing frequency; PVI, peri-vascular inflammation.

Table 2.

d. Gliomatosis cerebri

This entity has been shifted to join astrocytic tumors in 2007 classification. By definition; it is an infiltrative tumor involving at least 2 lobes but lacking mass effect. When crossing from one side to the other it causes widening of the corpus callosum. Microscopically; there is an infiltrative glioma, usually corresponding to grade III anaplastic astrocytoma and occasionally to oligodendroglioma. Rarely grade II fibrillary astrocytoma or grade IV glioblastoma can be encountered. Characteristically; the infiltrating malignant cells preserve the underlying structures intact without destruction. P53 can highlight the tumor cells and MIB-1 labeling index is variable reflecting the grade of the tumor [38, 39].

2.1.2. Oligodendroglioma

This is characterized by proliferation of monotonous cells with regular round, uniform nuclei with delicate chromatin, sharply defined nuclear membrane and inconspicuous nucleoli, brining a "highly-uniform" appearance on low power examination. In formalin-fixed tissue there is clearing artifact creating "haloes" around tumor cell nuclei due to shrinkage of the cytoplasm; a useful diagnostic clue, although not an absolute criteria for diagnosis "Figure 10" [31].

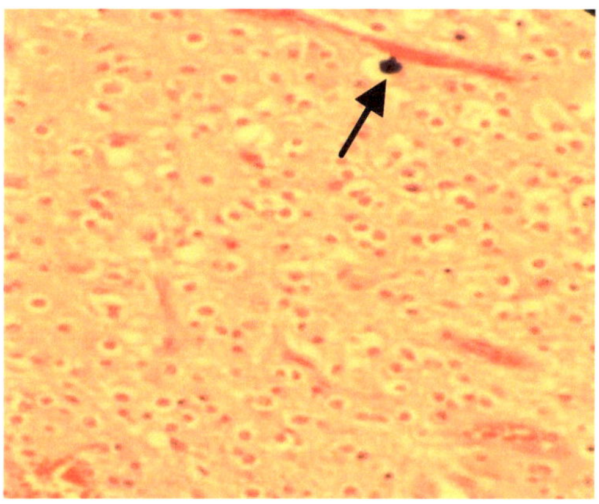

Figure 10. A case of oligodendroglioma with monotonous fried-egg appearance, chicken-wire vascularity and scattered calcification (arrow).

However; a small eccentric acidophilic cytoplasm can sometimes be appreciated. Hypertrophy of the cortical vessels leads to the development of the characteristic chicken-wire vascular proliferation [35].Micro-calcification, extensive infiltration of the cortical structures with perineural satellitosis and microcysts with basophilic mucinous contents are additional diagnostic features [20]. In the anaplastic variant; the vascularity becomes more prominent leading to the development of a nodular growth pattern at low power magnification. The cells become larger and exhibit more abundant cytoplasm with vesicular nuclei and prominent nucleoli; yet they retain their uniform appearance. There is increased cellularity with increased mitosis (≥6 MF/10HPFs), microvascular proliferation and necrosis. Important companions are the glio-fibrillary oligodendrocytes and the mini-gemistocytes "Figure 11".

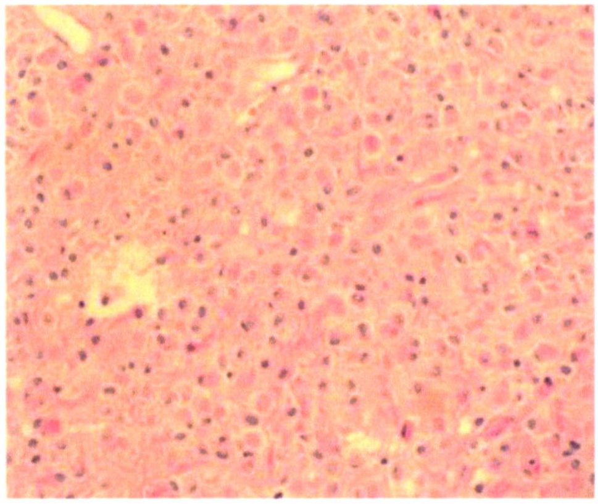

Figure 11. Minigemistocytes with whorling GFAP positive filaments. The tumor cells can be positive for GFAP. This is especially seen in the perinuclear staining in glio-fibrillary oligodendrocytes and the diffuse cytoplasmic staining in the mini-gemistocytes, thus potentiating confusion with infiltrating astrocytoma, or mixed oligo-astrocytoma [20]. In most case; P53 [25]and vimentin [40]stains are negative thus helping in sorting out the differential diagnosis with astrocytoma. A notable pitfall is the positivity of oligodendroglial tumors for neural markers including NeuN [41, 42], and synaptophysin which reacts with a para-nuclear dot-like positivity [31].

2.1.3. Mixed oligo-astrocytoma

Mixed oligo-astrocytoma is one of the most common tumors associated with considerable diagnostic difficulty and inter-observer variability [31]. A mixture of oligodendroglioma and infiltrative diffuse astrocytoma is seen. Both components can be spatially separated (compact variant) or they can be intermixed (diffuse variant). The minimum percentage of each component needed to establish the diagnosis is debatable, although a minimum of 10% astrocytic component of either fibrillary or gemistocytic morphology was used in some studies [43]. In the anaplastic variant; the tumors are highly cellular with pleomorphism and nuclear atypia, mitosis (≥6 MF/10HPFs) and/or microvascular proliferation [31] which could be identified in either or both components. Recent literature supports the up-grading into glioblastoma in the presence of necrosis (see above) [17, 35].

2.1.4. Ependymoma

a. Myxo-papillary ependymoma

This is a slowly growing tumor that is almost exclusively seen in the cauda equina and filum terminale of young adults. It is composed of hypo- and hypercellular areas. The hypocellular areas show abundant mucicarmine-positive mucinous matrix with scattered epithelioid-appearing cells. The hypercellular areas are formed of tumor cells arranged in papillary structures. Cystic spaces filled with alcian-blue, PAS positive mucin separate the tumor cells from the blood vessels "Figure 12".

http://dx.doi.org/10.5772/52356

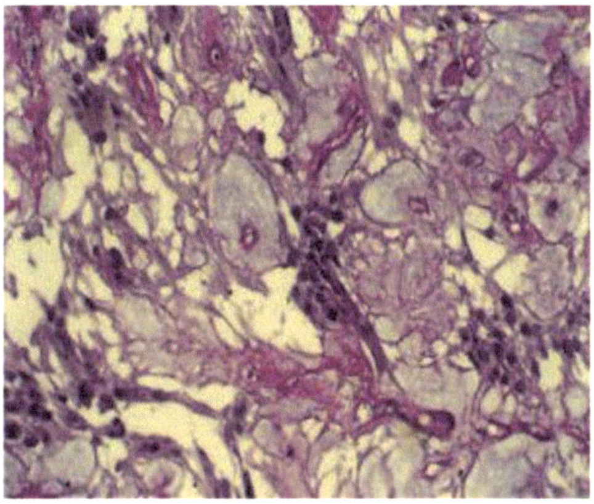

Figure 12. In myxo-papillary ependymoma, alcian-blue positive cores surround vessels and cells grow in between forming sheets and sometimes perivascular psuedorosettes.

The cells are bland with processes radiating to the walls of the vessels and are arranged in single or multiple layers. Cribriform areas, sheets of cells and cells with clear cytoplasm can occasionally be encountered, creating resemblance to metastatic carcinoma. Pleomorphic cellular features, proliferation of vascular spaces, mitosis or necrosis are not seen, even in more aggressive tumors [44].Tumor cells are reactive for GFAP and S-100 and MIB-1 labeling index is low. A potential pitfall is positivity of the cells for pancytokeratin (AE1/AE3), cam 5.2 and cytokeratin 7 [45]. EMA can show cytoplasmic positivity in few tumor cells, similar to the pattern seen in other ependymoma (see below).

b. Sub-ependymoma

This mostly arises in the 4th followed by lateral ventricles [46]. Many cases are asymptomatic and discovered incidentally, although symptoms of increased intra-cranial pressure are the presenting features in others [47]. Morphologically; this is a well-delineated tumor that is characterized by nodules of clustered isomorphic cells arranged against a fibrillary background alternating with hypocellular fibrillary areas. Vague perivascular rosettes can be seen "Figure 13".

Focal cystic degeneration is noted [48], as well as vascular hyalinization, nuclear pleomorphism and calcification [46]. This distinctive pattern may frequently be admixed with classical ependymoma (See below). No mitotic figures, vascular proliferation or necrosis is detected in most tumors. GFAP is diffusely positive in these cases. MIB-1 labeling index is extremely low approaching zero [46].

c. Cellular ependymoma;

This is characterized by the presence uniform monomorphic cells extending their fine processes radially to the walls of blood vessels creating a fibrillary cellular free zone around the

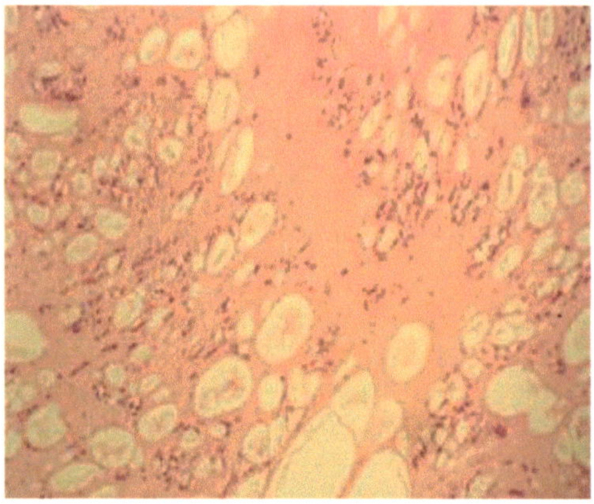

Figure 13. Sub-ependymoma shows the typical microcysts formation, aggregated nuclei with nuclear-free zones made up of fine fibrillary background.

vessels and forming perivascular pseudorosettes. True rosettes and ependymal canals, where clusters of ependymal cells are arranged around a lumen resembling spinal canal, are less commonly encountered "Figure 14".

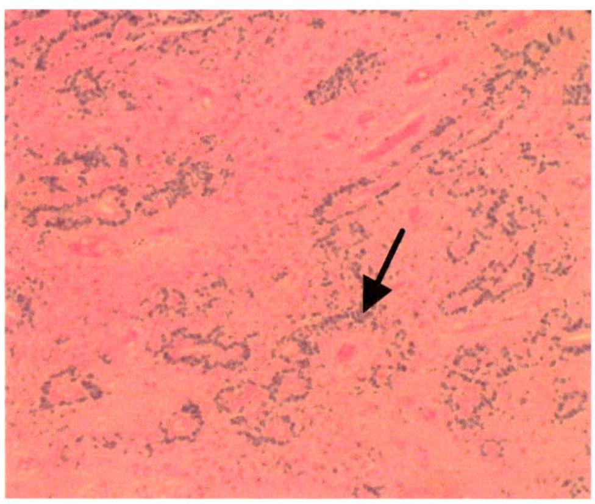

Figure 14. Ependymal rosettes and canals can be seen in few cases. They are less common than perivascular pseudorosettes (arrow).

Feature of anaplasia include diffuse hypercellularity with diffuse nuclear pleomorphism, vascular endothelial proliferation, palisading necrosis, increased mitosis (usually ≥5MF/10HPFs) and elevated MIB-1 labeling index (≥20.5%) [27, 49]. Necrosis, in the absence of palisading, is a common feature in posterior fossa tumors, and is not a poor prognostic feature [31]. Interestingly; the identification of sub-ependymoma like areas in infratentorial ependymoma seems to be associated with adverse outcome [14]. Another important microscopic feature is the focal hypercellular nodules, in which focal increase in cellularity is associated with nuclear pleomorphism and an increase in mitosis. In the absence of diffuse changes, these nodules are not associated with an adverse prognosis and as such may not warrant assigning a higher grade to the tumor [49]. GFAP is variably positive in tumor cells, especially in perivascular processes. EMA [50] and CD99 show charactersitic dot-like perinuclear cytoplasmic positivity [51]. Other positive stains include other intermediate filaments like vimentin and desmin [27].

d. Clear cell ependymoma

This is a tumor that predominates supratentorially and displays an enhancing cystic component in the majority of cases. It is characterized by proliferation of sheets of cells with round nuclei and prominent, clear haloes. Focal ependymal perivascular pseudorosettes may be seen but true rosettes and canals are not typical. Features of anaplasia including increased cellularity, mitosis and microvascular proliferation, and at least focal necrosis are frequent. Reactivity for GFAP with perivascular accentuation, dot-like cytoplasmic EMA and CD99 staining should all help in reaching the appropriate diagnosis. MIB-1 labeling index is increased especially in areas of increased mitosis. [52]. Clear cell ependymoma should be differentiated from oligodendroglioma [20, 52].

e. Tanycytic ependymoma

This is primarily a tumor of the spinal cord, but occasional cases may arise from the third ventricle or the hypothalamus. Tanycytic ependymoma posses an "astrocytoma-look", with solid proliferation of spindle cells with elongated processes and with at best focal ill-defined ependymal psuedorosettes. The nuclei are uniform, round to oval with salt and pepper chromatin, similar to other ependymoma "Figure 15".

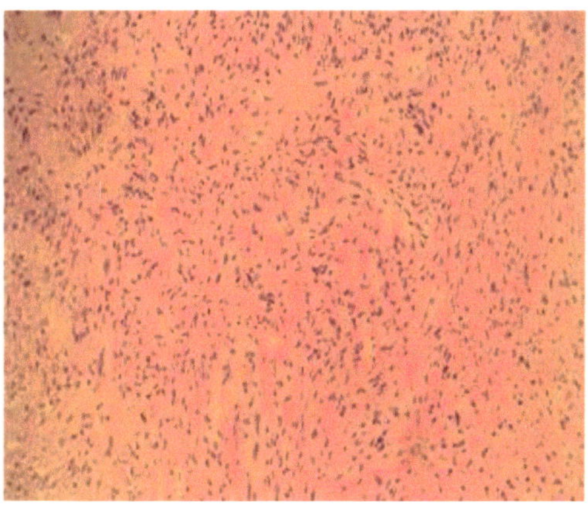

Figure 15. Tanycytic ependymoma is composed of "piloid" like tanycytes with only vague perivascular pseudorosettes noted.

Strong GFAP positivity is seen in the elongated processes. Other positive markers include S-100, vimentin and CD99 [20].

2.2. Embryonal tumors

They all share proliferation of small round blue cells with increased mitosis and apoptosis. This group includes

a. Medulloblastoma

This is a primitive neuroectodermal tumor that arises from the cerebellum. It is the most common malignant brain tumor in children and the most common embryonal tumor. Medulloblastoma is thought to originate from a primitive cell type in the cerebellum. The multipotent progenitor cells of ventricular zone that forms the innermost boundary of the cerebellum is the postulated origin of the classical medulloblastoma, while the external germinal layer that lines the outside of the cerebellum; the external granular layer, is the postulated origin of the desmoplastic medulloblastoma [53].

Several morphologic sub-types are recongized, some of which are prognostically relevant:

- Classic medulloblastoma; is the most common variant, and represents 66% of cases [54]. It is composed of densely-packed cells with hyperchromatic, round, oval or carrot-shaped nuclei with minimal cytoplasm "Figure 16".

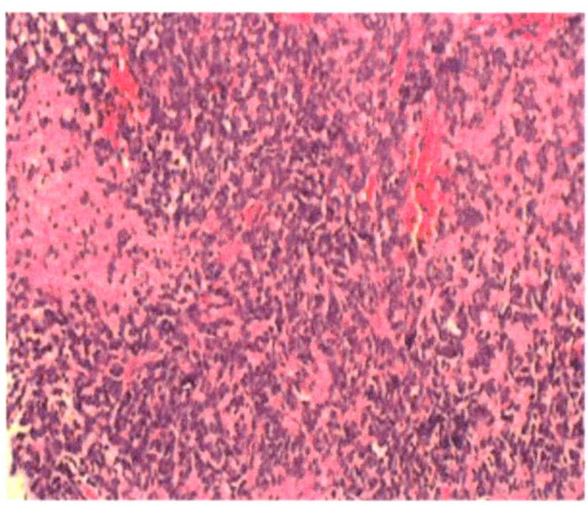

Figure 16. Sheets of tumor cells with Homer-Wright rosettes (right side) and neurocytic nodules (left) can be encountered in typical medulloblastoma.

The cells are usually arranged in diffuse sheets, but trabeculae, spongioblastic pattern, Homer-Wright rosettes and nodules can be identified. Necrosis, sometimes palisading, may be seen in some tumors, and has been identified as an adverse prognostic feature [55].

- Desmoplastic/nodular medulloblastoma(DNM) and medulloblastoma with extensive nodularity (MEN); both of these variants share the presence of reticulin-rich desmoplastic component and a reticulin-free, nodular component showing comparatively extensive neurocytic differentiation, fibrillary background, less mitoses and frequent apoptosis "Figure 17".

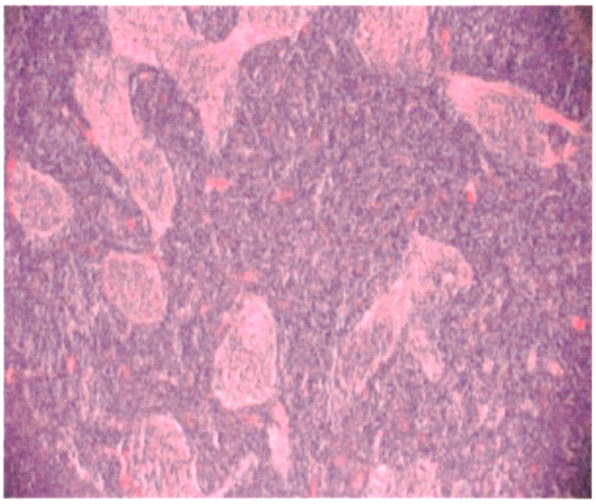

Figure 17. Desmoplastic medulloblastoma with pale islands and internodular area giving a reactive lymph node like appearance.

Both variants are claimed to be associated with better prognosis [54]. DNM can be seen in children and adults and represents 25% of cases of medulloblastoma. MEN, on the other hand, is characteristically seen in infants, where is accounts for 57% of medulloblastoma in this age group and is associated with excellent outcome. Whereas the reticulin-rich component predominates in DNM, and the presence of any percentage of nodularity and desmoplasia qualifies the tumor for DNM subtype [56], the reticulin-free differentiating component predominates in MEN, representing 96-100% of the tumor [57]. Thus MEN might be perceived as an exaggerated form of DNM [15]. Importantly; the borders between the nodules and the surrounding desmoplasia is usually sharp [54]. The presence of desmoplasia due to infiltration of the meninges in the absence of nodules does not qualify the tumor as DNM [57] and vice versa; the identification of less-delineated neurocytic nodules in the absence of desmoplasia i.e.biphasic medulloblastoma is considered a variation of classical or sometimes anaplastic/large cell medulloblastoma morphological patterns that is not assocaited with improved outcome in some [54], but not all studies [55]. Immunohistochemistry helps further confirming both growth patterns. The pale islands are synaptophysin positive with low MIB-1 labeling index, while the inter-nodular areas are at best focally positive for synaptophysin with high MIB-1 labeling index, in keeping with presence or absence of neuronal differentiation; respectively.

- Anaplastic/large cell medulloblastoma; these are closely related variants that frequently co-exist and account for17- 24 % of cases of medulloblastoma [54, 57]. In anaplastic medulloblastoma there is marked nuclear pleomorphism with angular, crowded pleomorphic cells with nuclear molding, cell-cell wrapping and numerous mitotic and apoptotic figures"Figure 18".

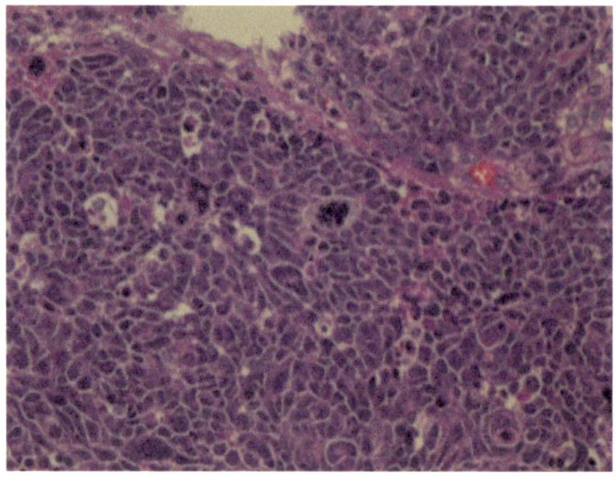

Figure 18. Anaplastic medulloblastoma with frequent cell wrapping (lower right), apoptosis and abnormal mitosis.

The nuclei are twice to three times the size of an RBC in moderate to severe anaplasia, thus varying in size from 18-21 micrometers; respectively [57, 58]. Hyperchromasia per se is not a defining feature of anaplasia. The large cell variant on the other hand is characterized by large spherical cells possessing round vesicular nuclei and prominent central nucleoli"Figure 19" [57, 58].

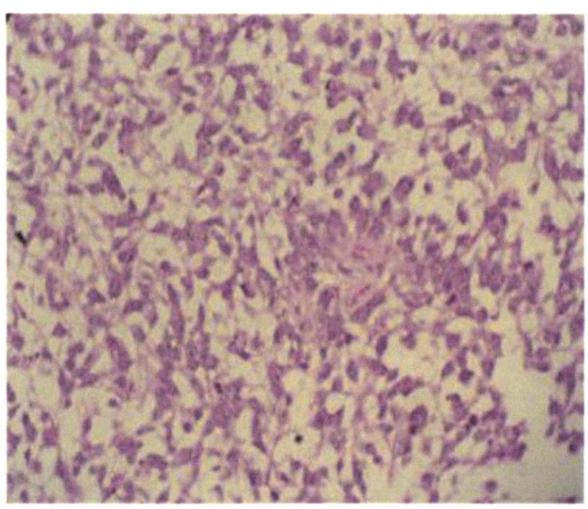

Figure 19. In large cell medulloblastoma; the cells have abudant cytoplasm, vesicular nuclei and prominent nucleoli.

Anaplasia is considered diffuse when seen involving every low power field, otherwise it is considered focal. It is the diffuse, moderate to severe anaplasia that is associated with poor prognosis. Anaplastic/large cell features can be detected in what appears to be DNM or in recurrent classical medulloblastoma. The presence of features of DNM, Homer-Wright rosettes or previously classical medulloblastoma is not incompatible with the diagnosis of anaplasia [31, 57, 58].

- "Medulloblastoma with myogenic differentiation" and "medulloblastoma with melanotic differentiation" are considered morphological patterns with divergent differentiation that can be seen in any of the medulloblastoma variants, but with no effect on prognosis. Respectively; desmin and myogenin positive rhabdomyoblasts and S-100 positive melanotic tumor cells are seen in both patterns, hence the nomenclature [15].

In medulloblastoma, the tumor cells are positive for synaptophysin in up to 80% of cases, while microtubule-associated protein 2 antibody (MAP2) is seen in cases with weak synaptophysin reactivity [27]. CD99 is usually negative in contrast to peripheral PNET [59]. GFAP reactivity can be seen in medulloblastoma cells in a perinuclear pattern and this might carry adverse prognosis [27]. Diffuse positivity for P53 (strong nuclear stain in > 50%), ErbB2 (strong membranous staining in ≥ 50% of tumor cells) and survivin (nuclear stain) is associated with poor prognosis [56, 60-62]. TrK-C (strong cytoplasmic staining in >50% of tumor cells) and beta-catenin (either diffuse, strong cytoplasmic and nuclear or nuclear staining in cell clusters of at least 10% of nuclei among others with negligible or weak staining) are associated with improved outcome [60, 63, 64]. MIB-1 labeling index is variable but with a mean that ranges between 46.5-59.03%. The prognostic importance of elevated MIB-1 labeling index varies from one study to another [56, 60], with higher figures reported among anaplastic/large cell variant, and correlating with poor outcome [65].

b. CNS-primitive neuroectodermal tumor (CNS-PNET)

This is a heterogeneous group of poorly-differentiated primitive small round blue cells that can be seen supratentorially, in the brainstem or in the spinal cord. Divergent differentiation along neuronal/ ganglio-neuronal, epithelial or ependymal lines can be seen occasionally, hence the neuroblastoma/ CNS ganglioneuroblastoma, medulloepithelioma and ependymoblastoma variants; respectively [15]. The presence of necrosis adversely affects the outcome [14]. Embryonal tumor with abundant neuropil and ependymoblastic rosettes (ETANTR) is a newly described variant that is considered a hybrid tumor where both neuroblastic and ependymoblastic differentiation co-exist. Characteristically; ETANTR has been reported to have extra-copies of chromosome 2 [66] and 19q amplification [67].

CNS-PNET can show positivity for synaptophysin, GFAP and occasionally dot-like cytoplasmic EMA, according to differentiation [68]. Of note is the total negativity for CD99 in contrast to the peripheral type PNET tumors [69].

c. Atypical teratoid/rhabdoid tumor (AT/RT)

This tumor predominates in infants and can be seen in supratentorial and infratentorial compartments. Growth pattern are predominantly diffuse in most cases with reticular and papillary patterns noticed in few [70]. The typical cell, "rhabdoid cell" is seen in most but not all tumors and is not an absolute prerequisite for establishing the diagnosis. It is a large cell with eccentric acidophilic cytoplasm, vesicular nucleus with prominent nucleolus, reminiscent of "rhabdomyoblasts" hence the name. Intra-cytoplasmic spherical filamentous inclusions are identified in a proportion of rhabdoid cells"Figure 20".

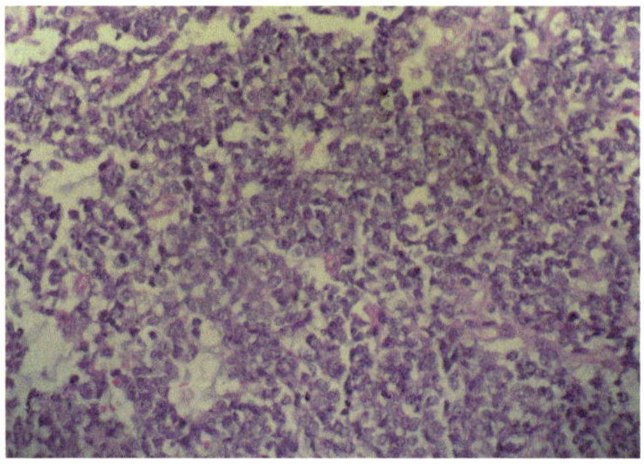

Figure 20. Typical case of AT/RT composed of cells with eccentric acidophilic cytoplasm and vesicular nuclei with prominent nucleoli. Note the myxoid background in the lower left corner.

Other common cellular components included large pale cells and primitive small round blue cells. Pale cells are characterized by vesicular nuclei, prominent nucleoli, and granular vacuolated wispy or water clear cytoplasm lacking intra-cytoplasmic inclusions, while small cells are cells with high nuclear: cytoplasmic ratio reminiscent of medulloblastoma/PNET [42, 71]. Admixture of all three cell components is noted in most cases. However; cases composed entirely of one cell type are not uncommon. Variable mesenchymal structures including myxoid changes, chondroid, lipoblastic and spindle cells elements can be seen. Occasional cases may contain glandular or papillary structures as an evidence of epithelial differentiation. Dystrophic calcifications and necrosis can be identified in some tumors.

Nowadays; the diagnosis of AT/RT can be confirmed by loss of INI1/BAF47 immunostain in tumor cells nuclei with appropriate positive normal endothelial and mononuclear cell control in the background [42]. In the rare instances of retained INI1/BAF47 nuclear stain, which is seen in 2% of cases, positivity for a panel of other markers can help in suggesting the diagnosis. A panel of EMA, synaptophysin, GFAP, vimentin, smooth muscle actin and pan-cytokeratin can show various combination of positive staining and thus can be of help in suggesting the diagnosis [27]. Confirmation by cytogenetics for monosomy 22 may be warranted in such cases. Notably is the absence of desmin [72]. MIB-1 labeling index ranges between 30-50%.

2.3. Neuronal and mixed neuronal-glial tumors

This is the most heterogeneous and rapidly expanding group of tumors with many newly recognized and added entities. As the name implies, many tumors are composed of a mixture of glial and neuronal components.

a. Ganglioglioma (GG) and gangliocytoma

Frequently presenting as long standing chronic seizure, this biphasic tumor is most commonly located in the temporal lobe and is seen mostly in children and young adults. This is a variably circumscribed tumor with intimate mixture of disfigured and dysplastic neurons and neoplastic glial cells of varying proportions. The ganglion cells are characterized by cyto-architectural disorientation with sub-cortical localization, abnormal aggregations and clustering. Morphologically; the neurons show abnormal forms with frequent cytomegaly, bi- and multinucleation, prominent nucleoli, and peri-membranous condensed Nissl substance [73]. The glial component can vary as well from pilocytic to diffuse astrocytoma to oligodendroglioma like component "Figure 21" [73, 74]. This is the proliferative component that ultimately determines the biological behavioral of GG. Tumors composed predominantly of ganglion cells, which are devoid of a glial component are termed gangliocytomas [73, 74]. Dysplastic calcification (globules or incrustation), eosinophilic granular bodies and increased reticulin meshwork can be seen in the background. Perivascular lymphocytes and scattered parenchymal plasma cells are common supportive features. An atypical or anaplastic ganglioglioma is rarely encountered and can arise either de novo or at recurrences of a previously diagnosed GG [74]. The presence of cellular atypia and pleomorphism, microvascular proliferation, necrosis and elevated MIB-1 labeling index supports the diagnosis of anaplastic ganglioglioma [17, 73]. It was suggested to lable tumors exhibiting features of anaplasia without necrosis as atypical GG [74]. Gemistocytes identified in some tumors might represent an additional feature of anaplasia [74].

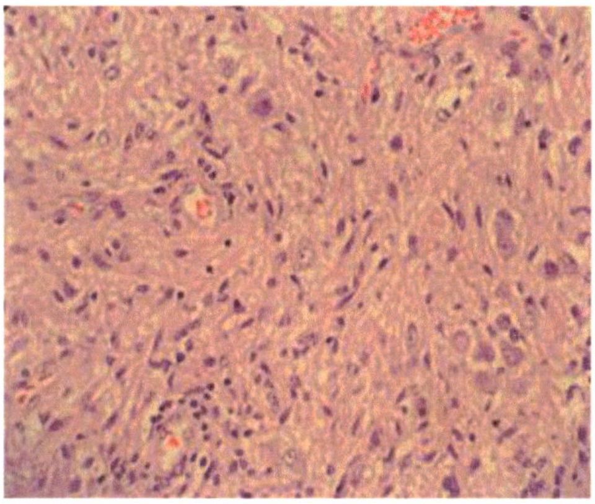

Figure 21. Ganglioglioma with dysplastic ganglion cells that are haphazardely oriented with abnormal aggregation of Nissl substance in the cytoplasm. Perivascular lymphocytic infiltrate is seen.

Immunohistochemically; the dysplastic ganglion cells are positive for synaptophysin, with peri-somatic synaptophysin reactivity, chromogranin A, neurofilament protein and MAP2 [74-76], while the glial component is positive for GFAP. Dysplastic ganglions frequently fail to react with NeuN, a potentially useful marker to differentiate dysplastic from normal neurons [42]. CD34 is reported to be positive in up to 80% of tumors; labeling the dysplastic neurons, being less frequently positive in atypical and anaplastic tumors [74]. MIB-1 labeling index is seen in the glial component and is usually <1% [77] and labeling index >5% is associated with a more aggressive behavior (see above). P53 is reported in only atypical/anaplastic tumors [74, 77].

b. Desmoplastic infantile ganglioglioma/astrocytoma (DIG/DIA)

DIG is a massive, supratentorial tumor that primarily affects infants, usually younger than 6 months of age. It is characterized by superficial leptomeningeal attachment, multiple conspicuous cysts, firm consistency and focal infiltration into adjacent brain parenchyma without clear plane of resection [78].Microscopically; there is admixture of fibroblasts, neuroastroglial cells and primitive cells, all enmeshed within a desmoplastic stoma, that can be highlighted by reticulin and Massons's trichrome stains [79]. The proportion of the different cellular components varies from one tumor to the other. The astroglial cells are the most abundant cell component, especially in regions of desmoplasia, are characterized by strap-like to polygonal, GFAP positivity. The neuronal cells; on the other hand are more frequently seen in the less desmoplastic areas, with proliferation of small abortive neurons to occasional polygonal ganglioid cells with prominent nucleoli and Nissl substance that are reactive with synaptophysin and NFP. The proportion of the small primitive cells can vary from scattered to a considerable amount in some tumors. It is within these areas that rare mitosis and foci of micronecrosis, but not endothelial proliferation can be detected [78, 79]. However; regardless of their amount; this tumor continues to carry a favorable prognosis in most cases. MIB-proliferative index is low with a mean of 6.5% [79]. There has been reported cases in the literature in which the prognosis was not as favorable and resulted occasionally in patient's death [80]. DIA shares with DIG the desmoplasia and the astrocytic components, but not the neuronal or the primitive cells [78].

c. Dys-embryoplastic neuroectodermal tumor (DNET)

The essential diagnostic features of this peculiar epilepsy-associated tumor are the combination of cortical localization, multi-nodular architectures with nodules composed of glial cells of either astrocytic or oligodendroglial or a mixture of both, foci of dysplasia in the adjacent cortex and the "specific glioneuronal elements" [81]. These are composed of bundles of axons lined by small S-100 positive, GFAP-negative oligodendrocytes with normal appearing neurons floating within pale eosinophilic interstitial fluid i.e."floating neurons", all arranged in columns perpendicular to the overlying cortex, and is strikingly similar from one case to another. Thin capillaries run within the columns. When sectioned perpendicular to the columns; the capillaries are seen to be rosetted by the oligodendroglial cells with the "floating neurons" in between. Calcification can sometimes be seen. Two morphological forms exist; the simple and complex forms [81]. In the simple form; only the "specific glioneuronal elements" are seen within the cortex. The complex form, on the other hand; features the glial nodules and/or cortical dysplasia in addition to the "specific glioneuronal elements". The nuclei of the oligodendrocytes within the nodules are frequently voluminous and multilobated "fleurettes-like", while the astrocytic component is usually in the form of pilocytic astrocytoma, sometimes accompanied by the "vascular arcade" proliferation typically seen in cerebellar pilocytic astrocytoma. Fibrillary astrocytoma, of both grades II and III like features can also be seen. The presence of morphological features of anaplasia in the form of rare mitosis and necrosis can occasionally be seen. MIB-1 labeling index is mostly negative in the simple form with rare reactive cells in the complex form, although higher labeling index can be seen in some cases according to the type and grade of the glioma seen within the nodules [81]. Cases can still be

http://dx.doi.org/10.5772/52356

diagnosed as DNET even in the absence of histological appearances previously described, if all of the following clinical and radiological features are fulfilled including 1)partial seizure with or without secondary generalization beginning before the age of 20 years, 2)no neurological deficit or stable congenital deficits, 3)cortical topography of the lesion as demonstrated by MRI and 4) absence of mass effect on imaging. The underlying spectrum of histopathologic entities that can be seen include mostly pilocytic and fibrillary astrocytoma [82].

d. Central neurocytoma

This tumor typically occupies the lateral ventricles or less commonly the third ventricle in young adults without significant invasion into the adjacent brain tissue [83]. It is characterized by proliferation of uniform round cells, embedded within and focally separated by a fibrillary background, the "neuropil" giving an overall monotonous appearance "Figure 22".

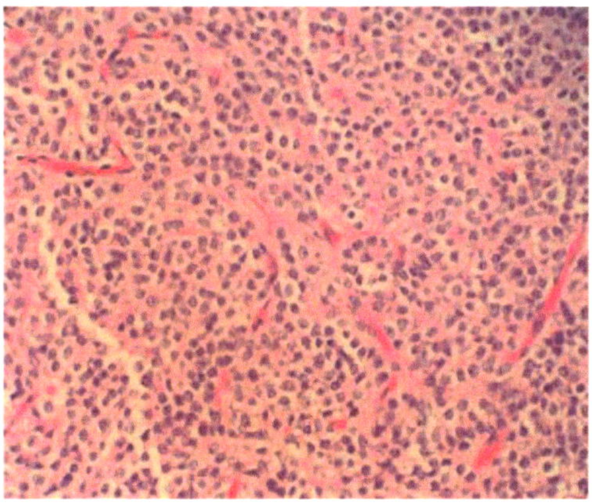

Figure 22. Typical neurocytoma with monotonous tumor cells with vesicular chromatin and delicate capillary-sized vessels. The background is fibrillary.

The tumor cells grow in sheets, clusters, "Indian filing" but rarely rosettes. The fibrillary areas can be seen to form acellular aggregates, bringing resemblance to pineocytomatous rosettes (see below). The nuclei are round to oval with finely speckled chromatin and occasional prominent nucleoli. The cytoplasm is scanty and can be acidophilic or rarely clear. Calcification, which is seen throughout the tumor, and delicate-branching capillaries bring resemblance to oligodendroglioma. Occasional cases show ganglion cells [17]. Mitosis is scarce and there is usually no necrosis [15]. When present such features warrant the diagnosis of atypical neurocytoma. Synaptophysin is strongly and diffusely positive in both the neurocytes and neuropil. NeuN shows strong nuclear stain in tumor cells [42]. Other positive neural markers include neurofilament protein and MAP2. Leu-7 can be positive but it is not specific as is staining for neuron-specific enolase (NSE). Chromogranin is typically negative in both the neurocytoma cells and neuropil [84]. Occasional positivity for GFAP can be seen in some tumors [83]. MIB-1 labeling index is $<2\%$ in typical cases [83]. An elevated MIB-1 labeling index $>3\%$ correlates with poorer outcome [14].

e. Extra-ventricular neurocytoma (EVN)

EVN shares morphologic and immunophenotypic features with central neurocytoma. It arises, however from the parenchyma, mostly in the cerebral hemispheres in adults [15, 84]. In addition, Ganglion cell differentiation is a more frequent occurrence, being described in more than half of the cases and can be either focal or diffuse [17, 84]. Frequent reactivity for GFAP is seen in nearly half of cases [84].

f. Cerebellar liponeurocytoma

This is another biphasic tumor that occurs in adults. Originally described in the posterior fossa mostly in the cerebellar hemispheres, cases with identical morphological features are also being reported supratentorially, arising from the lateral ventricle [85]. Morphologically a well differentiated neurocytic component composed of uniform round nuclei and minimal cytoplasm is admixed with mature lipomatous component. Thin and occasionally hyalinized vessels can be detected in the tumor as well as dispersed foci of neuropil. The tumor is diffusely reactive for synaptophysin, NSE and NeuN. Other neuronal markers including chromogranin and NFP can be focally positive. The lipomatous component shows cytoplasmic reactivity for NFP, chromogranin, occasionally for GFAP and S-100 rimming the vacuoles. MIB-1 labeling index is low (<1%) in the majority of cases [17].

g. Papillary glio-neuronal tumor (PGNT)

This tumor is characterized by pseudopapillae and less frequently by papillae, with hyalinized cores lined by a single or multiple layers of hyperchromatic GFAP positive, S-100 positive astrocytes that exhibit acidophilic cytoplasm. These are separated by sheets of synaptophysin positive, Neu-N positive mature neuronal cells in the inter-papillary areas. The neurocytic component includes neurocytes with vesicular nuclei and clear cytoplasm, ganglionoid cells and ganglion cells [15]. A fibrillary or mucoid matrix is seen in the background and can form nodules outside the papillary regions [30]. Sharp demarcation from the adjacent brain is seen. Mitoses is rare or absent and microvascular proliferation and necrosis are not seen. MIB-1 labeling index is low usually in the range of 1-2%.

h. Rosette forming tumor of the 4th ventricle (RGNT)

This is another example of hybrid glial/neuronal tumor, that arises in midline structures, mostly but not exclusively the 4th ventricle. It often shows involvement of the surrounding periventricular tissue [30]. The neural component shows neuropil-rich rosettes and perivascular pseudorosettes that are lined by synaptophysin-positive neurocytes with clear cytoplasm. A microcystic component with blue mucinous extracellular matrix is sometimes described [17]. The glial component is in the form of pilocytic astrocytoma with Rosenthal fibers and eosinophilic granular bodies [15]. No nuclear atypia or mitosis is seen. However; vascular proliferation of the type seen in pilocytic astrocytoma can be encountered and should not lead to the suggestion of anaplasia [30]. Reactivity for NSE and MAP2 can be seen in the neural component, while GFAP and S-100 are positive in glial component. MIB-1 labeling index is low.

http://dx.doi.org/10.5772/52356

2.4. Choroid plexus tumors

These tumors originate within the ventricular system, and are composed of "epithelial-like" cells reminiscent of choroid plexus [86].

a. Choroid plexus papilloma (CPP)

This is the most frequent entity in this group of tumors and is characterized by papillae lined by a single layer of bland looking cuboidal to columnar epithelial-like cells with abundant acidophilic cytoplasm, bland basal, round to oval nuclei [15]. Tubular or solid growths may occasionally be encountered [86]. Rare mitotic figures, microscopic infiltration into adjacent brain but not necrosis can be seen [14, 17]. Oncocytic changes, melanin deposition, calcification, ossification, and xanthogranulomatous changes may occasionally be encountered [86].

b. Atypical choroid plexus papilloma (atypical CPP)

This recent addition is characterized by preservation of the papillary architecture similar to papilloma, but with increased mitotic activity of ≥ 2 mitoses per 10 high power fields "Figure 23" [15, 87].

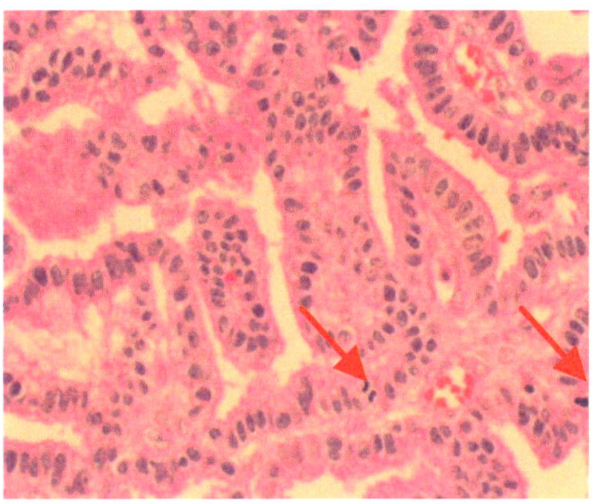

Figure 23. Atypical Choroid plexus tumor with typical papillary arrangement but several mitotic figures per high power field (arrows).

The additional presence of at least 2 of the following features might warrant the diagnosis of atypical CPP including increased cellularity, nuclear pleomorphism, solid growth and necrosis [17]. However; these are not necessary for the diagnosis.

c. Choroid plexus carcinoma

This is the most aggressive entity in this group of tumors and is characterized microscopically by blurring of the papillae with increased cellularity and pleomorphism in addition to features of frank malignancy including brisk mitosis of >5 MF/10HPFs, and necrosis [15]. Diffuse invasion into brain parenchyma is often seen [17]. PAS positive, diastase resistant variably-sized hyaline globules can be seen that are positive for alpha-1-antitrypsin [14].

The choroid plexus tumors are positive for cytokeratins, especially Cam 5.2, vimentin, S-100, transthyretin, and GFAP, with stains being more positive in papilloma versus carcinoma. Two recently described markers, stanniocalcin 1 and Kir 7.1 are claimed to be specific for choroid plexus tumors. EMA is typically negative in choroid plexus tumors [17], while CK7/CK20 show variable patterns and should be interpreted with caution [86]. MIB-1 proliferative index ranges between 1.9% in CPP to 13.8% in CPC, with higher indices correlating with poor outcome [14].

2.5. Tumors of the pineal region

a. Pineocytoma

This is a histologically bland tumor composed of mature-looking pinealocytes [17]. The cells are bland looking with amphophilic cytoplasm and round nuclei. Large fibrillary pineocytomatous rosettes and pseudorosettes can be seen. A pleomorphic variant is described with giant cells and abnormally-shaped hyperchromatic nuclei and gangliocytic cells [88]. No mitosis is seen in both variants. Immunostains are typically positive for NSE, synaptophysin, chromogranin A and neurofilaments [89]. MIB labeling index is usually zero [90].

b. Pineal parenchymal tumor of intermediate differentiation (PPTID)

This group accounts for at least 20% of tumors of the pineal gland and shows intermediate differentiation between pineocytoma and pineoblastoma [17]. They grow in sheets or lobules and are composed of uniform cells with moderate nuclear atypia. Although occasional Homer –Wright rosettes can be seen, pineocytoma-like rosettes are not reported. On the other hand; this tumor lacks the primitive cell appearance and necrosis typically seen in pineoblastoma [35]. According to the number of mitosis, proliferative index labeling and neurofilament immunostains, these tumors are divided into two prognostically different groups [17, 89]. MIB labeling index ranges between 5.2-11.2% [90].

c. Pineoblastoma

This is a small primitive tumor similar to CNS-PNET. It is hypercellular with proliferation of primitive cells with scant cytoplasm, hyperchromatic nuclei, nuclear pleomorphism and occasional prominent nucleoli. Frequent mitoses, necrosis and calcification can all be encountered [91]. Immunostains for NSE, synaptophysin, chromogranin A and neurofilaments are typically weak or negative [89]. MIB labeling index is around 36.4%-50% [90, 91].

d. Papillary tumor of the pineal region (PTPR)

This is the most recent addition to this group of tumors. It is seen both in children and adults. It grows in papillae with hyalinized cores that are lined by epithelial-like cells. The cells are large columnar to cuboidal, with pale to acidophilic cytoplasm and vesicular round nuclei, thus being different from pineal parenchymal tumors. These tumors are positive for cytokeratin, S-100 and vimentin with only focal positivity for GFAP [15]. EMA is usually negative or at best focally positive; an important feature in the differential diagnosis with ependymoma [17].

http://dx.doi.org/10.5772/52356

2.6. Other neuroepithelial tumors

a. Angiocentric glioma

This is probably a benign tumor that occurs in young adults with history of epilepsy. It is cortically based and is characterized by monomorphous bipolar cells with an angiocentric growth pattern, hence the name [15]. In most cases the cells tend to arrange themselves radially around blood vessels. Additionally 2 important distinct growth patterns can be seen in a subset of cases; the arrangement of the elongated tumor cells parallel to blood vessels causing sometimes expansion of the perivascular spaces and the tendency of the tumor cells to accumulate perpendicularly beneath the pia [17]. Immunostains are positive for EMA, GFAP, S-100 and vimentin. Neuronal markers are negative.

b. Chordoid glioma of the third ventricle

This tumor usually arises from the anterior third ventricle and is characterized by cohesive clusters and cords of epithelial-like cells growing in a myxoid background [92], hence the close resemblance to chordoma and chordoid meningioma [93], from which it should be differentiated. The presence of lympho-plasmacytic infiltrate which can sometimes be heavy with abundant Russell bodies is seen at the periphery and is helpful in supporting the diagnosis. Chondroid metaplasia can occasionally be encountered [94]. Reactivity for GFAP and vimentin is the rule but with variable reactivity for S-100. EMA is positive in the infiltrating plasma cells [20, 92].

c. Astroblastoma

A well circumscribed tumor that involves mostly the cerebral hemispheres, astroblastoma is characterized by perivascular pseudorosettes with sclerosed fibrovascular cores, on which broad cytoplasmic processes of astroblasts rest "Figure 24".

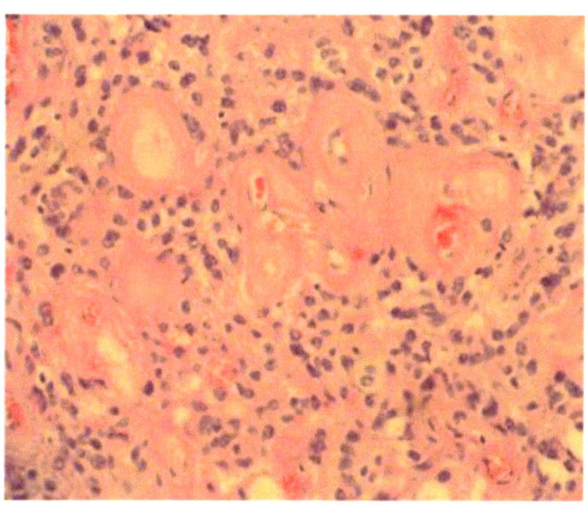

Figure 24. In astroblastoma hyalinized blood vessels are surrounded by cells with broad-based cytoplasmic processes.

This is in contrast to the fine tapering processes of classical ependymoma [20, 95]. A high grade "malignant" variant is diagnosed when hypercellularity, increased mitoses, vascular proliferation and palisading necrosis are seen, otherwise the tumor is considered a low grade or "benign" [14]. The tumor cell processes are strongly positive for vimentin and S-100, but focally for GFAP with focal membranous EMA reactivity.

2.7. Recently described tumor entities that are not included in the most recent WHO classification

a. Cribriform Neuroepithelial Tumor (CRINET)

This recently described tumor is composed of proliferation of a relatively small undifferentiated cells, arranged in cribriform, trabeculae, strands and focal compact areas exhibiting rosette formation [96]. Well defined surfaces characterize the cellular strands, which exhibit elongated nuclei but with no stratification. The cytoplasm is ill-defined and slightly acidophilic and the nuclei posses dense chromatin and lack prominent nucleoli. Mitoses and necrosis are seen. The tumor cells are immunoreactive for EMA highlights the surface as well as for vimentin, and synaptophysin with focal expression of cytokeratin and S-100. Other markers including GFAP, neurofilament, NeuN, chromogranin are negative. MIB-1 labeling index is elevated. Characteristically this tumor lack INI-1/Baf47 nuclear immunoreactivity, despite of lacking the typical features of AT/RT including eccentric acidophilic cytoplasm, cytoplasmic inclusions and vesicular nuclei with prominent nucleoli [96, 97]. CRINET seems to be associated with a better prognosis than AT/RT.

Author details

Maysa Al-Hussaini*

Address all correspondence to: mhussaini@khcc.jo

Department of Pathology and Laboratory Medicine, King Hussein Cancer Center, Amman, Jordan

References

[1] Rorke, L. B. *Pathologic diagnosis as the gold standard.* Cancer, (1997)., 665-667.

[2] Coons, S. W, et al. *Improving diagnostic accuracy and interobserver concordance in the classification and grading of primary gliomas.* Cancer, (1997)., 1381-1393.

[3] Pollack, I. F, et al. *The influence of central review on outcome associations in childhood malignant gliomas: results from the CCG-945 experience.* Neuro Oncol, (2003)., 197-207.

[4] Grisold, W, Oberndorfer, S, & Hitzenberger, P. *Editorial: Brain tumour treatment: the concept of inter- and multidisciplinary treatment.* Wien Med Wochenschr, (2006). , 329-331.

[5] Wharton, S. B, Ironside, H. D, Grant, J. W, & Collins, R. VP., *Dataset for tumours of the central nervous system, including the pituitary gland* R.C.o. Pathologists, Editor (2011). Londan.

[6] Qaddoumi, I, et al. *Closing the survival gap: implementation of medulloblastoma protocols in a low-income country through a twinning program.* Int J Cancer, (2008). , 1203-1206.

[7] Qaddoumi, I, et al. *Impact of telemedicine on pediatric neuro-oncology in a developing country: the Jordanian-Canadian experience.* Pediatr Blood Cancer, (2007). , 39-43.

[8] Louis, D. N. O, Wiestler, H, & Cavenee, O. D. W.K., *WHO Classification of Tumours of the Central Nervous System*. Fourth ed. (2007). Lyon: International Agency for Research on Cancer (IARC).

[9] Koeller, K. K, & Rushing, E. J. *From the archives of the AFIP: pilocytic astrocytoma: radiologic-pathologic correlation.* Radiographics, (2004). , 1693-1708.

[10] Tihan, T, et al. *Pathologic characteristics of pediatric intracranial pilocytic astrocytomas and their impact on outcome in 3 countries: a multi-institutional study.* Am J Surg Pathol, (2012). , 43-55.

[11] Tomlinson, F. H, et al. *The significance of atypia and histologic malignancy in pilocytic astrocytoma of the cerebellum: a clinicopathologic and flow cytometric study.* J Child Neurol, (1994). , 301-310.

[12] Cheng, Y, et al. *Pilocytic astrocytomas do not show most of the genetic changes commonly seen in diffuse astrocytomas.* Histopathology, (2000). , 437-444.

[13] Horbinski, C, et al. *Interplay among BRAF, 16p53, and MIB1 in pediatric low-grade gliomas.* Neuro Oncol, (2012). p. 777-89.

[14] Rickert, C. H, & Paulus, W. *Prognosis-related histomorphological and immunohistochemical markers in central nervous system tumors of childhood and adolescence.* Acta Neuropathol, (2005). , 69-92.

[15] Louis, D. N, et al. *The 2007 WHO classification of tumours of the central nervous system.* Acta Neuropathol, (2007). , 97-109.

[16] Ceppa, E. P, et al. *The pilomyxoid astrocytoma and its relationship to pilocytic astrocytoma: report of a case and a critical review of the entity.* J Neurooncol, (2007). , 191-196.

[17] Brat, D. J, et al. *Surgical neuropathology update: a review of changes introduced by the WHO classification of tumours of the central nervous system, 4th edition.* Arch Pathol Lab Med, (2008). , 993-1007.

[18] Kepes, J. J. *Pleomorphic xanthoastrocytoma: the birth of a diagnosis and a concept.* Brain Pathol, (1993). , 269-274.

[19] Tonn, J. C, et al. *Pleomorphic xanthoastrocytoma: report of six cases with special consideration of diagnostic and therapeutic pitfalls.* Surg Neurol, (1997). , 162-169.

[20] Dunbar, E, & Yachnis, A. T. *Glioma diagnosis: immunohistochemistry and beyond.* Adv Anat Pathol, (2010). , 187-201.

[21] Marton, E, et al. *Malignant progression in pleomorphic xanthoastrocytoma: personal experience and review of the literature.* J Neurol Sci, (2007). , 144-153.

[22] Buccoliero, A. M, et al. *Subependymal giant cell astrocytoma (SEGA): Is it an astrocytoma? Morphological, immunohistochemical and ultrastructural study.* Neuropathology, (2009). , 25-30.

[23] Grajkowska, W, et al. *Subependymal giant cell astrocytomas with atypical histological features mimicking malignant gliomas.* Folia Neuropathol, (2011). , 39-46.

[24] Kumar, R, & Singh, V. *Subependymal giant cell astrocytoma: a report of five cases.* Neurosurg Rev, (2004). , 274-280.

[25] Gupta, M, Djalilvand, A, & Brat, D. J. *Clarifying the diffuse gliomas: an update on the morphologic features and markers that discriminate oligodendroglioma from astrocytoma.* Am J Clin Pathol, (2005). , 755-768.

[26] Lind-landstrom, T, et al. *Prognostic value of histological features in diffuse astrocytomas WHO grade II.* Int J Clin Exp Pathol, (2012). , 152-158.

[27] Takei, H, et al. *New immunohistochemical markers in the evaluation of central nervous system tumors: a review of 7 selected adult and pediatric brain tumors.* Arch Pathol Lab Med, (2007). , 234-241.

[28] Camelo-piragua, S, et al. *Mutant IDH1-specific immunohistochemistry distinguishes diffuse astrocytoma from astrocytosis.* Acta Neuropathol, (2010). , 509-511.

[29] Johannessen, A. L, & Torp, S. H. *The clinical value of Ki-67/MIB-1 labeling index in human astrocytomas.* Pathol Oncol Res, (2006). , 143-147.

[30] Edgar, M. A, & Rosenblum, M. K. *Mixed glioneuronal tumors: recently described entities.* Arch Pathol Lab Med, (2007). , 228-233.

[31] Trembath, D, Miller, C. R, & Perry, A. *Gray zones in brain tumor classification: evolving concepts.* Adv Anat Pathol, (2008). , 287-297.

[32] Miller, C. R, & Perry, A. *Glioblastoma.* Arch Pathol Lab Med, (2007). , 397-406.

[33] Galloway, M. *CD34 expression in glioblastoma and giant cell glioblastoma.* Clin Neuropathol, (2010). , 89-93.

[34] Nagaishi, M, et al. *Transcriptional Factors for Epithelial-Mesenchymal Transition Are Associated with Mesenchymal Differentiation in Gliosarcoma.* Brain Pathol, (2012).

[35] Scheithauer, B. W, & Fuller, G. N. and S.R. VandenBerg, *The 2007 WHO classification of tumors of the nervous system: controversies in surgical neuropathology.* Brain Pathol, (2008). , 307-316.

[36] Perry, A, et al. *Malignant gliomas with primitive neuroectodermal tumor-like components: a clinicopathologic and genetic study of 53 cases.* Brain Pathol, (2009). , 81-90.

[37] Rodriguez, F. J, et al. *Epithelial and pseudoepithelial differentiation in glioblastoma and gliosarcoma: a comparative morphologic and molecular genetic study.* Cancer, (2008). , 2779-2789.

[38] Herrlinger, U, et al. *Gliomatosis cerebri: molecular pathology and clinical course.* Ann Neurol, (2002). , 390-399.

[39] Glas, M, et al. *NOA-05 phase 2 trial of procarbazine and lomustine therapy in gliomatosis cerebri.* Ann Neurol, (2011). , 445-453.

[40] Ikota, H, et al. *Systematic immunohistochemical profiling of 378 brain tumors with 37 antibodies using tissue microarray technology.* Acta Neuropathol, (2006). , 475-482.

[41] Perry, A, et al. *Oligodendrogliomas with neurocytic differentiation. A report of 4 cases with diagnostic and histogenetic implications.* J Neuropathol Exp Neurol, (2002). , 947-955.

[42] Edgar, M. A, & Rosenblum, M. K. *The differential diagnosis of central nervous system tumors: a critical examination of some recent immunohistochemical applications.* Arch Pathol Lab Med, (2008). , 500-509.

[43] Buckner, J. C, et al. *Prognosis in patients with anaplastic oligoastrocytoma is associated with histologic grade.* J Neurooncol, (2007). , 279-286.

[44] Al-hussaini, M, & Herron, B. *Metastasizing myxopapillary ependymoma.* Histopathology, (2005). , 469-470.

[45] Hussein, S. A, & Sur, M. *Cytokeratin positivity in myxopapillary ependymoma--a potential diagnostic pitfall.* Diagn Pathol, (2008). , 40.

[46] Rushing, E. J, et al. *Subependymoma revisited: clinicopathological evaluation of 83 cases.* J Neurooncol, (2007). , 297-305.

[47] Maiuri, F, et al. *Symptomatic subependymomas of the lateral ventricles. Report of eight cases.* Clin Neurol Neurosurg, (1997). , 17-22.

[48] Limaiem, F, et al. *Subependymomas: a clinicopathological study of 6 symptomatic cases.* Pathologica, (2008). , 401-404.

[49] Tihan, T, et al. *The prognostic value of histological grading of posterior fossa ependymomas in children: a Children's Oncology Group study and a review of prognostic factors.* Mod Pathol, (2008). , 165-177.

[50] Hasselblatt, M, & Paulus, W. *Sensitivity and specificity of epithelial membrane antigen staining patterns in ependymomas.* Acta Neuropathol, (2003). , 385-388.

[51] Choi, Y. L, Chi, J. G, & Suh, Y. L. *CD99 immunoreactivity in ependymoma.* Appl Immunohistochem Mol Morphol, (2001). , 125-129.

[52] Fouladi, M, et al. *Clear cell ependymoma: a clinicopathologic and radiographic analysis of 10 patients.* Cancer, (2003). , 2232-2244.

[53] Packer, R. J, & Mac, T. Donald, and G. Vezina, *Central nervous system tumors.* Pediatr Clin North Am, (2008). xi., 121-145.

[54] Mcmanamy, C. S, et al. *Nodule formation and desmoplasia in medulloblastomas-defining the nodular/desmoplastic variant and its biological behavior.* Brain Pathol, (2007). , 151-164.

[55] Verma, S, Tavare, C. J, & Gilles, F. H. *Histologic features and prognosis in pediatric medulloblastoma.* Pediatr Dev Pathol, (2008). , 337-343.

[56] Haberler, C, et al. *Histopathological prognostic factors in medulloblastoma: high expression of survivin is related to unfavourable outcome.* Eur J Cancer, (2006). , 2996-3003.

[57] Eberhart, C. G, et al. *Histopathologic grading of medulloblastomas: a Pediatric Oncology Group study.* Cancer, (2002). , 552-560.

[58] Eberhart, C. G, & Burger, P. C. *Anaplasia and grading in medulloblastomas.* Brain Pathol, (2003). , 376-385.

[59] Ishii, N, et al. *Alternative EWS-FLI1 fusion gene and MIC2 expression in peripheral and central primitive neuroectodermal tumors.* Neuropathology, (2001). , 40-44.

[60] Ray, A, et al. *A clinicobiological model predicting survival in medulloblastoma.* Clin Cancer Res, (2004). , 7613-7620.

[61] Gajjar, A, et al. *Clinical, histopathologic, and molecular markers of prognosis: toward a new disease risk stratification system for medulloblastoma.* J Clin Oncol, (2004). , 984-993.

[62] Tabori, U, et al. *Universal poor survival in children with medulloblastoma harboring somatic TP53 mutations.* J Clin Oncol, (2010). , 1345-1350.

[63] Ellison, D. W, et al. *Definition of disease-risk stratification groups in childhood medulloblastoma using combined clinical, pathologic, and molecular variables.* J Clin Oncol, (2011). , 1400-1407.

[64] Ellison, D. W, et al. *beta-Catenin status predicts a favorable outcome in childhood medulloblastoma: the United Kingdom Children's Cancer Study Group Brain Tumour Committee.* J Clin Oncol, (2005). , 7951-7957.

[65] Das, P, et al. *Medulloblastomas: a correlative study of MIB-1 proliferation index along with expression of c-Myc, ERBB2, and anti-apoptotic proteins along with histological typing and clinical outcome.* Childs Nerv Syst, (2009). , 825-835.

[66] Gessi, M, et al. *Embryonal tumors with abundant neuropil and true rosettes: a distinctive CNS primitive neuroectodermal tumor.* Am J Surg Pathol, (2009)., 211-217.

[67] Pfister, S, et al. *Novel genomic amplification targeting the microRNA cluster at 19q13.42 in a pediatric embryonal tumor with abundant neuropil and true rosettes.* Acta Neuropathol, (2009)., 457-464.

[68] Nishio, S, et al. *Supratentorial primitive neuroectodermal tumours: a report of four cases with an unusual clinical course in one patient.* Acta Neurochir (Wien), (1998)., 207-213.

[69] Theeler, B. J, et al. *Ewing's sarcoma family tumors mimicking primary central nervous system neoplasms.* J Neurol Sci, (2009)., 186-189.

[70] Athale, U. H, et al. *Childhood atypical teratoid rhabdoid tumor of the central nervous system: a meta-analysis of observational studies.* J Pediatr Hematol Oncol, (2009)., 651-663.

[71] Haberler, C, et al. *Immunohistochemical analysis of INI1 protein in malignant pediatric CNS tumors: Lack of INI1 in atypical teratoid/rhabdoid tumors and in a fraction of primitive neuroectodermal tumors without rhabdoid phenotype.* Am J Surg Pathol, (2006). , 1462-1468.

[72] Mohapatra, I, et al. *Histological and immunohistochemical characterization of AT/RT: a report of 15 cases from India.* Neuropathology, (2010)., 251-259.

[73] Blumcke, I, & Wiestler, O. D. *Gangliogliomas: an intriguing tumor entity associated with focal epilepsies.* J Neuropathol Exp Neurol, (2002)., 575-584.

[74] Luyken, C, et al. *Supratentorial gangliogliomas: histopathologic grading and tumor recurrence in 184 patients with a median follow-up of 8 years.* Cancer, (2004)., 146-155.

[75] Hirose, T, et al. *Ganglioglioma: an ultrastructural and immunohistochemical study.* Cancer, (1997)., 989-1003.

[76] Diepholder, H. M, et al. *A clinicopathologic and immunomorphologic study of 13 cases of ganglioglioma.* Cancer, (1991)., 2192-2201.

[77] Wolf, H. K, et al. *Ganglioglioma: a detailed histopathological and immunohistochemical analysis of 61 cases.* Acta Neuropathol, (1994)., 166-173.

[78] VandenBergS.R., *Desmoplastic infantile ganglioglioma and desmoplastic cerebral astrocytoma of infancy.* Brain Pathol, (1993)., 275-281.

[79] Gelabert-gonzalez, M, Serramito-garcia, R, & Arcos-algaba, A. *Desmoplastic infantile and non-infantile ganglioglioma. Review of the literature.* Neurosurg Rev, (2010). , 151-158.

[80] De Munnynck, K, et al. *Desmoplastic infantile ganglioglioma: a potentially malignant tumor?* Am J Surg Pathol, (2002)., 1515-1522.

[81] Daumas-duport, C. *Dysembryoplastic neuroepithelial tumours.* Brain Pathol, (1993). , 283-295.

[82] Daumas-duport, C, et al. *Dysembryoplastic neuroepithelial tumors: nonspecific histological forms-- a study of 40 cases.* J Neurooncol, (1999). , 267-280.

[83] Hassoun, J, et al. *Central neurocytoma: a synopsis of clinical and histological features.* Brain Pathol, (1993). , 297-306.

[84] Brat, D. J, et al. *Extraventricular neurocytomas: pathologic features and clinical outcome.* Am J Surg Pathol, (2001). , 1252-1260.

[85] Chakraborti, S, et al. *Supratentorial and cerebellar liponeurocytomas: report of four cases with review of literature.* J Neurooncol, (2011). , 121-127.

[86] Ikota, H, et al. *Clinicopathological and immunohistochemical study of 20 choroid plexus tumors: their histological diversity and the expression of markers useful for differentiation from metastatic cancer.* Brain Tumor Pathol, (2011). , 215-221.

[87] Jeibmann, A, et al. *Prognostic implications of atypical histologic features in choroid plexus papilloma.* J Neuropathol Exp Neurol, (2006). , 1069-1073.

[88] Fevre-montange, M, et al. *Prognosis and histopathologic features in papillary tumors of the pineal region: a retrospective multicenter study of 31 cases.* J Neuropathol Exp Neurol, (2006). , 1004-1011.

[89] Fauchon, F, et al. *Parenchymal pineal tumors: a clinicopathological study of 76 cases.* Int J Radiat Oncol Biol Phys, (2000). , 959-968.

[90] Fevre-montange, M, et al. *Utility of Ki67 immunostaining in the grading of pineal parenchymal tumours: a multicentre study.* Neuropathol Appl Neurobiol, (2012). , 87-94.

[91] Gilheeney, S. W, et al. *Outcome of pediatric pineoblastoma after surgery, radiation and chemotherapy.* J Neurooncol, (2008). , 89-95.

[92] Brat, D. J, et al. *Third ventricular chordoid glioma: a distinct clinicopathologic entity.* J Neuropathol Exp Neurol, (1998). , 283-290.

[93] Ricoy, J. R, et al. *Suprasellar chordoid glioma.* Acta Neuropathol, (2000). , 699-703.

[94] Castellano-sanchez, A. A, et al. *Pediatric chordoid glioma with chondroid metaplasia.* Pediatr Dev Pathol, (2001). , 564-567.

[95] Brat, D. J, et al. *Astroblastoma: clinicopathologic features and chromosomal abnormalities defined by comparative genomic hybridization.* Brain Pathol, (2000). , 342-352.

[96] Hasselblatt, M, et al. *Cribriform neuroepithelial tumor (CRINET): a nonrhabdoid ventricular tumor with INI1 loss and relatively favorable prognosis.* J Neuropathol Exp Neurol, (2009). , 1249-1255.

[97] Park, J. Y, et al. *Cribriform neuroepithelial tumor in the third ventricle: A case report and literature review.* Neuropathology, (2012).

Section 3

Brain Metastases

Chapter 8

Surgical Treatment for Multiple Brain Metastases

Takeshi Okuda and Amami Kato

Additional information is available at the end of the chapter

http://dx.doi.org/10.5772/52353

1. Introduction

Brain metastasis occurs with a fairly high frequency, in 25–35% of cancer patients [1]. Because brain metastasis directly affects prognosis, quality of life (QOL), and performance status (PS), treatment is crucial. Survival time is reported to be 1 month in the case of untreated brain metastasis [2], 2 months with steroid treatment alone [3], and 3-6 months with whole-brain radiotherapy (WBRT) [4-7]. This shows that brain metastasis is a seriously life-threatening condition. Therapeutic approaches have become more varied with the appearance of stereotactic radiosurgery (SRS), and establishment of multiple treatment plans has become possible. In addition to surgical resection (SR), WBRT, and SRS, systemic chemotherapy (SC) is also an option. The ideal treatment is to control the brain metastasis and prevent destruction of the central nervous system using combinations of these therapeutic approaches. Among these multiple approaches, SR is effective in that it enables treatment of large tumors and early improvement of symptoms, which are not possible with other approaches. The indications for SR are expanded with the early improvement of symptoms, leading particularly to improved QOL from the palliative viewpoint. However, SR is also highly invasive compared with other treatments, and the indications are strict. The standard surgical indication is single brain metastasis, and patients with fairly good prognosis, such as those with good general condition, are selected [8]. Recently, however, partly as a result of advances in imaging, the number of cases of multiple brain metastases has been trending upward. This means that there are patients in whom SR is excluded as an indication because of findings for multiple brain metastases, and who cannot obtain the benefits of surgery. We provide aggressive treatment using the same surgical indications for cases of multiple brain metastases as for single metastasis. The present study therefore investigated treatment outcomes and reported on the effectiveness of SR for multiple brain metastases.

2. Methods

Subjects were 100 patients with brain metastasis who underwent craniotomy and surgical removal of tumors in the Department of Neurosurgery at Kinki University Hospital between 2004 and 2011. They included 54 patients with single brain metastasis and 46 with multiple brain metastases. Details are shown in Table 1.

Characteristic	Single	Multiple
No. of cases	54	46
Age (mean)	63.3	61.3
Range	39-81	46-81
Male-to-female ratio	31:23	22:24
Primary site		
Lung	29	22
Breast	9	13
Rectum	2	3
Colon	3	1
Kidney	2	1
Other	9	6
RPA classification		
I	18	10
II	21	12
III	15	24
Size (mm, mean)	34.1	28.7

Table 1. Clinical characteristics of patients with single and multiple brain metastases

Surgical indications are shown in Figure 1, and treatments following surgery were done in close conference with departments related to cancer, such as the Department of Radiation Oncology and the Department of Medical Oncology. Each case was treated using a tailor-made approach.

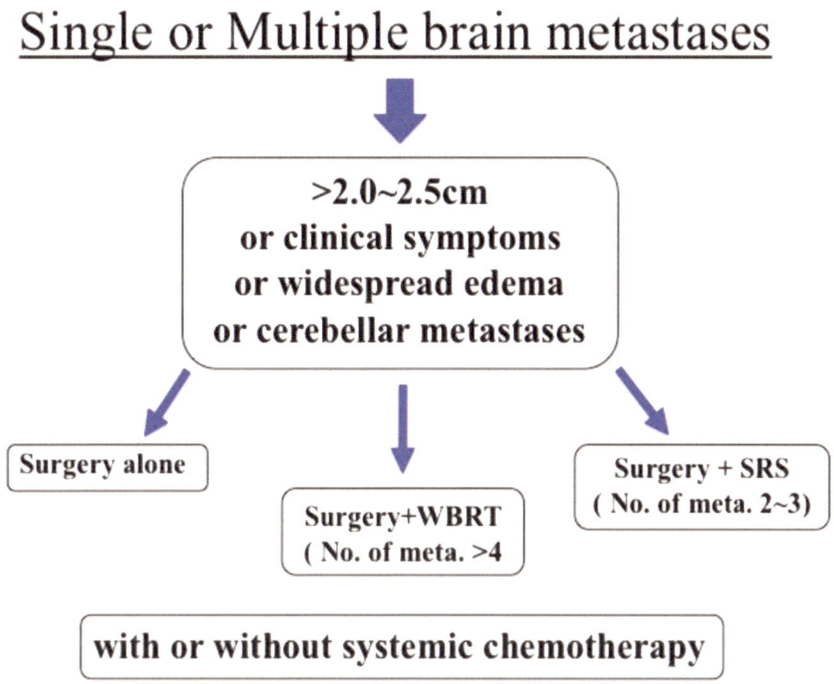

Figure 1. Therapeutic strategies in brain metastases

The basic surgery was en bloc resection, with resection of a single site even in cases of multiple metastases. During removal, we used fluorescence-guided surgery using fluorescein sodium with transformation to a solid-type tumor by hydrofiber dressing for cystic lesions [9-11]. In comparing survival time, duration of survival from the day of surgery until death was obtained using the Kaplan-Meier method, and significant differences were determined with the log-rank test. For all tests, a significance level of 5% was applied.

3. Results

Among the 100 patients, gross total resection was performed in 89%. Reasons for sub-total resection were invasion into blood vessels or dura mater, huge tumor size, or tumor involving an eloquent area. Follow-up treatments are shown in Figure 2. SC was also performed in 45 cases.

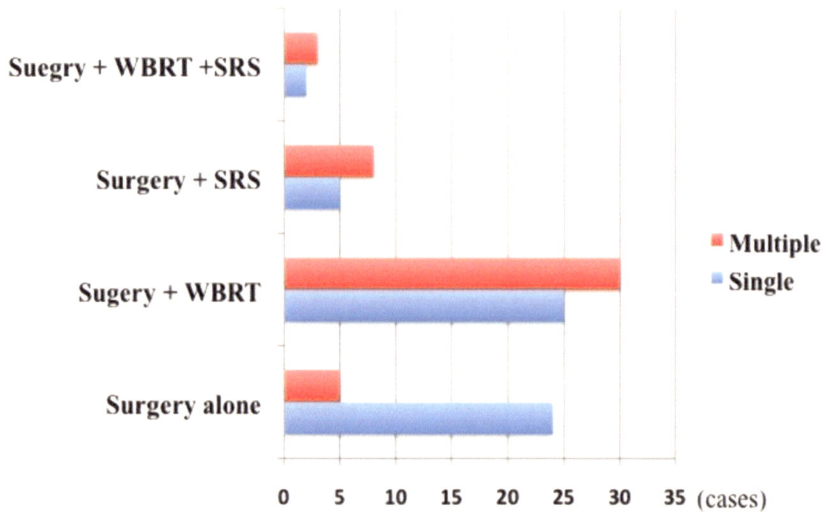

Figure 2. Postoperative treatments. Concurrent systematic chemotherapy was used in 45% of cases.

Central nervous system death occurred in 9% and 6 patients died within 3 months of surgery. Three of these patients showed exacerbation of the primary cancer and three showed poor control of brain metastases. For all 100 patients median survival time (MST) was 9.3 months, the 1-year survival rate was 45%, the 2-year survival rate was 10%. A comparison of single and multiple metastases is shown in Table 2.

	Single	Multiple
Median survival time (mo)	9.8	8.1
1- year survival rate (%)	44	46
2- year survival rate (%)	11	9

Table 2. Survival rate of single and multiple metastases

In this comparison by number of metastases, no significant differences were seen in survival time, including 1-year survival rate, 2-year survival rate, or MST (Fig. 3).

http://dx.doi.org/10.5772/52353

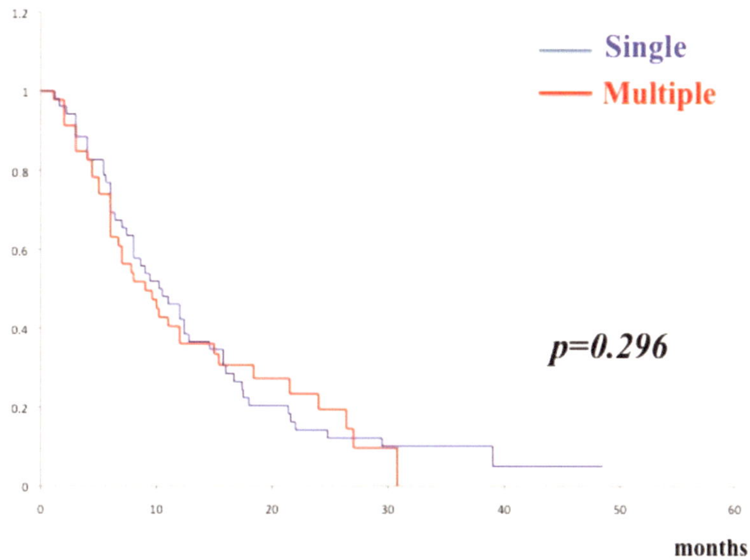

Figure 3. Comparison of survival times with single and multiple brain metastases. No statistically significant difference was confirmed between the 2 groups (p=0.296).

In a comparison by number of metastases in patients with multiple metastases, no significant difference in survival time was seen between patients with 2-3 metastases (MST, 8.8 months; n=32) and those with ≥4 metastases (MST, 8.0 months; n=14) (Fig. 4).

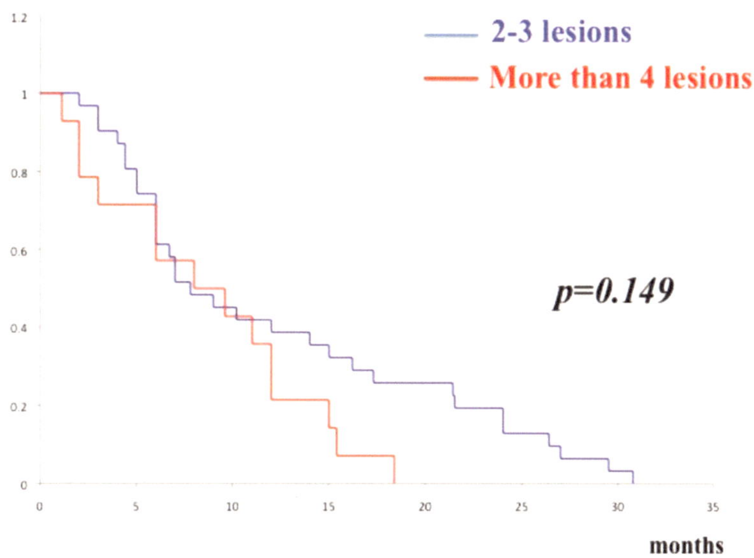

Figure 4. Comparison of survival times according to number of metastases in cases of multiple brain metastases. No statistically significant difference was confirmed between the 2 groups (p=0.149).

In addition, new pathological findings were revealed through pathological diagnosis obtained with SR, and the treatment strategy was changed in some cases. The case of a typical patient is described below.

This patient was a 49-year-old woman who was undergoing chemotherapy for lung cancer (adenocarcinoma). SC was continued for 4 courses, when she was switched to best supportive care because of a lack of efficacy. In screening tests for headache and visual impairment, six brain metastases were seen. At this point, multiple metastases to other organs were identified and she was expected to live less than 3 months (Fig. 5A-C).

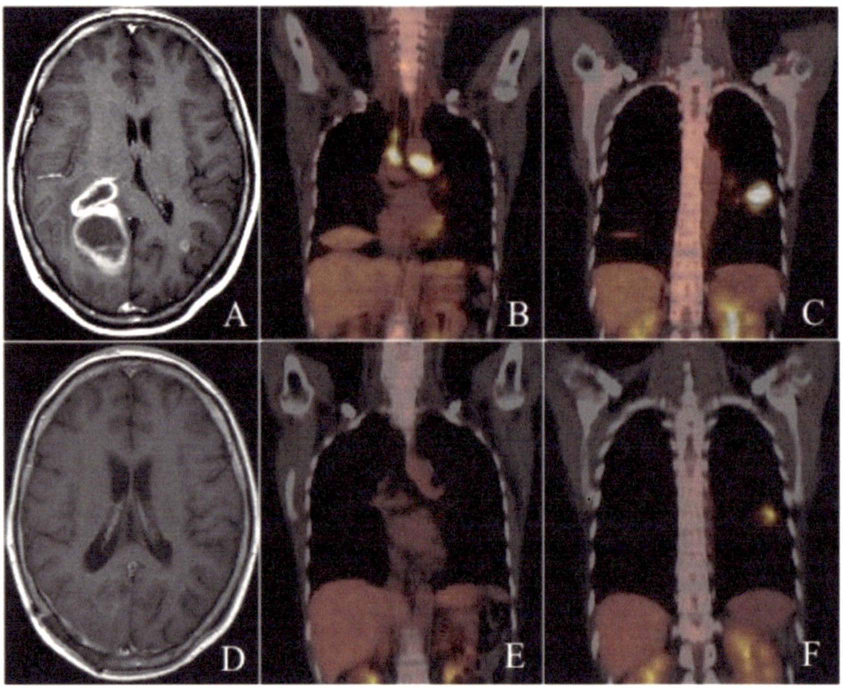

Figure 5. A) Contrast-enhanced MRI findings before treatment. A total of six metastases are seen, including a lesion ≥4 cm in diameter with ventricular invasion in the right occipital lobe. (B,C) Preoperative FDG-PET examination. Multiple metastases are seen in the lungs. (D) Contrast-enhanced MRI after treatment. All of the multiple lesions have disappeared. (E,F) FDG-PET examination following systemic chemotherapy. The lesions in the lungs are markedly reduced in size.

Headache associated with increased intracranial pressure is difficult to treat, and SR was performed for the right occipital lobe lesion with the aim of relieving symptoms. Symptoms rapidly improved after surgery, and the pathological diagnosis was small cell cancer. Initially, the diagnosis had been adenocarcinoma based on adenocarcinomatous tissue obtained from bronchoscopic biopsy of the primary lung cancer. In fact, however, the tumor represented mixed-type lung cancer with small cell cancer, and these brain metastases was thought to represent a recurrence of the small cell cancer. WBRT was performed postoperatively and SC

http://dx.doi.org/10.5772/52353

was applied using the approach used for small cell lung cancer. A marked decrease in systemic lesions was seen (Fig. 5D-F). Ultimately, the patient survived 19 months after surgery. This patient obtained a greater-than-expected benefit from surgery.

4. Discussion

Various biases are inherent in the treatment for brain metastasis, according to factors such as the primary cancer or general condition. Moreover, because of the problem of brain function, establishing a treatment plan can be difficult. In such circumstances, many reports with a fairly high evidence level have described results for single brain metastasis. Reports on level I include those of Patchell et al. [12] and Noordijk et al. [13] in the 1990s. SR + WBRT was established for single brain metastasis based on these reports. In a report by Bindal et al. [14], SR for multiple brain metastases was seen to be effective only in cases when all of the multiple brain metastases could be removed. However, when all lesions could not be removed, no significant difference was seen compared with WBRT alone, and SR was not considered effective. Based on these findings, the priority came to be placed on WBRT monotherapy in cases of multiple brain metastases, but treatment later diversified with active SRS intervention for brain metastasis and in 1999 Kondziolka et al. [15] reported WBRT + SRS combination radiotherapy for cases of multiple brain metastasis. With this approach, significantly longer survival times were obtained compared with WBRT alone, and WBRT + SRS became the general therapy for multiple brain metastases. In 2006, Aoyama et al. [16] also reported the efficacy of SRS monotherapy for brain metastasis with ≤4 lesions. Various treatment strategies have thus been reported, including not only conventional WBRT, but also combination with SRS and SRS monotherapy. Recent reports have also suggested the efficacy of SC for multiple brain metastases [17]. Up to this time, there has been little recognition of the efficacy of SC for brain metastasis. A response rate of 60% has been reported, but the effect is temporary and MST is less than 6 months in the majority of cases [18-20]. However, striking advances have recently been made in SC, with the emergence of molecularly targeted drugs as a major breakthrough. Drugs for lung cancer include gefitinib and erlotinib. The response rate to erlotinib is in cases of brain metastasis with EGFR mutation, showing very high efficacy. In breast cancer, the appearance of lapatinib is also reported to be effective against brain metastasis. SC will thus likely become necessary as one therapeutic approach in brain metastasis, particularly for patients with multiple brain metastases.

As mentioned above, various therapeutic approaches can be used for brain metastasis, including SR, WBRT, SRS, and SC, and various combinations. In this situation, at our hospital, we do not consider it necessary to select treatment based on the number of metastases, such as single or multiple, and aggressively perform SR in cases of multiple metastases just as in cases of single metastasis. Likewise in follow-up treatment, we implement tailor-made treatment strategies matched to the individual patients. The results have shown no differences in either MST or survival rate depending on the number of metastases, and good treatment outcomes have been obtained in cases of multiple brain metastases. Today, when various therapeutic approaches are available, performing SR to eliminate lesions at an early stage is highly effective. Early improvement of symptoms leads to improved PS and QOL, producing new treatment opportunities. In addition, early elimination of brain metastatic lesions reduces the steroid dosage as well as the possibility of radiation necrosis. The result is thought to lead ultimately to longer survival times. In our investigation, prognosis tended to be better for the group with fewer brain metastases (2-3 lesions), but the difference did not reach the level of statistical significance. This suggests that there is no correlation between prognosis and the number of metastases, including even single brain metastases. This is also supported by the low probability of central nervous system death. The total number of patients in this study was low (100 patients) and it was not a randomized controlled trial, so the results of evaluation are not definitive. However, the advances in cancer treatment in recent years may necessitate a rethink of the policy of determining treatment plans based on the number of metastases.

5. Conclusions

The efficacy of SR in multiple brain metastases was investigated. Survival time and survival rate were not significantly different compared with single brain metastasis, and no significant difference was seen in a comparison of survival time according to number of metastases. The reasons are thought to be that tailor-made therapeutic strategies using the multimodalities advanced in recent years are effective. It may be time to rethink the approach of determining treatment plans based on the number of metastases in therapeutic strategies for brain metastases.

Author details

Takeshi Okuda and Amami Kato

*Address all correspondence to: okuda@neuro-s.med.kindai.ac.jp

Department of Neurosurgery, Kinki University School of Medicine, Osaka, Japan

References

[1] Paek SH, Audu PB, Sperling MR, Cho J, Andrews DW. Reevaluation of surgery for the treatment of brain metastases: Review of 208 patients with single or multiple brain metastases treated at one institution with modern neurosurgical techniques. Neurosurgery 2005;56: 1021-1034.

[2] Markesbery WR, Brooks WH, Gupta GD, Young AB. Treatment for patients with cerebral metastases. Arch Neurol 1978;35: 754-756.

[3] Ruderman NB, Hall TC. Use of glucocorticoids in the palliative treatment of metastatic brain tumors. Cancer 1965;18: 298-306.

[4] Cairncross JG, Kim JH, Posner JB. Radiation therapy for brain metastases. Ann Neurol 1980;7: 529-541.

[5] Kurtz JM, Gelber R, Brady LW, Carella RJ, Cooper JS. The palliation of brain metastases in a favorable patient population: A randomized clinical trial by the Radiation Oncology Group. Int J Radiat Oncol Biol Phys 1981;7: 891-895.

[6] Patchell RA, Tibbs PA, Regine WF, Dempsey RJ, Mohiuddin M, Kryscio RJ, Markesbery WR, Foon KA, Young B. Postoperative radiotherapy in the treatment of single metastases to the brain: A randomized trial. JAMA 1998;280: 1485-1489.

[7] Sause WT, Crowley JJ, Morantz R, Rotman M, Mowry PA, Bouzaglou A, Borst JR, Selin H. Solitary brain metastasis: Results of an RTOG/SWOG protocol evaluation surgery plus RT versus RT alone. Am J Clin Oncol 1990;13: 427-432.

[8] Mut M. Surgical treatment of brain metastasis: A review. Clin Neurol Neurosurg 2012;114(1): 1-8.

[9] Okuda T, Kataoka K, Taneda M. Metastatic brain tumor surgery using fluorescein sodium: technical note. Minim Invas Neurosurg 2007;50: 382-384.

[10] Okuda T, Teramoto Y, Yugami H, Kataoka K, Kato A. Surgical technique for a cystic-type metastatic brain tumor: transformation to a solid-type tumor using hydrofiber dressing. Surg Neurol 2009;72: 703-706.

[11] Okuda T, Kataoka K, Yabuuchi T, Yugami H, Kato A. Fluorescence-guided surgery of metastatic brain tumors using fluorescein sodium. J Clin Neurosci 2010;17: 118-121.

[12] Patchell RA, Tibbs PA, Walsh JW, Dempsey RJ, Maruyama Y, Kryscio RJ, Markesbery WR, Macdonald JS, Young B. A randomized trial of surgery in the treatment of single metastases to the brain. N Engl J Med 1990;322: 494-500.

[13] Noordijk EM, Vecht CJ, Haaxma-Reiche H, Padberg GW, Voormolen JH, Hoekstra FH, Tans JT, Lambooij N, Metsaars JA, Wattendorff AR. The choice of treatment of single brain metastasis shoud be based on extracranial tumor activity and age. Int J Radiat Oncol Biol Phys 1994;29: 711-717.

[14] Bindel RK, Sawaya R, Leavens ME, Lee JJ. Surgical treatment of multiple brain metastases. J Neurosurg 1993;79: 210-216.

[15] Kondziolka D, Patel A, Lunsford LD, Kassam A, Flickinger JC. Stereotactic radiosurgery plus whole brain radiotherapy versus radiotherapy alone for patients with multiple brain metastases. Int J Radiat Oncol Biol Phys 1999;45: 427-434.

[16] Aoyama H, Shirato H, Tago M, Nakagawa K, Toyoda T, Hatano K, Kenjyo M, Oya N, Hirota S, Shioura H, Kunieda E, Inomata T, Hayakawa K, Katoh N, Kobayashi G.

Stereotactic radiotherapy plus whole-brain radiation therapy vs stereotactic radiosurgery alone for treatment of brain metastases: a randomized controlled trial. JAMA 2006;295: 2483-2491.

[17] Grimm SA. Treatment of brain metastases: chemotherapy. Curr Oncol Rep 2012;14(1): 85-90.

[18] Drappatz J, Wen PY. Chemotherapy and targeted molecular therapies for brain metastases. Expert Rev Neurother 2006;6(10): 1465-1479.

[19] van den Bent MJ. The role of chemotherapy in brain metastases. Eur J Cancer 2003;39(15): 2114-2120.

[20] Walbert T, Gilbert MR. The role of chemotherapy in the treatment of patients with brain metatstases from solid tumors. Int J Clin Oncol 2009;14(4): 299-306.

Chapter 9

Metastatic Brain Tumors

Steven N. Kalkanis and Sanjay Patra

Additional information is available at the end of the chapter

http://dx.doi.org/10.5772/51041

1. Introduction

The 2008 American Cancer Society Registry data show that approximately 1.4 million Americans are diagnosed with cancer every year of which 40% will go onto to develop brain metastases. Consequently, the incidence of these secondary brain tumors is about four to five times that of primary brain tumors [1, 2].

The past two decades have seen a large increase in treatment options, resulting in longer life expectancy and better quality of life to a point where metastatic lesions are no longer the major cause of mortality in this patient group. This has made decision making on treatment modality more complex. Evidence for local aggressive control through surgery and stereotactic radiosurgery (SRS) [3–5] has resulted in a paradigm shift since the mid 1990's when whole brain radiation therapy (WBRT) was the mainstay of treatment. Now, treatment of metastatic tumors includes a full spectrum of medical providers including neurosurgeons, medical oncologists, radiation oncologists, neurologists, and neuro-oncologists. This Chapter will focus on the contemporary management of metastatic brain tumors using surgery, radiosurgery, conventional radiation therapy, chemotherapy, steroids, anti-epileptics, and emerging modalities. Given the myriad of treatment options and the multiple providers utilizing them, the substantiation for these treatments are vital for the clinician to make an evidence-based decision. The information in this chapter will not only serve to guide the clinician in treatment options, but also to focus the researcher on areas that need further investigation.

2. Radiation Therapy

Historically, whole brain radiation therapy (WBRT) was the mainstay for treatment of metastatic brain tumors. Today, it remains an important part of the treatment regime, although in a more complimentary role.

In the randomized control trial (RTC) of Patchell [6] a total of 48 patients were treated with WBRT and either biopsy or complete surgical resection. The surgical group had a statistically significant increase in survival (40 weeks) compared to the biopsy group (15 weeks) (Ib/A). Freedom from death due to neurologic compromise, duration of functional independence and time to recurrence of a new brain lesion were all increased significantly as well. All patients had a Karnofsky performance score (KPS) of at least 70 and patients with acute neurological deterioration and radiosensitive tumors (SCLC, lymphoma, germ cell tumors, multiple myeloma or leukemia) were excluded from the study.

Another RCT done in Canada done by Mitz et al looked at 84 patients treated with WBRT and surgery or WBRT alone [7]. This trial included patients who spent greater than 50% of day in bed and MRI scans were not mandatory. They did not find any statistically significant difference in causes of death, quality of life, or overall survival. The lack of mandatory MRI scans raised the possibility of patients with multiple lesions being included in the study population.

Finally, a RTC done by Vecht et al [8] in the Netherlands looked at 63 patients and compared surgical resection plus WBRT to WBRT alone. Survival in the surgical group was significantly longer (10 months) compared with the non-surgical group (6 months). The patients included in the trial were younger than 60 years, within 6 months of diagnosis, and without progressive systemic disease.

In total, there are three randomized controlled trials (RCTs) [6-8] and three level II studies [9-11] that show surgical resection plus WBRT is superior to WBRT alone for surgically accessible single brain (verified by MRI) metastatic lesions in patients with limited extra cranial disease who spend less than 50% of the day in bed. Taken together, there is level Ia/A evidence supporting the use of surgical resection plus WBRT rather than WBRT alone.

3. WBRT dosing and fractionation schedule

There are 10 level I studies [12-20] including 9 RCT that have shown deviating from the standard 30Gy in 10 fractions does not significantly change local control, neurocognitive outcome or median survival in newly diagnosed adults with brain metastasis (Ia/A).

4. Surgical Resection

In the previous section we described the evidence for improved mortality outcomes in patients with newly diagnosed single metastatic lesions undergoing surgical resection plus WBRT compared to WBRT alone in terms of overall survival. Various groups have compared the effects of surgery alone to surgery plus WBRT given the known side effects of radio therapy.

Patchel et al [3] studied 95 patients who underwent MRI verified complete surgical resection and randomized them to receive WBRT or no further treatment. Tumor recurrence was 70%

in the surgery alone group compared to 18% in the WBRT group (p<0.001). Recurrences were lower for both the resection site and de novo lesions. There were fewer deaths from neurologic causes in the WBRT (14% vs. 44%) but the study was not powered to analyze overall survival. This RCT along with three retrospective cohort studies [21-23] provide level Ib/A evidence for improved tumor control with surgical resection and WBRT compared to surgical resection alone.

With the emergence of high dose single fraction radiotherapy groups have compared surgical resection plus WBRT to stereotactic radiosurgery (SRS) alone. There has been one small multicenter RCT in Germany by Muacevic et al [24] that enrolled a total of 64 patients with KPS scores greater than 70 with single, small (<3cm) metastatic lesion into a surgical resection plus WBRT group and a SRS group. Their primary outcome was overall survival but they also looked at time of freedom from local recurrence. The only outcome that was statistically different between the groups was distant recurrence, which was higher in the SRS alone group.

There have been four retrospective cohort studies [25-28] comparing surgical resection and WBRT to SRS and WBRT. Taken together these studies provide level III/B evidence that surgical resection with WBRT is comparable to SRS with WBRT in terms of survival and local recurrence. These studies also show that lesions larger than 3cm or those with significant mass effect have better outcomes with surgical resection and WBRT.

5. Stereotactic radiosurgery

SRS has emerged as a less invasive focal treatment modality to treat metastatic lesion. There have been two RCTs comparing single dose SRS and WBRT to WBRT alone.

Kondziolka et al [4] evaluated a total of 27 patients (KPS<70) with 2-4 solid metastatic lesions less than 2.5cm in diameter and randomized them to receive SRS and WBRT or WBRT alone. The primary outcome was image-defined local tumor control with median survival being the secondary outcome. The study showed the local failure rate was 8% in the SRS plus WBRT group compared to 100% in the WBRT group. The study was stopped prematurely due to this significant benefit. This did not give the study enough power to look at survival.

The other multicenter RCT [5] looked at a total of 272 patients with 1-3 solid metastatic lesions (<4cm in diameter) and KPS of more than 70. They randomized patients into a group undergoing WBRT plus SRS and WBRT alone. Their primary endpoint was median survival which was statistically improved in the group receiving SRS (6.5 vs. 5.7 months). Superior one year local control and improved KPS was also evident in the group receiving SRS.

There have also been three other retrospective series [29-31] looking at the above comparisons which have supported the findings of the RCTs in regards to improved overall survival, thus providing level Ia/A evidence for using single dose SRS with WBRT rather than WBRT alone for single metastatic lesions in patients with a KPS greater than 70. There is level IIa/B evidence that SRS plus WBRT is superior in local tumor control and maintaining functional status compared with WBRT alone in patients with less than 4 lesions.

There has been one RCT that compared SRS alone to WBRT plus SRS. This was a multi-institutional study by Aoyama et al [32] that randomized patients with 1-4 solid brain metastatic lesions (diameter <3cm) and KPS greater than 70 to received SRS alone or SRS with WBRT. Median survival, which was the primary end point, was not statistically different between the groups (8vs7.5 months). No difference was found in 1 year local control or neurologic cause of death. Distant brain recurrence and the requirement for salvage therapy were significantly greater in the SRS alone group. There has also been a prospective cohort study [30] along with 9 retrospective cohort studies [33-41] that have addressed this question. Together, there is level IIa/B evidence that SRS alone provides a similar survival advantage to SRS and WBRT. There is also Ia/B evidence that WBRT provides improved distant site control. For this reason patients only undergoing SRS require close monitoring so salvage therapy can be delivered early to a de novo lesion.

A three arm prospective cohort study by Li et al [30] provides a comparison between SRS alone and WBRT alone. The SRS alone group had improved neuroimaging response (87% vs. 38%), median time to progression (6.9 vs. 4 months) and longer median survival (9.3 vs. 5.7) months. Although there have been no RCTs addressing this question data from the Li et al trial and four other retrospective cohorts studies [42-45] provides level II/B evidence for SRS alone being superior to WBRT alone in terms of survival for patients with up to 3 lesions.

6. Chemotherapy

Chemotherapy has remained the primary treatment modality for systemic metastases. However, it is believed that brain metastases are selected to be chemoresistent because only resistant cells are able to survive systemic chemotherapy and make it to the brain. Furthermore, the effectiveness of chemotherapy in the brain has remained a concern due to the blood-brain barrier and active efflux pumps [46] limiting the effective dose in the central nervous system. For this reason, chemotherapy has been less effective in treating CNS metastases. This is evident from a study [47] that involved treatment of metastatic SCLC which showed decreased effectiveness from chemotherapy of CNS compared to system lesions.

There have been four RCTs [48-51] comparing WBRT plus chemotherapy to WBRT alone. A multi-institutional RCT [48] studied patients who had histologically proven NSCLC and a WHO performance status of 0, 1, or two and at least one brain metastasis on CT or MRI. These patients either refused surgery or were deemed inoperable. The patients were randomized to receive WBRT and Carboplatin or WBRT alone and the primary end point was overall survival. The median survival was similar in both groups. The trial was halted for poor accrual and did not show improved survival (Ib/A).

Another RCT was performed by Ushio et al [49] where patients with all lung cancer subtypes and projected survivals of greater than 4 months were randomized to WBRT, WBRT plus chloroethyl nitrosourea (CCNU), and WBRT plus CCNU plus tegafur. Patients were excluded if they received any prior chemotherapy. The primary end point of tumor response rates were 36%, 69%, and 74% respectively. The only statistically significant difference was between WBRT and WBRT plus CCNU plus tegafur. The secondary end point of survival showed no statistically significant difference (Ib/A).

The two other RCTs [50, 51] looked at temazolamide (TMZ) and radiotherapy and did not show any statistically significant differences.

Taken together these studies provide level Ia/A evidence that adding chemotherapy to WBRT does not improve survival. However, these trials did not take into account all histologies, focusing on NSCLC and breast cancer and their results cannot be applied to chemo sensitive tumors such as germinomas.

7. Re-treatment

There is very little data on managing recurrent metastasis. Detailed guidelines on this were published by Ammirati et al in 2010 [52].

There have been three retrospective case series looking at the effects of repeating WBRT in patients with brain recurrence following previous therapy. Post WBRT survival was 4-5 months in all series [53-55] (III/B).

Four case series [56-59] evaluated the effects of surgery on patients with recurrent or progressive brain metastases. Median time to recurrence at local and distant sites was 5-8.4 months with survival ranging from 8.9-11.5 months (III/B).

There has been one prospective Phase/II study [59] that investigated the effects of SRS for recurrent brain metastases. Twelve patients with progressive metastatic lesions, with at least 3 months of projected survival and who were previously treated with WBRT were given SRS. The median survival was 6 months.

Currently, there is only enough evidence to give a level III/B recommendation for individualization of care based on functional status, extent of systemic and intracranial disease, previous treatment type, primary cancer type, progression at original or distant site, and enrollment in clinical trials. Taking this into consideration no further treatment of WBRT, SRS or surgical excision can be recommended.

8. Prophylactic anticonvulsants

It is thought that brain metastases are unlikely to be as epileptogenic as primary gliomas due to their less infiltrative nature. However, the role of prophylactic antiepileptic drugs (AEDs) remains unclear. Mikklesen et al [60] has published evidence-based guidelines on this topic in 2010.

Forsyth et al [61] performed a RCT and studied anticonvulsant use in 100 patients with all types of brain tumors and stratified them into primary and metastatic groups. Exclusion criterions were known seizures, life expectancy less than 4 weeks, allergies to AEDs, history of substance abuse, and pregnancy. Most patients were treated with phenytoin. The primary outcome was seizure occurrence at 3 months. The trial was halted early because the anticipated seizure rate in the non AED arm was only 10% and the 3 month mortality was higher than expected (30 vs. 15%). This lowered the power of the study and the authors reported no difference between treatment groups.

Taking into account the known side effects of AEDs there is level III/B evidence for not using them routinely for seizure prophylaxis in patients with newly diagnosed brain metastases. Further studies are needed in this area and are currently underway.

9. Steroids

Steroids have an established role in controlling cerebral edema with dexamethasone typically chosen due to its minimal mineralocorticoid activity. They are however not without side effects including myelopathy, insulin resistance, and gastrointestinal bleeding. The role of steroid use and timing are discussed in this section. Ryken et al [62] has published the evidence based guidelines on this topic in 2010.

Vechet et al [63] performed a RCT in patients with metastatic disease and a KPS of less than 80. This study evaluated the minimal effective dose of oral dexamethasone. The author found no evidence for higher doses in patients who were not in immediate danger of herniation. In moderately symptomatic patients doses of 4-8mg/day were equivalent to 16mg/day.

Given the minimal data, a level III/B recommendation can be made for the use of corticosteroids with dexamethasone (4-8mg/day) as the glucocorticoid of choice, to provide temporary symptomatic relief of elevated intracranial pressure. In patients experiencing severe symptoms of elevated intracranial pressure a dose of 16mg/day can be recommended. Doses should be tapered off over a 2 week period.

10. Emerging and investigational therapies

Plainly, successful control of brain tumors has not been uniformly achieved given the efficacy and toxicity profile of the currently used modalities. Several new treatment modalities are emerging including radiation sensitizers, local irradiation with balloon-based brachytherapy, local chemotherapy with BCNU-impregnated polymers, and molecular targeting. The evidence based guidelines for these modalities have been reviewed by Olson et al [64].

11. Motexafin gadolinium

Motexafin gadolinium (MGd) is a metallotexaphrin that concentrates within tumors at higher levels than within normal tissues. It is detectable on MRI scanners and although its exact mechanism of action is unclear, it is thought to act as a radiation sensitizer. Two RCTs and one prospective single arm study have studied this agent.

Carde et al studied the dosing of MGd and found 5mg/day with 30Gy of WBRT in 10 fractions to be best tolerated [65]. This led to a RCT of 410 patients that compared WBRT with WBRT plus MGd in patients with brain metastasis [66]. Although the study showed no difference in median survival or tumor response there was a 0.5 month delay in neurologic progression in the MGd group. A Phase III RCT was then conducted that included 554 patients with NSCLC. They were randomized to WBRT or WBRT plus MGd. No statistically significant difference was found in neurologic progression between groups.

12. Efaproxiral

Efaproxiral is a radiation sensitizer that is thought to change the conformation of hemoglobin. This is thought to increased free radical formation by decreasing oxygen binding. The two phase II studies done did not show any benefit in survival. There is level IIa/B evidence that early use of efaproxiral with WBRT does not prolong survival.

13. Interstitial modalities

Interstitial modalities are defined as brachytherapy placed inside or next to the areas being treated. There has been one retrospective cohort study by Ostertab and Kreth who implanted ^{125}I seeds in spherical brain metastases with a diameter of 4cm or less, giving 60Gy to the rim of the lesion [67]. No difference was found between WBRT and ^{125}I to ^{125}I alone. Two other case [68, 69] series supported the feasibility of the modality but did not offer any evidence for increased efficacy.

A phase II study by Rogers et al [70] evaluated the Glia Site Radiation Therapy System in post resection surgical beds in patients with metastatic lesions. The system involved liquid ^{125}I that could be injected via a balloon system from a subcutaneous reservoir. The median survival was 40 weeks at 1 year of follow-up with tumor progression only being involved in 4 of the 35 total deaths. Although the data was prospectively obtained, there was no comparison group.

Two single-arm studies evaluated surgery plus local chemotherapy with or without WBRT. Nakagawa et al [71] used the DNA synthesis inhibitor 5-fluro-d-deoxyuridine (FdUrd) in post resection tumor cavities via an Ommaya reservoir. This study only included 6 patients and no comparative data were given. Ewend et al [72] prospectively studied 25 patients with newly diagnosed solitary brain metastases treated with surgical resection. They used the Gliadel Wafer and WBRT. Median survival was 33 weeks but again there was no comparative data (III/B).

Two case series [73, 74] investigated interstitial radiosurgery with the Photon Radiosurgery System. Neither study had comparative data but showed a median survival of 8 months and 1-year survival of 53% (III/B).

Based on the current data there is no evidence to support the use of interstitial radiation, chemotherapy or other modalities outside of clinical trials.

14. Molecularly targeted therapy

Currently there is no level 1 evidence for the use of molecularly targeted therapies in brain metastasis. Given the promising theoretical advantage of these therapies prospective trials focusing on survival, tumor control, and quality of life are warranted.

There have been a few case reports and single arm prospective studies [75-79] showing tumor response or stabilization in patients with metastatic NSCLC being treated with the receptor tyrosine kinase inhibitor Gefitinib. Angiogenesis inhibitors such as bevacizumab, a monoclonal antibody against vascular epidermal grown factor, is also being vigorously investigated but no evidence based recommendation can yet be made.

15. Conclusion

Current treatment of brain metastasis is complex involving multiple specialists and modalities. Evidence based recommendations can be extremely helpful in making sense of the vast array of treatment modalities when properly understood and utilized. They allow for contemporary treatment regimens affording maximal patient survival and delayed neurologic progression while pointing out gaps in current knowledge to direct future research. A key knowledge gap is in quality of life outcomes. Also, little data exists for creative combination treatments such as post-operative SRS to the operative bed without WBRT with frequent surveillance imaging and for resection of 2+ metastatic lesions. The complete evidence based guidelines [80] for metastatic brain tumors has recently been published and should be reviewed by all clinicians who treat patients with brain metastasis.

http://dx.doi.org/10.5772/51041

Author details

Steven N. Kalkanis* and Sanjay Patra

*Address all correspondence to: kalkanis@neuro.hfh.edu

Department of Neurosurgery, Henry Ford Health System, Detroit, Michigan, USA

References

[1] Gavrilovic, IT., & Posner, JB. (2008). Brain metastases: epidemiology and pathophysiology. *J Neurooncol*, 75(1), 5-14.

[2] American Cancer Society. (2008). Cancer Facts and Figures. Available from:, http://www.cancer.org/docroot/stt/content/stt_1x_cancer_facts_and_figures_2008.asp.

[3] Patchell, RA., Tibbs, PA., Regine, WF., et al. (1998). Postoperative radiotherapy in the treatment of single metastases to the brain: a randomized trial. *JAMA*, 280(17), 1485-9.

[4] Kondziolka, D., Patel, A., Lunsford, L. D., Kassam, A., & Flickinger, J. C. (1999). Stereotactic radiosurgery plus whole brain radiotherapy versus radiotherapy alone for patients with multiple brain metastases. *Int J Radiat Oncol Biol Phys*, 45(2), 427-34.

[5] Andrews, DW., Scott, CB., Sperduto, PW., et al. (2004). Whole brain radiation therapy with or without stereotactic radiosurgery boost for patients with one to three brain metastases: Phase III results of the RTOG 9508 randomized trial. *Lancet*, 363(9422), 1665-672.

[6] Patchell, RA., Tibbs, PA., Walsh, JW., et al. (1990). A randomized trial of surgery in the treatment of single metastases to the brain. *N Engl J Med*, 322(8), 494-500.

[7] Mintz, A. H., Kestle, J., Rathbone, M. P., et al. (1996). A randomized trial to assess the efficacy of surgery in addition to radiotherapy in patients with a single cerebral metastasis. *Cancer*, 78(7), 1470-6.

[8] Vecht, C. J., Haaxma-Reiche, H., Noordijk, E. M., et al. (1993). Treatment of single brain metastasis: radiotherapy alone or combined with neuro-surgery? *Ann Neurol*, 33(6), 583-90.

[9] Ampil, F. L., Nanda, A., Willis, B. K., Nandy, I., & Meehan, R. (1996). Metastatic disease in the cerebellum. The LSU experience. *Am J Clin Oncol*, 19(5), 509-11.

[10] Sause, W. T., Crowley, J. J., Morantz, R., et al. (1990). Solitary brain metastasis: results of an RTOG/SWOG protocol evaluation surgery + RT versus RT alone. *Am J Clin Oncol*, 13(5), 427-32.

[11] Rades, D., Kieckebusch, S., Haatanen, T., Lohynska, R., Dunst, J., & Schild, S. E. (2008). Surgical resection followed by whole brain radiotherapy versus whole brain radiotherapy alone for single brain metastasis. *Int J Radiat Oncol Biol Phys*, 70(5), 1319-24.

[12] Borgelt, B., Gebler, R., Larson, M., Hendrickson, F., Griffin, T., & Roth, R. (1981). Ultra-rapid high dose irradiation schedules for the palliation of brain metastases: final results of the first two studies by Radiation Therapy Oncology Group. *Int J Radiat Oncol Biol Phys*, 7(12), 1633-8.

[13] Chatani, M., Matayoshi, Y., Masaki, N., & Inoue, T. (1994). Radiation therapy for brain metastases from lung carcinoma. Prospective randomized trial according to the level of lactate dehydrogenase. *Strahlenther Onkol*, 170(3), 155-61.

[14] Chatani, M., Teshima, T., Hata, K., Inoue, T., & Suzuki, T. (1985). Whole brain irradiation for metastases from lung carcinoma. A clinical investigation. *Acta Radiol Oncol*, 24(4), 311-14.

[15] Davey, P., Hoegler, D., Ennis, M., & Smith, J. (2008). A Phase III study of accelerated versus conventional hypofractionated whole brain irradiation in patients of good performance status with brain metastases. *Radiother Oncol*, 88(2), 173-6.

[16] Haie-Meder, C., Pellae-Cosset, B., Laplanche, A., et al. (1993). Results of a randomized clinical trial comparing two radiation schedules in the palliative treatment of brain metastases. *Radiother Oncol*, 26(2), 111-16.

[17] Komarnicky, L. T., Phillips, T. L., Martz, K., Asbell, S., Isaacson, S., & Urtasun, R. (1991). A randomized Phase III protocol for the evaluation of misonidazole combined with radiation in the treatment of patients with brain metastases (RTOG-7916). *Int J Radiat Oncol Biol Phys*, 20(1), 53-8.

[18] Kurtz, J. M., Gleber, R., Brady, L. W., Carella, R. J., & Cooper, J. S. (1981). The palliation of brain metastases in a favorable patient population: a randomized clinical trial by the Radiation Therapy Oncology Group. *Int J Radiat Oncol Biol Phys*, 7(7), 891-5.

[19] Murray, K. J., Scott, C., Greenberg, H. M., et al. (1997). A randomized Phase III study of accelerated hyperfractionation versus standard in patients with unresected brain metastases: a report of the Radiation Therapy Oncology Group (RTOG) 9104. *Int J Radiat Oncol Biol Phys*, 39(3), 571-4.

[20] Priestman, T. J., Dunn, J., Brada, M., Rampling, R., & Baker, P. G. (1996). Final results of the Royal College of Radiologists trial comparing two different radiotherapy schedules in the treatment of cerebral metastasis. *Clin Oncol (R Coll Radiol)*, 8(5), 308-15.

[21] Armstrong, JG., Wronski, M., Galicich, J., Arbit, E., Leibel, SA., & Burt, M. (1994). Postoperative radiation for lung cancer metastatic to the brain. *J Clin Oncol*, 12(11), 2340-4.

[22] Hagen, N. A., Cirrincione, C., Thaler, H. T., & De Angelis, L. M. (1990). The role of radiation therapy following resection of single brain metastasis from melanoma. *Neurology*, 40(1), 158-60.

[23] Skibber, J. M., Soong, S. F., Austin, L., Balch, C. M., & Sawaya, R. E. Cranial irradiation after surgical excision of brain metastases in melanoma patients. *Ann Surg Oncol*, 3(2), 118.

[24] Muacevic, A., Wowra, B., Siefert, A., Tonn, J. C., Steiger, H. J., & Kreth, F. W. (2008). Microsurgery plus whole brain irradiation versus Gamma Knife surgery alone for treatment of single metastases to the brain: a randomized controlled multicentre Phase III trial. *J Neurooncol*, 87(3), 299-307.

[25] Garell, P. C., Hitchon, P. W., Wen, B. C., Mellenberg, D. E., & Torner, J. (1999). Stereotactic radiosurgery versus microsurgical resection for the initial treatment of metastatic cancer to the brain. *J Radiosurg*, 2(1), 1-5.

[26] Schöggl, A., Kitz, K., Reddy, M., et al. (2000). Defining the role of stereotactic radiosurgery versus microsurgery in the treatment of single brain metastases. *Acta Neurochir (Wien)*, 142(6), 621-6.

[27] O'Neill, BP., Iturria, NJ., Link, MJ., Pollock, BE., Ballman, KV., & O'Fallon, JR. (2003). A comparison of surgical resection and stereotactic radiosurgery in the treatment of solitary brain metastases. *Int J Radiat Oncol Biol Phys*, 55(5), 1169-76.

[28] Bindal, AK., Bindal, RK., Hess, KR., et al. (1996). Surgery versus radiosurgery in the treatment of brain metastasis. *J Neurosurg*, 84(5), 748-54.

[29] Sanghavi, S. N., Miranpuri, S. S., Chappell, R., et al. (2001). Radiosurgery for patients with brain metastases: a multi-institutional analysis, stratified by the RTOG recursive partitioning analysis method. *Int J Radiat Oncol Biol Phys*, 51(2), 426-34.

[30] Li, B., Yu, J., Suntharalingam, M., et al. (2000). Comparison of three treatment options for single brain metastasis for lung cancer. *Int J Cancer*, 90(1), 37-45.

[31] Want, L. G., Guo, Y., Zhang, X., et al. (2002). Brain metastasis: experience of the Xi-Jing Hospital. *Stereotact Funct Neurosurg*, 78(2), 70-83.

[32] Aoyama, H., Shirato, H., Tago, M., et al. (2006). Stereotactic radiosurgery plus whole-brain radiation therapy vs stereotactic radiosurgery alone for treatment of brain metastases: a randomized controlled trial. *JAMA*, 295(21), 2483-91.

[33] Aoyama, H., Tago, M., Kato, N., et al. (2007). Neurocognitive function of patients with brain metastasis who received either whole brain radiotherapy plus stereotactic radiosurgery or radiosurgery alone. *Int J Radiat Oncol Biol Phys*, 68(5), 1388-95.

[34] Chidel, MA., Suh, JH., Reddy, CA., Chao, ST., Lundbeck, MF., Barnett, GH., et al. (2000). Application of recursive partitioning analysis and evaluation of the use of whole brain radiation among patients treated with stereotactic radiosurgery for newly diagnosed brain metastases. *Int J Radiat Oncol Biol Phys*, 47(4), 993-9.

[35] Combs, S. E., Schulz-Ertner, D., Thilmann, C., Edler, L., & Debus, J. (2004). Treatment of cerebral metastases from breast cancer with stereotactic radiosurgery. *Strahlenther Onkol*, 180(9), 590-6.

[36] Hoffman, R., Sneed, P. K., McDermott, M. W., et al. (2001). Radiosurgery for brain metastases from primary lung carcinoma. *Cancer J*, 7(2), 121-31.

[37] Jawahar, A., Willis, B. K., Smith, D. R., Ampil, F., Datta, R., & Nanda, A. (2002). Gamma Knife radiosurgery for brain metastases: do patients benefit from adjuvant external-beam radiotherapy? An 18 -month comparative analysis. *Stereotact Funct Neurosurg*, 79(3-4), 262-71.

[38] Noel, G., Medioni, J., Valery, CA., et al. (2003). Three irradiation treatment options including radiosurgery for brain metastases from primary lung cancer. *Lung Cancer*, 41(3), 333-43.

[39] Pirzkall, A., Debus, J., Lohr, F., et al. (1998). Radiosurgery alone or in combination with whole-brain radiotherapy for brain metastases. *J Clin Oncol*, 16(11), 3563-9.

[40] Sneed, PK., Lamborn, KR., Forstner, JM., et al. (1999). Radiosurgery for brain metastases: is whole brain radiotherapy necessary? *Int J Radiat Oncol Biol Phys*, 43(3), 549-58.

[41] Sneed, PK., Suh, JH., Goetsch, SJ., et al. (2002). A multi-institutional review of radiosurgery alone vs radiosurgery with whole brain radiotherapy as the initial management of brain metastases. *Int J Radiat Oncol Biol Phys*, 53(3), 519-26.

[42] Varlotto, J. M., Flickinger, J. C., Niranjan, A., Bhatnagar, A., Kondziolka, D., & Lunsford, L. D. (2005). The impact of whole-brain radiation therapy on the long-term control and morbidity of patients surviving more than one year after Gamma Knife radiosurgery for brain metastases. *Int J Radiat Oncol Biol Phys*, 62(4), 1125-32.

[43] Lee, YK., Park, NH., Kim, JW., Song, YS., Kang, SB., & Lee, HP. (2008). Gamma-Knife radiosurgery as an optimal treatment modality for brain metastases from epithelial ovarian cancer. *Gynecol Oncol*, 108(3), 505-9.

[44] Rades, D., Pluemer, A., Veninga, T., Hanssens, P., Dunst, J., & Schild, SE. (2007). Whole-brain radiotherapy versus stereotactic radiosurgery for patients in recursive partitioning analysis classes 1 and 2 with 1 to 3 brain metastases. *Cancer*, 110(10), 2285-92.

[45] Datta, R., Jawahar, A., Ampil, F. L., Shi, R., Nanda, A., & D'Agostino, H. (2004). Survival in relation to radiotherapeutic modality for brain metastasis: whole brain irradiation vs Gamma Knife radiosurgery. *Am J Clin Oncol*, 27(4), 420-4.

[46] Mehta, M. P., Paleologos, N. A., Mikkelsen, T., et al. (2010). The role of chemotherapy in the management of newly diagnosed brain metastases: a systematic review and evidence-based clinical practice guideline. *J Neurooncol*, 96(1), 71-83.

[47] Seute, T., Leffers, P., Wilmink, JT., ten Velde, GP., & Twijnstra, A. (2006). Response of asymptomatic brain metastases from small-cell lung cancer to systemic first-line chemotherapy. *J Clin Oncol*, 24(13), 2079-83.

[48] Guerrieri, M., Wong, K., Ryan, G., Millward, M., Quong, G., & Ball, D. L. (2004). A randomised Phase III study of palliative radiation with concomitant carboplatin for brain metastases from non-small cell carcinoma of the lung. *Lung Cancer*, 46(1), 107-11.

[49] Ushio, Y., Arita, N., Hayakawa, T., et al. (1991). Chemotherapy of brain metastases from lung carcinoma: a controlled randomized study. *Neurosurgery*, 28(2), 201-5.

[50] Antonadou, D., Paraskevaidis, M., Sarris, G., et al. (2002). Phase II randomized trial of temozolomide and concurrent radiotherapy in patients with brain metastases. *J Clin Oncol*, 20(17), 3644-50.

[51] Verger, E., Gil, M., Yaya, R., et al. (2005). Temozolomide and concomitant whole brain radiotherapy in patients with brain metastases: a Phase II randomized trial. *Int J Radiat Oncol Biol Phys*, 61(1), 185-91.

[52] Ammirati, M., Cobbs, C. S., Linskey, ME., et al. (2010). The role of retreatment in the management of recurrent/progressive brain metastases: a systematic review and evidence-based clinical practice guideline. *J Neurooncol*, 96(1), 85-96.

[53] Cooper, JS., Steinfeld, AD., & Lerch, IA. (1990). Cerebral metastases: value of reirradiation in selected patients. *Radiology*, 174(3: Pt 1), 883-5.

[54] Sadikov, E., Bezjak, A., Yi, Q. L., et al. (2007). Value of whole brain re-irradiation for brain metastases- single centre experience. *Clin Oncol (R Coll Radiol)*, 19(7), 532-8.

[55] Wong, WW., Schild, SE., Sawyer, TE., & Shaw, EG. (1996). Analysis of outcome in patients reirradiated for brain metastases. *Int J Radiat Oncol Biol Phys*, 34(3), 585-90.

[56] Arbit, E., Wroski, M., Burt, M., & Galicich, J. H. (1995). The treatment of patients with recurrent brain metastases. A retrospective analysis of 109 patients with nonsmall cell lung cancer. *Cancer*, 76(5), 765-73.

[57] Bindal, R. K., Sawaya, R., Leavens, ME., Hess, K. R., & Taylor, S. H. (1995). Reoperation for recurrent metastatic brain tumors. *J Neurosurg*, 83(4), 600-4.

[58] Truong, MT., St Clair, EG., Donahue, BR., et al. (2006). Results of surgical resection for progression of brain metastases previously treated by Gamma Knife radiosurgery. *Neurosurgery*, 59(1), 86-97.

[59] Vecil, G. G., Suki, D., Maldaun, M. V., Lang, F. F., & Sawaya, R. (2005). Resection of brain metastases previously treated with stereotactic radiosurgery. *J Neurosurg*, 102(2), 209-15.

[60] Mikkelsen, T., Paleologos, N. A., Robinson, P. D., et al. (2010). The role of prophylactic anticonvulsants in the management of brain metastases: a systematic review and evidence-based clinical practice guideline. *J Neurooncol*, 96(1), 97-102.

[61] Forsyth, P. A., Weaver, S., Fulton, D., et al. (2003). Prophylactic anticonvulsants in patients with brain tumour. *Can J Neurol Sci*, 30(2), 106-12.

[62] Ryken, T. C., McDermott, M., Robinson, P. D., et al. (2010). The role of steroids in the management of brain metastases: a systematic review and evidence-based clinical practice guidelines. *J Neurooncol*, 96(1), 103-14.

[63] Vecht, C. J., Hovestadt, A., Verbiest, H. B., Vliet, J. J., & Putten, W. L. (1994). Dose-effect relationship of dexamethasone on Karnofsky performance in metastatic brain tumors: a randomized study of doses of 4, 8, and 16 mg per day. *Neurology*, 44(4), 675-80.

[64] Olson, JJ., Paleologos, NA., Gaspar, LE., et al. (2010). The role of emerging and investigational therapies for metastatic brain tumors: a systematic review and evidence-based clinical practice guideline of selected topics. *J Neurooncol*, 96(1), 115-42.

[65] Carde, P., Timmerman, R., Mehta, MP., et al. (2001). Multicenter Phase Ib/II trial of the radiation enhancer motexafin gadolinium in patients with brain metastases. *J Clin Oncol*, 19(7), 2074-83.

[66] Mehta, M. P., Rodrigus, P., Terhaard, C. H., et al. (2003). Survival and neurologic outcomes in a randomized trial of motexafin gadolinium and whole-brain radiation therapy in brain metastases. *J Clin Oncol*, 21(13), 2529-36.

[67] Ostertag, CB., & Kreth, FW. (1995). Interstitial iodine-125 radiosurgery for cerebral metastases. *Br J Neurosurg*, 9(5), 593-603.

[68] Alesch, F., Hawliczek, R., & Koos, W. T. (1995). Interstitial irradiation of brain metastases. *Acta Neurochir*, 63(Suppl.), 29-34.

[69] Bernstein, M., Cabantog, A., Laperriere, N., Leung, P., & Thomason, C. (1995). Brachytherapy for recurrent single brain metastasis. *Can J Neurol Sci*, 22(1), 13-16.

[70] Rogers, LR., Rock, JP., Sills, AK., et al. (2006). Results of a Phase II trial of the GliaSite radiation therapy system for the treatment of newly diagnosed, resected single brain metastases. *J Neurosurg*, 105(3), 375-84.

[71] Nakagawa, H., Maeda, N., Tsuzuki, T., et al. (2001). Intracavitary chemotherapy with 5-fluoro-2′-deoxyuridine (FdUrd) in malignant brain tumors. *Jpn J Clin Oncol*, 31(6), 251-8.

[72] Ewend, M. G., Brem, S., Gilbert, M., et al. (2007). Treatment of single brain metastasis with resection, intracavity carmustine polymer wafers, and radiation therapy is safe and provides excellent local control. *Clin Cancer Res*, 13(12), 3637-41.

[73] Curry, W. T. Jr., Cosgrove, G. R., Hochberg, F. H., Loeffler, J., & Zervas, N. T. (2005). Stereotactic interstitial radiosurgery for cerebral metastases. *J Neurosurg*, 103(4), 630-5.

[74] Nakamura, O., Matsutani, M., Shitara, N., et al. (1994). New treatment protocol by intra-operative radiation therapy for metastatic brain tumours. *Acta Neurochir*, 131(1-2), 91-6.

[75] Hotta, K., Kiura, K., Ueoka, H., et al. (2004). Effect of gefitinib ('Iressa', ZD1839) on brain metastases in patients with advanced non-small-cell lung cancer. *Lung Cancer*, 46(2), 255-61.

[76] Namba, Y., Kijima, T., Yokota, S., et al. (2004). Gefitinib in patients with brain metastases from non-small-cell lung cancer: review of 15 clinical cases. *Clin Lung Cancer*, 6(2), 123-8.

[77] Shimato, S., Mitsudomi, T., Kosaka, T., et al. (2006). EGFR mutations in patients with brain metastases from lung cancer: association with the efficacy of gefitinib. *Neuro-Oncol*, 8(2), 137-44.

[78] Ceresoli, G. L., Cappuzzo, F., Gregorc, V., Bartolini, S., Crino, L., & Villa, E. (2004). Gefitinib in patients with brain metastases from non-small-cell lung cancer: a prospective trial. *Ann Oncol*, 15(7), 1042-7.

[79] Chiu, CH., Tsai, CM., Chen, YM., Chiang, SC., Liou, JL., & Perng, RP. (2005). Gefitinib is active in patients with brain metastases from non-small cell lung cancer and response is related to skin toxicity. *Lung Cancer*, 47(1), 129-38.

[80] Kalkanis, SN., & Linskey, ME. (2009). Evidence-based clinical practice parameter guidelines for the treatment of patients with metastatic brain tumors: introduction. *J Neurooncol*, 96(1), 7-10.

Section 4

Tumor Induced Epilepsy

Chapter 10

Tumor Associated Epilepsy

Edward K. Avila

Additional information is available at the end of the chapter

http://dx.doi.org/10.5772/55491

1. Introduction

Epilepsy in the general population occurs with an incidence of 44 per 100,000 person-years in a population based study [1]. Symptomatic etiologies such as vascular injuries, infection, and neoplasm are usually associated with a higher incidence of seizures and epilepsy. In the cancer population, seizures arise mainly as a result of an infiltrative neoplastic process in the brain. However, cancer treatment, metabolic causes, and paraneoplastic disease can also cause seizures in this population despite the absence of a structural lesion. The etiology of epilepsy in brain tumor patients includes primary malignancies and metastatic disease to the brain. A multifaceted approach is required for treatment of seizures including surgery, radiation treatment, chemotherapy, and antiepileptic drugs. A combination of treatments has the potential of adverse effects and generally requires a multidisciplinary team.

This chapter will review the causes of epilepsy in cancer patients, incidence, treatment, the role of electroencephalogram (EEG) and antiepileptic prophylaxis in this group of patients. The factors which predispose seizures in these patients will also be reviewed, such as tumor grade, histology and brain tumor morphology.

2. Incidence

The cumulative incidence of seizures in the general population is almost 10% by age 74. More than 4% of the population has one unprovoked seizure by age 74 and 3% will develop epilepsy [2]. Symptomatic etiologies such as brain tumors account for a higher percentage (30%-49%) of all unprovoked seizures and epilepsy. Although brain tumors account for 4% of all epilepsies, symptomatic seizures can occur in up to 85% of patients depending on tumor type and location. In 30%-50% of patients with brain tumors a seizure is the presenting clinical sign.

However, up to 30% will develop seizures later in the course of their disease [2]. In the cancer population seizures can occur for numerous reasons including primary brain tumors, brain metastasis, paraneoplastic syndromes, and other etiologies such as toxic/metabolic, infection, or from a reaction to cancer treatment [3]. Drug interactions and adverse drug effects are important considerations in this population as many treatments may have neurologic adverse effects and seizures are one such problem.

Incidence rates of epilepsy based on etiology including brain tumors, traumatic brain injuries, central nervous system (CNS) infections, cerebrovascular disease, and other causes have been determined [4]. Symptomatic etiologies such as brain injuries and brain tumors account for a higher percentage (30%-50%) of all unprovoked seizures and epilepsy.

The incidence of seizures in patients with systemic cancer is estimated to be 5%, but for patients with an intracranial neoplasm, seizure incidence may be as high as 30% [5,6]. There are several factors which affect the incidence of seizures in brain tumor patients and these include age, location of the lesion, histology, and the grade of the tumor. With regard to age, there is a higher incidence in young patients and those over age 65 which mirrors the incidence of epilepsy in the general population [7,8]. The reason for this finding is likely the higher incidence of low grade brain tumors in children versus adults and the subsequent longer survival rate [9].

3. Etiology

Location, grade, histology and tumor morphology are important contributors to seizure incidence.

Cortical location is an important determinant for the development of seizures as neural generators are located in the cortex. Rarely do subcortical or infratentorial lesions cause seizures. Location in the temporal, frontal, and parietal lobes are more likely to result in seizures than occipital or subcortical lesions. Location near the rolandic fissure can also result in seizures [8,10].

Grade of the tumor is an important determinant as low-grade lesions are more likely to be associated with seizures. Chronicity of the lesion and subsequent secondary epileptogenesis appear to play a role in the devolvement of seizures. Morphological characteristics of low-grade lesions portend higher seizure incidence when compared to high-grade tumors. In one study examining morphological characteristics, low grade gliomas tended to be larger in patients presenting with seizures. This contrasted with patients with high grade gliomas where patients who presented with seizures had smaller tumors. Location in the temporal lobe was associated with higher seizure incidence for low-grade tumors [11].

Histology is an important contributor to the development of seizures and subsequent tumor associated epilepsy as low-grade tumors are more often epileptogenic. Chronicity of the tumor has been shown to be directly correlated with the incidence of seizures [12]. There are several reasons for this: slow-growing tumors may isolate and deafferentate focal regions of normal tissue and prevent normal regulation. Low-grade brain tumors such as gangliogliomas and dysembryoplastic neuroepithelial tumors can have an almost 100% incidence of seizures whereas the incidence rate is 60%-85% in low-grade astrocytomas and oligodendrogliomas (Fig. 1) [13].

4. Causes of seizures

4.1. Brain tumors

Primary brain tumors. As discussed, tumor histology and grade of tumor are important contributors to the development of seizures in primary brain tumor patients.

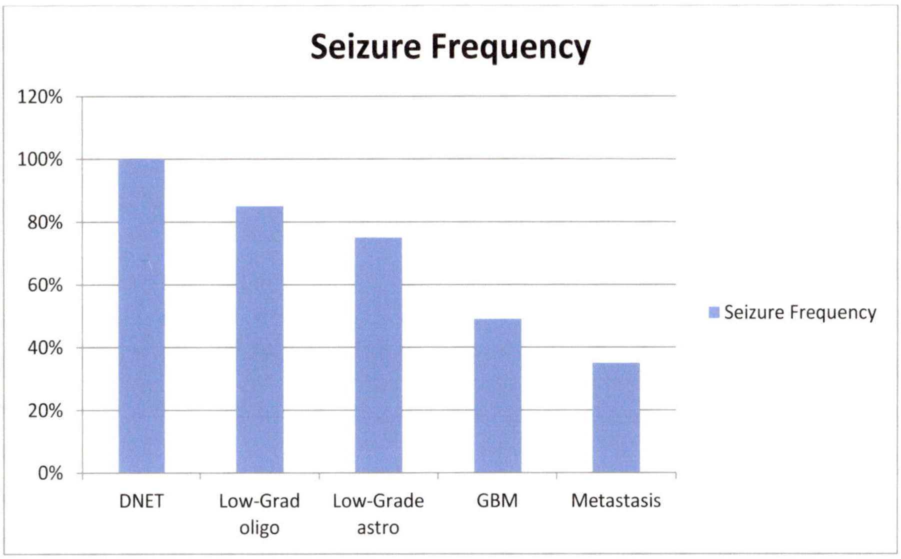

Figure 1. Seizure Frequency Based on Tumor Type

Neuronal tumors have a higher incidence of seizures. One possible reason is that the population of neurons could be epileptogenic within the tumor whereas in the glial tumors the seizure focus is generally in the peritumoral brain tissue [8].

Glial neuronal tumors also have a high incidence of seizures which is more likely due to cortical involvement of the tumor. Secondary epileptogenesis can occur in up to one-third of brain tumor patients where the epileptogenic focus does not correspond to the tumor location. The process by which this occurs can be described as an actively discharging epileptogenic region that induces a similar paroxysmal activity in the region distant from the original site. This phenomenon has been seen in animal models and it is believed that it occurs in humans as well. Secondary epileptogenesis can be seen in low-grade brain tumors in the temporal lobe which have associated hippocampal sclerosis [14].

Several other factors can affect epileptogenesis including imbalance between excitatory and inhibitory pathways. Higher levels of excitatory neurotransmitters such as glutamate can result in excitability of cortical neurons and therefore seizures [15]. Alkaline pH levels in peritumoral brain tissue can also lead to epileptogenesis by disrupting levels of intracellular and extracellular Na.

Morphologic changes in the peritumoral brain tissue such as aberrant neuronal migration, persistent neurons and white matter, and changes in synaptic vesicles can result in seizures in brain tumor patients. Changes in receptor binding sites for excitatory and inhibitory neurotransmitters (GABA, NMDA) can affect epileptogenicity [16]. One example of this phenomenon is seen in gliomas as they have been shown to have higher concentrations of inotropic glutamate receptors which can lead to neuronal hyperexcitability with resultant seizures and possible cell death [17].

Metastatic lesions account for a smaller percentage of patients with intracranial neoplasms who go on to develop seizures and epilepsy. Systemic cancers which occur more commonly, such as lung and breast cancer, tend to have a higher incidence of brain metastasis and subsequent seizures. Some cancers have a higher predilection for central nervous system metastasis such as melanoma and, depending on location, may have a higher seizure frequency [18].

4.2. Treatment-related causes of seizures

Chemotherapy. Various chemotherapeutic agents can be toxic to the central nervous system either directly or through other mechanisms which result in epileptogenesis or lower seizure threshold.

Agents such as cytarabine, methotrexate, high-dose cisplatin, bevacizumab, ifosfamide, vincristine, and nitrosoureas can cause seizures by direct central nervous system toxicity when given systemically or in the case of methotrexate when given intrathecally [19].

Radiation therapy. For patients undergoing whole brain radiation for brain metastasis, leptomeningeal disease, and for primary brain tumors, seizures can occur as a direct result of radiation. Complications can occur acutely such as during radiation treatment. They can occur early within weeks to months after radiation or they can occur late, 1-2 years after receiving radiation treatment from radiation necrosis [19, 20].

4.3. Toxic/metabolic

Medication toxicity or withdrawal can result in symptomatic seizures. This can occur with numerous different agents including antimicrobials, antipsychotic medication, antidepressant medication, and, of course, antiepileptic drug medication.

Conditions which can cause seizures even in patients without cancer can also contribute to seizures in those with a brain tumor such as renal or liver failure. Electrolyte disturbance including disturbances of sodium, calcium, magnesium and glucose can precipitate seizures.

http://dx.doi.org/10.5772/55491

Glucose disturbances in particular can also result in focal neurologic disturbances such as seizures or stroke-like syndromes [21].

4.4. Paraneoplastic syndromes

There are several paraneoplastic syndromes which have been characterized and which seizures are one symptom. Paraneoplastic limbic encephalitis has been associated with numerous antibodies including anti-Hu, anti-Ma2, CRMP5, and amphiphysin. Recently, antibodies have been associated with encephalitis and seizures in patients who may or may not have a neoplasm. One such antibody has been the NMDA receptor antibody which was initially described in women with ovarian teratoma but has also been found in children without cancer [22].

5. Treatment

Treatment will be discussed for patients with brain tumor epilepsy. In general, treatment for patients with systemic cancer without intracranial lesions will consist of antiepileptic drugs only. In patients with intracranial lesions, there is a multifaceted approach which includes antiepileptic drugs, surgery, chemotherapy, and radiation therapy.

5.1. Antiepileptic drugs

Antiepileptic drugs are a mainstay of treatment for seizures of any etiology. In patients with cancer this is also true, but a consideration of drug interactions and drug metabolism is important as patients receiving chemotherapy, with or without corticosteroids, can have untoward drug interactions in combination with antiepileptic drugs [23]. This is usually the case for some of the first generation antiepileptic drugs which can be hepatic enzyme inducers, specifically of the cytochrome P-450 pathway. Drug interactions can also occur with antiepileptic drugs that are enzyme inhibitors. A benefit of the second and third generation antiepileptic drugs is that many are not metabolized through the same hepatic pathways as chemotherapy agents or corticosteroids. In addition, there is less protein binding with these agents which makes them more suitable for treatment in patients receiving concurrent chemotherapy (Table 1).

Enzyme-inducing antiepileptic drugs can decrease the effects of corticosteroids and in turn corticosteroids can also alter the metabolism of antiepileptic drugs resulting in decreased serum levels [24]. Enzyme-inducing antiepileptic drugs can also have an effect on the serum drug levels of chemotherapeutic agents such as nitrosureas, paclitaxel, cyclophosphamide, etoposide, doxorubicin, and methotrexate. Temozolomide, an alkylating agent commonly used for treating high-grade gliomas, has minimal CYP metabolism. One study documented no effect of temozolomide on levels of topiramate or oxcarbazepine [25].

Treatment of seizures with antiepileptic drug therapy in brain tumor patients has been evaluated in several retrospective trials (Table 2). Use of older antiepileptic drugs with

Enzyme inducers (CYP 450)	Non-enzyme inducers
Phenytoin	Gabapentin
Carbamazepine	Lamotrigine
Phenobarbital	Valproic acid (enzyme inhibitor)
Primidone	Felbamate (enzyme inhibitor)
Oxcarbazepine	Levetiracetam
	Pre-gadolinium
	Tiagabine
	Topiramate
	Zonisamide
	Lacosamide

Table 1. List of antiepileptic drugs comparing those metabolized through the CYP 450 pathway and those that are not

adjunctive treatment with agents such as levetiracetam, lamotrigine, or topiramate have been reviewed and shown to be safe and efficacious in the brain tumor population. There are varying degrees of success with reports of seizure reduction in many patients and a smaller percentage achieving seizure freedom. Follow-up in these studies has been variable and difficult to compare.

Side effects of antiepileptic drug treatment are an important consideration. In patients with brain tumors who have undergone craniotomy, radiation treatment, and who may or may not be receiving chemotherapy, additional toxicity from antiepileptic drugs can be additive. Common side effects such as cognitive impairment, bone marrow suppression, liver dysfunction, electrolyte abnormalities, and dermatologic reactions are important considerations in patients receiving this antiepileptic drug therapy. Side effects are more frequent in patients with brain tumors compared to the overall population with epilepsy as was noted in the 2000 AAN Practice Parameter [33].

A benefit to the newer antiepileptic drugs is that there are fewer interactions with chemotherapy, they can be used in clinical trials aimed at treatment of brain tumors, and at times there can be a better side effect profile. However, side effects from antiepileptic drugs can be seen more often in patients with brain tumors. This is likely because patients with brain tumors have fixed neurologic deficits which can be worsened in the setting of drug toxicity of any kind.

Treatment with antiepileptic drugs in the cancer population should be similar to treatment for anyone with localization related epilepsy. Monotherapy should be the goal with the lowest possible dose to control seizures and to avoid adverse side effects. Drugs which control focal seizures with secondary generalization are desired and agents such as lamotrigine, carbamazepine, and oxcarbazepine are generally well-tolerated [34]. Other agents which can have an

http://dx.doi.org/10.5772/55491

Author	N	Type	Grade	Primary AED	Add-on AED	Seizure Free (%)	Seizure reduction (%)
Hildebrand et al[26]	234	R	HGG	VPA, CBZ, GBP, LMT, others		13	NA
Maschio et al.[27]	14	P	HGG, LGG	LEV, VPA, LTG, others	LCS	43	78
Wick et al.[28]	107	R	HGG, LGG	PHT, VPA, CBZ		30	
Wagner et al.[27]	26	P	HG	VPA	LEV	20	65
Mashio et al.[30]	19	P	HG	LTG, VPA, TPM, OXC	LEV	47	72
Newton et al[31]	41	R	HG	PHT, CBZ	LEV	59	90
Mashio et al.[25]	47	P	HG, LG, BM	PHT, CBZ, PB	TPM	56	76
Perry et al.[32]	14	P	HG	PHT, CBZ, Clobazam	GBP	57	100

N- number of patients; R- retrospective; P- prospective; HGG- high grade glioma; LGG-low grade glioma; HG- High grade; LG- low grade; BM-brain metastases; LEV-levetiracetam; VPA-valproic acid; LTG- lamotrigine; GBP-gabapentin; CBZ-carbamazepine; OXC-oxcarbazepine; LCS-lacosamide; TPM-topiramate; PB-phenobarbital

Table 2. AED drug trials in brain tumor patients

effect on this population such as topiramate or valproic acid can be used. However, cognitive side effects with topiramate may limit its dosing and therefore its efficacy. Valproic acid would appear to be a good agent; however, it can cause drug interactions and liver toxicity. In patients already receiving chemotherapy, the potential for liver toxicity and thrombocytopenia can be a problem with valproic acid [35]. Valproic acid does have possible antitumor effects due to inhibition of histone deacetylase (HDAC) [36]. There is recent evidence that in patients with glioblastoma undergoing standard treatment, radiation treatment with concurrent temozolomide, receiving valproic acid for the treatment of seizures may be a survival benefit [35]. However, prospective studies examining this issue have yet to be performed. Whether this survival benefit was seen due to HDAC effects or hepatic enzyme inhibitory properties was unclear. In contrast, a study examining 620 patients with newly diagnosed glioblastoma found an overall survival benefit and progression-free survival in patients who received an enzyme inducing agent versus those who did not [37]. The role of enzyme inducing AEDs on survival has not been established in the brain tumor population but is something that should be prospectively analyzed in new clinical trials.

Levetiracetam and gabapentin have ideal properties in that neither is liver metabolized and there are few if any drug interactions. In several retrospective studies, levetiracetam has been well-tolerated in brain tumor patients but can be associated with mood disturbances [29, 30, 38]. Cognitive side effects and fatigue are also seen with use of this agent which can be compounded in patients who have received brain radiation.

5.2. Surgery

There are generally two approaches to surgery for brain tumor patients. The first and most important is gross total resection of either the primary brain tumor or a metastatic lesion. A secondary consideration can be additional removal of a seizure focus (lesionectomy) for patients who present with seizures as a symptom of their brain tumor. Circumstances which can limit lesionectomy are the location of the seizure focus in an eloquent area of cortex. In the brain tumor population, surgery is almost always geared towards gross total resection which has shown on its own to improve outcomes from a seizure standpoint [39]. However, there remains a significant population of patients who undergo brain tumor surgery and continue to have seizures postoperatively. Patients with lesions near the motor cortex are more likely not to be surgically "cured" as the lesion causing seizures is unlikely to be amenable to surgical resection. Therefore, these patients remain with symptomatic partial epilepsy.

In tumor associated epilepsy, seizures generally arise from the peritumoral brain tissue and not from the mass. Tumor tissue is generally electrically inert and does not give rise to seizures. Electrocorticography (Ecog) performed intraoperatively may assist in identifying a seizure focus and aid the neurosurgeon in removal of the lesion. A study reviewing 35 patients with intractable temporal lobe epilepsy due to benign lesions (ganglioglioma, DNET, cavernoma) found 3-year post-operative seizure rates to be improved in patients who underwent Ecog with additional removal of spike-positive areas [40]. However, there is no universal standard established.

For temporal lobe lesions, the additional resection of mesial structures may be beneficial in some cases. A series with patients with low grade temporal lobe tumors (DNET, ganglioglioma) with associated hippocampal sclerosis suggest that lobectomy with hippocampectomy is preferable to tumor resection alone [41]. Overall, prognostic factors which favor control of epilepsy with surgery are a shorter duration of epilepsy prior to surgery, a single focus on EEG, a single lesion on neuroimaging, and complete tumor resection [10,41,39].

5.3. Chemotherapy

Chemotherapy is one of the primary treatment modalities for all types of metastatic and primary central nervous system tumors. The use of chemotherapy can result in seizure reduction for patients with primary brain tumors. Recent studies retrospectively reviewing the use of temozolomide or nitrosoureas in patients with low grade glioma have shown a reduction in seizures with some patients achieving seizure freedom [42-44].

Additionally, in patients with subependymal giant cell astrocytomas with tuberous sclerosis complex, the mTor inhibitor, everolimus, has been associated with reduction of subependymal tumors and subsequent improvement in seizures. Whether this agent is antiepileptogenic in itself or causes a reduction of tumor bulk which improves seizures remains to be seen [45].

5.4. Radiation therapy

Treatment for glioblastoma with surgery followed by radiation with concurrent temozolomide has been established as a standard of care. There have been small studies which have shown that radiation treatment for malignant lesions has also resulted in improvement in seizures independent of antiepileptic drug adjustment [46, 47]. The EORTC 22845 randomized trial of long-term efficacy of early versus delayed radiation treatment for low grade brain tumors revealed an improvement in seizure frequency at one year post treatment. Although later data points were not collected, this study shows what has been evident in clinical practice which is that radiation treatment for low-grade brain tumors can improve seizure frequency [48].

6. Antiepileptic drug prophylaxis

6.1. Postsurgical patients

The role of prophylactic anticonvulsant medications in the perioperative period has been reviewed for numerous tumor types including primary brain tumors and brain metastasis. Prophylaxis appears effective for preventing early postoperative seizures but does not appear to affect the delayed development of epilepsy [49]. Current practice is to use prophylactic anticonvulsants during the first week after surgery and then to discontinue after that time period [50]. The data on these recommendations are derived from the older anticonvulsants, phenytoin, phenobarbital, and valproic acid. The newer generation antiepileptic drugs have not been studied as rigorously in this setting and therefore recommendations for their use is limited. However, recent studies using levetiracetam in this setting have been promising in that there are few if any drug interactions and minimal adverse effects related to the use of this drug [51,52]. Certain tumor types may not benefit from the use of prophylactic anticonvulsants in the perioperative period, such as meningioma, as seen in a recent meta analysis [53]. Prospective studies are needed to determine the validity and efficacy of prophylactic anticonvulsants in the perioperative period with newer generation antiepileptic drugs. In view of the minimal drug interactions and favorable side effect profile of these drugs, they may have a role in early seizure prophylaxis after craniotomy.

6.2. Brain tumor patients

Both the American Academy of Neurology and the Association for Neurologic Surgeons/ Congress of Neurologic Surgeons recommend against routine prophylaxis with antiepileptic drugs for patients with primary brain tumors or brain metastasis without a history of seizures [33,54]. Treatment is recommended only after patients with brain tumors experience a seizure.

7. Role of Electroencephalogram in brain tumor patients

Altered mental status is a common clinical manifestation in patients with brain tumors and seizures are one cause of altered mental status. In patients with overt clinical seizures, the diagnosis is usually not in question and therefore treatment can be started immediately for this potentially life-threatening problem. However, in patients with subtle clinical signs of seizures or nonconvulsive seizures, the diagnosis is often not clear without the use of an EEG.

The workup in patients in whom seizures are suspected can be accomplished with routine bedside EEG or long-term monitoring (LTM) with continuous video EEG recording. The use of LTM has increased, especially in intensive care unit (ICU) settings. One study reported seizures in 110 (19%) of 570 critically ill patients who had continuous video EEG, most of whom were in an ICU setting. Of note, 101 of these patients had nonconvulsive seizures. Therefore, in that setting, seizures would have been missed had EEG not been used [55]. Clinical suspicion should be high in patients with structural brain lesions with altered mental status and an EEG may be beneficial for evaluating these patients.

8. Conclusion

Epilepsy in cancer patients can be from numerous causes including the cancer itself, cancer treatment, or toxic metabolic etiologies. Numerous factors contribute to the development of epilepsy in these patients. Adverse effects due to cancer treatment and antiepileptic drugs should be recognized early as patients with brain tumors and epilepsy are more likely to experience adverse effects. Treatment will be multifaceted and include antiepileptic drugs, surgery, chemotherapy, and radiation treatment. A multidisciplinary approach is usually needed for treatment of these complicated patients.

Author details

Edward K. Avila[1,2]

Address all correspondence to: avilae@mskcc.org

1 Department of Neurology, Memorial Sloan-Kettering Cancer Center, New York, NY, USA

2 Department of Neurology and Neuroscience, Weill College of Medicine of Cornell University, New York, NY, USA

References

[1] Hauser WA, Annegers JF, Rocca WA (1996) Descriptive epidemiology of epilepsy: Contributions of population studies from Rochester, Minnesota. Mayo Clin Proc 71:576-586.

[2] Herman ST (2002) Epilepsy after brain insult. Neurology 59:S21-26.

[3] Grewal J, Grewal HK, Forman AD (2008) Seizures and epilepsy in cancer: etiologies, evaluation, and management. Curr Oncol Rep 10:63–71.

[4] Banerjee PN, Filippi D, Hauser WA (2009) The descriptive epidemiology of epilepsy —a review. Epilepsy Res 85:31–45.

[5] Clouston PD, DeAngelis LM, Posner JB (1992) The spectrum of neurologic disease in patients with systemic cancer. Ann Neurol 1992, 31:268–273.

[6] Hauser WA, Annegers JF, Kurland LT (1993) Incidence of epilepsy and unprovoked seizures in Rochester, Minnesota. Epilepsia 34:453–468.

[7] Epilepsy Foundation: Epilepsy and seizure statistics. Available at http://www.epilepsyfoundation.org/about/statistics.cfm. Accessed October 2009.

[8] van Breemen MS, Wilms EB, Vecht CJ (2007) Epilepsy in patients with brain tumours: epidemiology, mechanisms, and management. Lancet Neurol 6:421–430.

[9] Lote K, Egeland T, Hager B, et al (1997) Survival, prognostic factors, and therapeutic efficacy in low-grade glioma: a retrospective study in 379 patients. J Clin Oncol 15:3129–3140.

[10] Chang EF, Potts MB, Keles GE, et al (2008) Seizure characteristics and control following resection in 332 patients with low grade gliomas. J Neurosurg 108:227-235.

[11] Lee JW, Wen PY, Hurwitz S, et al (2010) Morphological characteristics of brain tumors causing seizures Arch Neuro 67:336-342.

[12] Samji MF, Fric-Shamji EC, Benoit BG (2009) Brain tumors and epilepsy: pathophysiology of peritumoral changes. Neurosurg Rev 32:275–285.

[13] Villemure JG, de Tribolet N (1996) Epilepsy in patients with central nervous system tumors. Curr Opin Neurol 9:424–428.

[14] Gilmore R, Morris H, Van Ness P, Gilmore-Pollak W, Estes M (1994) Mirror focus: Function of seizure frequency and influence on outcome after surgery. Epilepsia 35: 258-263.

[15] Rajneesh KF, Binder DK (2009) Tumor-associated epilepsy. Neurosurg Focus 27:1-4.

[16] Wolf HK, Roos D, Blümcke I, Pietsch T, Wiestler OD (1996) Perilesional neurochemical changes in focal epilepsies. Acta Neuropathol 91:376-84.

[17] Maas S, Patt S, Schrey M, Rich A (2001) Underediting of glutamate receptor GluR-B mRNA in malignant gliomas. Proc Nat Acad Sci 98:14687-14692.

[18] Bafaloukos D and Gogas H (2004) The treatment of brain metastases in melanoma patients. Cancer Treat Rev 30: 515–520.

[19] DeAngelis LM, Posner JB (2009) Side Effects of Radiation Therapy. In: DeAngelis LM, Posner JB, editors. Neurologic Complications of Cancer (2nd Ed), Oxford University Press. pp 511-555.

[20] Sheline G (1977) Radiation therapy of brain tumors. Cancer 39: 873–81.

[21] Singh G, Rees JH, Sander JW (2007) Seizures and epilepsy in oncological practice: causes, course, mechanisms and treatment. JNNP 78:342-49.

[22] Darnell RB, Posner JB (2006) Paraneoplastic syndromes affecting the nervous system. Semin Oncol 33:270-298.

[23] Yap KY, Chui WK, Chan A (2008) Drug interactions between chemotherapeutic regimens and anticonvulsants. Clin Ther 30:1385–1407.

[24] Chalk JB, Ridgeway K, Tro'r B, et al (1984) Phenytoin impairs the bioavailability of dexamethasone in neurological and neurosurgical patients. JNNP 47:1087-1090.

[25] Maschio M, Albani F, Jandolo B, et al (2008) Temozolomide treatment does not affect topiramate and oxcarbazepine plasma concentrations in chronically treated patients with brain tumor-related epilepsy. J Neurooncol 90:217–221.

[26] Hildebrand Lecaille C, Perennes J, Delattre JY (2005) Epileptic seizures during during follow-up of patients treated for primary brain tumors. Neurology 65:212-215.

[27] Maschio M, Dinapoli L, Mingoia M, et al (2011) Lacosamide as add-on in brain tumor-related epilepsy: preliminary report on efficacy and tolerability. J Neurol 258(11):2100-4.

[28] Wick W, Menn O, Meisner C, et al (2005) Pharmacotherapy of epileptic seizures in glioma patients: who, when, why and how long? Onkologie 28:391-396.

[29] Wagner GL, Wilms EB, Van Donselaar CA, Vecht ChJ (2003) Levetiracetam: preliminary experience in patients with primary brain tumours. Seizure 12(8):585-6.

[30] Mashio M, Dinapoli L, Jandolo B (2010) In reference to Usery JB et al. J Neurooncol 100:491-2.

[31] Newton HB, Dalton J, Goldlust S, Pearl D (2007) Retrospective analysis of the efficacy and tolerability of levetiracetam in patients with metastatic brain tumors. J Neurooncol 84:293-6.

[32] Perry JR, Sawka C (1996) Add-on gabapentin for refractory seizures in patients with brain tumours Can J Neurol Sci 23:128-131.

[33] Glantz MJ, Cole BF, Forsyth PA, et al (2000) Practice parameter: anticonvulsant prophylaxis in patients with newly diagnosed brain tumors. Report of the quality standards subcommittee of the American Academy of Neurology. Neurology 54(10):1886–1893.

[34] Karceski S, Morrell MJ, Carpenter D (2005) Treatment of epilepsy in adults: Epilepsy Behav7:S1-64.

[35] Weller M, Gorlia T, Cairncross JG, et al (2011) Prolonged survival with valproic acid use in the EORTC/NCIC temozolomide trial for glioblastoma. Neurology 77:1156-64.

[36] Eyal S, Yagen B, Sobol E, Altschuler Y, Shmuel M, Bialer M (2004) The activity of antiepileptic drugs as histone deacetylase inhibitors. Epilepsia 45:737–744.

[37] Jaeckle K, Ballman K, Furth A, Buckner JC (2009) Correlation of enzyme-inducing anticonvulsant use with outcome of patients with glioblastoma. Neurology 73:1207-1213.

[38] Newton HB, Dalton J, Goldlust S, Pearl D (2007) retrospective analysis of the efficacy and tolerability of levetiracetam in patients with metastatic brain tumors. J Neurooncol 84:293–296.

[39] Englot DJ, Berger MS, Barbaro NM, Chang EF (2011) Predictors of seizure freedom after resection of supratentorial low-grade gliomas. A review. J Neurosurg 115:240-244.

[40] Sugano H, Shimizu H, Sunaga S (2007) Efficacy of intraoperative electrocorticography for assessing seizure outcomes in intractable epilepsy patients with temporal-lobe-mass lesions Seizure 16:120-127.

[41] Chan CH, Bittar RG, Davis GA, Kalnins RM, Fabinyi GC (2006) Long-term seizure outcome following surgery for dysembryoplastic neuroepithelial tumor. J Neurosurg 104:62-69.

[42] Brada M, Viviers L, Abson C, et al (2003) Phase II study of primary temozolomide chemotherapy in patients with WHO grade II gliomas. Ann Oncol 14:1715–1721.

[43] Frenay MP, Fontaine D, Vandenbos F, Lebrun C (2005) First-line nitrosourea-based chemotherapy in symptomatic non-resectable supratentorial pure low-grade astrocytomas. Eur J Neurol 12:685–690.

[44] Sherman JH, Moldovan K, Yeoh HK, Starke RM, Pouratian N, Shaffrey ME, Schiff D (2011) Impact of temozolomide chemotherapy on seizure frequency in patients with low-grade gliomas. J Neurosurg 114:1617-1621.

[45] Krueger DA, Care MM, Holland K, et al (2010) Everolimus for subependymal giant-cell astrocytomas in tuberous sclerosis. NEJM 363:1801-11.

[46] Rogers LR, Morris HH, Lupica K (1993) Effect of cranial irradiation on seizure frequency in adults with low-grade astrocytoma and medically intractable epilepsy. Neurology 43:1599-1601.

[47] Chalifoux R, Elisevich K. Effect of ionizing radiation on partial seizures attributable to malignant cerebral tumors. Stereotact Funct Neurosurg 1996–1997, 67:169-182. Review.

[48] van den Bent, MJ, Afra D, de Witte O; EORTC Radiotherapy and Brain Tumor Groups and the UK Medical Research Council (2005). Long-term efficacy of early versus delayed radiotherapy for low-grade astrocytoma and oligodendroglioma in adults: the EORTC 22845 randomised trial. Lancet 366:985-90.

[49] Temkin N (2002) Prophylactic anticonvulsants after neurosurgery. Epi Curr 2; 105-107.

[50] Klimek M, Dammers R (2010) Antiepileptic drug therapy in the perioperative course of neurosurgical patients. Curr Opin Anaesthesiol 23:564-7.

[51] Bähr O, Hermisson M, Rona S (2012) Intravenous and oral levetiracetam in patients with a suspected primary brain tumor and symptomatic seizures undergoing neurosurgery: The HELLO trial. Acta Neurochir 154:229-35.

[52] Zachenhofer I, Donat M, Oberndorfer S, Roessler K (2011) Perioperative levetiracetam for prevention of seizures in supratentorial brain tumor surgery. J Neurooncol. 101:101-106.

[53] Komotar RJ, Raper DM, Starke RM, Iorgulescu JB, Gutin PH (2011) Prophylactic antiepileptic drug therapy in patients undergoing supratentorial meningioma resection: a systematic analysis of efficacy. J Neurosurg 115:483-490.

[54] Mikkelsen T, Paleologos NA, Robinson PD, et al (2010) The role of prophylactic anticonvulsants in the management of brain metastases: a systematic review and evidence-based clinical practice guideline. J Neurooncol 96:97-102.

[55] Hirsch L (2004) Continuous EEG monitoring in the intensive care unit: an overview. J Clin Neurophysiol 21:332–340.

Chapter 11

Glioma-Associated Epilepsy

Kost Elisevich

Additional information is available at the end of the chapter

http://dx.doi.org/10.5772/52355

1. Introduction

Hughlings Jackson, in the nineteenth century, first noted that epilepsy could be the only clinical manifestation of a primary brain tumour [1] (Figure 1). Among patients with epilepsy, the incidence of brain tumours is about 4% [2] whereas the prevalence of epilepsy among patients with brain tumours is over 30% [3] Seizures will herald the presence of a cerebral glioma in 20-45% of patients [4,5] and another 15-30% of patients will develop seizures during the course of the condition [6]. In particular, epilepsy occurs in over 80% of patients with low-grade gliomas [7] and 30-60% of those with high-grade gliomas [8]. Factors which favour epileptogenesis in low-grade tumours appear related to slow growth kinetics coupled with cerebral location [9,10]. The relative risk for a cerebral tumour following a diagnosis of epilepsy approaches 20-fold overall compared with control and, when differentiated between malignant and benign tumours, it is about 26-fold and 10-fold, respectively [11]. It is highest for those aged 15-44 years at the time of diagnosis of the epileptic condition and will persist for several years afterward.

Apart from the adversity brought about by the growth of a cerebral tumour, a tumour-associated epilepsy adds further disadvantage for the patient with its impact on the quality of life and on the course of treatment. Epilepsy in brain tumour patients is often refractory to pharmacological therapy. The unpredictability of seizure occurrence, particularly those associated with a loss of consciousness, denies patients the ability to move freely in society, promoting a sense of isolation. Adverse effects of antiepileptic medications, particularly when taken in combination in those cases that are difficult to bring under control, may add to the burden of those imposed by therapy dedicated to the tumour itself. Debate has also arisen over the effect of some enzyme-inducing antiepileptic medications upon such therapy as certain of these agents will induce hepatic P450 microsomal enzymes that could accelerate the metabolism of chemotherapeutic agents. Particular attention must be given to the view that, in addition to the optimal removal of tumour, surgical intervention should be dedicated, as best

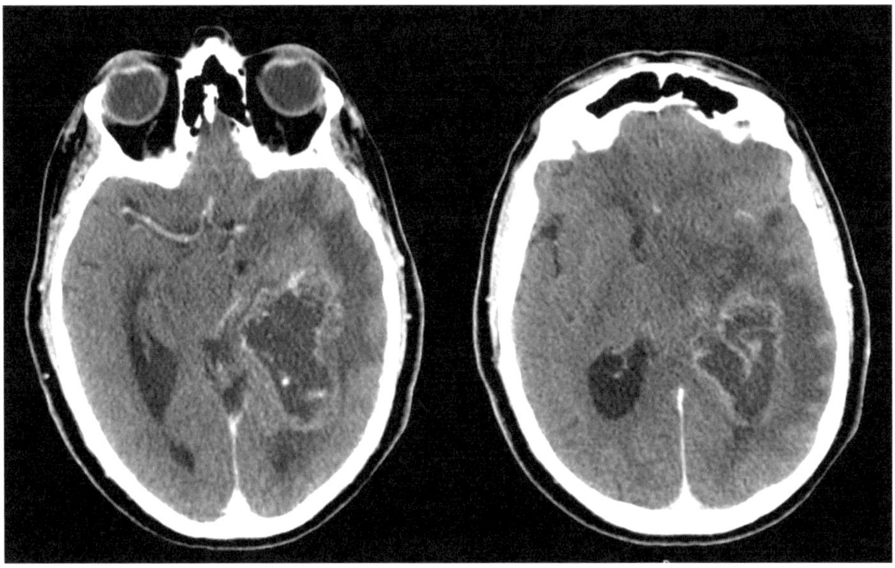

Figure 1. Axial contrast-enhanced computed tomography (CT) images identify a large left temporo-occipital glioblastoma. This 58 year old man acquired a medically intractable complex partial epilepsy 3 years previously and was investigated then by noncontrast CT imaging which showed no abnormality. The presence of an implanted cardiac defibrillator precluded magnetic resonance imaging.

as possible, to the elimination of the associated epilepsy with the ultimate aim of withdrawing the antiepileptic medical regimen altogether. This requires a greater perspective upon the neurobiology of this attendant condition in order to effect as best an outcome as possible for the patient.

As more is becoming known of tumor biology and the putative factors underlying epileptogenesis, a periodic review of the current status of glioma-associated epilepsy in this context is mandatory. This chapter will review the principal clinical features of the epileptic condition, its neurobiology as it pertains to etiological mechanisms, in particular, and the therapeutic options, both medical and surgical, that seek to control it.

2. Neurobiology

The fundamental characteristic of epilepsy is the presence of recurrent, usually unprovoked seizures that, when viewed electrographically, consist of paroxysmal, self-limiting, excessive and synchronous discharge of a population of neuronoglial elements comprising a coherent network, often limited in its topography. These elements are contained predominantly in the cerebral cortex and, at the cellular level, manifest as unrestrained excitation attributable to deregulatory mechanisms affecting membrane depolarization and repolarization. It is important that we attempt to understand the phenomenon of epilepsy from a cellular and molecular level by addressing the constituent elements that give rise to a region of excitability and from a network perspective to establish the relatedness of neuronoglial populations that interact with one another to perpetuate the condition.

Previous literature regarding localization-related epileptogenicity referred to irritative and ictal onset zones wherein the former designated the cerebrocortical area that generated interictal spikes and the latter, that area responsible for initiating actual seizure activity. The two zones, although related, were not necessarily congruent as in a perilesional environment. This conceptualization is being supplanted by the realization of multiple limited functional connectivities that exist in the brain which itself is seen as a complex integrated master network. These connectivities are defined by statistical interdependencies or coherences as identified by neurophysiological time series, particularly by electroencephalography (EEG) and magnetoencephalography (MEG) [12,13]. In essence, the strength of connections among network nodes and their directionality may define for us the extent of epileptogenic territory. An altered functional connectivity has been proposed in the case of both mesial temporal lobe epilepsy [14] and tumour-associated epilepsy [15] patients. A pathologically increased theta or low frequency band connectivity was found to be related to increased seizure activity in brain tumour patients raising some consideration as to whether such findings may shed light on peritumoural epileptogenesis. Greater appreciation of such local network behavior and the integration of EEG, MEG and resting state functional MRI will allow a more definitive interpretation of seizure vulnerability and a better disclosure of perilesional epileptogenicity as it relates to network topology for use in the planning of surgical intervention.

At the cellular level, it is insufficient to describe epileptogenicity as a neuronal phenomenon as the intimacy of neuronoglial interaction declares an inseparability of function of these two essential cell types. The impact of astrocytes on neuronal function through influences upon synaptic function and plasticity, provision of energy and regulation of local blood flow and blood-brain integrity is profound [16]. Protoplasmic astrocytic processes surround neuronal synapses and form gap junctions among one another [17] allowing electrotonic communication through a local syncytium. Astrocytes bear sodium and potassium channels and demonstrate excitability through regulated increases in intracellular calcium concentration [18,19]. These elevations can be triggered by glutamate released during neuronal activity propagated to neighbouring astrocytes via gap junctions and, in turn, cause the release of glutamate from astrocytes into the extracellular space triggering receptor-mediated currents in neurons remote from the original site of stimulation [20-24]. Higher concentrations of glutamine have been found in gliomas [25] and glioma cells have been shown to take up and release glutamine [26, 27] providing a potential reservoir of precursor for glutamate production in the peritumoural area. Otherwise, glutamate uptake has been demonstrated to be 100-fold lower in human glioma cells compared to that in astrocytes and has been attributed to a reduction of sodium-dependent glutamate transporters and an upregulation of cystine-glutamate exchange [28].

In fact, marked glutamate release in murine brain slices implanted with human-derived glioma cells has been shown to induce epileptiform hyperexcitability in adjacent brain tissue [29]. Administration of sulfasalazine, an inhibitor of glutamate release, to tumour-bearing mice reduced ictal behavior compared with untreated controls. Certain antiepileptic agents will also block astrocytic calcium signaling pointing to a mechanism underlying epileptogenicity [30].

Synaptic interstitial homeostasis is provided by astrocytic processes through the maintenance of fluid, pH and transmitter balance. The aquaporin 4 (AQP4) water channel and transporters for potassium uptake [31, 32], proton shuttling mechanisms [33] and transporter-mediated clearance of synaptic glutamate, glycine and gamma aminobutyric acid (GABA) [34] coupled with the ability for an astrocytic gap junction-mediated syncytium to dissipate detrimental accumulation of all such elements [35] argues for the essential nature of the neuonoglial relationship. Glutamate also modulates astrocytic glycogen storage [36] and neuronal activity may influence the passage of glucose metabolites through this same syncytium [37]. Reactive astrocytosis in a peritumoural environment may contribute to epileptogenesis through the release of glutamate [38, 30], compromise of blood-brain barrier integrity through production of vascular endothelial growth factor [39], production of excess reactive oxygen species [40], accentuation of inflammation through cytokine production [41, 139] and through AQP4 overactivity [32]. In the end, there are several putative epileptogenic mechanisms involving the neuronoglial relationship which, individually or in concert, may promote and sustain ictal behavior. Both the local infiltrative and structurally disruptive process of gliomatous invasion and the altered neurochemistry of the peritumoral environment undoubtedly combine to bring about the epileptogenicity.

Reduced numbers of both GABA- and somatostatin-containing interneurons in the area adjacent to low-grade gliomas [42] suggests a change in peritumoural neuronal phenotype and an alteration in the excitatory-inhibitory balance. A similar reduction in somatostatinergic neurons has been demonstrated in the human hippocampus in mesial temporal epileptogenicity [43, 44] and in animal models of experimental epilepsy [45]. Other cellular alterations demonstrated in animal models have raised suspicion regarding similar evolution in human peritumoural epileptogenicity. Particular attention has been given to synaptic vesicle protein 2A, a membrane glycoprotein present in synaptic vesicles of neurons and a calcium regulator in neurotransmitter release [46], as it is the binding site for the antiepileptic, levetiracetam [47]. It has been shown to have a low distribution in the cerebral cortex and hippocampus of spontaneously epileptic rats [48] and its removal in knockout mice promotes severe seizure development [49]. Expression of SV2A in human peritumoural cortex in both low- and high-grade gliomas, however, was no different between those patients identified with epilepsy and those without, suggesting different mechanisms of regulation of SV2A than in the models examined (50).

Further attention has turned to signaling pathways that trigger epileptogenesis following a cerebral insult. In particular, serine/threonine kinase (mTOR) activates several downstream processes involved in protein synthesis, ribosomal biogenesis, cell growth and proliferation [51]. As a consequence, it will respond to aberrant events in order to initiate a cellular reaction and, indeed, has been found to be dysregulated in neurological disease including brain tumours [52, 53]. Inhibition of mTOR by rapamycin attenuates the development of epilepsy and interferes with epileptogenesis in the kainate model [54]. Its delivery even following an induced status epilepticus succeeded in blocking the chronic phase of mTOR activation demonstrating not only an antiepileptic but an antiepileptogenic effect.

The influence of inflammatory factors in the mediation of epileptogenesis has also been addressed in recent years. Seizures themselves are known to induce an upregulation of cyclooxygenase-2 (COX-2) in neurons and, particularly, in non-neuronal cells [55]. This agent is known to promote neurodegeneration of somatostatin-expressing GABAergic interneurons, intensify cytokine reactivity and underlie the loss of integrity of the blood-brain barrier after seizure activity [56]. Its involvement in the peritumoural region may explain the loss of GABAergic neurons [42], in particular, and suggest a role in the mechanism for the epileptogenic process here.

3. Clinical presentation

The standardized mortality ratio (SMR; ratio of observed and expected deaths) for patients with recurrent seizures attributed to an acquired lesion such as a brain tumour during the first two years is 4.3 [57]. The frequency of status epilepticus, with its attendant risk of morbidity and mortality, increases from 3.8% in all patients with epilepsy to 9% in those with an underlying lesion. Three primary factors influence the risk of acquiring epilepsy in the presence of a cerebral glioma – glioma type, location and proximity to the cerebral mantle [10, 58]. As many as 80% of patients with oligodendrogliomas or gangliogliomas experience seizures. Anaplastic astrocytomas carry a risk of 68% [59], similar to astrocytomas, and the risk for glioblastomas is 29% to 37% [59, 10, 58]. The transitional histopathology of astrocytomas and anaplastic astrocytomas, with the latter likely to retain regional features of the more epileptogenic low-grade neoplasm, may explain the similarity in risk.

The propensity toward epileptogenicity by cerebral region varies considerably with the motor-sensory region most susceptible and the occipital region less so [10, 60]. The motor-sensory cortical region substantially raises the general risk of seizure occurrence for both the astrocytoma (83%) and glioblastoma (53%) [59].

The semiology of partial epilepsy may, at times, provide useful lateralizing or localizing information as to the whereabouts of a cerebral glioma. One of the more characteristic of such occurrences is the classic uncinate fit or olfactory aura brought about by a lesion situated in the uncus or lateral olfactory area in which the patient commonly experiences the recurrent spontaneous sensation of a bad odour. Lateralized elementary visual hallucinations originate typically in the vicinity of the calcarine cortex [61, 62] and gustatory hallucinations in the parietal operculum and/or insula [3, 63]. Focal motor or sensory manifestations as simple partial seizures, with or without a Jacksonian march, will also indicate the presence of a centrally located tumour as will periods of speech arrest in cases of tumours in the dominant hemisphere occupying the frontal opercular and inferior premotor or posterior temporal convexity region. In these latter circumstances, certain subtle aspects of the clinical presentation will shed further localizing information as in some loss of contralateral manual dexterity, a widening of the contralateral palpebral fissure and lapses in the proficiency of speech. Postictal manifestations may accentuate these features for variable periods of time. Although versive head deviation at ictal onset has been shown to be unreliable as a lateralizing feature [64, 65], combined contralateral head and eye deviation may have lateralizing significance [66].

A detailed rendering of lobar-specific ictal manifestations may best be presented in a tabular form for completeness (Table 1); however, as the majority of both low- and high-grade gliomas appear in the fronto-temporal distribution, our particular attention may be drawn to the anterior cerebral hemispheres to review some of the more common ictal features.

Frontal	**Orbitofrontal**: olfactory hallucinations, experiential sensations, gestural automatisms, autonomic features, speech arrest (likelihood of spread to mesial temporal area) **Dorsolateral**: generalized event without warning, possible contraversive tonic head and eye motion (likelihood of spread to rolandic area and transcallosally) **Cingulate**: complex motor gestural and sexual automatisms, mood changes, urinary incontinence (likelihood of spread transcallosally and to temporal lobe) **Supplementary**: abduction and lateral rotation of upper arm with elbow flexion and tonic head rotation to involved limb, vocalization, bicycling, scissoring of legs (likelihood of spread transcallosally) **Perirolandic**: focal clonic motor activity, possible Jacksonian march
Temporal	**Mesiobasal**: experiential sensations with epigastric features, déjà vu, memory flashes, behavioural arrest, staring with oroalimentary automatisms (likelihood of spread to frontal and insular areas) **Opercular**: auditory hallucinations, focal motor and sensory symptoms, vertigo (likelihood of spread to insula and parietal area) **Convexity**: complex visual hallucinations, vertigo, speech arrest (likelihood of spread to mesial temporal and parietal areas)
Parietal	**Inferior**: speech arrest/dysphasia, vertigo, arm/facial sensory and motor activity, tonic posturing, head deviation **Superior**: metamorphosia, asomatognosia, arm/leg sensory and motor activity, tonic posturing, vertigo
Occipital	Elementary contralateral visual phenomena – scotoma, hemianopia, phosphenes, object distortion

Table 1. Semiologies of Lobar Epilepsies

In the case of frontal lobe ictal origin, the tendency for rapid dissemination of discharge both ipsi- and contralaterally and to generalize confounds our ability to localize or even lateralize the condition. The seizure may manifest in a variety of forms – primary generalized, absence, simple and complex partial [67-71]. Auras tend to be less frequent then in temporal lobe epilepsy and, when present, rather nonspecific [72,70]. Prominent motor features with focal tonic-clonic activity, adversive head and eye deviation and stereotypic motor automatisms (i.e., fencing posture, scissoring) may develop [73, 74, 69, 63, 71, 70] and secondary generalization without evidence of focal onset occurs often, particularly in the case of seizures arising in the dorsolateral frontal convexity [75, 63, 72]. There is also some vulnerability toward status epilepticus of the convulsive [76] or of the complex partial [71] variety. By contrast, brief tonic and absence-like seizures may occur [77]. Frontopolar seizures without spread are commonly clinically silent whereas posterior spread may result in a loss of consciousness, focal tonic motor activity and generalization [71]. Orbitofrontal seizures are typically complex partial in nature and may be mixed with motor and gestural automatisms, olfactory hallucinations and autonomic signs, perhaps through connections with the mesial temporal structure via the uncinate fasciculus. Seizures of cingulate origin may also be complex partial in nature with similar motor and gestural automatisms in addition to sexual automatisms, mood changes and urinary incontinence [78, 71]. Finally, supplementary motor seizures tend to be brief but frequent and may manifest as an abduction and external rotation of the contralateral arm and flexion of the elbow with the head directed toward the postured arm while the legs may be flexed, extended or elevated [63]. Either vocalization or speech arrest may be apparent while the patient remains conscious. Alternating locomotor activity, as in bicycling, may also be witnessed. Many frontal lobe seizures, particularly of convexity origin and exclusive of generalized events, are characterized by a rapid postictal recovery with little evidence of fatigue.

Epilepsy of temporal lobe origin is commonly of a complex partial variety and, in the case of a mesial origin, may be heralded by an aura of an experiential sort, followed or accompanied by impaired consciousness, behavioural arrest, staring and subsequent automatic behaviour as with oroalimentary automatisms (i.e., chewing, lip-smacking, swallowing) [79]. A postictal fatigue of variable duration, sometimes profound, often follows. Those complex partial events arising from an extratemporal source often begin with semipurposeful motor activity and commonly do not manifest a behavioural arrest or stereotypical automatisms [80, 81]. Auras appear in 80% of patients with a mesial temporal epileptogenicity and may be characterized by epigastric sensations, déjà vu experiences and memory flashes [82]. Additional features to those described above include uni- and bilateral tonic-clonic or dystonic posturing. Seizures arising in the temporal opercular area may cause auditory hallucinations in addition to focal motor or sensory experiences, depending upon subsequent spread of activity. Vestibular and complex visual hallucinations may characterize the more posteriorly situated temporal convexity ictal semiology. Language disturbance in the form of speech arrest, in particular, in the ictal or postictal state, will often declare dominant hemispheric involvement.

4. Antiepileptic medical management

Apart from the issue of refractory seizures, patients with epilepsy attributable to a glioma are threatened by potential interactions between antiepileptic and chemotherapeutic agents and risks associated with toxicity of either.

All gliomas, whether low- or high grade, must be assessed for surgical resection in order to optimize survival [83, 84, 85]. The literature has supported the notion of aggressive removal, to the extent allowable, in any region of the brain and, to this end, the inclusion of the immediate peritumoural region in the resection volume affords the opportunity of removing sufficient epileptogenic tissue to reduce or eliminate the presenting epilepsy or deny its further evolution (*Figure 2).* Postoperative antiepileptic medical prophylaxis is advised for patients with supratentorial gliomas. In a study of anaplastic gliomas, 36% of patients without preoperative indication of epileptogenicity experienced a postoperative seizure [86]. In a nonrandomized study, the incidence of all seizure types was lower in the early postoperative stage (21% vs 39%) in patients receiving antiepileptic treatment compared with those left untreated [87]. Moreover, no impairment of consciousness was witnessed in those treated compared to 18% of those untreated, suggesting that a putative subclinical epileptogenicity was averted. Postoperative complications (i.e., hemorrhage, worsening edema) raise the likelihood of seizures during the initial 48 hour period by over two-fold, including status epilepticus even in the presence of antiepileptic medical coverage [9]. Late postoperative seizures were found to occur in 34% of those patients who had presented preoperatively with seizure activity. Although a significant difference was not substantiated, the incidence of late-onset epilepsy appeared lower in the treated patients (12% vs 21%) in the same study. The interval between surgery and the first postoperative seizure was less than six months in 52% of patients and the majority harboured a malignant glioma. Maintenance of therapeutic levels is essential in judging the efficacy of treatment and maximizing serum levels to individual tolerability is required before consideration is given to adding a second agent.

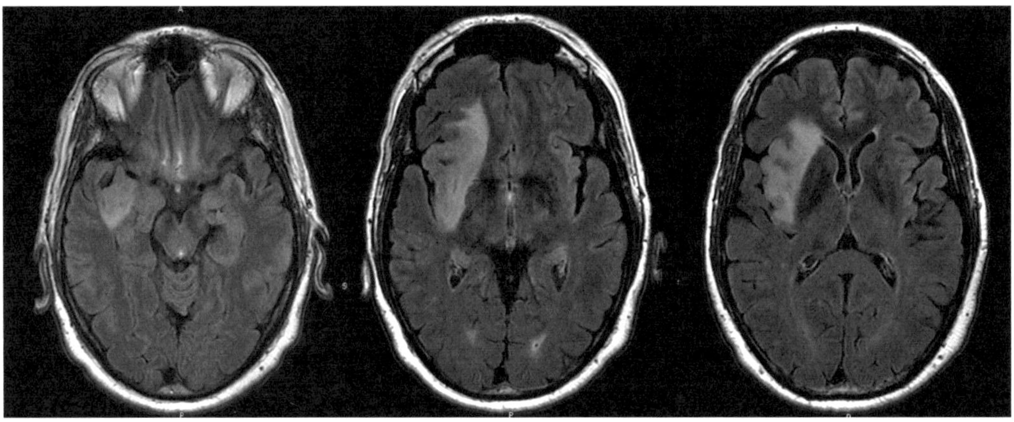

Figure 2. Axial magnetic resonance imaging identifies a predominant right insular tumour in a 62 year old man with a 3 year history of medically intractable complex partial epilepsy. Acute nausea followed by behavioural arrest, oroalimentary automatisms and a postictal drowsiness began manifesting at an almost daily frequency with no distinct electroencephalographic features. Resection of this grade 2 oligoastrocytoma resulted in cessation of seizures

The risk of late postoperative seizure recurrence and a declared epileptogenicity may be judged by a number of factors. These include, primarily, the extent of glioma removal with the consequent reduction of tumour burden and elimination or reduction of vasogenic edema. The proximity to cortical regions prone toward epileptogenicity where such regions have been left intact (i.e., dominant mesial temporal region, motor-sensory region) must also be taken into consideration. Exclusive of the inability to optimally remove the tumour and/or a sufficient portion of the peritumoural region, the duration of preoperative epileptogenicity, postoperative complications (i.e., cerebrovascular compromise, intracerebral hemorrhage) and difficulties in maintaining adequate serum antiepileptic medication levels will also influence the outcome.

Several antiepileptic agents have appeared over the past two decades that have shown efficacy and greater tolerability in patients with brain tumour-related epilepsy [88-92]. The side effect profile of the traditional antiepileptic medications such as phenobarbital, phenytoin, carbamazepine and valproic acid was such [93, 94, 5, 95] that it seemed often to take precedence over the desire to reduce seizure activity [96]. The administration of phenobarbital, phenytoin or primidone can markedly lower serum levels of carbamazepine and both valproic acid and lamotrigine will increase the serum concentrations of an active metabolite, carbamazepine-10,11-epoxide. On the other hand, the half-life of phenytoin can be significantly shortened and the serum level of valpoic acid may be reduced when delivered with carbamazapine. Finally, agents such as calcium channel blockers, erythromycin and propoxyphene may elevate plasma levels of carbamazepine when given concurrently. The incidence of severe rash (14%) accompanying therapy with these agents is higher in patients undergoing radiation and chemotherapy [93] and cognitive decline more pronounced [95]. Moreover, phenobarbital, phenytoin and carbamazepine are potent inducers of P450 microsomal enzymes, particularly, CYP 3A4 and CYP 2D6, and will putatively enhance metabolism of chemotherapeutic agents degraded by these enzymes resulting in the reduction of plasma levels and reduced efficacy [97, 98]. Some controversy regarding this effect has arisen, however, with some studies declaring improved outcomes in the presence of enzyme-inducing antiepileptic medications [99, 100]. Nevertheless, a decline in the use of the latter has occurred in recent years in favour of the newer non-enzyme-inducing antiepileptics such as levetiracetam, lamotrigine and vigabatrin which are relatively devoid of P450 microsomal enzyme induction or inhibition. Oxcarbazepine and topiramate are weak inducers of CYP 3A4 and weak inhibitors of CYP 2C19 and zonisamide has shown variability but overall weak inducing and inhibiting effects [101]. Valproic acid has been shown to be a potent inhibitor of microsomal enzymes and may increase the toxicity of chemotherapy [101].

A total of 14 new antiepileptic medications have been approved by the Federal Drug Administration (FDA) since 1992. These newer medications are safer, more tolerable, have, in general, fewer interactions with one another and require less monitoring. Moreover, several medications are under development which target other mechanisms underlying epileptogenicity other than those which currently effect voltage-gated Na and Ca channels and GABA inhibition. For instance, 2-deoxyglucose inhibits glycolysis and appears to have both antiepileptic and antiepileptogenic effects. Both ezogabine and ICA-105665 affect voltage-activated (KCNQ) potassium channels and are the first such agents dedicated to this ion channel. Targetting receptors for the neuropeptide, galanin, also shows promise as an antiepileptic. An AMPA (alpha-amino-3-hydroxy-5-methyl-4-isoxazolepropropionic acid) receptor antagonist, perampanel, appears effective in patients with refractory partial epilepsy and is in the late stages of clinical development. Because of the interest in neuroinflammation as a promoter of epileptogenicity, an active inhibitor (VX-765) of caspase 1, the enzyme responsible for the production of interleukin-1-beta, has been investigated and found to show longterm antiepileptic effects that may be relevant.

Of particular interest has been the discovery of an antiepileptic effect brought about by topoisomerase inhibition [102]. Given the antineoplastic efficacy of DNA topoisomerase 1 inhibition, such an agent would be particularly useful in patients with cerebral glioma-associated epilepsy. Type 1 DNA topoisomerase (Top1) binds with DNA and relaxes the helix at the time of torsional stresses associated with its replication and transcription [103]. In a situation where transcription is generating supercoiled DNA to sustain high levels of RNA synthesis, as in an area of excitability, such inhibition would be detrimental to the epileptic process. Reduced Top1 activity could result in the inhibition of gene transcription critical for efficient synaptic transmission or possibly result in an enhanced apoptosis of those cellular elements involved in epileptogenic circuitry [104].

In the absence of postoperative seizure occurrence or recurrence for a period of 3 – 6 months and in the absence of both imaging evidence of tumour recurrence and EEG evidence of epileptiform features, a tapering regimen for the antiepileptic medication may be contemplated. Where a patient has presented with a single ictal event preoperatively, the decision, as dictated above, may be reached comfortably. In the case where there is uncertainty regarding the veracity of a patient's statement as to the absence of clinical seizure activity, the presence of artefactual changes that may obscure tumour recurrence in potentially epileptogenic territory on followup imaging and/or an inability by the electroencephalographer to adequately survey the cerebral cortex for hidden epileptogenicity, the decision to taper medication must be tempered accordingly.

5. Surgery

Tumour resection alone results in good postoperative seizure control in those patients presenting with a glioma-associated epilepsy [105, 9, 106]. As is often the case, a variable amount of epileptogenic cortical tissue is removed in the process of optimizing the removal of a glioma with its ill-defined border, affording the patient a good seizure outcome postoperatively. When the peritumoural tissue removal is not satisfactory, postoperative seizure control remains effectively unchanged [107, 108, 9, 106, 109, 58]. Image-guided stereotactic lesional resection achieves a longterm seizure-free outcome in 57% of cases [108] whereas the inclusion of peritumoural tissues in the resection volume raised this metric beyond 80% [110, 111]. The realization that the peritumoural environment is critical in the promotion of most epileptic manifestations has prompted the use of intraoperative electrocorticography in cases of low grade gliomas, in particular, to increase the likelihood of capturing those responsible cortical areas in the resection volume [112-116]. In a review of 45 patients with low grade gliomas and intractable epilepsy, 53% were rendered seizure-free and no longer requiring antiepileptic medical management after a mean followup of 54 months [112]. An additional 38% were seizure-free but still required medical management, although reduced. A meta analysis of studies addressing the benefit of resecting additional epileptogenic tissues showed that, in the case of low grade gliomas, seizure-free outcome was 63%, in marked contrast to the 18% seizure-free outcome achieved by lesionectomy alone [117]. Persistence of epileptiform activity following resection of an epileptogenic area is associated with seizure recurrence [118] and, hence, postresection electrocorticography has been promoted also [112]. When addressing specifically complex partial epilepsy in the context of temporal lobe tumors, the use of

http://dx.doi.org/10.5772/52355

electrocorticography clearly favoured outcome [119]. When a lesionectomy alone was performed, a seizure-free status of 18.8% was achieved compared with a 92.8% seizure-free outcome when electrocorticography was used.

At times, in cases of low grade gliomas, the source of some of the epileptogenicity may be remote from the tumor [106, 120]. Such occurrences may only be documented, in most circumstances, with prolonged inpatient extraoperative electrocorticography and reflect the engagement of an epileptogenic network type of activity in which remote nodes of epileptic activity may attain sufficient independence to perpetuate clinical manifestations despite removal of the original offending lesion. Indeed, resection of a remote epileptogenic site in the presence of an unresectable tumour has resulted in the relief of the epileptic condition [121].

Both the glioma type and its cerebral location typically determines its epileptogenic potential. Although oligodendrogliomas are found more commonly in the frontal region (35%), their epileptogenicity is better expressed in the temporal and temporoparietal regions where about 80% will promote an epilepsy [122]. A distinct clinicopathological group of patients with a protracted history of epilepsy attributable to the occurrence of a limbic or neocortical glioma has been identified [123]. Most such gliomas were confined to the temporal (63%) and occipital (18%) lobes and occupied limbic or perilimbic locations. The majority (61%) were identified as low grade tumors although 17% were anaplastic despite a stable clinical history of epilepsy with a mean of 15 years duration. Following resection of the tumour, 82% of the group of 60 patients studied were seizure-free after one year. A similar group, consisting typically of low grade gliomas, has been studied more recently [124] and characterized by a low cellularity, lack of mitoses and the absence of certain protein expression, such as the microtubule-associated protein (MAP2) which is critical in neurogenesis. The protein stabilizes microtubules that are enriched in dendrites, implicating a role in stabilizing dendritic shape during neuronal development. Microtubular assembly is therefore an essential step in neurogenesis. Patients are reported to have 50% fewer recurrences at 7.5 years followup and an 80% ten year survival.

Complex partial epilepsy in the context of a temporal lobe tumour must always raise suspicion of a dual pathology with an associated atrophy of the ipsilateral hippocampus resulting from cell loss, particularly in the CA4 region [125, 126]. In a series of 17 patients harbouring temporal lobe tumours presenting with complex partial epilepsy, 12 were found to have gliomas of which four were mixed gliomas (astrocytoma-oligodendroglioma), three were low grade astrocytomas and two were classed as cellular astrocytomas [126]. Neuronal densities throughout all the hippocampal subfields including the granule cell layer were diminished. Medially placed tumours were associated with the more dramatic changes than laterally placed tumours. Where an atrophic hippocampus has been identified, resection of both the lesion and the hippocampus is more likely to result in a seizure-free outcome [127].

6. Effect of ionizing radiation

Experience over the last several decades has indicated that ionizing radiation is capable of reducing both the clinical and electrographic expression of partial epilepsy [128-132]. The radiosurgical treatment of cerebral arteriovenous malformations with an associated epilepsy has been shown to have an antiepileptic effect even in the absence of angiographic evidence of obliteration of the malformation [129]. In this latter series, seizures had ceased altogether in 55% of cases and a seizure-free interval had been maintained for a duration of followup of 2 – 8 years. In a review of patients presenting with glioma-associated epilepsy of long term, three of four patients with frontal lobe tumours who had undergone biopsy and conventional radiation therapy were found to be seizure-free during a followup of four years [106]. In the same series, 83% of 23 patients who had undergone a resection followed by radiation therapy also became seizure-free. In the shorter interval, recurrent seizures attributable to malignant gliomas have been shown responsive to ionizing radiation [133]. Five of nine patients harbouring a biopsy-proven malignant glioma and manifesting an intractable partial epilepsy responded to treatment with a seizure-free outcome for the duration of their survival and the remainder showed a reduction in frequency of greater than 75%.

Radiosurgical application in the case of nonlesional partial epilepsy has also been shown to be beneficial in the longterm [134, 135], enough so that its use in the treatment of partial epilepsies remains an option. Whether lesionally-associated or not, there is much yet to be understood regarding the radiobiology of the effect upon the epileptic condition [136- 138].

7. Summary

Importantly, seizures will herald the presence of an underlying glioma, particularly in the adult, and will result in intervention before any other clinical manifestation is realized. This alone may afford the patient an opportunity to delay or avoid the inevitable loss of function that occurs with the further growth of the tumour and its further malignant transformation. Surgical intervention constitutes the most effective means by which an often intractable glioma-associated epilepsy may be brought under control. The extent of peritumoural resection is critical in this intervention and the use of intraoperative electrocorticography, particularly in the case of a longstanding epilepsy, provides the necessary objective criteria by which the surgeon will appreciate the location and extent of the epileptogenic surround. Cerebrocortical mapping in the presence of electrographic monitoring allows the surgeon to optimally perform such a resection by avoiding eloquent structure and concurrently reduce the tumour burden further in the infiltrative zone.

There is great promise in future antiepileptic pharmaceutical applications as they apply specifically to glioma therapy. Dual antiepileptic-antineoplastic effects may be realized. Better understanding of the biology underlying the antiepileptic effect of ionizing radiation may ultimately be used to guide therapy specifically to certain peritumoural areas where epileptogenicity is expressed.

The presence of epilepsy diminishes the quality of life for the patient with a glioma and dedicated effort is required to assure that the patient benefits maximally from intervention not only to reduce tumour burden but to eliminate the epileptogenicity.

http://dx.doi.org/10.5772/52355

Author details

Kost Elisevich*

Michigan State University, Department of Clinical Neurosciences, Division of Neurosurgery, Spectrum Health Medical Group, Grand Rapids, Michigan, USA

References

[1] Jackson JH. Localized convulsions from tumour of the brain. Brain (1882) 5: 364 - 374.

[2] Herman ST. Epilepsy after brain insult: targeting epileptogenesis. Neurology 2002; 59(9 Suppl 5): S21-S26.

[3] Hausser-Hauw C, Bancaud J. Gustatory hallucinations in epileptic seizures: electrophysiological, clinical and anatomical correlates. Brain (1987) 110: 339 – 359.

[4] Krouwer HG, Pallagi JL, Graves NM. Management of seizures in brain tumor patients at the end of life. J Palliat Med (2000) 3: 465 – 475.

[5] Glantz MJ, Cole BF, Forsyth PA, Recht LD, Wen PY, Chamberlain MC, Grossman SA, Cairncross JG. Practice parameter: anticonvulsant prophylaxis in patients with newly diagnosed brain tumors. Report of the Quality Standards Subcommittee of the American Academy of Neurology. Neurology (2000) 54: 1886 -1893.

[6] Beaumont A, Whittle IR. The pathogenesis of tumour associated pilepsy. Acta Neurochir (Wien) (2000) 142: 1 – 15.

[7] Vertosick FT, Jr, Selker RG, Arena VC. Survival of patients with well-differentiated astrocytomas diagnosed in the era of computed tomography. Neurosurgery (1991) 28: 496 – 501.

[8] Scott GM, Gibberd FB. Epilepsy and other factors in the prognosis of gliomas. Acta Neurol Scand (1980) 61: 227 – 239.

[9] Franceschetti S, Binelli S, Casazza M, Lodrini S, Panzica F, Pluchino F, Solero CL, Avanzini G. Influence of surgery and antiepileptic drugs on seizures symptomatic of cerebral tumors. Acta Neurochir (Wien) (1990) 103: 47 – 51.

[10] Penfield W, Erickson TC, Tarlov I. Relation of intracranial tumors and symptomatic epilepsy. Arch Neurol Psychiatry (1940) 44: 300 – 315.

[11] Khan T, Akhtar W, Wotton CJ, Hart Y, Turner MR, Goldacre MJ. Epilepsy and the subsequent risk of cerebral tumour: record linkage retrospective cohort study. J Neurol Neurosurg Psychiatry (2011) 82: 1041 – 1045.

[12] Stephan KE, Riera JJ, Deco G, Horwitz B. The Brain connectivity Workshops: moving the frontiers of computational systems neuroscience. Neuroimage (2008) 42: 1 – 9.

[13] Reijneveld JC, Ponten SC, Berendse HW, Stam CJ. The application of graph theoretical analysis to complex networks in the brain. Clin Neurophysiol (2007) 118: 2317 – 2331.

[14] Liao W, Zhang Z, Pan Z, Mantini D, Ding J, Duan X, Luo C, Lu G, Chen H. Altered functional connectivity and small-world in mesial temporal lobe epilepsy. PLoS One 2009; 5: e8525.

[15] Douw L, van Dellen E, de Groot M, Heimans JJ, Klein M, Stam CJ, Reijneveld JC. Epilepsy is related to theta band brain connectivity and network topology in brain tumor patients. BMC Neurosci (2010) 11: 103.

[16] Sofroniew MV, Vinters HV. Astrocytes: biology and pathology. Acta Neuropathol (2010) 119: 7 – 35.

[17] Peters A, Palay SL, Webster HD. The fine structure of the nervous sytem. 3rd Ed, 1991, Oxford University Press, New York.

[18] Charles AC, Merrill JE, Dirksen ER, Sanderson MJ. Intercellular signaling in glial cells: calcium waves and oscillations in response to mechanical stimulation and glutamate. Neuron (1991) 6: 983 – 992.

[19] Cornell-Bell AH, Finkbeiner SM, Cooper MS, Smith SJ. Glutamate induces calcium waves in cultured astrocytes: long-range glial signaling. Science (1990) 247: 470 – 473.

[20] Halassa MM, Fellin T, Haydon PG. The tripartite synapse: roles for gliotransmission in health and disease. Trends Mol Med (2007) 13: 54 – 63.

[21] Nedergaard M, Ransom B, Goldman SA. New roles for astrocytes: redining the functional architecture of the brain. Trends Neurosci (2003) 26: 523 – 530.

[22] Perea G, Navarrete M, Araque A. Tripartite synapses: astrocytes process and control synaptic information. Trends Neurosci (2009) 32: t421 – t431.

[23] Shigetomi E, Browser DN, Sofroniew MV, Khakh BS. Two forms of astrocyte calcium excitability have distinct effects on NMDA receptor-mediated slow inward currents in pyramidal neurons. J Neurosci (2008) 28: 6659 – 6663.

[24] Volterra A, Meldolesi J. Astrocytes, from brain glue to communication elements: the revolution continues. Nat Rev Neurosci (2005) 6: 626 – 640.

[25] Bateman DE, Hardy JA, McDermott JR, Parker DS, Edwardson JA. Amino acid neurotransmitter levels in gliomas and their relationship to the incidence of epilepsy. Neurol Res (1988) 10: 112 – 114.

[26] Nicklas WJ, Browning ET. Amino acid metabolism in glial cells: homeostatic regulation of intra- and extracellular milieu by C6 glioma cells. J Neurochem (1978) 30: 955 – 963.

[27] Walum E. Counter transport of glutamine and choline in cultures of human glioma cells. Biochem Biophys Res Comm (1979) 88: 1271 – 1274.

[28] Ye ZC, Rothstein JD, Sontheimer H. Compromised glutamate transport in human glioma cells: reduction-mislocalization of sodium-dependent glutamate transporters

and enhanced activity of cystine-glutamate exchange. J Neurosci (1999) 19: 10767 – 10777.

[29] Buckingham SC, Campbell SL, Haas BR, Montana V, Robel S, Ogunrinu T, Sontheimer H. Glutamate release by primary brain tumors induces epileptic activity. Nat Med (2011) 17: 1269 – 1274.

[30] Tian GF, Azmi H, Takano T, Xu Q, Peng W, Lin J, Oberheim N, Lou N, Wang X, Zielke HF, Kang J, Nedergaard M. An astrocytic basis of epilepsy. Nat Med (2005) 11: 973 – 981.

[31] Simard M, Nedergaard M. The neurobiology of glia in the context of water and ion homeostasis. Neuroscience (2004) 129: 877 – 896.

[32] Zador Z, Stiver S, Wang V, Manley GT. Role of aquaporin-4 in cerebral edema and stroke. Handb Exp Pharmacol (2009) 190: 159 – 170.

[33] Obara M, Szeliga M, Albrecht J. Regulation of pH in the mammalian central nervous system under normal and pathological conditions: facts and hypotheses. Neurochem Int (2008) 52: 905 – 919.

[34] Sattler R, Rothstein JD. Regulation and dysregulation of glutamate transporters. Handb Exp Pharmacol (2006) 175: 277 – 303.

[35] Seifert G, Schilling K, Steinhauser C. Astrocyte dysfunction in neurological disorders: a molecular perspective. Nat Rev Neurosci (2006) 7: 194 – 206.

[36] Brown AM, Ransom BR. Astrocyte glycogen and brain energy metabolism. Glia (2007) 55: 1263 – 1271.

[37] Rouach N, Koulakoff A, Abudara V, Willecke K, Giaume C. Astroglial metabolic networks sustain hippocampal synaptic transmission. Science (2008) 322: 1551 – 1555.

[38] Takano T, Kang J, Jaiswal JK, Simon SM, Lin JH, Yu Y, Li Y, Yang J, Dienel G, Zielke HR, Nedergaard M. Receptor-mediated glutamate release from volume sensitive channels in astrocytes. Proc Natl Acad Sci USA (2005) 102: 16466 – 16471.

[39] Argau AT, Gurfein BT, Zhang Y, Zameer A, John GR. VEGF-mediated disruption of endothelial CLN-5 promotes blod-brain barrier breakdown. Proc Natl Acad Sci USA (2009) 106: 1977 – 1982.

[40] Hamby ME, Hewett JA, Hewett SJ. TGF-beta1 potentiates astrocytic nitric oxide oxide production by expanding the population of astrocytes that express NOS-2. Glia (2006) 54: 566 – 577.

[41] Brambilla R, Bracchi-Ricard V, Hu WH, Frydel B, Bramwill A, Karmally S, Green EJ Bethea JR. Inhibitiion of astroglial nuclear factor kappaB reduces inflammation and improves functional recovery after spinal cord injury. J Exp Med (2005) 202: 145 – 156.

[42] Haglund MM, Berger MS, Kunkel DD, Franck JE, Ghatan S, Ojemann GA. Changes in gamma-aminobutyric acid and somatostatin in epileptic cortex associated with low-grade gliomas. J Neurosurg (1992) 77: 209 – 216.

[43] de Lanerolle NC, Kim JH, Robbins RJ, Spencer DD. Hippocampal interneuron loss and plasticity in human temporal lobe epilepsy. Brain Res (1989) 495: 387 – 395.

[44] Kim JH, Guimaraes PO, Shen MY, Masukawa LM, Spencer DD. Hippocampal neuronal density in temporal lobe epilepsy with and without gliomas. Acta Neuropathol (1990) 80: 41 – 45.

[45] Sloviter RS. Decreased hippocampal inhibition and selective loss of interneurons in experimental epilepsy. Science (1987) 235: 73 – 76.

[46] Custer KL, Austin NS, Sullivan JM, Bajjalieh SM. Synaptic vesicle protein 2 enhances release probability at quiescent synapses. J Neurosci (2006) 26: 1303 – 1313.

[47] Lynch BA, Lambeng N, Nocka K, Kensel-Hammes P, Bajjalieh SM, Matagne A, Fuks B. The synaptic vesicle protein SV2A is the binding site for the antiepiltpic drug levetiracetam. Proc Natl Acad Sci USA (2004) 101: 9861 – 9866.

[48] Hanaya R, Hosoyama H, Sugata S, Tokudome M, Hirano H, Tokimura H, Kurisu K, Serikawa T, Sasa M, Arita K. Low distribution of synaptic vesicle protein 2A and synaptotagmin-1 in the cerebral cortex and hippocampus of spontaneously epileptic rats exhibiting both tonic convulsion and absence seizure. Neuroscience (2012) http://dx.doi.org/10.1016/j.neuroscience.2012.06.058

[49] Crowder KM, Gunther JM, Jones TA, Hale BD, Zhang HZ, Peterson MR, Scheller RH, Chavkin C, Bajjalieh SM. Abnormal neurotransmission in mice lacking synaptic vesicle protein 2A (SV2A). Proc Natl Acad Sci USA (1999) 96: 15268 – 15273.

[50] de Groot M, Toering ST, Boer K, Spliet WGM, Heimans JJ, Aronica E, Reijneveld JC. Expression of synaptic vesicle protein 2A in epilepsy-associated brain tumors and in the peritumoral cortex. Neuro Oncol (2010) 12: 265 – 273.

[51] Sandsmark DK, Pelletier C, Weber JD, Gutmann DH. Mammalian target of rapamycin: master regulator of cell growth in the nervous system. Histol Histopathol (2007) 22: 895 – 903.

[52] Inoki K, Corradetti MN, Guan KL. Dysregulation of the TSC-mTOR pathway in human disease. Nat Genet (2005) 37: 19 – 24.

[53] Tsang CK, Qi H, Liu LF, Zheng XF. Targeting mammalian target of rapamycin (mTOR) for health and diseases. Drug Discov Today (2007) 12: 112 – 124.

[54] Zeng L-H, Rensing NR, Wong M. The mammalian target of rapamycin (mTOR) signaling pathway mediates epileptogenesis in a model of temporal lobe epilepsy. J Neurosci (2009) 29: 6964 – 6972.

[55] Friedman A, Dingledine R. Molecular cascades that mediate the influence of inflammation on epilepsy. Epilepsia (2011) 52: S33 – S39.

[56] Serrano GE, Lelutiu N, Rojas A, Cochi S, Shaw R, Makinson CD, Wang D, Fitzgerald GA, Dingledine R. Ablation of cyclooxygenase-2 in forebrain neurons is neuroprotective and dampens brain inflammation after status epilepticus. J Neurosci (2011) 31: 14850 – 14860.

[57] Hauser WA, Annegers JF, Elveback LR. Mortality in patients with epilepsy. Epilepsia (1980) 21: 339 – 412.

[58] White JC, Liu CT, Mixter WJ. Focal epilepsy: a statistical study of its causes and the results of surgical treatment. I. Epilepsy secondary to intracranial tumors. N Engl J Med (1948) 238: 891 – 899.

[59] Lund M. Epilepsy in association with intracranial tumors. Acta Psychiatr Neurol Scand Suppl (1952) 8: 1 – 149.

[60] Rasmussen T, Blundell J. Epilepsy and brain tumor. Clin Neurosurg (1961) 7: 138 – 158.

[61] Salanova V, Andermann F, Olivier A, Rasmussen T, Quesney LF. Occipital lobe epilepsy: electroclinical manifestations, electrocorticography, cortical stimulation and outcome in 42 patients treated between 1930 and 1991. Brain (1992) 115: 1655 – 1680.

[62] Williamson PD, Thadani VM, Darcey TM, Spencer DD, Spencer SS, Mattson RH. Occipital lobe epilepsy: clinical characteristics, seizure spread patterns, and results of surgery. Ann Neurol (1992) 31: 3 – 13.

[63] Penfield W, Jasper H. Epilepsy and the functional anatomy of the human brain. Boston: Little, Brown, 1954.

[64] Ochs R, Gloor P, Quesney LF, Ives J, Olivier A. Does head-turning during a seizure have lateralizing or localizing significance? Neurology (1984) 34: 884 – 890.

[65] Robillard A, Saint-Hilaire JM, Mercier M, Bouvier G. The lateralizing and localizing value of adversion in epileptic seizures. Neurology (1983) 33: 1241 – 1242.

[66] Wyllie E, Luders H, Morris HH, Lesser RP, Dinner DS. The lateralizing significance of versive head and eye movements during epileptic seizures. Neurology (1986) 36: 606 – 611.

[67] Bladin PF, Woodward J. Epilepsy and the frontal lobe. Proc Aust Assoc Neurol (1974) 11: 229 – 237.

[68] Geier A, Bancaud J, Talairach J, Bonis A, Szikla G, Enjelvin M. Clinical note: clinical and tele-stereo-EEG findings in a patient with psychomotor seizures. Epilepsia (1975) 16: 119 - 125.

[69] [69] Geier S, Bancaud J, Talairach J, Bonis A, Szikla G, Enjelvin M. The seizures of frontal lobe epilepsy: a study of clinical manifestations. Neurology (1977) 27: 951 – 958.

[70] Mazars G. Cingulate gyrus epileptogenic foci as an origin for generalized seizures. In: Gastaut H, Jasper H, Bancaud J, Waltregny A, eds. The physiopathogenesis of the epilepsies. Springfield, IL: Charles C Thomas, 1969; pp 186 – 189.

[71] Williamson PD, Spencer DD, Spencer SS, Novelly RA, Mattson RH. Complex partial seizures of frontal lobe origin. Ann Neurol (1985) 18: 497 – 504.

[72] Rasmussen T. Characteristics of a pure culture of frontal lobe epilepsy. Epilepsia (1983) 24: 482 – 493.

[73] Fegerstein L, Roger A. Frontal epileptogenic foci and their clinical correlations. Electroencephalogr Clin Neurophysiol (1961) 13: 905 – 913.

[74] Geier S, Bancaud J, Talairach J, Bonis A, Enjelvin M, Hossard-Bouchaud H. Automatisms during frontal lobe epileptic seizures. Brain (1976) 99: 447 – 458.

[75] Niedermeyer E, Laws ER Jr, Walker AE. Depth EEG findings in epileptics with generalized spike-wave complexes. Arch Neurol (1969) 21: 51 – 58.

[76] Janz D. Status epilepticus and frontal lobe lesions. J Neurol Sci (1964) 1: 446 – 457.

[77] Delgado-Escueta AV, Bacsal FE, Treiman DM. Complex partial seizures on closed-circuit television and EEG: a study of 691 attacks in 79 patients. Ann Neurol (1981) 11: 292 – 300.

[78] Stoffels C, Munari C, Bonis A, Bancaud J, Talairach J. Manifestations gênitales et sexuelles lors des crises épileptiques partielles chez l'homme. Rev electroencephalogr Neurophysiol Clin (1981) 10: 386 – 392.

[79] Gastaut H. Clinical and electroencephalographic classification of epileptic seizures. Epilepsia (1970) 11: 102 - 113.

[80] Delgado-Escueta AV, Walsh GO. Type I complex partial seizures of hippocampal origin: excellent results of anterior temporal lobectomy. Neurology (1985) 35: 143 – 154.

[81] Walsh GO, Delgado-Escueta AV. Type II complex partial seizures: poor results of anterior temporal lobectomy. Neurology (1984) 34: 1 – 13.

[82] Wieser HG. Psychomotor seizures of hippocampal-amygdalar origin. In: Pedley TA, Meldrum BS, eds. Recent advances in epilepsy. Edinburgh: Churchill Livingstone, 1986; pp 57 – 79.

[83] Keles GE, Lamborn KR, Berger MS. Low-grade hemispheric gliomas in adults: a critical review of extent of resection as a factor influencing outcome. J Neurosurg (2001) 95: 735 – 745.

[84] Lacroix M, Abi-Said D, Fourney DR, Gokaslan ZL, Shi W, DeMonte F, Lang FF, McCutcheon IE, Hassenbusch SJ, Holland E, Hess K, Michael C, Miller D, Sawaya R. A multivariate analysis of 416 patients with glioblastoma multiforme: prognosis, extent of resection, and survival. J Neurosurg (2001) 95: 190 – 198.

[85] Chang EF, Clark A, Smith JS, Polley M-Y, Chang SM, Barbaro NM, Parsa AT, McDermott MW, Berger MS. Functional mapping-guided resection of low-grade gliomas in eloquent areas of the brain: improvement of long-term survival. J Neurosurg (2011) 114: 566 – 573.

[86] Mahaley MS, Dudka L. The role of anticonvulsant medication in the management of patients with anaplastic gliomas. Surg Neurol (1981) 16: 399 – 401.

[87] Boarini DJ, Beck DW, Van Gilder JC. Postoperative prophylactic anticonvulsant therapy in cerebral gliomas. Neurosurgery (1985) 16: 290 – 292.

[88] Maschio M, Albani F, Baruzzi A, Zarabla A, Dinapoli L, Pace A, Pompili A, Carapella CM, Occhipinti E, Jandolo B. Levetiracetam therapy in patients with brain tumor and epilepsy. J Neurooncol (2006) 80: 97 – 100.

[89] Maschio M, Dinapoli L, Vidiri A, Pace A, Fabi A, Pompili A, Carapella MC, Jandolo B. The role side effects play in the choice of antiepileptic therapy in brain tumor-related epilepsy: a comparative study on traditional antiepileptic drugs versus oxcarbazepine. J Exp Clin Canc Res (2009) 28: 60 – 66.

[90] Maschio M, Dinapoli L, Zarabla A, Pompili A, Carapella CM, Pace A, Giannarelli D, Occhipinti E, Jandolo B. Outcome and tolerability of topiramate in brain tumor associated epilepsy. J Neurooncol (2008) 86: 61 – 70.

[91] Mauro AM, Bomprezzi C, Morresi S, Provinciali L, Formica F, Iacoangeli M, Scerrati M. Prevention of early postoperative seizures in patients with primary brain tumors: preliminary experience with oxcarbazepine. J Neurooncol (2007) 81: 279 – 285.

[92] Newton HB, Goldlust SA, Pearl D. retrospective analysis of the efficacy and tolerability of levetiracetam in brain tumor patients. J Neurooncol (2006) 78: 99 – 102.

[93] Aguiar D, Pazo R, Durán I, Terrasa J, Arrivi A, Manzano H, Martin J, Rifá J. Toxic epidermal necrolysis in patients receiving anticonvulsants and cranial irradiation: a risk to consider. J Neurooncol (2004) 66: 345 – 350.

[94] Arif H, Buchsbaum R, Weintraub D, Koyfman S, Salas-Humara C, Bazil CW, Resor SR Jr, Hirsch LJ. Comparison and predictors of rash associated with 15 antiepileptic drugs. Neurology (2007) 68: 1701 – 1709.

[95] Klein M, Engelberts NH, van der Ploeg HM, Kasteleijn-Nost Trenité DG, Aaronson NK, Taphoorn MJ, Baaijen H, Vandertop WP, Muller M, Postma TJ, Heimans JJ. Epilepsy in low-grade gliomas: the impact on cognitive function and quality of life. Ann Neurol (2003) 54: 514-520.

[96] Hildebrand J. Management of epileptic seizures. Curr Opin Oncol (2004) 16: 314 – 317.

[97] Prados MD, Lamborn K, Yung WK, Jaeckle K, Robins HI, Mehta M, Fine HA, Wen PY, Cloughesy T, Chang S, Kelly Nicholas M, Schiff D, Greenberg H, Junck L, Fink K, Hess K, Kuhn J. A phase 2 trial of irinotecan (CPT-11) in patients with recurrent malignant glioma: a North American Brain Tumor Consortium study. Neuro Oncol (2006) 8: 189 – 193.

[98] Cloughesy TF, Wen PY, Robins HI, Chang SM, Groves MD, Fink KL, Junck L, Schiff D, Abrey L, Gilbert MR, Lieberman F, Kuhn J, DeAngelis LM, Mehta M, Raizer JJ, Alfred Yung WK, Aldape K, Wright J, Lamborn KR, Prados MD. Phase II trial of tipifarnib in

patients with recurrent malignant glioma either receiving or not receiving enzyme-inducing antiepileptic drugs: a North American Brain Tumor Consortium Study. J Clin Oncol (2006) 24: 3651 – 3656.

[99] Groves MD, Puduvalli VK, Conrad CA, Gilbert MR, Alfred Yung WK, Jaeckle K, Liu V, Hess KR, Aldape KD, Levin VA. Phase II trial of temozolomide plus marimastat for recurrent anaplastic gliomas: A relationship among efficacy, joint toxicity and anticonvulsant status. J Neurooncol (2006) 80: 83 – 90.

[100] Jaeckle KA, Ballman K, Furth A, Buckner JC. Correlation of enzyme-inducing anticonvulsant use with outcome of patients with glioblastoma. Cancer Res Treat (2011) 43: 160 – 169.

[101] Benedetti MS. Enzyme induction and inhibition by new antiepileptic drugs: a review of human studies. Fundam Clin Pharmacol (2000) 14: 301 – 319.

[102] Song J, Hu J, Tanouye MA. Seizure suppression by top1 mutations in Drosophila. J Neurosci (2007) 27: 2927 – 2937.

[103] Champoux JJ. DNA topoisomerases: structure, function and mechanism. Annu Rev Biochem (2001) 70: 369 – 413.

[104] Song J, Parker L, Hormosi L, Tanouye MA. DNA topoisomerase I Inhibitors amerliorate seizure-like behaviors and paralysis in a Drosophila model of epilepsy. Neuroscience (2008) 156: 722 – 728.

[105] Cascino GD. Epilepsy and brain tumors: implications for treatment. Epilepsia (1990) 31(Suppl 3): 37 – 44.

[106] Goldring S, Rich KM, Picker S. Experience with gliomas in patients presenting with a chronic seizure disorder. Clin Neurosurg (1986) 33: 15 – 42.

[107] Awad IA, Rosenfeld J, Ahl J, Hahn JF, Luders H. Intractable epilepsy and structural lesions of the brain: mapping, resection strategies, and seizure outcome. Epilepsia (1991) 32: 179 – 186.

[108] Cascino GD, Kelly PJ, Sharbrough FW, Hulihan JF, Hirschorn KA, Trenerry MR. Long-term follow-up of stereotactic lesionectomy in partial epilepsy: predictive factors and electroencephalographic results. Epilepsia (1992) 33: 639 – 644.

[109] Spencer DD, Spencer SS, Mattson RH, Williamson PD. Intracerebral masses in patients with intractable partial epilepsy. Neurology (1984) 34: 432 – 436.

[110] Boon PA, Williamson PD, Fried I, Spencer DD, Novelly RA, Spencer SS, Mattson RH. Intracranial, intraaxial, space-occupying lesions in patients with intractable partial seizures: an anatomoclinical, neuropsychological and surgical correlation. Epilepsia (1991) 32: 467 – 476.

[111] Kirkpatrick PJ, Honavar M, Janota I, Polkey CE. Control of temporal lobe epilepsy following en bloc resection of low-grade tumors. J Neurosurg (1993) 78: 19 – 25.

[112] Berger MS, Ghatan A, Haglund MM, Dobbins J, Ojemann GA. Low-grade gliomas associated with intractable epilepsy: seizure outcome utilizing electrocorticography during tumor resection. J Neurosurg (1993) 79: 62 – 69.

[113] Gonzalez D, Elvidge AR. On the occurrence of epilepsy caused by astrocytomas of the cerebral hemispheres. J Neurosurg (1962) 19: 470 – 482.

[114] Pilcher WH, Silbergeld DL, Berger MS, Ojemann GA. Intraoperative electrocorticography during tumor resection: impact on seizure outcome in patients with gangliogliomas. J Neurosurg (1993) 78: 891 – 902.

[115] Ribaric I. Excision of two and three independent and separate ipsilateral potentially epileptogenic cortical areas. Acta Neurochir Suppl (1983) 33: 145 – 148.

[116] Van Buren JM, Ajmone-Marsan C, Matsuga N. Temporal lobe seizures with additional foci treated by resection. J Neurosurg (1975) 43: 596 – 607.

[117] Weber JP, Silbergeld DL, Winn HR. Surgical resection of epileptogenic cortex associated with structural lesions. Neurosurg Clin North Am (1993) 4: 327 – 336.

[118] Gloor P. Contributions of electroencephalography and electrocorticography to the neurosurgical treatment of the epilepsies. Acta Neurol (1975) 8: 59 – 105.

[119] Jooma R, Yeh HS, Privitera MD, Gartner M. Lesionectomy versus electrophysiologically guided resection for temporal lobe tumors manifesting with complex partial seizures. J Neurosurg (1995) 83: 231 – 236.

[120] Morris HH III, Luders H, Hahn JF, Lesser RP, Dinner DS, Estes ML. Neurophysiological techniques as an aid to surgical treatment of primary brain tumors. Ann Neurol (1986) 19: 559 – 567.

[121] Sperling MR, Cahan LD, Brown WJ. Relief of seizures from a predominantly posterior temporal tumor with anterior temporal lobectomy. Epilepsia (1989) 30: 559 – 563.

[122] Ketz E. Brain tumours and epilepsy. In: Vinken PJ, Bruyn GW, eds. Tumours of the Brain and Skull: Handbook of Clinical Neurology. Part I. Amsterdam: North-Holland, 1974: 254 – 269.

[123] Fried I, Kim JH, Spencer DD. Limbic and neocortical gliomas associated with intractable seizures: a distinct clinicopathological group. Neurosurgery (1994) 34: 815 – 823.

[124] Schramm J, Luyken C, Urbach H, Fimmers R, Blümcke I. Evidence for a clinically distinct new subtype of grade II astrocytomas in patients with long-term epilepsy. Neurosurgery (2004) 55: 340 – 348.

[125] Babb TL, Brown WJ, Pretorius J, Davenport C, Lieb JP, Crandall PH. Temporal lobe volumetric cell densities in temporal lobe epilepsy. Epilepsia (1984) 25: 729 – 740.

[126] Fried I, Kim JH, Spencer DD. Hippocampal pathology in patients with intractable seizures and temporal lobe masses. J Neurosurg (1992) 76: 735 – 740.

[127] Li LM, Cendes F, Watson C, Andermann F, Fish DR, Dubeau F, Free S, Olivier A, Harkness W, Thomas DGT, Duncan JS, Sander JWAS, Shorvon SD, Cook MJ, Arnold DL. Surgical treatment of patients with single and dual pathology: relevance of lesion and of hippocampal atrophy to seizure outcome. Neurology (1997) 48: 437 – 444.

[128] Baudoin MM, Stuhl L, Perrard AC. Un cas d'épilepsie focale traité par la radiothérapie. Rev Neurol (1951) 84: 60 – 63.

[129] Heikkinen ER, Yalynych N, Zubkov YN, Garmashov YA, Pak VA. Relief of epilepsy by radiosurgery of cerebral arteriovenous malformations. Stereotact Funct Neurosurg (1989) 53: 157 – 166.

[130] Rogers L, Morris H, Lupica K. Effect of cranial irradiation on seizure frequency in adults with low grade astrocytomas and medically intractable epilepsy. Neurology (1993) 43: 1599 – 1601.

[131] Rossi GF, Scerrati M, Roselli R. Epileptogenic cerebral low-grade tumors: effect of interstitial stereotactic irradiation on seizures. Appl Neurophysiol (1985) 48: 127 – 132.

[132] Von Wiezer W. Die roentgentherapie der traumatischen epilepsie. Monatsschr Psychiatr Neurol (1939) 101: 171 – 179.

[133] Chalifoux R, Elisevich K. Effect of ionizing radiation on partial seizures attributable to malignant cerebral tumors. Stereotact Funct Neurosurg (1996-97) 67: 169 – 182.

[134] Regis J, Bartolomei F, Rey M, Hayashi M, Chauvel P, Peragut JC. Gamma Knife surgery for mesial temporal epilepsy. J Neurosurg (2000) 93(Suppl 3): 141 – 146.

[135] Bartolomei F, Hayashi M, Tamura M, Rey M, Fischer C, Chauvel P, Regis J. Long-term efficacy of gamma knife radiosurgery in mesial temporal lobe epilepsy. Neurology (2008) 70: 1658 – 1663.

[136] Mori Y, Kondziolka D, Balzer J, Fellows W, Flickinger JC, Lundsford LD, Thulborn KR. Effects of stereotactic radiosurgery on an animal model of hippocampal epilepsy. Neurosurgery (2000) 46: 157 – 168.

[137] Cmelak A, Abou-Khalil B, Konrad PE, Duggin D, Maciunas RJ. Low dose stereotactic radiosurgery is inadequate for medically intractable mesial temporal epilepsy: a case report. Seizure (2001) 10: 442 – 446.

[138] Jenrow KA, Ratkewicz AE, Elisevich KV. Enhanced excitability induced by ionizing radiation in the kindled rat. Exp Neurol (2001) 169: 96 – 104.

[139] Brambilla R, Persaud T, Hu X, Karmally S, Shestopalov VI, Dvoriantchikova G, Ivanov D, Nathanson L, Barnum SR, Bethea JR. Transgenic inhibition of astroglial NF-kappaB improves functional outcome in experimental autoimmune encephalomyelitis by suppressing chronic central nervous system inflammation. J Immunol (2009) 182: 2628 - 2640.

Section 5

Photodynamic Therapy

Chapter 12

Current Applications of 5-ALA in Glioma Diagnostics and Therapy

Lei Teng, Mitsutoshi Nakada, Yutaka Hayashi, Takeshi Yoneyama, Shi-Guang Zhao and Jun-Ichiro Hamada

Additional information is available at the end of the chapter

http://dx.doi.org/10.5772/52428

1. Introduction

Gliomas, the most common primary brain tumors, are characterized by rapid proliferation, marked infiltration, and poor prognosis and are known for their dismal outcomes (Iacob & Dinca, 2009; Lefranc et al., 2006). The infiltrative nature of malignant glioma makes complete resection difficult, as tumor margins are unclear. Recurrence of glioma takes place within approximately 2 cm of the margins of the resected cavity owing to its invasive character (Aydin et al., 2001; Wallner et al., 1989). The use of fluorescence to delineate tumor margins intraoperatively has emerged as a safe and effective tool for increasing the extent of resection. Therefore, methods that easily detect tumor margins during surgery would be extremely beneficial. 5-aminolevulinic acid (5-ALA) fluorescence-guided glioma resection is a rapidly growing, novel approach to improve the extent of tumor resection with broad applications in both preclinical and clinical settings (Stummer et al., 2000; Stummer et al., 1998b; Stummer et al., 1998c). Intraoperative tumor fluorescence provided by the chemical compound 5-ALA assists surgeons in identifying the true tumor margin during resection of glial neoplasms, consequently increasing the extent of the resection. 5-ALA is the most studied fluorescer and has been used in many clinical trials, including a multicenter phase III randomized controlled trial. Recent controlled Phase III clinical trials have demonstrated that this surgical method enables more complete resection of contrast-enhancing lesions than conventional microsurgery and improves progression-free survival in patients with malignant glioma (Pichlmeier et al., 2008; Stummer et al., 2006).

Photodynamic therapy (PDT) is a treatment modality that takes advantage of the cytotoxic effects induced by a photosensitizer and light in the presence of oxygen (Norum et al., 2009). This photodamage may be due to direct cytotoxicity, vascular damage, and inflammatory and immunological responses (Castano et al., 2006). The relative importance of these pathways to the therapeutic effects depends on the tissue oxygenation, photosensitizer formulation, distribution, and light dosimeter (Norum et al., 2009). 5-ALA-induced protoporphyrin IX (PpIX) can also be used for 5-ALA-PDT rather than photodynamic diagnosis (PDD) by exposing the field to either blue or red laser light; however, a red light at 632 nm would target a much larger tumor volume owing to better light penetration (Eljamel et al., 2008). Activation of PpIX by red light in combination with oxygen causes cell death by apoptosis and necrosis through the release of cytotoxic singlet oxygen (Peng et al., 1997). This tool may aid in overcoming the hurdle of residual tumor cells after traditional neurosurgery. Application of 5-ALA-PDT has been emerging as a new field and is expected to create a major breakthrough in addressing several unsolved medical issues, especially photokilling of residual neoplastic cells.

Developing technologies such as fluorescence operation-systems to enhance endogenous fluorescence has fairly recently been shown to delineate brain tumor margins intraoperatively (Babu & Adamson, 2012). 5-ALA fluorescence-guided resection shows great promise for furthering our surgical abilities and will become the standard of care for patients diagnosed with malignant glioma in the foreseeable future. The following review analyzes the recent literature in an effort to describe how these modalities involving 5-ALA in glioma diagnostics and therapy can and should be used in the treatment of patients with glioma. This article reviews recent developments in the use of 5-ALA for simultaneous imaging and 5-ALA-triggered photodamage in glioma patients (Figure 1).

2. General knowledge of 5–ALA

5-ALA (molecular weight, 167.6) is a natural biochemical precursor for heme synthesis in living mammalian cells (Eljamel et al., 2008; Peng et al., 1997). Each cell metabolizes 5-ALA along a set pathway toward heme production, inducing the synthesis of the endogenous fluorescent molecule, PpIX, through metabolic conversion in the mitochondria (Bottomley & Muller-Eberhard, 1988). When PpIX emits peak fluorescence at 635 nm with a peak excitation wavelength at 405 nm, it is observed as a red light through a filter that allows this wavelength to pass. Clinical use of 5-ALA for PDT or PDD has also been reported in dermatology, urology, neurosurgery, otorhinolaryngology, gynecology, and gastroenterology for various epithelia and cancerous tissues (D'Hallewin et al., 1998; Guyon et al., 2012; Loning et al., 2004; Piotrowski et al., 2004). In the USA, it has been used with the approval of the Food and Drug Administration (FDA) as a therapeutic drug for solar keratosis. Its use has not yet been approved by the pharmaceutical authority in Japan, and it is only used after obtaining approval from the ethics committee of the respective institutes. The tumor tissue concentration of the fluorescent dye peaks at 2–6 hours after oral administration and disappears by 12 hours. Administration of antacid should be avoided at the time of oral administration because the dye is easily decomposed in the presence of alkali, and use of 5-ALA is contraindicated in cases of porphyria, a genetic disease. PpIX biosynthesized from 5-ALA is a phototoxic substance, although the incidence of skin photosensitivity is lower than that reported for conventional porphyrin derivatives (Stummer et al., 2006; Toda, 2008). When given orally, 5-ALA has been shown to produce fluorescence in glial neoplasms both *in vitro* and *in vivo* (Blake & Curnow, 2010). In addition, the fluorescence of PpIX is itself cytotoxic and has the potential for use as an adjuvant photodynamic therapy for neoplastic tissue that cannot be safely resected (Sherman et al., 2011). Since the administered 5-ALA is excreted into the urine within 24 hours after oral administration and does not remain in the skin, the occurrence of photosensitivity can be adequately prevented by avoiding sun exposure for approximately 24 hours after administration.

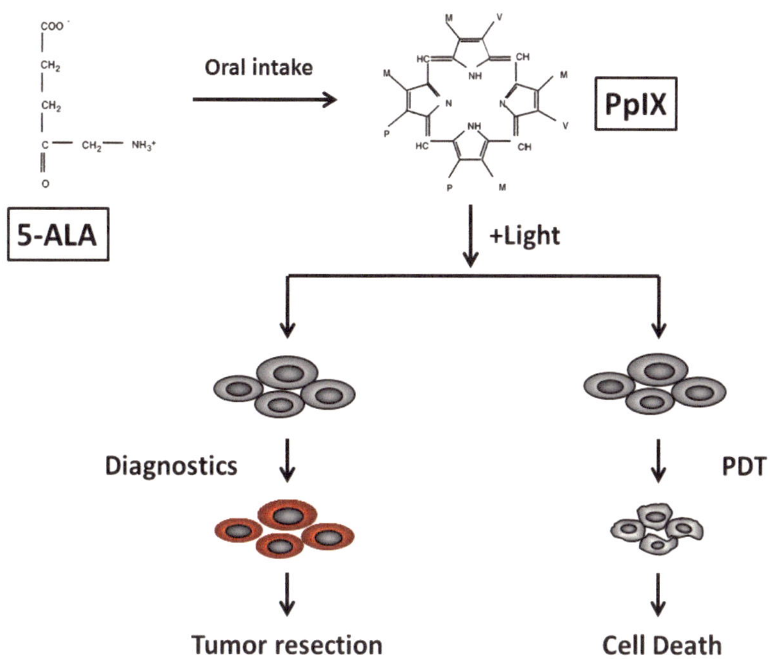

Figure 1. Schematic representation of diagnostics and PDT of 5-ALA for glioma cells. The figure illustrates 5-ALA is converted to PpIX in malignant gliomas via an oral-intake of exogenous 5-ALA. In the presence of an appropriate light source with the specific wavelength, PpIX fluorescence acts bimodal function; fluorescence diagnostic marker and 5-ALA-PDT. Red fluorescence acts as a discriminating marker to assist neurosurgeons to visualize the extent and margins of tumors; 5-ALA-PDT results in a series of irreversible photochemical and photobiological events that cause directly damage and killing glioma cells.

3. 5–ALA biology in glioma

5-ALA, the metabolic precursor of heme in the heme biosynthesis pathway, is not itself fluorescent, but is metabolized into endogenous fluorescent PpIX (Gossner et al., 1998; Inoue et al., 2007; Kennedy & Pottier, 1992; Loh et al., 1993; Peng et al., 1997). Heme biosynthesis consists of a series of enzyme-catalyzed steps, involving 5-aminolevulinate synthases 1 and 2,

5-aminolevulinate dehydratase, hydroxymethylbilane synthase, uroporphyrinogen III synthase, uroporphyrinogen decarboxylase, coproporphyrinogen oxidase (CPOX), protoporphyrinogen oxidase, and ferrochelatase (FECH). In addition to these enzymes, several transporters are also involved in the biosynthesis and catabolism of heme and porphyrin, including oligopeptide transporters 1 and 2 (PEPT1 and PEPT2) and the ABC transporters ABCB6 and ABCG2 (Takahashi et al., 2011) (Figure 2).

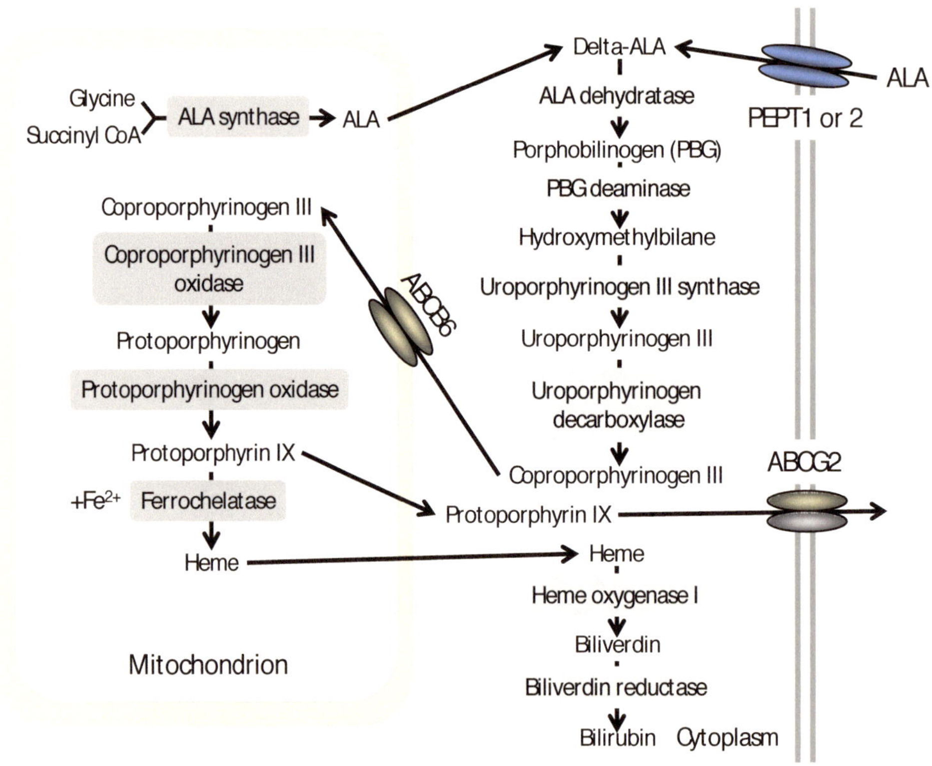

Figure 2. The porphyrin-heme biosynthetic pathway and putative mitochondrial transporters. The first step of heme synthesis occurs in the mitochondrial matrix with the condensation of succinyl CoA and glycine by ALA synthase to generate ALA. Oligopeptide transporters (PEPT1 or PEPT2) are responsible for the import of exogenous ALA from the extracellular space into the cytoplasm of target cells. ALA is converted to coproporphyrinogen III by 4 enzymatic reactions. Then, coproporphyrinogen III is transported back into the mitochondrial intermembrane space (IMS), possibly via ABCB6, where it is converted to protoporphyrinogen by protoporphyrinogen III oxidase. The conversion of protoporphyrinogen to PpIX by protoporphyrinogen oxidase, its transport into the matrix and the addition of Fe^{2+} by ferrochelatase (FECH) to generate heme are coupled processes. The transporter responsible for heme transfer across the outer mitochondrial membrane remains unidentified. Heme formed from porphyrin is catabolized to biliverdin by the microsomal enzyme heme oxygenase 1. Biliverdin is subsequently metabolized to bilirubin by biliverdin reductase. ABCG2 transports porphyrins across the plasma membrane to maintain intracellular porphyrin homeostasis.

Porphyrins are synthesized from glycine and succinyl CoA via a series of enzymatic reactions. The last enzymatic reaction is the conversion of PpIX to heme by FECH, which is located in the inner mitochondrial membrane (Ferreira et al., 1995; Kemmner et al., 2008). Heme formed from porphyrin is catabolized to biliverdin by the microsomal enzyme heme oxygenase 1.

Subsequently, biliverdin is metabolized to bilirubin by biliverdin reductase. The PEPT1/PEPT2 (influx transporters) can transport exogenous ALA from the extracellular space into the cytoplasm of target cells. ABCB6 is the ABC transporter responsible for the import of coproporphyrinogen III into the mitochondria, whereas ABCG2 transports PpIX across the plasma membrane to maintain intracellular PpIX homeostasis (Takahashi et al., 2011).

Oral-intake of 5-ALA results in the accumulation of PpIX in malignant gliomas. Because of the presence of the blood-brain barrier (BBB), 5-ALA given via the oral route does not usually enter the normal brain tissue. However, it can easily pass through the disrupted BBB found in the glioma tissue (Stummer et al., 2003). PpIX that accumulates in the intracellular compartments of tumor cells exhibits red fluorescence under excitation light of an appropriate wavelength (Takahashi et al., 2011). PpIX-accumulating tumor cells can be visually discerned intraoperatively from the surrounding normal cells that accumulate PpIX to a much lesser extent. To date, little is known about the molecular mechanisms underlying PpIX accumulation in malignant brain tumors after administration of 5-ALA; despite this, in the past decade, studies on ALA focusing on the mechanism of 5-ALA uptake in glioma tissue have been conducted by many research groups. Previously, our group revealed significantly greater down-regulation of FECH expression in glioblastomas than in normal brain tissues and that FECH plays a role in the metabolism of 5-ALA in glioma (Teng et al., 2011). In addition, Takahashi et al. demonstrated that the upregulated expression of the CPOX gene is correlated with the intensity of tumor fluorescence induced by 5-ALA; they also found that the mRNA level of ABCG2 was somewhat lower in the brain tumors with high ALA-induced fluorescence than in those without ALA-induced fluorescence (Takahashi et al., 2011). Therefore, they assumed that both the induction of the CPOX gene and the inhibition of ABCG2 would increase 5-ALA-induced PpIX accumulation and thereby enhance the efficacy of 5-ALA-PDT in malignant brain tumors. In agreement with this hypothesis, Zhao et al. demonstrated that ABCB6 expression levels were greatly elevated in human gliomas than in normal brain tissues and correlated with glioma histologic grade, indicating a crucial role for ABCB6 in ALA metabolism and accumulation of PpIX in gliomas (Zhao et al., 2012).

Further studies are required to explore the detailed mechanism of 5-ALA uptake and improve our knowledge concerning 5-ALA biology in gliomas.

4. 5–ALA guided neurosurgery

Many previous reports describing prognostic factors in patients with malignant gliomas indicate that outcome is associated with the completeness of tumor removal (Stummer et al., 1998a). Improving the prognosis of glioma patients cannot be achieved without considerable effort to remove as much as of the lesion as possible. Since glioma tissue is not easily recognized intraoperatively, methods that easily detect tumor margins during surgery would be extremely beneficial. 5-ALA fluorescence-guided resection is a rapidly growing, novel approach in treating glioma patients to improve the extent of tumor resection with broad applications in both preclinical and clinical settings (Stummer et al., 2000; Stummer et al., 1998b; Stummer et al., 1998c). In 1998, Stummer et al. first presented a detailed description of the technical principles for 5-ALA fluorescence-guided microsurgical resection of malignant glioma tissue (Stummer et al., 1998a). Subsequently, they performed a prospective study in 52 glioblastoma patients and identified the usefulness of 5-ALA-induced tumor fluorescence for guiding tumor resection. Recent controlled Phase III clinical trials have demonstrated that compared to conventional microsurgery, 5-ALA fluorescence-guided microsurgical resection enables more complete resection of contrast-enhancing lesions and improves progression-free survival in patients with malignant glioma (Pichlmeier et al., 2008; Stummer et al., 2006). After the rapid development of the neurosurgical fluorescence operation microscope, several investigators have recently demonstrated the feasibility of 5-ALA fluorescence-guided resection in patients with glioma (Kuroiwa et al., 1998; Kuroiwa et al., 2001; Sherman et al., 2011). Widhalm et al. also indicated that 5-ALA is a promising marker for intraoperative visualization of anaplastic foci in diffusely infiltrating gliomas without contrast enhancement and showed that the positive predictive value (PVV) of focal 5-ALA fluorescence for World Health Organization (WHO) grade III glioma was 100% (sensitivity 89%) (Widhalm et al., 2010). In addition, Nabavi's group investigated the feasibility and selectivity of 5-ALA-induced fluorescence to guide resection in recurrent gliomas (WHO grade III/IV) and found that 5-ALA fluorescence (weak and strong) had a high PPV (97.2%) in all pathological-appearing tissues obtained from 354 biopsies performed in 36 patients (Nabavi et al., 2009). Based on these findings, they suggested that 5-ALA fluorescence guidance is an effective surgical adjunct in the surgery of recurrent malignant gliomas, and many other trials have displayed similar successful results using 5-ALA fluorescence-guided resection in meningiomas to achieve optimal resection (Coluccia et al., 2010; Kajimoto et al., 2007).

Despite the advantages of 5-ALA fluorescence, successful glioma resection often depends on the neurosurgeon's ability to distinguish residual tumor tissue from surrounding brain tissue even with the assistance of PpIX fluorescence (Teng et al., 2011). The marginal area containing infiltrating glioma cells shows vague fluorescence because the density of the glioma cells in these areas is low and heterogeneous, resulting in insufficient 5-ALA uptake and PpIX accumulation (Utsuki et al., 2006). Conversely, because of the presence of reactive astrocytes and macrophages and leakage of PpIX into the extracellular matrix, false-positive (i.e., the area fluoresced, but no tumor was seen histologically) results in weakly fluorescing normal-appearing tissue are also common (Utsuki et al., 2007). Therefore, more objective and quantitative indicators need to be established for neurosurgeons to improve intraoperative identification of tumor margins. Recently, a quantitative method involving spectroscopic analysis for determining the amount of fluorescence present has been developed, which allows more precise visualization of quantitative fluorescence from tumor tissues (Utsuki et al., 2006; Valdes et al., 2011).

5. 5–ALA mediated-PDT

PDT is a tool for the treatment of certain cancerous and pre-cancerous conditions, especially in the field of dermatology (Buytaert et al., 2007). Among the many kinds of photosensitizers,

5-ALA has become widely accepted. 5-ALA-PDT is a novel treatment modality for early or superficial cancers, as well as a palliative treatment to a certain extent, that triggers a photodynamic effect similar to that of light in the visible range to produce a rapid PDT response in the targeted tissue. Three types of mechanisms have been identified in the literature as contributing to the rapid PDT response *in vivo*: (1) PDT can directly damage and kill the malignant tumor cells, either by apoptosis or a non-apoptotic mechanism; (2) PDT may produce profound changes in the tumor vasculature, including blood flow stasis, vascular collapse, and/or vascular leakage, that can result in indirect killing of malignant cells; and (3) PDT can promote the release of cytokines and other inflammatory mediators from target cells that induce an inflammatory response and recruit additional host cells to the tumor (MacDonald & Dougherty, 2001; Oleinick et al., 2002). Recent studies have shown that 5-ALA-PDT-induced photodamage causes mitochondrial and nuclear DNA damage. As a result, massive apoptosis occurs owing to mitochondrial release of cytochrome c and activation of caspase-3 and caspase-9 in glioma cells (Inoue et al., 2007; Karmakar et al., 2007). These results indicate that 5-ALA-PDT triggers apoptosis through a mitochondrial pathway.

Compared to the other modalities, 5-ALA-PDT has the advantage of better specificity and lower complication rates, and it is also a good alternative in tumor patients not eligible for surgery. Unfortunately, current 5-ALA-PDT protocols have yet to be widely established in clinical treatment for glioma. This may be partly due to limitations in current PDT regimens and partly due to the therapeutic efficacy of 5-ALA-PDT in preclinical settings (Teng et al., 2011). The reason for 5-ALA-PDT not being standard treatment in malignant glioma may be multifactorial, including the lack of randomized controlled trials and an optimal 5-ALA-PDT regimen. Generally, PDT efficacy depends on parameters such as the photosensitizing agent, irradiance and timing, oxygen, photosensitizer concentration, and different pathologic grade glioma tissue sensitivity to the PDT effect (Teng et al., 2011). Optimizing these parameters is difficult, expensive, and time consuming. The efficacy of 5-ALA-PDT may also be limited by reduced penetration of appropriate light through the target tissue and local acute phototoxicity to normal surrounding brain tissue (Norum et al., 2009). In addition, post-treatment edema and long-lasting skin photosensitivity after PDT of brain tumors are potentially challenging side effects that neurosurgeons have to deal with. Regarding the specificity of PDD for glioma surgery, new techniques allowing more specific accumulation of PpIX in target tumor cells need to be developed. Further studies are required for screening available and specific glioma antigens that are strongly expressed in glioma tissues, but not in normal brain tissues. 5-ALA labeled with antibodies against glioma-specific antigens may be useful in increasing the accumulation of PpIX and the specificity of PDD in glioma tissues. If the specificity and selectivity of 5-ALA-PDT could be improved in glioma tissue, 5-ALA-PDT would certainly be regarded as a promising and competitive alternative in glioma treatment.

6. Perspective

In this review, we focused on the 5-ALA agent as a potential treatment modality for patients with malignant glioma. 5-ALA-induced fluorescence is a useful intraoperative tool for the visualization of glioma tissue, and 5-ALA-PDT is a promising and alternative adjuvant therapy for photokilling residual neoplastic cells. Although impressive advances in the application of 5-ALA to glioma have been made from many clinical trials, this evolving field still faces important challenges. For example, single imaging in solid malignant glioma tissue with all of these features is not sufficient. Judgment of the extent of resection may still be treacherous within infiltrating parts of brain tumors, where the ratio of background noise of normal brain tissue to signal intensity of PpIX-saturated malignant glioma cells is less pronounced (Hefti et al., 2012; Liao et al., 2012). Recent efforts to boost target-to-background ratios have used a combination of intraoperative 5-ALA-induced fluorescence and 3D MRI imaging or neuronavigation imaging with some success (Liao et al., 2008; Panciani et al., 2012). Furthermore, more objective indicators to measure quantitative PpIX concentrations intraoperatively in the brain tumor margin need to be established. In the future, laboratory and clinical studies should be devoted to 5-ALA-PDT in conjunction with the use of other therapies, which will have maximal effect on the residual tumor after resection. This multiple adjuvant therapy should enhance specificity and allow lowering of the total PDT dose, while still increasing the therapeutic efficacy of PDT. Other proposals should adjust the current PDT treatment regimens, modify the existing photosensitizer, or develop new and more specific photosensitizers. Further studies are needed to elucidate possible mechanisms of 5-ALA uptake that could explain the diversity of intraoperative findings.

Author details

Lei Teng[1,2], Mitsutoshi Nakada[1*], Yutaka Hayashi[1], Takeshi Yoneyama[3], Shi-Guang Zhao[2] and Jun-Ichiro Hamada[1]

*Address all correspondence to: mnakada@med.kanazawa-u.ac.jp

1 Department of Neurosurgery, Graduate School of Medical Science, Kanazawa University, Kanazawa,, Japan

2 Department of Neurosurgery, The First Clinical College of Harbin Medical University, Harbin,, China

3 College of Science and Engineering, Kanazawa University, Kanazawa,, Japan

References

[1] Aydin, H, Sillenberg, I, & Von Lieven, H. (2001). Patterns of failure following CT-based 3-D irradiation for malignant glioma. Strahlenther Onkol. 0179-7158, 177(8), 424-431.

[2] Babu, R, & Adamson, C. (2012). Fluorescence-Guided Malignant Glioma Resections. Curr Drug Discov Technol. Vol. No. pp. 1875-6220, 1875-6220.

[3] Blake, E, & Curnow, A. (2010). The hydroxypyridinone iron chelator CP94 can enhance PpIX-induced PDT of cultured human glioma cells. Photochem Photobiol. 1751-1097, 86(5), 1154-1160.

[4] Bottomley, S. S, & Muller-eberhard, U. (1988). Pathophysiology of heme synthesis. Seminars in hematology. 0037-1963, 25(4), 282-302.

[5] Buytaert, E, Dewaele, M, & Agostinis, P. (2007). Molecular effectors of multiple cell death pathways initiated by photodynamic therapy. Biochim Biophys Acta. 0006-3002, 1776(1), 86-107.

[6] Castano, A. P, Mroz, P, & Hamblin, M. R. (2006). Photodynamic therapy and anti-tumour immunity. Nature reviews Cancer. 0147-4175X, 6(7), 535-545.

[7] Coluccia, D, Fandino, J, Fujioka, M, Cordovi, S, Muroi, C, & Landolt, H. (2010). Intraoperative 5-aminolevulinic-acid-induced fluorescence in meningiomas. Acta Neurochir (Wien). 0942-0940, 152(10), 1711-1719.

[8] Hallewin, D, Vanherzeele, M. A, & Baert, H. L. ((1998). Fluorescence detection of flat transitional cell carcinoma after intravesical instillation of aminolevulinic acid. American journal of clinical oncology. 0277-3732, 21(3), 223-225.

[9] Eljamel, M. S, Goodman, C, & Moseley, H. (2008). ALA and Photofrin fluorescence-guided resection and repetitive PDT in glioblastoma multiforme: a single centre Phase III randomised controlled trial. Lasers in medical science. 0268-8921, 23(4), 361-367.

[10] Ferreira, G. C, Franco, R, Lloyd, S. G, Moura, I, Moura, J. J, & Huynh, B. H. (1995). Structure and function of ferrochelatase. J Bioenerg Biomembr. 0014-5479X, 27(2), 221-229.

[11] Gossner, L, Stolte, M, Sroka, R, Rick, K, May, A, Hahn, E. G, & Ell, C. (1998). Photodynamic ablation of high-grade dysplasia and early cancer in Barrett's esophagus by means of 5-aminolevulinic acid. Gastroenterology. 0016-5085, 114(3), 448-455.

[12] Guyon, L, Ascencio, M, Collinet, P, & Mordon, S. (2012). Photodiagnosis and photodynamic therapy of peritoneal metastasis of ovarian cancer. Photodiagnosis Photodyn Ther. 1873-1597, 9(1), 16-31.

[13] Hefti, M, Albert, I, & Luginbuehl, V. (2012). Phenytoin reduces 5-aminolevulinic acid-induced protoporphyrin IX accumulation in malignant glioma cells. J Neurooncol. 1573-7373, 108(3), 443-450.

[14] Iacob, G, & Dinca, E. B. (2009). Current data and strategy in glioblastoma multiforme. J Med Life. 0184-4122X, 2(4), 386-393.

[15] Inoue, H, Kajimoto, Y, Shibata, M. A, Miyoshi, N, Ogawa, N, Miyatake, S, Otsuki, Y, & Kuroiwa, T. (2007). Massive apoptotic cell death of human glioma cells via a mito-

chondrial pathway following 5-aminolevulinic acid-mediated photodynamic therapy. J Neurooncol. 0016-7594X, 83(3), 223-231.

[16] Kajimoto, Y, Kuroiwa, T, Miyatake, S. I, Ichioka, T, Miyashita, M, Tanaka, H, & Tsuji, M. (2007). Use of 5-aminolevulinic acid in fluorescence-guided resection of meningioma with high risk of recurrence- Case report. Journal of Neurosurgery. 0022-3085, 106(6), 1070-1074.

[17] Karmakar, S, Banik, N. L, Patel, S. J, & Ray, S. K. (2007). Aminolevulinic acid-based photodynamic therapy suppressed survival factors and activated proteases for apoptosis in human glioblastoma U87MG cells. Neurosci Lett. 0304-3940, 415(3), 242-247.

[18] Kemmner, W, Wan, K, Ruttinger, S, Ebert, B, Macdonald, R, Klamm, U, & Moesta, K. T. (2008). Silencing of human ferrochelatase causes abundant protoporphyrin-IX accumulation in colon cancer. FASEB J. 1530-6860, 22(2), 500-509.

[19] Kennedy, J. C, & Pottier, R. H. (1992). Endogenous protoporphyrin IX, a clinically useful photosensitizer for photodynamic therapy. J Photochem Photobiol B. 1011-1344, 14(4), 275-292.

[20] Kuroiwa, T, Kajimoto, Y, & Ohta, T. (1998). Development of a fluorescein operative microscope for use during malignant glioma surgery- A technical note and preliminary report. Surgical Neurology. 0090-3019, 50(1), 41-48.

[21] Kuroiwa, T, Kajimoto, Y, & Ohta, T. (2001). Development and clinical application of near-infrared surgical microscope: preliminary report. Minim Invasive Neurosurg. 0946-7211, 44(4), 240-242.

[22] Lefranc, F, Sadeghi, N, Camby, I, Metens, T, Dewitte, O, & Kiss, R. (2006). Present and potential future issues in glioblastoma treatment. Expert Rev Anticancer Ther. 1744-8328, 6(5), 719-732.

[23] Liao, H, Shimaya, K, Wang, K, Maruyama, T, Noguchi, M, Muragaki, Y, Kobayashi, E, Iseki, H, & Sakuma, I. (2008). Combination of intraoperative 5-aminolevulinic acid-induced fluorescence and 3-D MR imaging for guidance of robotic laser ablation for precision neurosurgery. Med Image Comput Comput Assist Interv. No. Pt 2, ISSN:, 11, 373-380.

[24] Liao, H. E, Noguchi, M, Maruyama, T, Muragaki, Y, Kobayashi, E, Iseki, H, & Sakuma, I. (2012). An integrated diagnosis and therapeutic system using intra-operative 5-aminolevulinic-acid-induced fluorescence guided robotic laser ablation for precision neurosurgery. Med Image Anal. 1361-8415, 16(3), 754-766.

[25] Loh, C. S, & Vernon, D. MacRobert, A.J., Bedwell, J., Bown, S.G. & Brown, S.B. ((1993). Endogenous porphyrin distribution induced by 5-aminolaevulinic acid in the tissue layers of the gastrointestinal tract. J Photochem Photobiol B. 1011-1344, 20(1), 47-54.

[26] Loning, M, Diddens, H, Kupker, W, Diedrich, K, & Huttmann, G. (2004). Laparoscopic fluorescence detection of ovarian carcinoma metastases using 5-aminolevulinic acid-induced protoporphyrin IX. Cancer. 0000-8543X, 100(8), 1650-1656.

[27] MacDonaldI.J. & Dougherty, T.J. ((2001). Basic principles of photodynamic therapy. J Porphyr Phthalocya. 1088-4246, 5(2), 105-129.

[28] Nabavi, A, Thurm, H, Zountsas, B, Pietsch, T, Lanfermann, H, Pichlmeier, U, Mehdorn, M, & Glioma, A. L. A. R. (2009). Five-Aminolevulinic Acid for Fluorescence-Guided Resection of Recurrent Malignant Gliomas: A Phase Ii Study. Neurosurgery. 0014-8396X, 65(6), 1070-1076.

[29] Norum, O. J, Selbo, P. K, Weyergang, A, Giercksky, K. E, & Berg, K. (2009). Photochemical internalization (PCI) in cancer therapy: from bench towards bedside medicine. J Photochem Photobiol B. 1873-2682, 96(2), 83-92.

[30] Oleinick, N. L, Morris, R. L, & Belichenko, T. (2002). The role of apoptosis in response to photodynamic therapy: what, where, why, and how. Photoch Photobio Sci. 0147-4905X, 1(1), 1-21.

[31] Panciani, P. P, Fontanella, M, Garbossa, D, Agnoletti, A, Ducati, A, & Lanotte, M. (2012). aminolevulinic acid and neuronavigation in high-grade glioma surgery: results of a combined approach. Neurocirugia. 1130-1473, 23(1), 23-28.

[32] Peng, Q, Warloe, T, Berg, K, Moan, J, Kongshaug, M, Giercksky, K. E, & Nesland, J. M. (1997). Aminolevulinic acid-based photodynamic therapy. Clinical research and future challenges. Cancer. 0000-8543X, 79(12), 2282-2308.

[33] Pichlmeier, U, Bink, A, Schackert, G, & Stummer, W. (2008). Resection and survival in glioblastoma multiforme: an RTOG recursive partitioning analysis of ALA study patients. Neuro Oncol. 1522-8517, 10(6), 1025-1034.

[34] Piotrowski, W. J, Marczak, J, Nawrocka, A, Antczak, A, & Gorski, P. (2004). Inhalations of 5-ALA in photodynamic diagnosis of bronchial cancer. Monaldi Arch Chest Dis. 1122-0643, 61(2), 86-93.

[35] Sherman, J. H, Hoes, K, Marcus, J, Komotar, R. J, Brennan, C. W, & Gutin, P. H. (2011). Neurosurgery for brain tumors: update on recent technical advances. Current neurology and neuroscience reports. 1534-6293, 11(3), 313-319.

[36] Stummer, W, Novotny, A, Stepp, H, Goetz, C, Bise, K, & Reulen, H. J. (2000). Fluorescence-guided resection of glioblastoma multiforme by using 5-aminolevulinic acid-induced porphyrins: a prospective study in 52 consecutive patients. J Neurosurg. 0022-3085, 93(6), 1003-1013.

[37] Stummer, W, Pichlmeier, U, Meinel, T, Wiestler, O. D, Zanella, F, Reulen, H. J, Group, A. L, & Fluorescence-guided, G. S. surgery with 5-aminolevulinic acid for resection of malignant glioma: a randomised controlled multicentre phase III trial. Lancet Oncol. 1470-2045, 7(5), 392-401.

[38] Stummer, W, Reulen, H. J, Novotny, A, Stepp, H, & Tonn, J. C. (2003). Fluorescence-guided resections of malignant gliomas--an overview. Acta Neurochir Suppl. No. 0065-1419, 88, 9-12.

[39] Stummer, W, Stepp, H, Moller, G, Ehrhardt, A, Leonhard, M, & Reulen, H. J. (1998a). Technical principles for protoporphyrin-IX-fluorescence guided microsurgical resection of malignant glioma tissue. Acta Neurochir (Wien). 0001-6268, 140(10), 995-1000.

[40] Stummer, W, Stocker, S, Novotny, A, Heimann, A, Sauer, O, Kempski, O, Plesnila, N, Wietzorrek, J, & Reulen, H. J. (1998b). In vitro and in vivo porphyrin accumulation by C6 glioma cells after exposure to 5-aminolevulinic acid. J Photochem Photobiol B. 1011-1344, 45(2-3), 160-169.

[41] Stummer, W, Stocker, S, Wagner, S, Stepp, H, Fritsch, C, Goetz, C, Goetz, A. E, Kiefmann, R, & Reulen, H. J. (1998c). Intraoperative detection of malignant gliomas by 5-aminolevulinic acid-induced porphyrin fluorescence. Neurosurgery. discussion 525-526, 0014-8396X, 42(3), 518-525.

[42] Takahashi, K, Ikeda, N, Nonoguchi, N, Kajimoto, Y, Miyatake, S, Hagiya, Y, Ogura, S, Nakagawa, H, Ishikawa, T, & Kuroiwa, T. (2011). Enhanced expression of coproporphyrinogen oxidase in malignant brain tumors: CPOX expression and 5-ALA-induced fluorescence. Neuro Oncol. 1523-5866, 13(11), 1234-1243.

[43] Teng, L, Nakada, M, Zhao, S. G, Endo, Y, Furuyama, N, Nambu, E, Pyko, I. V, Hayashi, Y, & Hamada, J. I. (2011). Silencing of ferrochelatase enhances 5-aminolevulinic acid-based fluorescence and photodynamic therapy efficacy. Br J Cancer. 1532-1827, 104(5), 798-807.

[44] Toda, M. (2008). Intraoperative navigation and fluorescence imagings in malignant glioma surgery. The Keio journal of medicine. 1880-1293, 57(3), 155-161.

[45] Utsuki, S, Oka, H, Sato, S, Shimizu, S, Suzuki, S, Tanizaki, Y, Kondo, K, Miyajima, Y, & Fujii, K. (2007). Histological examination of false positive tissue resection using 5-aminolevulinic acid-induced fluorescence guidance. Neurol Med Chir (Tokyo). 0470-8105, 47(5), 210-213.

[46] Utsuki, S, Oka, H, Sato, S, Suzuki, S, Shimizu, S, Tanaka, S, & Fujii, K. (2006). Possibility of using laser spectroscopy for the intraoperative detection of nonfluorescing brain tumors and the boundaries of brain tumor infiltrates. Technical note. J Neurosurg. 0022-3085, 104(4), 618-620.

[47] Valdes, P. A, Leblond, F, Kim, A, Harris, B. T, Wilson, B. C, Fan, X. Y, Tosteson, T. D, Hartov, A, Ji, S. B, Erkmen, K, Simmons, N. E, Paulsen, K. D, & Roberts, D. W. (2011). Quantitative fluorescence in intracranial tumor: implications for ALA-induced PpIX as an intraoperative biomarker. Journal of Neurosurgery. 0022-3085, 115(1), 11-17.

[48] Wallner, K. E, Galicich, J. H, Krol, G, Arbit, E, & Malkin, M. G. (1989). Patterns of failure following treatment for glioblastoma multiforme and anaplastic astrocytoma. Int J Radiat Oncol Biol Phys. 0360-3016, 16(6), 1405-1409.

[49] Widhalm, G, Wolfsberger, S, Minchev, G, Woehrer, A, Krssak, M, Czech, T, Prayer, D, Asenbaum, S, Hainfellner, J. A, & Knosp, E. (2010). Aminolevulinic Acid Is a Promising Marker for Detection of Anaplastic Foci in Diffusely Infiltrating Gliomas With Nonsignificant Contrast Enhancement. Cancer. 0000-8543X, 116(6), 1545-1552.

[50] Zhao, S. G, Chen, X. F, Wang, L. G, Yang, G, Han, D. Y, Teng, L, Yang, M. C, Wang, D. Y, Shi, C, Liu, Y. H, Zheng, B. J, Shi, C. B, Gao, X, & Rainov, N. G. (2012). Increased Expression of ABCB6 Enhances Protoporphyrin IX Accumulation and Photodynamic Effect in Human Glioma. Annals of surgical oncology. Vol. No. pp. 1534-4681, 1534-4681.

Photodynamic Therapy Using Talaporfin Sodium and Diode Laser for Newly Diagnosed Malignant Gliomas

Jiro Akimoto

Additional information is available at the end of the chapter

http://dx.doi.org/10.5772/53485

1. Introduction

Wilson et al. [1] investigated the progression of glioblastoma (Grade 4) at the cellular level and showed that cells from tumors of 4 cm or greater in diameter on diagnostic imaging are considered to be present in both normal and affected brain tissues, with a distribution of 92% of tumor cells in the tumor bulk, 6% in areas within a 2-cm margin around the tumor, and 1.8% within an additional 2-cm area surrounding this margin. The majority of recurrent malignant gliomas develop in this marginal area, and therefore, controlling infiltrating cells in this region while protecting normal brain cells is critical to inhibit tumor recurrence.

In photodynamic therapy (PDT), a photosensitizer taken up in tumor tissues and neovascularized tumor vessels is administered to cancer patients. Tumor tissues are then later irradiated using a laser to induce a photochemical reaction in the photosensitizer, thereby selectively causing tumor cell apoptosis and necrosis. This tumor cell apoptosis and necrosis result from the strong oxidative effect of singlet oxygen (active oxygen) produced by the photochemical reaction in the photosensitizer, induced by a laser at a specific wavelength [2].

We previously reported that PDT using talaporfin sodium (TS), a second-generation photosensitizer, induced tumor coagulation necrosis and tumor cell-selective apoptosis in rats in which C6 glioma cells had been transplanted into the brain [3]. In the present study, we evaluated the safety and efficacy of PDT in areas with tumor invasion following tumor removal in patients with malignant glioma.

2. Materials

Eligible subjects were patients with a first time diagnosis of adult intracranial malignant glioma (Grade 3 or 4) based on preoperative diagnostic imaging and with a tumor bulk adjacent to the eloquent areas of the brain associated with language, motor, sensation and vision, for which a wide resection of the tumor much larger than the tumor bulk was impossible. Selective treatment of the infiltrating tumor cells by PDT was considered necessary because of tumor invasion into the eloquent areas, despite the fact that the tumor bulk had been removed as extensively as possible. PDT was performed after a rapid intraoperative pathological diagnosis confirmed malignant glioma. We excluded patients who had received radiotherapy or chemotherapy within 3 weeks prior to the surgery, patients with bleeding or abnormal coagulation test results, and patients with porphyria or porphyrin hypersensitivity. This clinical study was approved by the Institutional Review Board of our institution. All subjects provided written informed consent. The subjects were consecutive 8 patients (7 men and 1 woman) treated at our hospital between May 2006 and Mar 2009 and aged 48 to 82 years (median, 58 years). The tumors were localized in the frontal lobe in 4 patients, temporal lobe in 2 patients, insular gyrus in 1 patient and parietal lobe in 1 patient. Preoperative Karnofsky Performance Scale (KPS) was 50 to 80 (median 60). The extent of tumor resection was subtotal in 7 patients and partial in 1 patient. The final pathological diagnosis was Grade 3 in 3 patients, and Grade 4 glioblastoma in 5 patients. As postoperative adjuvant therapy, 4 patients received irradiation in combination with temozolomide (TMZ) and 2 patients received irradiation and ACNU-based multidrug chemotherapy.

3. Methods

3.1. Talaporfin sodium and diode laser

Talaporfin sodium (TS: Laserphyrin®, Meiji Seika Pharma Co., Ltd., Tokyo, Japan) is a photosensitizer utilized in PDT which was approved for use in Japan in 2003 as treatment for early-stage lung cancer, in conjunction with a diode laser (PD Laser®, Panasonic HealthCare Co., Ltd., Ehime, Japan) at a wavelength of 664 nm [4]. (Fig. 1A and B) Talaporfin sodium is a second-generation photosensitizer which is more quickly excreted from the body than the first-generation porfimer sodium (Photofrin®, Pfizer Japan Inc.,Tokyo, Japan). It is characterized by the rapid resolution of a skin photosensitive reaction, which is important with the use of photosensitizers. This has enabled the period of necessary light shielding in a room with measurement of < 500 lux to be reduced to 2 weeks for talaporfin sodium, whereas porfimer sodium requires patients to stay in a semi-dark(< 300 lux) room for 1 month after administration. The diode laser instrument is a compact system weighing 14 kg, has low power consumption, and can be easily maintained without the need for dye exchange. (Fig. 2A).

3.2. Operating microscope equipped with diode laser

The PD Laser® (Panasonic HealthCare Co., Ltd.), installed in the MM30 microscope (Mitaka Kohki Co., Ltd., Tokyo, Japan), is combined into a system which provides laser irradiation from the operating microscope from a plane nearly coaxial to the surgical view. The laser is introduced into the microscope by a quartz fiber, and providing a laser transmission path close to an observation light path using a conventional halogen light. This allows surgeons to accurately identify an irradiation target area during surgery. (Fig. 2A, B)

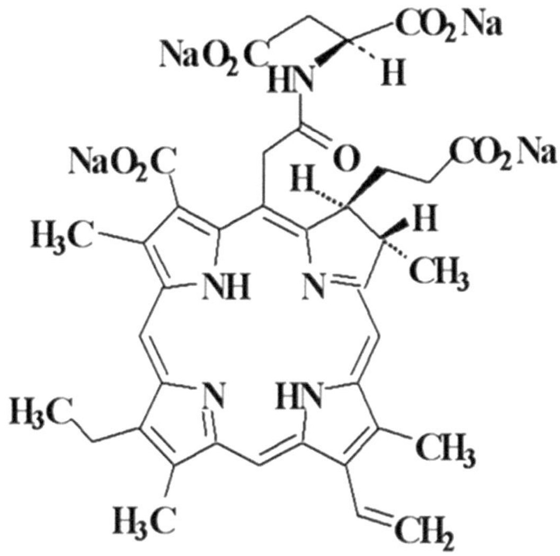

(a)

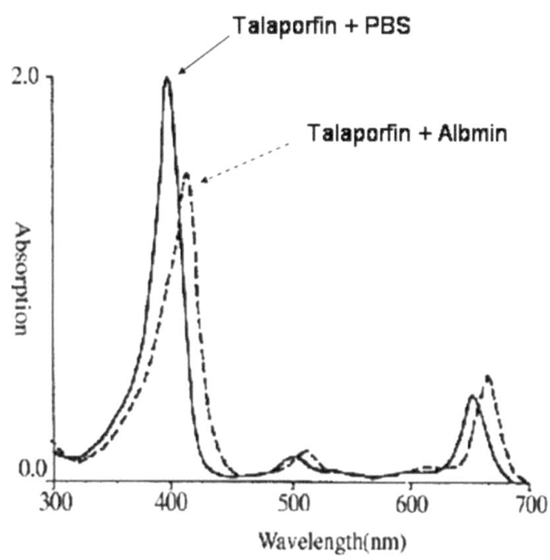

(b)

Figure 1. Second-generation photosensitizer, Talaporfin sodium. A:Chemical structures of talaporfin sodium (mono-L-aspartyl chlorine e6, NPe6) *N*-[[(2S,3S)-18-carboxy-2-(2-carboxyethyl)-13-ethyl-2,3-dibydro-3,7,12,17-tetramethyl-8-vinylporphyrin-20-yl]-L-asparatic acid. B:Absorption spectrum of talaporfin sodium and change in absorption wavelength following conjugation with albumin (solid line; talaporfin sodium and phosphate buffer solution, dotted line; talaporfin sodium conjugated with albumin) talaporfin sodium has absorption peaks in the Soret band (398nm) and Q bands (502, 530, 620 and 654nm) in pH 7.4 phosphate buffer solution (PBS). When it conjugates with albumin, its absorption band wavelength becomes approximately 10nm longer (bathochromic shift).

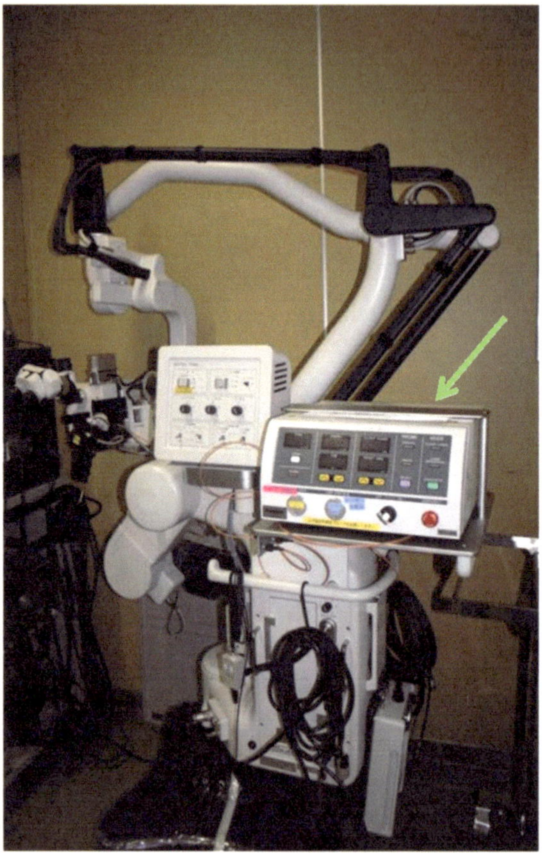

(a)

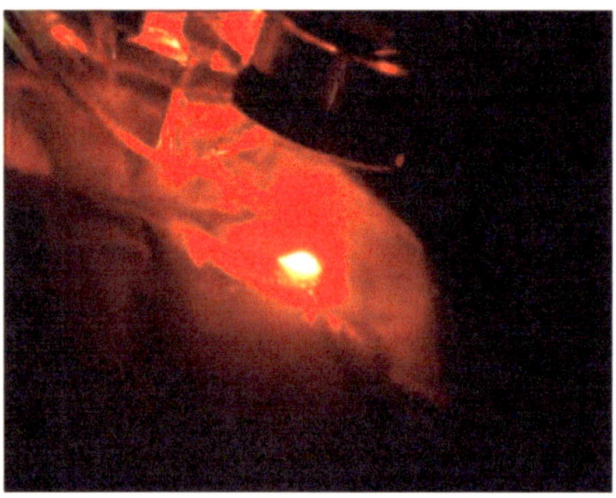

(b)

Figure 2. Diode laser with a neurosurgical operating microscope. A: MM80® microscope (Mitaka Kohki Co., Ltd.) equipped with a compact-size diode laser (PD Laser®, Panasonic Health Care Ltd., arrow). B: From the operating microscope, the diode laser irradiates the surgical field with an irradiation diameter of 1.5 cm^2.

3.3. Photodynamic therapy (PDT)

TS was administered bolus intravenously at a dose of 40mg/m^2 in shielded conditions 24 hours prior to surgery. At surgery, maximal resection of the tumor was performed usually utilizing optical navigation system and electrophysiological monitoring leaving a tumor bed area to be irradiated. The surface area of tumor bed was observed under operative microscope and optimal navigation system, and identified the optimal target for PDT. PDT covering an area of 1.5 cm^2 diameter was used for any tumor growth in these area. When 2 sites were to be irradiated, we took care to avoid overlapping the irradiated areas under operative microscope. Irradiation energy density of 27 J/cm^2 (power density of 150mW/cm^2, irradiation time of 180 seconds) of 664nm diode laser for PDT was irradiated superficially to one or two targets of tumor bed.

3.4. Skin photosensitive reaction test

The administration of TS enhances sensitivity to light, and which may produce a photosensitive reaction. Patients should therefore avoid direct sunlight immediately after the administration of talaporfin sodium and stay in a room where the illumination intensity is adjusted to < 500 lux using a shading curtain. After surgery, patients were required to expose the back of the palm of the hand to direct sunlight for 5minutes every day between 11:00 and 14:00 to evaluate the development of erythema. However, even when the result of this skin photosensitivity test confirmed the resolution of a photosensitive reaction (defined by the absence of evident erythema) and the restriction for shading at < 500 lux could be removed, patients were advised to avoid further direct sunlight for 2 weeks after the administration of talaporfin sodium. In particular, we recommended that special shading eye goggles should be used worn 7 days after the administration of talaporfin sodium to avoid exposing the retinas to direct sunlight.

4. Results

4.1. Selected case

A 65-year-old man presented with 2 months history of headache and gradually worsened. Head MRI showed a tumor in the right frontal lobe, and edema extending as far as the premotor area at the posterior edge of the tumor bulk. On a sagittal view, part of the posterior edge of the tumor bulk extended posteriorly, and this part was determined to have invaded the supplemental motor area(SMA) (Fig. 3A and B). Using optical navigation system and motor evoked potential (MEP) monioring, we performed craniotomy in order to resect the tumor, and rapid pathological diagnosis confirmed that the tumor was a glioblastoma. From the optical navigation images, the posterior margin of the tumor bulk was confirmed to have reached the pre-motor area (SMA-proper) (Fig.3C), and a single session of PDT at 27 J/cm^2 (diameter of the irradiated area: 1.5 cm^2) was performed at this site (Fig 3.D and E). Under a pathological diagnosis of glioblastoma, the patient given postoperative irradiation and chemotherapy with oral TMZ. On day 3 after surgery, MRI showed remaining contrast-enhanced tumor growth in the pre-motor area, but by the end of radiotherapy (on day 51 after surgery, Fig. 3F), complete response was confirmed at this site. His headache was disappeared and he enjoyed a play of weekly golf until 3 years after operation.

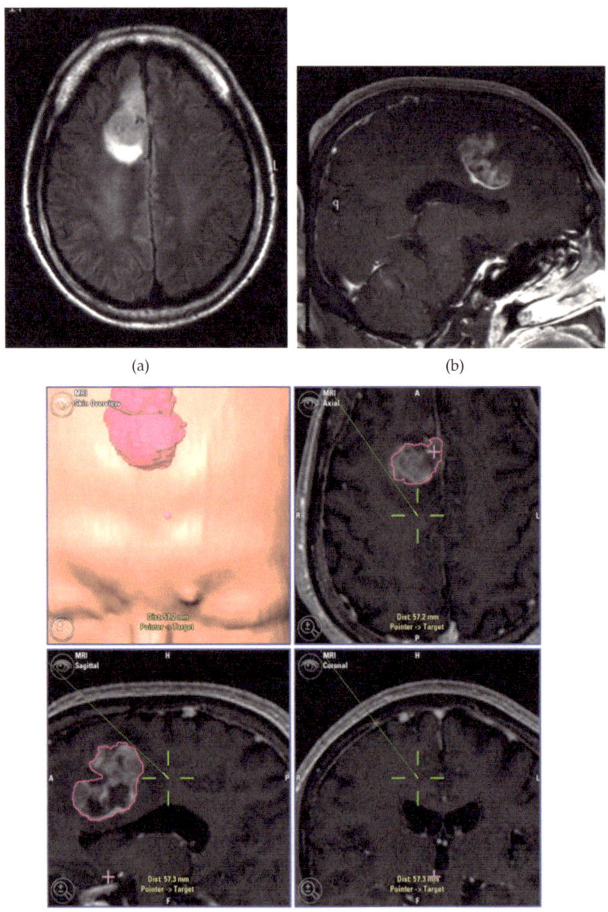

(a) (b) (c)

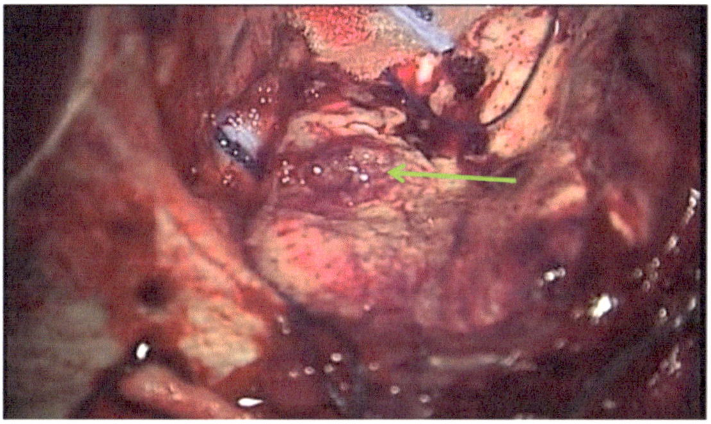

(d)

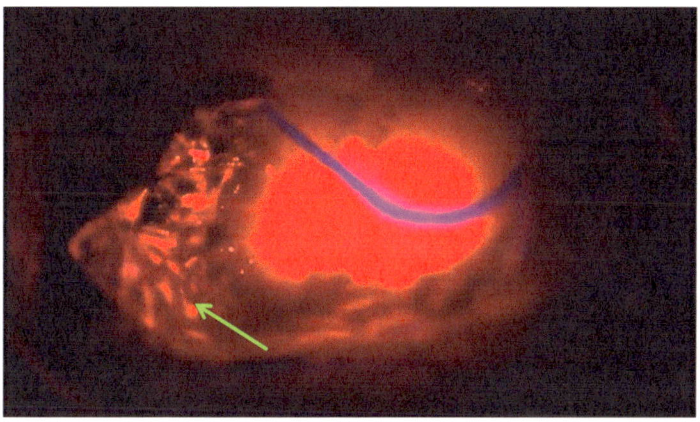

(e)

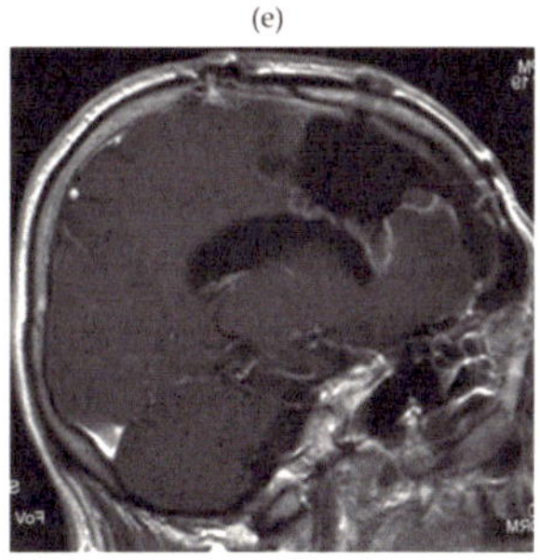

(f)

Figure 3. PDT and changes over time on postoperative magnetic resonance imaging (MRI) in Case 3. A: Preoperative axial FLAIR image showed the right frontal tumor and the peri-tumoral edema extending to the right pre-motor cortex. B: Preoperative gadolinium-enhanced T1-weighted sagittal imaging showed a heterogeneously enhanced tumor was present in the right superior frontal gyrus to supplementary motor cortex. C: Based on intra-operative optical navigation images, it was determined that the tumor had reached a portion adjacent to the ambulatory motor area (green cross). D: The tumor was remained in this area (arrow). E: PDT at 150 mW/cm^2 and 27 J/cm^2 (diameter of the irradiation area: 1.5 cm^2) was performed for tumor infiltration into this area. (aluminum foil protected the anterior cerebral arteries, arrow). F: Gadolinium-enhanced T1-weighted sagittal imaging on days 51 after surgery showed that gadolinium-enhancement at the site of PDT had disappeared.

4.2. Summary

In the evaluation of patients, of the 6 patients who were assessable after surgery, 3 achieved complete response, 2 achieved partial response, and 1 had progressive disease. The response rate was high at 83.3%. Regarding adverse events associated with PDT, brain edema involving a large part of the middle cerebral artery perforator region occurred during PDT after insular glioma resection in Case 1. While it remains uncertain whether this was associated with the surgical procedure or PDT, the effect on normal capillary vessels should be closely monitored. No other obvious adverse events were observed. In most patients, postoperative chemo-radiation therapy was initiated, but recurrence was observed at the site of PDT in 7 patients. Despite recurrence, the progression-free survival time was 1 to 34 months (median: 22 months), and in cases receiving treatment after recurrence, 5 patients had a survival time of 6 to 14 months (median: 6 months). A further 3 patients of Grade 3 were alive during a follow-up period of 42 to 74 months (median: 50 months). An evaluation of 5 patients with glioblastoma also showed a median progression-free survival time of 14 months and a median survival time of 26 months.

While it was possibly an adverse event associated with the surgical procedure, a causal relationship with the PDT could not be excluded. In terms of photosensitivity, the photosensitive reaction resolved within 3 days after surgery (within 4 days after the intravenous injection) in all patients, at which point light shading at 500 lux was discontinued.

5. Discussion

The objective of PDT is to selectively kill infiltrating tumor cells via a photochemical reaction, and this selectivity facilitates optimal local control therapy [2], making it possible to maintain brain function. PDT is designed to cause damage at the cellular level in the form of apoptosis [2]. There are numerous studies which have reported that the main mechanism of PDT is the induction of vascular occlusion from fibrin thrombus formation due to vascular endothelial cell damage [5]. In particular, it has been assumed that the main mechanism on cellular damage induced by PDT using TS in conjunction with a diode laser irradiation is indirect damage in the form of coagulation necrosis by tumor vascular occlusion [5]. In our basic experimental study, C6 glioma tissue showed coagulation necrosis in tissues located in a portion near the tumor surface that was laser irradiated, and cellular death in the distal portion [3]. However, in the actual area of tissue damage, 80% of the area was considered to be tissue damage caused by the coagulation necrosis. Yamamoto et al. [5] reported that factor XIII was activated by vascular endothelial cell damage within 20 seconds following PDT of cancer tissue. A fibrin thrombus formed as a consequence, which appeared to be the main mechanism of PDT.

Our strategy was to optimally reduce vascular damage caused by PDT, and to ensure safety to avoid ischemic damage to normal brain tissues. Madsen et al. [6] reported that the factors which influence the effects of PDT were tissue factors and irradiation laser factors. The tissue factors included the tissue concentrations of the photosensitizer, the level of tissue oxygenation, and the depth from the site of laser irradiation. The irradiation laser factors included irradiation level and duration. How the cytotoxic effects can be enhanced while minimizing the vascular effects, and how ischemic damage to normal brain tissues can be minimized may well be the keys to determining whether or not PDT can be developed for the treatment of malignant glioma.

In the present study, we selected a dose of 40 mg/m^2 of TS and performed PDT approximately 24 hours after the administration of TS. The practice of the PDT was performed on the diode laser (664nm) irradiation at a power density of 150 mW/cm^2 for 180 seconds (27 J/cm^2). We previously reported that this PDT protocol was considered safe in terms of the protection of early vascular endothelial cell damage and normal brain tissues, and could induce the selective tumor cell damage by singlet oxygen [7].

Although there were only consecutive 8 patients of newly diagnosed malignant glioma in this series, PDT achieved a response rate of 83.3% and a median progression-free survival time of 14 months, a median survival time of 26 months in the glioblastoma patients who eventually died, and all 3 cases of Grade 3 patients were survived for 50 months median follow up period. In the 5 patients who achieved complete or partial response, preoperative KPS was improved. None of the patients had adverse events unequivocally attributable to PDT. The brain edema observed in Case 1 was possibly due to the surgical procedure, but the possibility of direct laser irradiation of brain blood vessels inducing vascular occlusion due to PDT could not be completely excluded. Therefore, normal blood vessels should be covered with aluminum foil whenever possible.

Response	RTx	Chemo Tx	KPS after treatment	Progression	PFS	Prognosis, Survival period
NE	60Gy	ACNU/VCR/IFN	50	(+)	22 mon.	Dead: 36 mon.
CR	60Gy	IFN	70	(+)	24 mon.	Alive: 74 mon.
CR	60Gy	TMZ	90	(+)	34 mon.	Dead: 40 mon.
PR	60Gy	TMZ	90	(+)	14 mon.	Dead: 26 mon.
PR	60Gy	(-)	50	(+)	24 mon.	Alive: 50 mon.
PD	(-)	TMZ	40	(+)	1 mon.	Dead: 7 mon.
CR	60Gy	PCZ/ACNU/VCR	80	(+)	6mon.	Dead: 12mon.
NE	60Gy	TMZ	90	(-)		Alive: 42mon.

KPS: Karnofsky Performance Scale, PDT: photodynamic therapy, RTx: radiation therapy, Chemo Tx: chemotherapy, PFS: progression-free survival, Rt: right, Lt: left, Bil: bilateral, Anapl: anaplastic, CR: complete response, PR: partial response, PD: progression disease, NE: not evaluable, TMZ: temozolomide, VCR: vincristine, IFN: interferon-beta, PCZ: procarbazine, mon. months

Table 1. Clinical summary of patients with newly diagnosed malignant glioma who received photodynamic therapy (PDT)

The present study of PDT using talaporfin sodium in conjunction with diode laser irradiation for malignant glioma supports the validity of PDT for malignant glioma in Japan. Laser irradiation used to activate TS has a longer wavelength (664 nm) than that used with other photosensitizers, such as Porfimer sodium [8-11], 5-ALA [12-14] and m-THPC [15, 16], and theoretically, it can penetrate brain tissue to a greater depth. We believe that our strategy will demonstrate a therapeutic effect not to be inferior to those of previous reports [17] using other photosensitizers. In future, it is necessary to perform the larger-scale prospective clinical study to confirm the clinical feasibility of this novel therapeutic option to malignant gliomas.

6. Conclusions

We performed PDT using TS in conjunction with diode laser irradiation in areas of tumor invasion, following resection of adult malignant glioma which had infiltrated the eloquent areas. We selected a 24 hours interval after the administration of TS before commencing PDT and reduced irradiation energy intensity of the diode laser to 27 J/cm^2 to preserve normal brain function. The therapy achieved with no adversed event directly attributable to PDT and a response rate of 83.3% in patients with a newly diagnosed malignant gliomas.

Author details

Jiro Akimoto

Address all correspondence to: jakimoto@tokyo-med.ac.jp

Department of Neurosurgery, Tokyo Medical University, Tokyo, Japan

The authors report no conflict of interest concerning the materials or methods used in this study and findings specified in this paper.

References

[1] Wilson CB. Glioblastoma: the past, the present, and the future. Clin Neurosurg 1992, 38, 32-48

[2] Castano AP, Demidova TN, Hambrin MR. Mechanism of photodynamic therapy: Part three - Photosensitizer pharmacokinetics, biodistribution, tumor localization and modes of tumor destruction. Photodiag Photodyn Therapy 2005, 2(2), 91-106

[3] Namatame H, Akimoto J, Matsumura H, Haraoka J, Aizawa K. Photodynamic therapy of C6 implanted glioma cells in the rat brain employing Talaporfin sodium. Photodiag Photodyn Therapy 2008, 5, 198-209

[4] Kato H, Furukawa K, Sato M, Okunaka T, Kusunoki Y, Kawahara M, Fukuoka M, Miyazawa T, Yana T, Matsui K, Shiraishi T, Horinouchi H. Phase II clinical study of photodynamic therapy using mono-L-aspartyl chlorine e6 and diode laser for early squamous cell carcinoma of the lung. Lung Cancer 2003, 42, 103-111

[5] Yamamoto Y, Shibuya H, Okunaka T, Aizawa K, Kato H. Fibrin plugging as a cause of microcirculatory occlusion during photodynamic therapy. Lasers Med Sci 1999, 14,129-135

[6] Madsen SJ, Angell-Petersen E, Spetalen S, Carper SW, Ziegler SA, Hirschberg H. Photodynamic therapy of newly implanted glioma cells in the rat brain. Lasers Surg Med 2006, 38, 540-548

[7] Akimoto J, Haraoka J, Aizawa K. Preliminary clinical report on safety and efficacy of photodynamic therapy using Talaporfin sodium for malignant gliomas. Photodiag Photodyn Therapy 2012, 9, 91-99

[8] Muller PJ, Wilson BC. Photodynamic therapy for malignant newly diagnosed supratentorial gliomas. J Clin Laser Med Surg 1996, 14, 263-270

[9] Muller PJ, Wilson BC. Photodynamic therapy for recurrent supratentorial gliomas. Semin Surg Oncol 1996, 14, 263-270

[10] Popovic EA, Kaye AH, Hill JS. Photodynamic therapy of brain tumors. Semin Surg Oncol 1995, 11, 335-345

[11] Stylli SS, Kaye AH, MacGregor L, Howes M, Rajendra P. Photodynamic therapy of high grade glioma - long term survival. J Clin Neurosci 2005, 12(4), 389-398

[12] Beck TJ, Kreth FW, Beyer W, Mehrkens JH, Obermeier A, Stepp H, Stummer W, Baumgartner R. Interstitial photodynamic therapy of nonresectable malignant glioma recurrences using 5-aminolevulinic acid induced protoporphyrin IX. Lasers Surg Med 2007, 39, 386-393

[13] Stummer W, Beck T, Beyer W, Mehrkens JH, Obermeier A, Etminan N, Stepp H, Tonn JC, Baumgartner R, Herms J, Kreth FW. Long-sustaining response in a patient with non-resectable, distant recurrence of glioblastoma multiforme treated by interstitial photodynamic therapy using 5-ALA: case report. J Neurooncol 2008, 87,103-109

[14] Bisland SK, Ligle A, Lin A,Rusnow R, Wilson BC. Metronomic photodynamic therapy as a new paradigm for photodynamic therapy: rationale and preclinical evaluation of technical feasibility for treating malignant brain tumors. Photochem Photobiol 2004, 80, 22-30

[15] Kostron H, Fritsch E, Grunert V. Photodynamic therapy of malignant brain tumours: a phase I/II trial. Br J Neurosurg 1988, 2(2), 241-248

[16] Zimmermann A, Ritsch-Marte M, Kostron H. mTHPC-mediated photodynamic diagnosis of malignant brain tumors. Photochem Photobiol 2001, 74(4), 611-616

[17] Eljamel MS, Goodman C, Moseley H. ALA and Photofrin fluorescence-guided resection and repetitive PDT in glioblastoma multiforme: a single centre Phase III randomised controlled trial. Lasers Med Sci 2008, 23(4), 361-7

Section 6

Molecular Biology of Brain Tumors

Chapter 14

Epithelial to Mesenchymal Transition and Progression of Glioblastoma

Andrej Pala, Georg Karpel-Massler,
Christian Rainer Wirtz and Marc-Eric Halatsch

Additional information is available at the end of the chapter

http://dx.doi.org/10.5772/53183

1. Introduction

Glioblastoma multiforme (GBM) is the most common primary brain tumor among adults. Rapid tumor progression and diffuse invasion of brain tissue restrict the therapeutic options and result in poor prognosis despite advances in the understanding of this tumor's molecular biology and pathophysiology [1-4]. Current standard therapy consists of a combination of tumor resection, irradiation and temozolomide. Advances in the field of molecular biology have led to the development of targeted therapy, and the epidermal growth factor receptor (EGFR) has been introduced as one potential therapeutic target [5]. Although pre-clinical studies have shown promising effects, clinical applications yielded no significant benefit in comparison with standard therapy. This fact encouraged extensive investigations studying the molecular mechanisms underlying GBM resistance to EGFR-targeted therapy. Epithelial to mesenchymal transition (EMT) is considered an important factor contributing to resistance towards this therapy by diminishing the molecular target [1-6].

Epithelial to mesenchymal transition is a common process, taking part in organ development, wound healing, tissue remodelling, cancer progression and metastasis. The main features accompanying this mechanism are the loss of epithelial characteristics of cells and the acquisition of mesenchymal markers such as fibronectin, vimentin and N-cadherin. As a result, tumor cells develop increasing invasive and migratory potential. The loss of epithelial features mounts the resistance of tumor cells against targeted therapy directed towards the EGFR. Mesenchymal transition leads to disorganisation of the cytoskeleton, disruption of intercellular adhesions and changes in expression of transcriptional factors, resulting in the development of a more malignant cellular phenotype [1, 2, 7].

In embryogenesis, epithelial to mesenchymal transition appears during gastrulation and activates the formation of the mesodermal layer as the third germ layer after ectoderm and endoderm are built. In addition, EMT is involved in the development of neural crest cells, arising from the dorsal part of the neural tube [7]. This requires a highly specialised program that is necessary to allow the normal development of cells. On the other hand, under pathological conditions, EMT increases the invasiveness and migratory potential of tumor cells, supports their malignant transformation and may lead to resistance of tumor cells towards various therapeutic agents, especially in malignant gliomas.

2. EGFR

The EGFR is a transmembraneous glycoprotein belonging to the human EGFR (HER) family, which includes four members (HER 1-4) that share a similar structure. The EGFR/HER1 consists of external and internal domains. The extracellular part possesses a binding sequence for ligands such as EGF, hepatocyte growth factor (HGF), fibroblast growth factor (FGF), insulin-like growth factor-1 (IGF-1) or tumor growth factor-α (TGF-α). The internal domain contains a tyrosine kinase (TK), capable of phosphorylation and activation of a variety of downstream pathways such as phospholipase Cγ, phosphatidylinositol-3-kinase (PI3-K), Janus-activated kinase 2 (JAK-2) and mitogen-activated kinase (MAPK). Human epidermal growth factor family receptors are expressed on many cell types and mediate signal transduction to intracellular compartments and hereby regulate various functions of cells such as proliferation or differentiation [1, 5, 8, 9].

Phosphorylation and dephosphorylation are crucial pathophysiological events within intracellular interactions. A dysregulation of their balance contributes to the development of an invasive cellular phenotype. Upon activation, receptor tyrosine kinases dimerise and autophosphorylate on tyrosine residues, which in turn create complexes with proteins possessing SH2 domains such as GRB2, SHC or signalling proteins PI3-K and SRC [9].

Pathological activation of RAS occurs in numerous cancers. This signalling pathway integrates various diverse stimuli promoting cell transformation, gene expression and tumor progression. RAS is a small guanine triphosphate-binding protein that activates the serine-threonine kinase RAF. RAF phosphorylates the dual specificity kinase MEK, which in turn activates MAPK (ERK). The latter translocate into the nucleus and activate various transcription factors such as the ETS family factors FOS, JUN or SLUG (SNAI-2). Thereby RAS propagates the activation of EMT. Moreover, RAS is able to promote EMT by downstream activation of PI3-K or RHO/RAC. PI3-K is involved in cell cycle regulation via phosphorylation of cyclin-dependent kinase inhibitors. In addition, it controls the phosphorylation of proapoptotic proteins and survival of the cell. PI3-K can be activated either via RAS or directly via TK receptors. PI3-K is a lipide kinase, and its activation generates phosphatidylinositol-3,4,5-triphosphate (PIP3) at the inner side of plasma membrane, which furthermore mediates the signalling via the serine-threonine kinase AKT that is able to translocate into the nucleus and take part in gene regulation through phosphatidylinositol-dependent protein kinase-1 (PDK-1) [8, 9, 10].

Epidermal growth factor overexpression and/or mutational activation is the most common molecular alteration in primary GBM and can be detected in far more than 50% of glioblastoma cells [5]. There are several mechanisms that may cause dysfunction of the receptor. Epidermal growth factor receptor gene amplification is the most common reason leading to protein overexpression. Other mechanisms include constitutive receptor activation by deletion-mutation (EGFRvIII) or autocrine overproduction of EGFR ligands [5, 6, 9]. The presence of EGFRvIII is associated with EGFR gene amplification.

3. Therapeutic EGFR inhibitors

Several drugs that target EGFR have been introduced. The TK inhibitors erlotinib and gefitinib compete with adenosine triphosphate to bind to the intracellular TK domain and dissolve further signalling involving PI3-K/AKT and MAPK pathways. Erlotinib was approved in the treatment of metastatic non-small cell lung carcinoma (NSCLC) and in combination with gemcitabine for metastasized pancreatic cancer or pancreatic cancer without the possibility of gross total resection [11, 12]. Gefitinib is used for metastatic NSCLC. Another small molecule EGFR-TK inhibitor represents lapatinib, which affords dual inhibition of EGFR and HER-2 and has been approved for the treatment of advanced or metastatic breast cancer. Unfortunately, the clinical application in gliomas had shown no benefit in comparison to standard therapy [1, 5, 6, 8].

Another possibility to inhibit EGFR signalling consists in the prevention of ligand binding. Monoclonal antibodies such as cetuximab have been introduced and investigated for this purpose. However, their molecular weight impairs their penetration of the blood brain barrier. Often the concentration of the agent is insufficient to yield a significant therapeutic effect within the targeted tissue [13].

Antisense RNA has been introduced as an option to inhibit the EGFR pathway as well. Sense RNA hybridizes to antisense RNA which leads to inhibition of translation. Another strategy to switch off the EGFR cascade is the application of small interfering RNAs. These suppress the homolog genes and result in sequence-specific degradation of mRNA. Furthermore, ribozymes are small RNA molecules that are able to bind and cleave complementary RNA substrates. EGFRvIII-targeted ribozymes have been reported to reverse malignant phenotype of transformed fibroblasts and glioblastoma cells [14, 15]. However, the potential clinical value of these methods remains unknown [16].

4. Molecular principles of EMT

Tumor progression represents an integrated multistep complex of molecular changes that ultimately result in local invasion and dissemination of malignant cells. The cells invade the epithelial basement membrane, infiltrate the surrounding tissue, access the blood circulation and may create new tumor seeds. This dynamic and aggressive process demands cell-to-cell and cell-to-matrix interactions, degradation and remodelling of extracellular matrix, cytoskeleton reorganisation and gain of migratory behaviour of tumor cells. Epithelial to mesenchymal transition is a differentiation switch which promotes the loss of the epithelial phenotype and facilitates cell motility and invasiveness. One of the crucial steps promoting EMT is the repression of the epithelial marker E-cadherin, a transmembraneous calcium-dependent glycoprotein responsible for cell-cell adhesion, which plays a key role in embryonic development and homeostasis. The intracellular domain of E-cadherin associates with a protein complex involving α-catenin, β-catenin and p120-catenin. Actin proteins bind α-catenin and hereby allow the connection between E-cadherin and the actin microfilament network of the cytoskeleton that forms the shape of the cell. Epithelial cells are typically characterized by apicobasal difference. Thus, the apical compartment faces the lumen, whereas the basolateral surface is located on a basement membrane. Epithelial cells are anchored by specialized cell-to-cell connections, i.e. tight junctions, adherens junction and desmosomes. E-cadherin acts as a tumor suppressor by linking the epithelial cells and keeping them in a stationary rigid state [1, 2, 7, 8, 9, 17].

During EMT, tumor cells loose junctional contact and epithelial cell polarity and acquire typical properties of mesenchymal cells. E-cadherin is a central regulator of the epithelial phenotype, and its downregulation results in the destabilisation of the epithelial architecture. Dysregulation of E-cadherin may be located at various levels, and hypermethylation of the E-cadherin promoter is among the molecular mechanisms [1, 2, 8-10, 17].

Under normal physiological conditions, epithelial cells are separated from the extracellular matrix (ECM) by basement membranes. This barrier prevents the interaction between epithelial cells and their microenvironment. The destabilisation of the basement membrane enables contact between various signalling proteins of the ECM and epithelial cells. The resulting cellular signalling may enhance the progression of EMT by activating different intracellular signalling pathways [17]. Gene transcription regulated by transcription factors is an important mechanism involved in gene regulation. Some transcriptional repressors such as SNAI-1/2, zinc finger E-box binding homeobox-1 (ZEB-1) and ZEB-2 are able to bind directly to the E-cadherin promoter and repress its transcription. Overexpression of these proteins supports mesenchymal transformation and the change of behavioural characteristics and promotes the continuous acquisition of malignant features by tumor cells [18, 19]. Crucial transcription factors involved in EMT are TWIST-1 and signal transducers and activators of transcription-3/-5 (STAT-3/-5). TWIST-1 is a basic helix-loop-helix protein that forms heterodimers binding on DNA, hereby regulating the development and differentiation of cells. For instance, TWIST-1 inhibits p53-mediated apoptosis in rodent fibroblasts or stops normal skeletal muscle development by creating heterodimers with myogenic basic helix-loop-helix proteins (MyoD and myogen). Its function within EMT is repression of the epithelial marker E-cadherin, activation of N-cadherin and hereby promotion of mesenchymal transformation, resulting in a more aggressive phenotype and progression of glioblastoma. TWIST-1 is reported to be an important EMT regulator in other malignancies as well, such as breast, gastric, hepatocellular and prostate cancer. There is significant evidence that TWIST-1 is involved in regulation of programmed cell death and induction of apoptosis. Through inhibition of p53-mediated apoptosis, TWIST-1 enables cell survival by preventing growth arrest and promotes invasiveness of tumor cells [3, 4]. Moreover, this process may result in increased resistance to various chemotherapeutic agents.

Sex determining region Y-box-2, also known as SOX-2, is another transcription factor that is co-expressed with TWIST-1, playing an important role during the development of the nervous system and tumor progression. Knockdown of SOX-2 results in reduced expression of TWIST-1 [4], promoting EMT and potentially being essential for tumor progression and the development of tumor resistance to EGFR-targeted therapies.

Signal transducer and activator of transcription-3 activation is associated with more malignant tumors and poor prognosis. Its overexpression has been detected in malignant gliomas, and its activation correlates with glioma grade. The STAT protein family is phosphorylated by receptor-associated kinases and builds homo- or heterodimers that translocate to the cell nucleus and play a crucial role in cell cycle progression, EMT, anti-apoptosis and metastasis. Signal transducer and activator of transcription-3 is hereby considered an important factor mediating and converging many cellular pathways. Therefore, either direct or indirect inhibition of STAT-3 may represent an optional therapeutic target in gliomas. Moreover, STAT-3 interacts with EGFR and mediates TWIST-1 expression and TWIST-1-mediated EMT. In addition, there seems to be a correlation between EGFR/EGFR-vIII expression, activation of STAT-3 and glioma grade. Noteworthy, a nuclear interaction between EGFRvIII and STAT-3 leads to malignant transformation of glioma cells [20].

Another interesting point is a recent discovery, described by Lo. He found increased expression of the pro-inflammatory gene cyclooxygenase-2 (COX-2) activated by EGFR-EGFRvIII and STAT-3 cooperation [21]. These interactions represent potential factors contributing to increased resistance of GBM to EGFR-targeted therapy. The important inflammatory enzyme COX-2 is overexpressed in various malignancies. In NSCLC, it has been reported that increased levels of COX-2 contribute to apoptosis resistance, angiogenesis and invasiveness of tumor cells. The effector of COX-2 is prostaglandin E-2 (PGE-2) which is produced by tumorous stromal cells and reduces the expression of E-cadherin via ZEB-1 and SNAI-1. Prostaglandin E-2 activates four G-protein coupled receptors, also known as E-prostanoid receptors-1 to -4 (EP-1 to EP-4), and promotes signalling via the MAPK/ERK cascade, which finally upregulates SNAI-1 and ZEB-1 expression [1, 21, 23]. This loop enhances signalling in the same pathway that is activated by EGFR. In addition, low levels of E-cadherin have been reported to be associated with increased resistance to EGFR-TK inhibitors in NSCLC [21, 23].

Signal transducer and activator of transcription-5 represents an important transcription factor which is involved in the regulation of many genes, facilitating cellular growth, migration and motility. Dimers of STAT-5 bind to specific DNA promoter regions and mediate cellular gene responses. Dysregulation of STAT-5 has been recently described in many malignancies such as prostate, breast and squamous cell cancer of the head and neck (SCCHN). In SCCHN, the activity of STAT-5 results in increased resistance of tumor cells to erlotinib. Moreover, it confers decreased apoptosis following treatment with cisplatin, finally diminishing the clinical effect [19].

The SNAI family members (SNAI-1-3) are related transcriptional repressors. Their SNAG domain at the N-terminal region is responsible for their activity, and their zinc-finger C-terminal region enables the attachment to specific DNA sequences. The main role of SNAI genes is the regulation and promotion of E-cadherin expression. It has been reported that knockdown of SNAI-1 results in decreased invasion and migration of glioma cells. Moreover, SNAI-1 induces expression of matrix metalloprotease-2 (MMP-2), another contributor to EMT progression [18].

Zinc finger E-box binding homeobox-1 regulates transcription of E-cadherin by binding of two zinc finger domains to two E-boxes located in the E-cadherin promoter region. It has been shown that low levels of ZEB-1 improve the sensitivity of cells to erlotinib in head and neck squamous cell carcinoma cell lines [21].

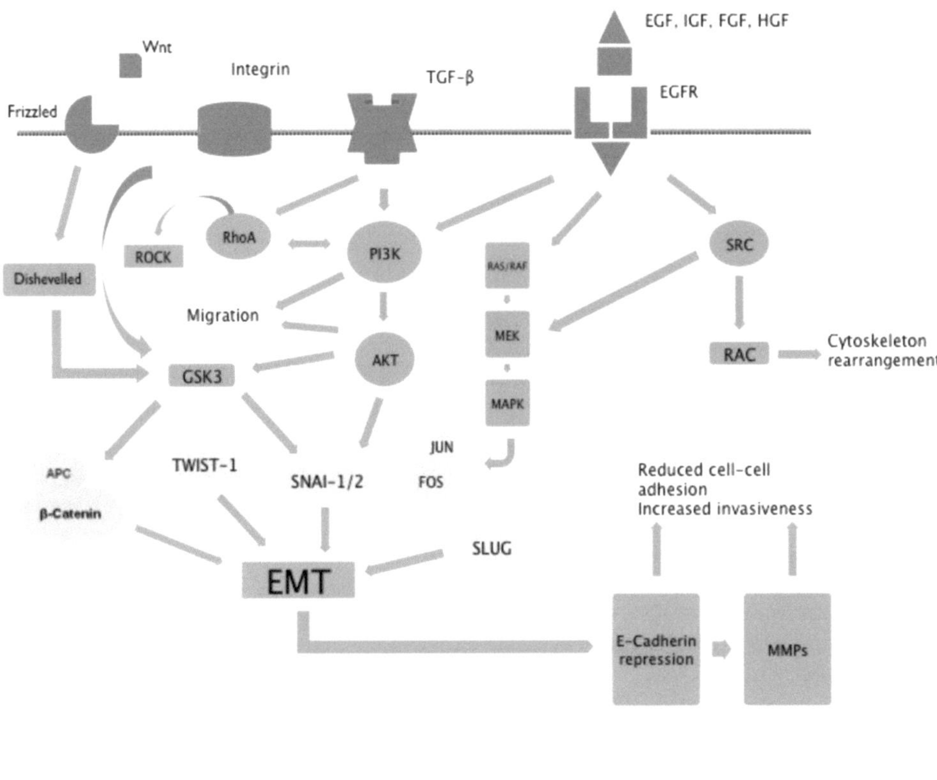

Figure 1. Signal transduction pathways associated with EMT. Abbreviations: APC – adenomatous polyposis coli, EMT - epithelial to mesenchymal transition, TGF-β – transforming growth factor β, EGF – epidermal growth factor, EGFR - epidermal growth factor receptor, FGF – fibroblast growth factor, GSK 3 – glycogen synthase kinase, HGF – hepatocyte growth factor, IGF – insulin-like growth factor, ILK – integrin-linked kinase, MAPK - mitogen-activated protein kinase, MEK - mitogen-activated protein kinase kinase, MMPs - matrix metalloproteases, PI3K – phosphoinositide 3-kinase, RTK – receptor tyrosine kinase.

Activator protein-1 (AP-1) is a protein complex consisting of JUN and FOS heterodimers or JUN homodimers. It plays an important role in the regulation of a variety of genes, resulting in the progression of EMT. Induction of AP-1 correlates with MAPK-activation and phosphorylation of the ETS family transcription factors such as E twenty-six-like transcription factor (ELK-1) which furthermore induces the transcription of FOS. Phosphorylated ETS factors result ultimately into the repression of E-cadherin and up-regulation of genes that lead to the transcription of MMPs [2].

As a result of downregulation of E-cadherin, loss of cell-to-cell adhesions and reorganisation of the actin cytoskeleton during EMT, cells acquire a mesenchymal identity. The expression of mesenchymal cytoskeleton proteins such as vimentin and the deposition of ECM proteins such as collagen or fibronectin become dominant and stimulate the activation of integrins and their signalling pathways that promote the migratory potential of cells. Moreover, it has been reported that the level of E-cadherin depends on the phosphorylation state of β-catenin. Tyrosine phosphorylation of β-catenin prevents the binding to E-cadherin and favours the loss of intercellular contact [1, 2, 17].

Endocytosis and proteolytic cleavage of the extracellular domain of E-cadherin are other factors contributing to destabilisation of intercellular adhesion complexes, cell dissociation and EMT. In addition, integrins together with TK receptor activity contribute to the acquisition of an invasive phenotype via SRC. SRC is a non-receptor, SH2-containing cytoplasmic TK which participates in the control of adhesion and migration. SRC signalling contributes to the alteration of the balance between the adhesive and migratory states of cells. SRC stimulates focal adhesion kinase (FAK) that in turn mediates MAPK signalling, leading to the phosphorylation of light chain kinase which ultimately creates phosphomyosin, resulting in increased cell motility and the disorganisation of cell-to-cell adhesions. In addition, SRC is involved in the regulation of numerous proteins of the ECM such as vinculin or paxillin [2, 17].

5. Cancer stem cells

Cancer stem cells have been introduced as cell colonies able to self-renew, proliferate and produce heterogeneous lineages of cancer cells. Hereby they are playing a crucial role in tumor initiation, growth, invasion and recurrence. Epithelial to mesenchymal transition promotes the development of cancer stem-like cells that exhibit mesenchymal phenotypes and acquire multipotent features. Recent studies have provided the evidence of glioma stem cells or brain tumor stem cells [22]. These exhibit a similar phenotype as neural stem cells and in the majority of cases are characterized by surface proteins such as CD133 or nestin [23, 24]. This type of cells exhibits radio-resistance and an abnormal growth pattern. Tumor recurrence is the primary consequence of treatment failure and cause of death in patients suffering from malignant gliomas. Glioma stem cells possess the potential to stimulate the survival of transformed cells and thereby may become a useful therapeutic target [23, 24]. However, a profound understanding of the biological features of these cells will require many more studies.

6. Extracellular matrix and EMT

Tumor cells express matrix metalloproteases (MMPs) which are able to dissolve the ECM and thereby promote tumor invasion, migration and metastasis. Matrix metaloproteases are a group of zinc-dependent endoproteases. Matrix metalloprotease-2 (MMP-2) and MMP-9 are regulated by SNAI-1 and SNAI-2 (SLUG). Epithelial to mesenchymal transition-mediated dysregulation of SNAI-1 and SLUG in turn promotes the activity of MMP-2 and MMP-9 and thereby increases the invasive and migratory activity of tumor cells. Thus, cancer cells undergoing EMT enhance the initiation of metastasis, often involving transforming growth factor-β (TGF-β) and SMAD, and represent a phenotypic subpopulation of cancer cells which promote the dissemination of the malignant disease. Stromelysin, known as MMP-3, promotes EMT through the induction of reactive oxygen species (ROS) that, in turn, results in overexpression of SNAI [2, 8-10, 17].

7. TGF–β

Transforming growth factor-β has been reported as a strong inducer of EMT. This protein belongs to the TGF-β superfamily and exhibits three isoforms, i.e. TGF-β1, TGF-β2 and TGF-β3, all of which are involved in cell proliferation and differentiation. Transforming growth factor-β is able to induce apoptosis in numerous cell types via the Smad pathway. In addition, TGF-β may recruit non-Smad signalling, for instance the MMP cascade, to promote the malignant transformation of cells. The TGF-β response results in Smad 2 and Smad 3 activation through C-terminal phosphorylation [7, 8].

Transforming growth factor-β signalling finally regulates the expression of SNAI, ZEB and TWIST proteins that, in turn, influence the expression of proteins such as claudin, desmoplakin, MMPs or fibronectin. In this context, TGF-β functions as an important regulator of EMT [7, 8].

Promoted by TGF-β, SNAI-1 and SNAI-2 (SLUG) levels are increased during EMT. Hepatocyte growth factor, FGF and EGF induce the RAS-MAPK or PI3K-AKT pathways that lead to the activation of SNAI expression. The increased expression of SNAI-1 or SNAI-2 enhances the expression of vimentin and fibronectin, reduces E-cadherin and plakoglobin levels and hereby switches on mesenchymal transformation. During embryological development, this process takes care of mesodermal layer and neural crest development. In addition, SNAI proteins inactivate a variety of epithelial proteins such as occludin and claudin. SNAI-1 represses the expression of claudin 3, claudin 4 and claudin 7 and regulates the expression of desmosome proteins such as desmoplakin. SNAI-1 and SNAI-2 decrease the expression level of claudin 1 and occludin. Furthermore, increased SNAI protein activity stimulates the expression of mesenchymal proteins such as Rho-like GTPases which are composed of RHO, RAC and CDC-42 proteins that influence cytoskeleton architecture and cell motility. RHO and RAC regulate E-cadherin activity and adhesiveness of cells, and their activity is among the important determinants of EMT. TGF-β activates the signalling cascade downstream of RHO. The main RHO effector in TGF-β response is ROCK activity which regulates different processes involved in cell migration such as cytoskeleton reorganisation [1, 2, 7, 8, 17, 18].

Transforming growth factor-β activates TK receptors via PI3-K that, in turn, controls AKT in diverse cells. AKT is an important regulator of various signalling cascades, controlling cell survival, migration and proliferation. Activation of the PI3K-AKT cascade plays a crucial role in EMT.

The WNT protein plays a significant role in the process of mesenchymal transformation as well. WNT is connected downstream to β-catenin, builds adherens junctions and connects E-cadherin to the cytoskeleton through α-catenin. The WNT glycoprotein binds to the transmembraneous Frizzled receptor that activates Dishevelled, which in turn prevents phosphorylation of β-catenin by inhibition of glycogen synthase kinase-3β (GSK-3β) and hereby stops its ubiquitination and degradation. This step increases the level of cytoplasmic β-catenin that ultimately translocates into the nucleus and builds complexes with T-Cell factor (TCF) and lymphoid enhancer factor-1 (LEF-1). These related transcription factors mediate the gene response by activating genes required for EMT such as SLUG, ETS and JUN or fibronectin and vimentin. In addition, the basic feature of EMT, downregulation of E-cadherin, increases the level of cytosolic free β-catenin itself. Similarly, the activation of PI3K-AKT and integrin-linked kinase (ILK) inhibits GSK-3β and leads to the accumulation of β-catenin. This inhibitory effect is responsible for the upregulation of SNAI, which normally is negatively regulated by the activation of GSK-3β. The process contributes significantly to the destabilisation of epithelial adhesiveness and promotes the acquisition of the mesenchymal phenotype with increased cell motility and invasiveness [2, 27].

8. Nuclear factor–κB

Nuclear factor-κB (NF-κB) belongs to a family of transcriptional factors, whose activity is important for the maintenance and promotion of the invasive phenotype in cancer cells. Nuclear factor-κB binds DNA sequences as hetero- or homodimers and consequently regulates various cellular processes. Several genes encoding proteins that are involved in the cell cycle (Cyclin D1, c-MYC), cell adhesion (vascular cell adhesion protein) or inflammation (interleukin-2, interleukin-6, interleukin-8) are regulated in this way. Even if NF-κB is ubiquitous, its activity is detected mostly in mature B-lymphocytes [28, 29].

The inhibitor protein IκB plays a crucial role in the degradation of NF-κB and has been discovered in breast cancer. Signalling via NF-κB results in increased expression of SNAI-1 and hereby contributes to EMT progression. Moreover, the activity of NF-κB correlates with the expression of ZEB-1, ZEB-2 and TWIST, which are other strong inducers of EMT [28].

Vimentin, a 56-kDa intermediate filament protein, contributes to mesenchymal transformation of the cell. Cells acquire a spindle-shape form and loosen their connections to neighbouring cells. Studies of vimentin-knockdown mice have shown significantly reduced wound healing abilities. In addition, vimentin expression promotes the migration of cancer cells. Nuclear factor-κB activates the vimentin promoter and thus increases the expression of vimentin [28].

9. Resistance to EGFR–targeted therapy

Epithelial to mesenchymal transition is considered an important factor contributing to the resistance of glioma cells against EGFR-targeted therapy. On the other hand, alternative potential explanations of this phenomenon have been suggested.

Glioblastomas exhibit a high degree of intrinsic heterogeneity with a variety of signalling pathways that mediate the subcellular actions. In the case of EGFR inhibition, alternative downstream pathways may be activated and potentiated. A functional-switch could lead to the survival of the cells and, by clonal selection, to the acquisition of resistance to specific therapeutic agents that inhibit one specific signalling pathway.

Phosphatase and tensin homolog is a tumor suppressor protein which dephosphorylates phosphatidylinositol (3, 4, 5)-triphosphate and hereby negatively regulates the AKT signalling axis. Phosphatase and tensin homolog is often mutated in GBM cells which promotes the activity of mTOR resulting in tumor progression. The inhibition of this dominant pathway may lead to alteration of the hierarchy in TKs such as platelet-derived growth factor receptor (PDGFR), JAK2 or cellular mesenchymal-epithelial transition factor (c-MET) [9, 29]. Platelet-derived growth factor receptor is the second most common TK receptor amplified in GBMs. Moreover, MET is also amplified in some GBMs. Concomitant presence of gene amplifications within GBMs may activate and potentiate alternative signalling pathways during inhibitory targeting of EGFR and hereby contribute to increased resistance of glioma cells to erlotinib or other TK-inhibitors [29].

10. Conclusion

The EGFR has been introduced as a therapeutic target in some malignancies. Unfortunately, in GBM, there has been no demonstrable benefit of this approach in comparison to standard therapy. Epithelial to mesenchymal transition is considered an important factor contributing to failure of this therapy by diminishing the molecular target. This phenomenon leads to the loss of epithelial characteristics of cells and to the expression of mesenchymal features. The acquisition of increased motility and invasiveness by glioma cells represents an essential prerequisite for subsequent tumor recurrence and malignant progression. Epithelial to mesenchymal transition is primarily regulated through signalling pathways affecting E-cadherin, a transmembraneous protein responsible for intercellular cell contact. Molecular changes are promoted by a variety of external stimuli. The identification and better understanding of these processes may enable the development of new therapeutic strategies

http://dx.doi.org/10.5772/53183

Author details

Andrej Pala*, Georg Karpel-Massler, Christian Rainer Wirtz and Marc-Eric Halatsch

*Address all correspondence to: andrej.pala@gmail.com; georg.karpel@uniklinik-ulm.de; marc-eric.halatsch@uniklinik-ulm.de

Department of Neurosurgery, University of Ulm School of Medicine, Albert-Einstein-Allee, Ulm, Germany

References

[1] Lo H.-W. EGFR-targeted therapy in malignant glioma: novel aspects and mechanisms of drug resistance. *Current Mol Pharm* 2010, *3*, 37-52.

[2] Guarino M.; Rubino B.; Ballabio G. The role of epithelial-mesenchymal transition in cancer pathology. *Pathology* 2007, *39*, 305-318.

[3] Mikheeva S.A.; Mikheev A.M.; Petit A.; Beyer R.; Oxford R.G.; Khorasani L.; Maxwell J.P.; Glackin C.A.; Wakimoto H.; González-Herrero I. Twist 1 promotes invasion through mesenchymal change in human glioblastoma. *Mol Cancer* 2010, *9*, 194–212.

[4] Elias M.C.; Tozer K.R.; Silber J.R.; Mikheeva S.; Deng M.; Morrison R.S.; Manning T.C.; Silbergeld D.L.; Glackin C.A.; Reh T.A.; Rostomily R.C. TWIST is expressed in human gliomas and promotes invasion. *Neoplasia* 2005, *9*, 824-837.

[5] Loew S.; Schmidt U.; Unterberg A.; Halatsch M.-E. The epidermal growth factor receptor as a therapeutic target in glioblastoma multiforme and other malignant neoplasms. *Anticancer Agents Med Chem* 2009, *9*, 703-715.

[6] Mellinghoff I.K.; Wang M.Y.; Vivanco I. Molecular determinants of the response of glioblastomas to EGFR kinase inhibitors. *N Engl J Med* 2005, *353*, 2012-2024.

[7] Xu J.; Lamouille S.; Derynck R. TGF-β-induced epithelial to mesenchymal transition. *Cell Res* 2009, *19*, 156-172.

[8] Pala A.; Karpel-Massler G.; Kast R.E.; Wirtz C.R.; Halatsch M.-E. Epidermal to mesenchymal transition and failure of EGFR-targeted therapy in glioblastoma. *Cancers* 2012, *4*, 523-530.

[9] Szerlip N.J.; Pedraza A.; Chakravaty D.; Azim M.; McGuire J.; Fang Y.; Ozawa T.; Holland E.C.; Huse J.T.; Jhanwar S.; Leversha M.A.; Mikkelsen T.; Brennan C.W. Intratumoral heterogeneity of receptor tyrosine kinases EGFR and PDGFRA amplification in glioblastoma defines subpopulations with distinct growth factor response. *Proc Natl Acad Sci* 2012, *109*, 3041-3046.

[10] Wever O.D.; Pauwels P.; Craene B.D.; Sabbah M.; Emami S.; Redeuilh G.; Gespach C.; Bracke M.; Berx G. Molecular and pathological signatures of epithelial-mesenchymal transitions at cancer invasion front. *Histochem Cell Biol* 2008, *130*, 481-494.

[11] Suda K.; Tomizawa K.; Fujii M, Murakami, H.; Osada H.; Maehara Y.; Yatabe Y.; Sekido Y.; Mitsudami T. Epithelial to mesenchymal transition in an epidermal growth factor receptor-mutant lung cancer cell line with acquired resistance to erlotinib. *J Thorac Oncol* 2011, *6*, 1152–1161.

[12] Thomson S.; Buck E.; Petti F.; Griffin G.; Brown E.; Ramnarine N.; Iwata KK.; Gibson N.; Haley J.D. Epithelial to mesenchymal transition is a determinant of sensitivity of non-small-cell lung carcinoma cell lines and xenografts to epidermal growth factor receptor inhibition. *Cancer Res* 2005, *65*, 9455-9462.

[13] Lu Y.; Li X.; Liang K.; Luwor R.; Siddik Z.H.; Mills G.B.; Mendelsohn J.; Fan Z. Epidermal growth factor (EGFR) ubiquitination as a mechanism of acquired resistance escaping treatment by the anti-EGFR monoclonal antibody cetuximab. *Mol Cancer Res* 2007, *67*, 8240-8247.

[14] Yamazaki H.; Kijima H.; Ohnishi Y. Inhibition of tumor growth by ribozyme-mediated suppression of aberrant epidermal growth factor receptor gene expression. *J Natl Cancer Inst* 1998, *90*, 581-587.

[15] Halatsch M.-E.; Schmidt U.; Bötefür I.C.; Holland J.F.; Ohnuma T. Overexpression of deletion-mutant epidermal growth factor receptor is assocated with altered genotoxic stress-provoked p53 mRNA induction in a human glioblastoma cell line. *Anticancer Res* 2001, *21*, 189-195.

[16] Halatsch M.-E.; Schmidt U.; Bötefür I.C.; Holland J.F.; Ohnuma T. Marked inhibition of glioblastoma target cell tumorigenicity in vitro by retrovirus-mediated transfer of a hairpin ribozyme against deletion-mutant epidermal growth factor receptor messenger RNA. *J Neurosurg* 2000, *92*, 297-305.

[17] Iwatsuki M.; Mimori K.; Yokobori T.; Ishi H.; Beppu T.; Nakamori S.; Baba H.; Mori M. Epithelial-mesenchymal transition in cancer development and its clinical significance. *Cancer Sci* 2010, *101*, 293-299.

[18] Han S.P.; Kim J.H.; Han M.E.; Sim H.E.; Kim K.S.; Yoon S.; Baek S.Y.; Kim B.S.; Oh S.O. Snai 1 is involved in the proliferation and migration of glioblastoma cells. *Cell Mol Neurobiol* 2011, *31*, 489–496.

[19] Koppikar P.; Lui, V.W.Y.; Man D.; Xi S.; Chai R.L.; Nelson E.; Tobey A.B.J.; Grandis J.R. Constitutive activation of signal tranducer and activator of transcription 5 contributes to tumor growth, epithelial-mesenchymal transition and resistance to epidermal growth factor receptor targeting. *Clin Cancer Res* 2008, *14*, 7682–7690.

[20] Lo H.-W.; Hsu S.-C.; Xia W.; Cao X.; Shih J.-Y.; Wei Y.; Abbruzzese J.L.; Hortobagyi G.N.; Hung M.-C. Epidermal growth factor receptor cooperates with signal transducer and activator of transcription 3 to induce epithelial-mesenchymal transition in can-

cer cells via up-regulation of TWIST gene expression. *Mol Cancer Res* 2007, *67*, 9066-9076.

[21] Lo H.-W.; Cao X.; Zhu H.; Ali-Osman F. COX-2 is a novel transcriptional target of the nuclear EGFR-STAT3 and EGFRvIII-STAT3 signaling axes. *Mol Cancer Res* 2010, *8*, 232-245.

[22] Sanai N.; Alvarez-Buylla A.; Berger M.S. Neural stem cells and the origin of gliomas. *N Engl J Med* 2005, *353*, 811-822.

[23] Krysan K.; Lee J.M.; Dohadwala M.; Gardner B.K.; Reckamp K.L.; Garon E.; John S.M.; Sharma S.; Dubinett S.M. Inflammation, epithelial to mesenchymal transition, and epidermal growth factor receptor tyrosine kinase inhibitor resistance. *J Thor Oncol* 2008, *3*, 107-110.

[24] Haddad Y.; Woonyoung C.; McConkey J.D. Delta-crystallin enhancer binding factor 1 controls the epithelial to mesenchymal transition phenotype and resistance to the epidermal growth factor receptor inhibitor erlotinib in human head and neck squamous cell carcinoma lines. *Clin Cancer Res* 2009, *2*, 532–542.

[25] Huang Q.; Zhang Q.-B.; Dong J.; Wu Y.-Y.; Shen Y.-T.; Zhao Y.-D.; Diao Y.; Wang A.-D.; Lan Q. Glioma stem cells are more aggressive in recurrent tumors with malignant progression than in the primary tumor, and both can be maintained long-term in vitro. *BMC Cancer* 2008, *8*, 304.

[26] Velpula K.K.; Dasari V.R. Tsung A.J.; Dinh D.H.; Rao J. Cord blood stem cells revert glioma cell EMT by down regulating transcriptional activation of SOX 2 and TWIST 1. *Oncotarget* 2011, *2*, 1028-1042.

[27] Xun J.; Hee-Young J.; Kveung M.J.; Kim J.K.; Jin J.; Kim S.H.; Kang B.G.; Beck S.; Lee S.J.; Kim J.K.; Park A.-K.; Park W.-Y.; Choi Y.-J.; Nam D.-H.; Kim H. Frizzled 4 regulates stemness and invasiveness of migrating glioma cells established by serial intracranial transplantation. *Cancer Res* 2011, *71*, 3066–3075.

[28] Min C.; Eddy S.F.; Sherr D.H.; Sonnenshein G.E. NF-κB and epithelial to mesenchymal transition of cancer. *J Cell Biochem* 2008, *104*, 733-744.

[29] Tanaka K.; Babic I.; Nathanson D. Oncogenic EGFR signalling activates an mTORC2-NF-κβ pathway that promotes chemotherapy resistance. *Cancer Discov* 2011, *1*, 525-538.

Chapter 15

Laboratory Testing for Prognostic and Predictive Markers in Gliomas

Milena Cankovic

Additional information is available at the end of the chapter

http://dx.doi.org/10.5772/52670

1. Introduction

Gliomas are the most common tumors of the brain. Normal glia includes astrocytes, oligodendrocytes, and ependyma. Gliomas are analogously designated as astrocytomas, oligodendrogliomas, and ependymomas to reflect the non-neoplastic cell types that they most closely resemble.

Gliomas can also be classified histologically as astrocytomas, oligodendrogliomas, or tumors with morphological features of both astrocytes and oligodendrocytes. The 2007 World Health Organization (WHO) classification recognizes three main histologic types of low grade diffuse glioma grade II: diffuse astrocytoma, oligoastrocytoma, and oligodendroglioma [1]. Diffuse astrocytomas account for approximately 40% of primary intracranial tumors. Their gross, microscopic, and biologic characteristics vary to a considerable degree according to their site. They occur at all ages, although the median age is 30 to 40 for astrocytoma (grade II), 40 to 50 for anaplastic astrocytoma (grade III), and 50 to 60 years for glioblastoma multiforme (grade IV). Diffuse astrocytomas tend to progress to more malignant histologic types, such as anaplastic astrocytoma (WHO grade III) and sometimes secondary glioblastoma (WHO grade IV). Oligodendrogliomas account for approximately 5% of intracranial gliomas. They are most often found in the cerebral hemispheres, where they usually involve the cortex and the white matter. Traditionally the prognosis of oligodendrogliomas has been regarded as relatively favorable, but in practice no valid correlation has been established between the microscopic appearances of these tumors and their clinical evolution. Progression of oligodendrogliomas to anaplastic oligodendrogliomas can be unpredictable. Glioblastomas are malignant, rapidly fatal, astrocytic neoplasms. Glioblastomamultiforme (GBM), account for 30% of primary brain tumors in adults [2, 3]. Patients with glioblastomamultiforme have a mean survival of about 12 months. They may occur in any region of the central nervous system, however, the cerebral hemispheres, in particular the frontal lobes or temporal lobes, the basal ganglia, and the commissural pathways are sites of predilection. Most GBMs are diagnosed as de novo or primary tumors and are more common in males. A subset of about 5% of GBM tumors, termed secondary GBM, progress from lower-grade tumors (grade II/III), are seen in younger patients, are more evenly distributed among the sexes, and exhibit longer survival times [4]. Depending on the grade and morphologic type of glioma, newly diagnosed patients receive watchful waiting, surgical resection, radiotherapy, or chemotherapy, or some combination of these therapies. Chemotherapy for GBM has very limited efficacy, however it has been shown that certain patients may respond to some treatments [5, 6]. Temozolomide is a novel alkylating agent that has demonstrated activity in recurrent gliomas [7-9]. Regardless of therapy, most patients will progress and have a high risk of mortality and reduced quality of life. For these reasons there has been a great deal of interest in understanding the biology and genetics of gliomas, to provide better diagnostic tools and new therapeutic approaches [10]. Molecular pathology markers are being identified that have been or will soon prove to be clinically useful in treatment of glioma patients.

Molecular genomic-based laboratory assays are often used for detection of prognostic and predictive markers in gliomas. Research efforts have identified a number of cytogenetic and molecular genetic alterations in gliomas [11] that may be exploited to facilitate glioma classification, especially in cases that exhibit inconclusive or borderline histologic features. This chapter will focus on those molecular biomarkers that have been established in glioma diagnostics, namely *MGMT* promoter methylation, 1p/19q Loss of Heterozygosity (LOH), *IDH*1 and *IDH*2 mutations, and epidermal growth factor variant III (*EGFR*vIII) mutations. Emphasis will be placed on clinical applications, most frequently used methods of detection, as well as issues involved in assay validation, specimen selection, and clinical laboratory oversight.

1.1. MGMT promoter methylation

Chemotherapy for GBM has very limited efficacy, however it has been shown that certain patients may respond to some treatments. Temozolomide is a novel alkylating agent that has demonstrated activity in recurrent gliomas. Alkylating agents cause cell death by forming cross-links between adjacent strands of DNA due to alkylation of the O^6 position of guanine. The O^6-methylguanine-DNA methyltransferase (*MGMT*) gene produces the cellular DNA repair protein O^6-alkylguanine DNA alkyltransferase (AGT) which is a key factor in resistance to alkylating agents. It functions as a DNA repair enzyme that removes the mutagenic alkyl-adducts from the O^6-poasition of guanine, and this transfer of alkyl groups to AGT prevents the formation of lethal cross links in DNA. Tumors appear to be heterogeneous with respect to MGMT expression, and in a subset of cancer cells, its expression is silenced due to abnormal promoter methylation. Aberrant methylation of CpG islands located in the promoter region of *MGMT* gene is associated with transcriptional inactivation of this gene, and consequent low levels of the MGMT DNA repair enzyme. Studies have shown that patients with low levels of this DNA repair enzyme are more likely to experience response to therapy and prolonged overall and disease free survival [12-15].

DNA methylation (for more detailed description and references please see [16]) is a mechanism by which the cell regulates gene expression. Methylation is an enzyme mediated modification that adds a methyl (-CH_3) group at a selected site on DNA or RNA. In humans, methylation occurs only at cytosine (C) bases followed by a guanosine (G), also known as CpGdinucleotides. The CpG dinucleotides are prone to spontaneous mutations and have been selectively depleted from mammalian genome. However, some regions of DNA have retained CpGdinucleotides and are referred to as CpG islands. The CpG islands are found primarily in the 5' region of expressed genes, often in association with promoters. When the promoter CpG island is methylated, the corresponding gene is silenced and transcription does not occur. Aberrant CpG island methylation of tumor suppressor genes is frequent in cancer and appears to be an important mechanism of neoplastic transformation.

Quantitative evaluation on methylated *MGMT* in tumors suggests that not all cells in a tumor positive for promoter methylation carry a methylated *MGMT* allele. This raises the question of what level of promoter methylation has clinical significance. A recent study [17] investigated the degree and pattern of *MGMT* promoter methylation in paired samples of glioblastoma tissue and glioblastoma-derived spheres. The degree and density of *MGMT* methylation was then compared with the chromatin structure of *MGMT*, gene dosage, gene expression and enzyme activity, and the tumor cell content of the patient samples. Ten paired samples were evaluated for the extent and density of methylation by clone sequencing 28 of 97 CpGs in the CpGisland of the *MGMT* promoter. This region of the promoter encompasses the enhancer element and, according to reporter assays, is associated with complete silencing of the gene when fully methylated [18]. Most assays interrogate CpG methylation in this region. For all glioblastomas with *MGMT* methylation, a band for unmethylated alleles was also detectable, which is expected since benign cells will always be present in the specimen. Sequencing of the original glioblastoma tissue revealed that 10% to 90% of all clones sequenced showed dense methylation, arbitrarily defined as at least 4 consecutive CpGs methylated in a given interrogated clone. The density of *MGMT* promoter methylation, defined as the number of methylated CpGs over 28 interrogated CPGs, ranged from 25% to 90%, never reaching 100%, and showing a characteristic pattern for each tumor.

The study [17] further showed that *MGMT* methylation is associated with no or low MGMT expression and closed chromatin structure. MGMT activity was below the limit of detection in glioblastoma spheres of completely methylated cases. Moderate activity was measured in the case with one unmethylated allele, and the unmethylated case showed the highest activity. MGMT activity was measurable in all respective original tissues likely due to contaminating normal cells. In accordance with lack of MGMT expression and MGMT activity, the closed chromatin pattern was also observed. Marks of active and inactive chromatin pattern were observed for unmethylated and partially methylated cases.

As combined chemoradiotherapy comprising the alkylating agent temozolomide has become the new standard of care [19], there has been growing interest to use *MGMT* promoter methylation status for individual patient management, and for patient stratification or selection in clinical trials. Knowledge of *MGMT* promoter methylation status is relevant for both prognostic and predictive considerations. Furthermore, *MGMT* promoter methylation status has been used as a stratifying factor or eligibility criterion in ongoing and accruing clinical trials [20].

Aberrant methylation of CpG islands in the promoter region of many genes has been recognized as an important epigenetic mechanism for gene silencing [21-24]. Inactivation of multiple tumor suppressor genes by aberrant hypermethylation is a fundamental process involved in the development of many malignant tumors [25, 26]. Mapping of methylation patterns in CpG islands has become an important tool in understanding tissue-specific gene expression in both normal and pathologic situations, and several protocols have been published for evaluating methylation status by methylation-specific PCR (MSP). Most of these protocols are based on bisulfite treatment of isolated DNA [27, 28]. Bisulfite treatment chemically changes unmethylated, but not methylated, cytosines to uracil. Methylated DNA can be distinguished from unmethylated DNA using sodium bisulfate treatment of DNA, which converts unmethylated C to uracil (U) but leaves methylated C intact. Detection of methylation or lack of it involves analysis of bisulfite-treated DNA using primer pairs that specifically identify either methylated or unmethylated DNA.

The methylated and unmethylated sequences are detected through the use of methylation-specific primers.

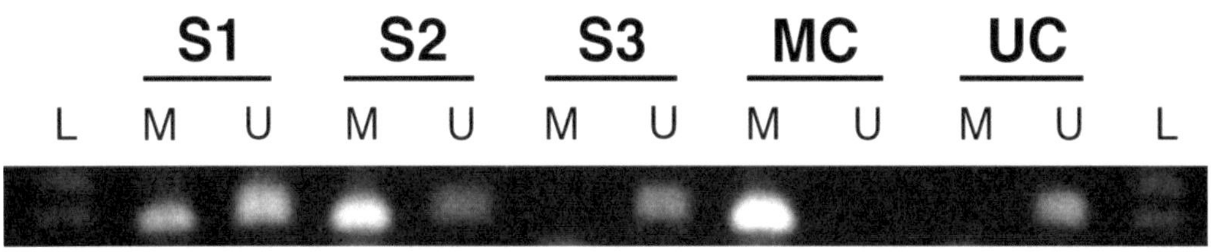

Figure 1. MGMT promoter methylation detection by methylation specific PCR. Methylated bands (M) can be seen in samples S1 and S2 and in methylated control (M). Unmethylated bands (U) are seen in S1, S2, S3, and in negative (unmethylated) control

Methylation Specific PCR (MSP): Methylation is a chemical modification that adds methyl (CH_3) groups at selected sites on protein, DNA and RNA. In humans, DNA methylation only affects the cytosine base (C) when it is followed by a guanine (G). Most CpG islands have been observed in the 5′ promoter regions of genes. When promoter CpG islands become methylated, the associated gene is silenced. Small amount of DNA, including those from paraffin embedded tissue, can be used for testing. DNA is first treated with bisulfite which converts unmethylated, but not methylated, cytosine to uracil. This modified DNA is then used as a template for PCR. The sequence differences between methylated and unmethylated DNA after bisulfite treatment allow the designing of PCR primers that are specific for each type. The primers are intended to amplify the identified region of the promoter mentioned above. PCR products are detected by gel electrophoresis or by capillary electrophoresis.

Methylight Protocol: The MethyLight assay utilizes the TaqMan PCR principle which requires forward and reverse primers as well as an oligomeric probe which emits fluorescence only after it is degraded by the 5′-3′ exonuclease activity of Taq polymerase. MethyLight protocol is a simple, real-time PCR method to determine the methylation status of CpG islands. Collagen 2A1 (COL2A1) gene is used as the internal reference (amplification control) to assess the quality and quantity of input DNA.

Pyrosequencing: This is a method of DNA synthesis based on sequencing by synthesis principle. The procedure involves taking a single strand of the DNA to be sequenced and then synthesizing its complementary strand enzymatically. The pyrosequencing method is based on detecting the activity of DNA polymerase with another chemiluminescent enzyme [29, 30]. The pyrosequencing reaction occurs in 5 steps. In step 1, a sequencing primer is hybridized to a single-stranded amplicon that serves as a template, and incubated with the enzymes DNA polymerase, ATP sulfurylase, luciferase, and apyrase, as well as substrates adenosine 5' phosphosulfate and luciferin. In subsequent steps triphosphates are added to reaction and each incorporation event is accompanied by release of pyrophosphate PPi). The PPi is subsequently converted to ATP which then drives conversion of luciferin to oxyluciferin that generates visible light. Addition of dNTPs is performed sequentially. As the process continues, the complementary DNA stand is built up and the nucleotide sequence is determined from the signal peaks in the pyrogram trace.

Methylation-Specific MLPA (MS-MLPA): The multiplex ligation-dependent probe amplification (MLPA) method allows for multiplex detection of gene copy number aberrations in a routine laboratory. The methylation-specific MLPA (MS-MLPA) can detect changes in both CpG methylation as well as copy number of up to 40 chromosomal sequences in a simple reaction. In MS-MLPA, the ligation of MLPA probe oligonucleotides is combined with digestion of the genomic DNA-probe hybrid complexes with methylation-sensitive endonucleases [31, 32]. MS-MLPA is not based on bisulfite conversion of unmethylatedcytosines, can provide methylation status, is semiquantitative, and can be used to evaluate methylation status of multiple sequences simultaneously. Furthermore, it allows for a combined copy number detection and methylation-specific analysis.

1.2. 1p/19q Loss of heterozygosity(LOH)

Among the major subtypes of gliomas, oligodendrogliomas are distinguished by their remarkable sensitivity to chemotherapy, with approximately 70% of anaplastic (malignant) oligodendrogliomas responding dramatically to treatment with procarbazine, lomustine, and vincristine (termed PCV) [33]. Unfortunately, no clinical or pathologic feature allows accurate prediction of chemotherapeutic response. The prognosis for grade II oligodendrogliomas is significantly better than that for grade II astrocytomas, with average survival times of 10 to 15 years. As with astrocytomas, there is considerable individual variability in time to progression and overall survival. The average survival for anaplastic grade III oligodendrogliomas is 3 to 5 years, although some patients with genetically favorable subset may survive 10 years or longer. The histologic distinction between oligodendroglioma and astrocytoma is often highly subjective, and there has been significant interobserver variation.

Patients with oligodendroglial tumors are often stratified into therapeutic groups according to age, extent of resection, tumor grade, and 1p/19q status. The current national Comprehensive Cancer Network (NCCN) guidelines for central nervous tumor cancers recommend testing for 1p/19q codeletion or unbalanced translocation, for cases of suspected oligodendroglioma. The test is also recommended to distinguish anaplastic oligodendroglioma from anaplastic astrocytomas and glioblastomas. Recent studies [34-36] have shown that: (1) - allelic loss (loss of heterozygosity) of chromosome arm 1p is a statistically significant and currently the best predictor of chemosensitivity; (2) combined loss involving chromosome arms 1p and 19q predicts both chemotherapeutic response and longer survival in patients with oligodendrogliomas; and (3) combined allelic loss of chromosomes 1p and 19q can be considered a molecular signature of oligodendroglioma (present in approximately 70-80% of oligodendroglial tumors and in only 10% of astrocytomas). Anaplastic oligodendrogliomas with loss on 1p, or combined loss on 1p and 19q usually respond favorably to chemotherapy, with about half of such tumors showing complete neuroradiological response. Owing to the major prognostic significance of the 1p/19q status in patients with anaplastic gliomas treated with radio and/or chemotherapy, ongoing prospective trials are no longer stratifying anaplastic glioma patients according to histological types but according to the 1p/19q deletion status [37]. Detection methods for 1p and 19q deletion include polymerase chain reaction (PCR), fluorescent in situ hybridization (FISH), array comparative genomic hybridization, and multiplex ligation-dependent probe amplification (MPLA) [38-40].

Primary Markers		Back up markers	
Microsatellite Locus	**Abbreviation**	**Microsatellite Locus**	**Abbreviation**
D1S548	1-1	D1S468	1-2
D1S592	1-3	D1S1612	1-5
D1S552	1-4	D1S496	1-6
D19S219	19-1		
D19S412	19-2	D19S606	19-3
PLA2G4C	19-5	D19S1182	19-4

Table 1. Primary and back up microsatellite markers for detection 1p and 19q deletion

1.3. 1p/19q LOH - Microsatellite-based method of detection

Allelic loss is assessed by PCR assay in normal DNA / tumor DNA pairs using markers at both 1p and 19q. For this type of testing, a patient's blood sample is needed to accurately assess patient's genotype and establish the normal DNA baseline. Because there might be partial as well as complete deletions, any reductions in tumor peaks can then accurately be interpreted as deletions. The 6 markers on 1p and the 5 markers on 19q are microsatellites (2 or 4 nucleotide repeats) except PLA2G4C which is a minisatellite (26 nucleotide repeat) polymorphism. The markers were selected based on heterozygosity score, amplicon size, and ease of interpretation. LOH at all informative loci on each chromosomal arm represents the typical finding in oligodendrogliomas with 1p and 19q deletion. To streamline the work

http://dx.doi.org/10.5772/52670

flow process, a set of primary markers in tested first. If at least two markers for 1p and two marker for 19q show either no deletion or clear deletion, the results can be considered valid. If the results with primary markers are not clear, either because the markers are not informative (homozygosity), or they did not amplify, then the back up markers are used in subsequent PCR reaction.

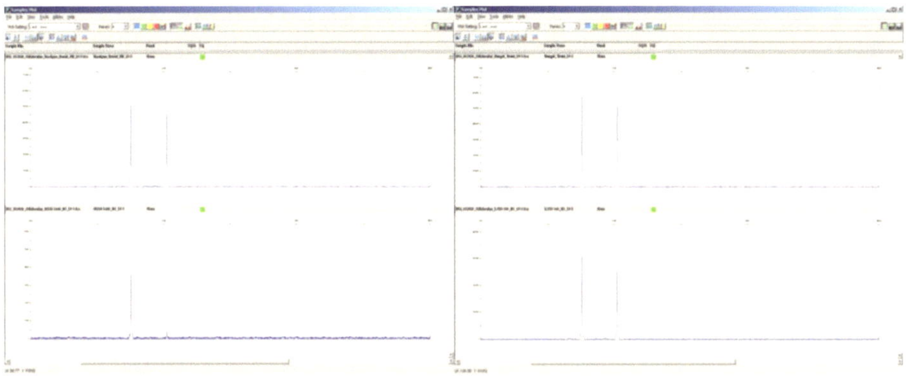

Figure 2. The tumor sample on the left demonstrates 1p deletion. Normal DNA baseline is on the top.

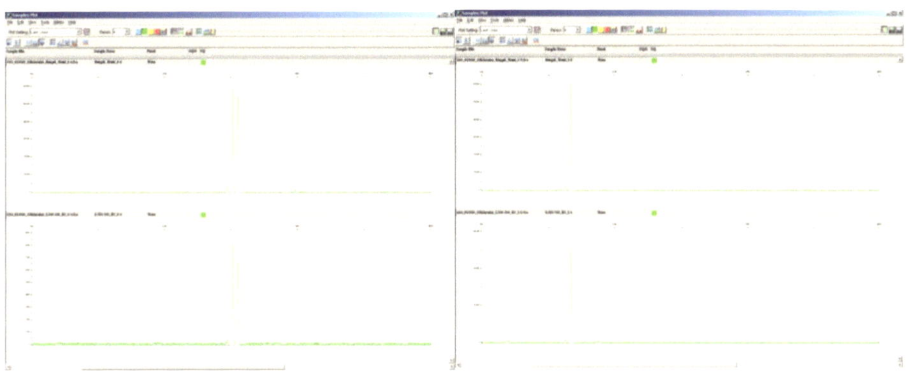

Figure 3. Sample on the left demonstrates two alleles both in base line sample and in tumor sample. The sample on the right has a non-informative microsatellite marker.

Array Comparative Genomic Hybridization (aCGH) - aCGH is a technique to detect genomic copy number variations at a higher resolution level than chromosome-based comparative genomic hybridization (CGH). DNA from a test sample and normal sample are labeled differentially, using different fluorophores, and hybridized to several thousand probes. The probes are derived from known genomic sequences and are printed on glass slides. The fluorescence intensity of the test and of the reference DNA is then measured to calculate the ratio between them and subsequently the copy number changes for a particular location in the genome. This method allows one to detect microdeletions and chromosomal duplications and is used with increasing frequency for loss of heterozygosity detection [41].

1.4. IDH1 and IDH2 mutations

Point mutations in the cytosolic isocitrate dehydrogenase enzyme gene (*IDH*1) or the mitochondrial version of the same gene (*IDH*2) are frequently detected in low grade astrocytomas, oligodendrogliomas and in secondary glioblastomas. *IDH*1 is involved in the metabolic conversion of isocitrate to alpha-ketoglutarate, which reduces NADP to NADPH. In gliomas, mutations in this gene were discovered through large scale DNA sequencing of tumor samples [42]. Among WHO grade II and grade III gliomas, 50% to 80% have mutated *IDH*1, whereas 5% to 10% of WHO grade IV gliomas carry *IDH*1 mutation. Studies of clinical trial samples of low grade gliomas showed that mutated *IDH1* may be both prognostic and predictive, because it was associated with longer survival times and better response to temozolomide therapy [43, 44]. Another study with astrocytoma showed an association with improved survival but not with response to temozolomide [45]. Further clarification of the correlation of chemotherapy response and *IDH*1 mutational status will be needed for this marker to receive broad clinical use. At present, lack of *IDH*1 mutation can not be considered strong enough evidence to alter therapy.

Because the presence of an *IDH* mutation is considered tumor specific, it has a role as a diagnostic marker when morphologic features are inconclusive and a non neoplastic (reactive) condition is possible.

Nt#		Nucleotide Change	Amino Acid Change	Frequency (%) (Hartman, 2009)
395	**IDH1**	G395A CGT à CAT	Arg132His, R132H	92.7
394	"	C394T CGT à TGT	Arg132Cys, R132C	4.2
394	"	C394A CGT à AGT	Arg132Ser, R132S	1.5
394	"	C394G CGT à GGT	Arg132 Gly, R132G	1.4
395	"	G395T CGT à CTT	Arg132Leu, R132L	0.2
515	IDH2	G515A AGG à AAG	Arg172Lys, R172K	64.5
515	"	G515T AGG à ATG	Arg172Meth, R172M	19.3
514	"	A514T AGG à TGG	Arg172Trp, R172W	16.2

Table 2. *IDH* 1 and *IDH*2 mutations and resulting amino acid changes

http://dx.doi.org/10.5772/52670

Sanger Sequencing - The ability to sequence DNA has been essential to the field of molecular pathology because sequence information is needed for primer design in PCR-based assays, for determination of target sequence, and for detection of any changes such as mutations, insertions and deletions in DNA sequence. The method for DNA sequencing developed by Sanger [46] is the basis for most DNA sequencing currently performed in clinical molecular laboratories. The Sanger sequencing reaction (for more detailed description see [16]) uses a single DNA primer and DNA polymerase with linear amplification rather than the exponential amplification of PCR. Components essential to the Sanger sequencing reaction include: (1) an electrophoresis technique capable of clearly distinguishing single nucleotide length differences in DNA strands dozens or hundreds nucleotides in length, (2) sequence-specific complementary primers, with one primer used in the forward reaction and the other used in reverse reaction for each DNA template strand, and (3) the addition of small proportions of dideoxynucleoside triphosphates (ddNTPs) in addition to the conventional deoxyribonucleoside triphosphates (dNTPs) used in polymerase chain reaction. Dideoxynucleotides differ from deoxynucleotides by having a hydrogen atom attached to the 3' carbon rather than an OH group, which is present on the deoxynucleotide. Because the ddNTPs lack a 3'-hydroxyl group, elongation of the newly polymerized chain cannot occur once a ddNTP has been incorporated. The end result is a set of fragments of different lengths complementary to the parent DNA strand. The sequencing reaction products are most frequently detected by capillary electrophoresis on a DNA sequencing instrument.

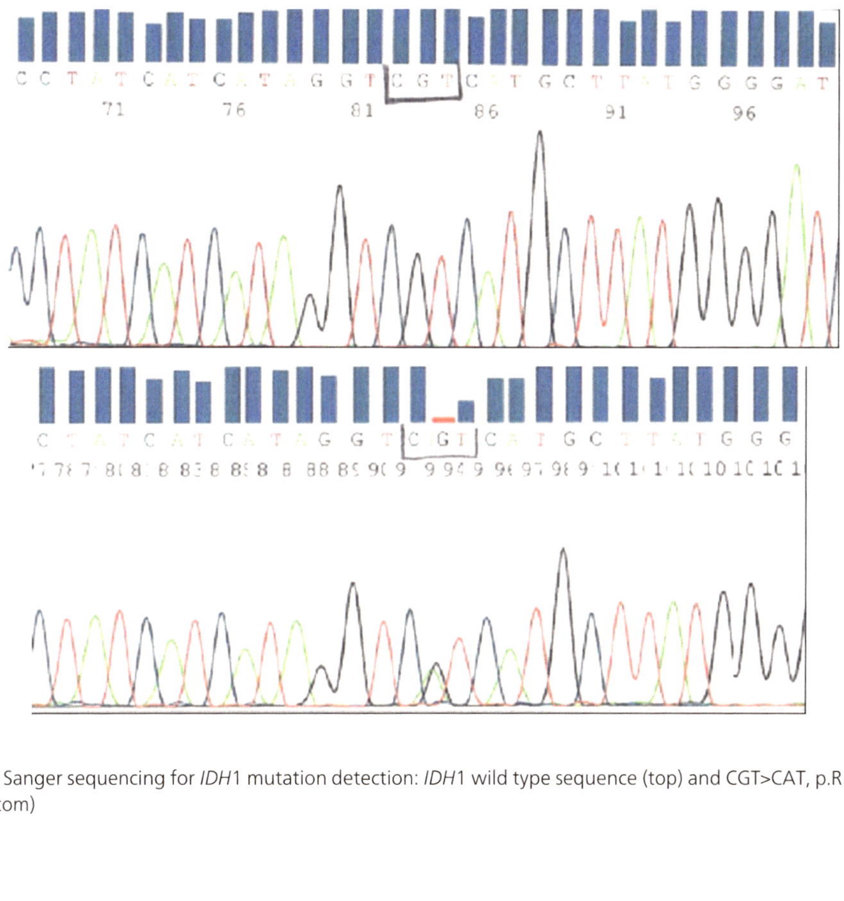

Figure 4. Sanger sequencing for *IDH*1 mutation detection: *IDH*1 wild type sequence (top) and CGT>CAT, p.R132H mutant (bottom)

Immunohistochemistry: Approximately 90% of IDH1 mutated proteins can be detected by using immunohistochemistry with a monoclonal antibody that detects p.R132H, the most common IDH1 mutation [47].

1.5. EGFRvIII mutation detection in glioblastomamultiforme

The epidermal growth factor receptor (EGFR) is an attractive molecular target in glioblastoma because it is amplified, overexpressed, and/or mutated in up to 40% to 50% of patients. EGFR variant III (EGFRvIII) is an oncogenic, constitutively active mutant form of EGFR that is commonly expressed in glioblastoma. *EGFR*vIII is generated by in-frame genomic deletion of 801bp from exons 2 to 7 of the coding region of *EGFR* which produces a truncated receptor lacking a portion of extracellular ligand binding domain. *EGFR*vIII mutations in gliomas typically lead to unique signal transduction properties to the receptor, particularly enhanced downstream activation of a phosphatidylinositol 3'-kinase (PI3K) signaling pathway with concurrent loss of PTEN. Cell culture and in vivo models of glioblastoma have demonstrated *EGFR*vIII as defining prognostically distinct subgroups of glioblastomas. Additionally, the presence of *EGFR*vIII has been shown to sensitize tumors to EGFR tyrosine kinase inhibitors when the tumor suppressor protein PTEN is intact [48, 49].

Expression of EGFRvIII is associated with favorable clinical response to the EGFR kinase inhibitors gefitinib and erlotinib when the tumor suppressor protein PTEN is intact

EGFRvIII also presents a unique antigenetic target on tumor cells that is currently being therapeutically used with anti- EGFRvIII vaccines as a molecularly targeted treatment approach. In addition to its recently shown relevance for defining prognostically distinct subgroups, *EGFR*vIII detection is likely to be increasingly important for determining treatment decisions for patients with glioblastoma and potentially for those with other types of cancer.

RT-PCR-Based Detection - Reverse transcription-polymerase chain reaction (RT-PCR) is an RNA-based PCR assay [50]. Reverse transcriptase catalyzes DNA synthesis using RNA as the template, producing a DNA strand complementary to the RNA template, called complementary DNA (cDNA). Because cDNA is not subject to RNase degradation, it is much more stable in laboratory environment than corresponding RNA. For EGFRvIII detection, RNA is extracted from FFPE tissue and reverse transcribed into cDNA. PCR is performed and PCR products are detected by gel electrophoresis. PCR primers are designed to detect EGFRvIII sequences but not unmutated sequences. A portion of a control gene is amplified in parallel to test for RNA/cDNA yield and integrity.

2. Testing and quality control issues

2.1. Specimen types

Formalin-fixed paraffin-embedded tissue - most frequently used in clinical testing, both for DNA-based and RNA-based analysis. Fresh and frozen tissue can be used to extract DNA or RNA, however it is less frequently used in clinical molecular laboratories.

http://dx.doi.org/10.5772/52670

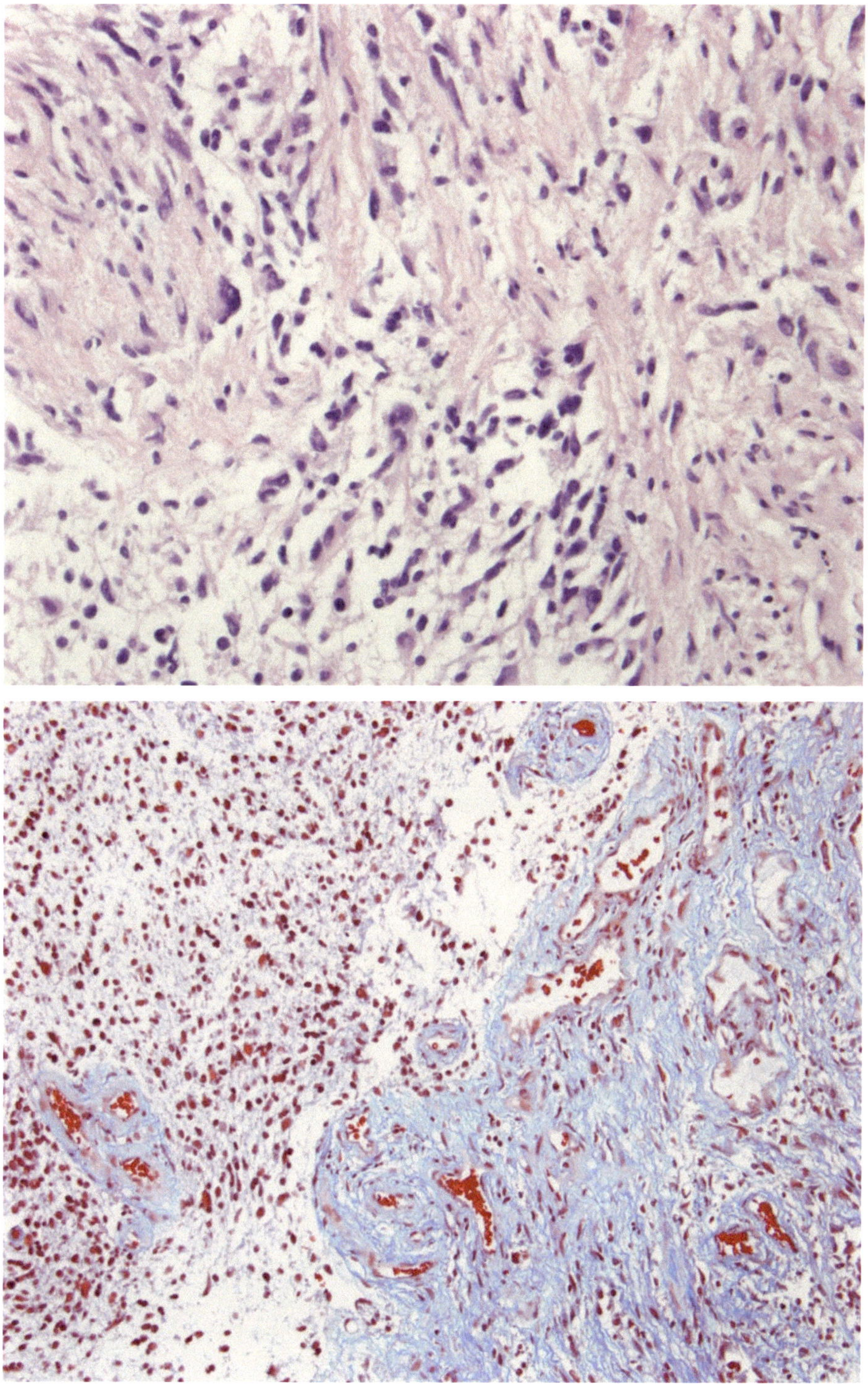

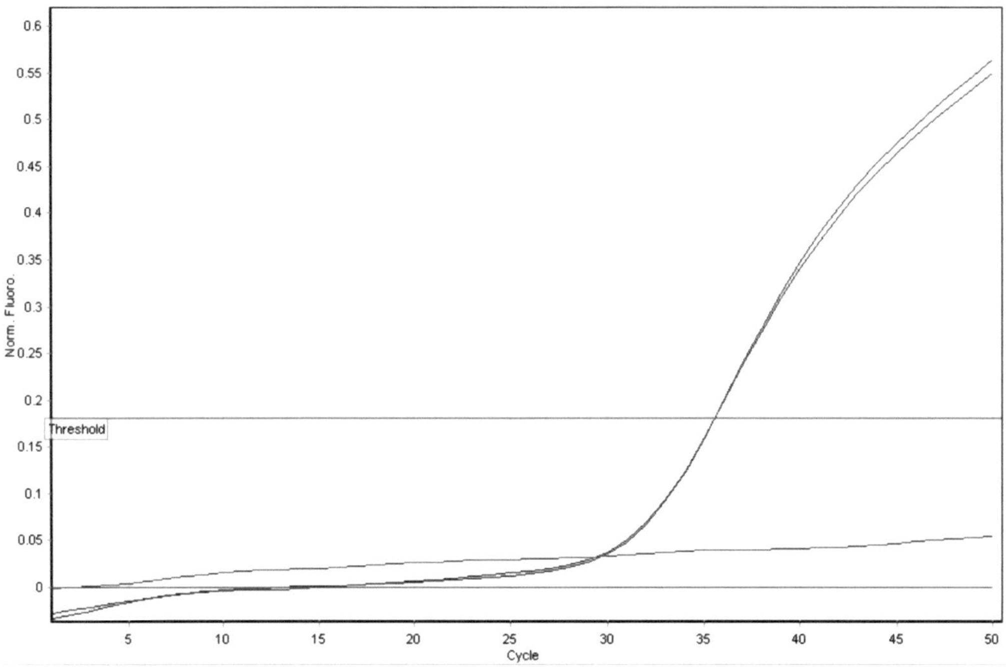

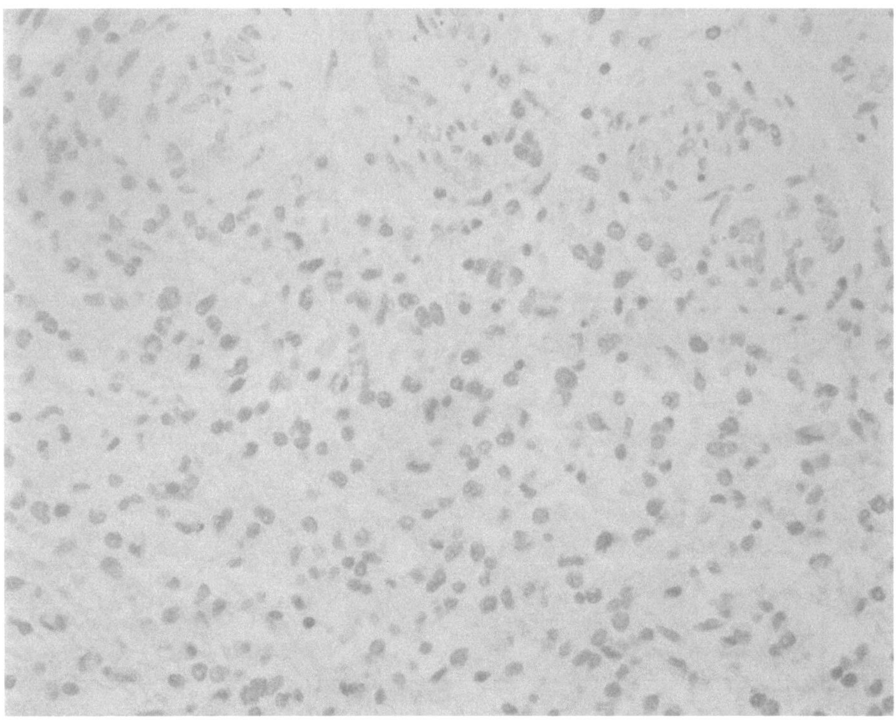

Figure 5. Gliosarcoma, WHO grade IV. (A and B) Sections show a moderately pleomorphic, biphasic glial tumor. Tumor tissue tested positive for MGMT promoter methylation (C) and negative for IDH1 mutation (D).

http://dx.doi.org/10.5772/52670

Microdissection may need to be performed to enrich for tumor content. If a specimen contains too few tumor cells or too many background reactive cell types, the sensitivity of the test may be diminished. In the past 15 years, various techniques of microdissection have been employed to isolate cells of interest in order to increase test sensitivity. Most frequently, a pathologist will examine an H&E stained tissue section and mark areas of tumor involvement. Tissues from tumor rich areas are then manually scrapped off the slides and used for nucleic acid extraction. Less frequently, laser capture microdissection might be performed, however this method is not practical for use in routine clinical molecular laboratories.

2.2. Nucleic acid extraction

Nucleic acid purification begins with lysis of the cells in the sample. Cell lysis liberates cellular macromolecules including proteins, lipids, and nucleic acids. Cell lysis can be accomplished using a detergent solution to break cell membranes and remove lipids. Proteins are enzymatically degraded with protease, usually proteinase K, or selectively precipitated. Protein digestion is performed at about 56°C and will permanently denature many proteins but does not affect nucleic acids. This process is followed by selective extraction that takes advantage of the physical and chemical differences between nucleic acids and other cellular molecules, forming the basis for their isolation. The nucleic acid is then purified from the soluble contaminants produced in the extraction process by precipitation in an ethanol-salt solution. The isolated nucleic acid is then resuspended in a dilute salt buffer.

2.3. DNA

PCR-based genetic analyses most frequently require isolated genomic DNA. Molecular analyses of nucleic acids have traditionally required DNA derived from blood, bone marrow aspirate, and fresh or frozen tissues. New developments in DNA extraction methods now make it possible to also use DNA extracted from formalin-fixed, paraffin-embedded (FFPE) tissues. The purpose of DNA isolation/extraction procedures is to obtain useful samples of DNA that are free of contaminating molecules which could hinder downstream DNA analysis. DNA is a hardy molecule present at stable cellular levels. It is relatively easy to isolate and store because deoxyribonucleases (DNases) that could potenitially degrade isolated DNA are easily denatured by heating or inhibited by sequestration of divalent cations.

2.4. RNA

Gene expression protocols (RT-PCR based genetic analyses) require isolated human RNA. RNA analysis depends on successful RNA isolation and preservation. Total RNA is purified with the use of RNA purification kits by first adding the white blood cells or tissue samples to a detergent/salt solution to lyse and homogenize the cells and eliminate endogenous RNase activity. Homogenization disrupts the cell membranes releasing RNA into the lysing solution, and shears the genomic DNA to reduce its ability to bind to the purification column with the RNA. The lysates are then passed through a purification column to bind the RNA and wash away proteins, DNA and other contaminants. Residual DNA is removed by an on-column DNase treatment. Finally, the purified RNA is eluted with DEPC-treated water.

2.5. Limitations of nucleic acid-based procedures

The following can affect the quality of lab results and should ideally be addressed during assay validation:

1. The accumulation of normal cells in the tumor, including infiltrating lymphocytes, may complicate accurate assessment of *MGMT* promoter methylation. Review of tissue morphology by a pathologist prior to testing will ensure that best suited tissue block are examined.
2. Excessive necrosis of tumor tissue will complicate analysis; a different tissue block needs to be selected, when available.
3. Bisulfite treatment of DNA is technically the most challenging part of this protocol. Since DNA loss routinely occurs during bisulfite treatment; it is important to select cases with minimal necrosis to ensure adequate yield of DNA. In order to control for bisulfite effect, methylated and unmethylated controls must be treated in parallel to patient samples to ensure that complete conversion occurred.

Appropriate specimen handling is critical to ensure specimen integrity and the accuracy of quantitative and qualitative nucleic acid detection. Inappropriate specimen handling can result in nucleic acid degradation, which can lead to erroneous quantitation of target from the patient. For example, RNA is rapidly degraded by a variety of ribonuclease (RNase) enzymes that are abundantly present within cells, on the skin surfaces, and possibly laboratory bench tops and equipment. RNases are very stable, active in virtually any aqueous environment, and can regain their activity after denaturation, and steps need to be developed to prevent RNA degradation by exposure to contaminating RNases.

2.6. Contamination prevention measures in a PCR laboratory

Millions of copies of target DNA are generated when PCR and other in vitro nucleic acid amplification techniques are used. If precautions are not taken, amplicons from previous reactions can be introduced into new amplification reactions and act as substrates for new DNA synthesis. The contaminating amplicons, amplified along with the patient samples will produce false positive results. Clinical molecular laboratories must have strict policies regarding contamination prevention and unidirectional work flow. Amplicon contamination and false positive results are prevented by using physical barriers and chemical and ultraviolet (UV) techniques to destroy amplicons or make them unsuitable for amplification. The physical barriers involve doing separate procedure steps in specially designated areas. For example, DNA isolation and PCR set-up are done in areas, separated by a wall, from areas used in downstream processing (thermal cycling, data analysis). This is also known as unidirectional work flow. Each area must have designated equipment and supplies to avoid cross contamination. Laminar flow hoods and other biological containment boxes equipped with UV light must be available in pre-PCR areas. Small scale physical separation techniques also include the use of barrier pipette tips, frequent glove changes, designated lab coats, and PCR tube openers or careful, slow opening of tubes to prevent aerosolization of contents. Chemical techniques include daily cleansing with bleach and other specialized de-

http://dx.doi.org/10.5772/52670

contaminants of work areas before and after use. Use of UV light will further degrade any residual nucleic acids on work surfaces. A no template PCR reaction must be included with every assay as a quality control check for amplicon contamination.

3. Assay validation

For a test to become generally useful, it must have demonstrated analytic validity and clinical utility. Analytic validation focuses on determining how accurately and reliably the assay measures the molecular event of interest. The assay must be reliable in routine laboratory setting using a variety of specimen types. Even assays that are routinely performed in the laboratory require analytic validation within the clinical setting of each laboratory when test results are used for clinical decisions. To ensure reproducible findings, clinical laboratories need to understand the impact that preanalytic variables and specimen processing have on assay performance. Analytic validation ensures that the same answer will be produced for the same sample within predefined technical variation. In recognition of the critical importance of analytic validation for biomarkers, multiple groups have developed recommendations and frameworks with which to standardize the assessment.

Clinical validation assesses the strength of association between the assay results and the clinical outcome of interest, whether it is diagnostic, prognostic, or predictive. A large number of measures are used to assess these associations. These analyses address whether one can be sure the clinical state is positive if the test is positive (positive predictive power) and that the clinical state is negative if the test is negative (negative predictive power).

Evaluation of new biomarkers can be aided if tumor biomarker studies and the journals reporting them adhere to the Reporting Recommendations for Tumor Marker Prognostic Studies (REMARK). These guidelines were produced by a working group convened as part of the NCI-EORTC joint meeting on Cancer Diagnostics in Nyborg, Denmark, in 2000 [51]. REMARK criteria include specifications of patient populations, biological specimen under study, assay methods, study design, and statistical methods, and detailed guidelines for analysis and presentation of data. This reporting standard is now requested for manuscripts being submitted to many journals. Although the tissue sources are not always available to allow the most rigorous validation of assays, providing a standardized means to communicate the level of clinical validation is critical to biomarker development. Using the above reporting standards should help establish the clinical validity of new biomarkers being used in cancer research and treatment.

An emerging standard for the adoption of new molecular tests is the demonstration of clinical utility. Clinical utility refers to the ability of the assay to improve clinical decision making and patient outcomes. Clinical utility depends on the clinical situation, availability of effective therapies, magnitude of clinical benefit, and relative value the patient, caregiver, and society place on the differences in benefits and risks in these separate groups. For example, if a marker clearly distinguishes differences between positive and negative results but the evidence for differential treatment is not available, there is no reason to test for the marker. Likewise, if therapy is effective regardless whether the patient tests positive or negative, the marker does not have clinical utility. Additionally, a novel assay might have outstanding analytic validity and proven clinical validity but there is already an established method to test for the same parameters, which makes the new assay unnecessary.

Associations such as Clinical Laboratory Standards Institute (CLSI) have published several guidelines dealing with molecular genomic testing in clinical laboratories. As more molecular tests are being introduced for patient management, CLSI will likely continue to publish new and expanded guidelines addressing current and possibly future considerations and best practices.

3.1. Issues with MGMT assay validation

Molecular markers in general are developed to address a variety of indications [52]. Diagnostic markers are a large category of molecular tests that aid in the diagnosis or subclassification of a particular disease state. Diagnostic subclassification may result in different management of the disease, but the marker is used primarily to establish the particular disease that is present in the patient sample. An example of a diagnostic marker is BCR/ABL t(9;22) translocation in chronic myelogenous leukemia. Prognostic markers have an association with some clinical outcomes, such as overall survival or recurrence-free survival, independent of the treatment rendered. An example of a prognostic marker is the *FLT3* IDT mutation in acute myeloid leukemia, which identifies a subset of patients who will have a more aggressive disease course regardless of current treatment options. Predictive markers predict the activity of a specific class or type of therapy, and are used to help make more specific treatment decisions. They are used as indicators of the likely benefit of a specific treatment to a specific patient. Human epidermal growth factor receptor (EGFR) is an example of a predictive marker. Patients with lung cancers whose tumors exhibit adenocarcinoma histology and carry one of the sensitizing *EGFR* mutations are likely to respond well to treatment with tyrosine kinase inhibitors erlotinib and gefitinib. Some of these markers may also be used as companion markers to identify a subgroup of patients that are likely to respond to a specific therapy. One example of a companion diagnostic is the *BRAF* V600E mutation test which is coapproved with the kinase inhibitor vemurafenib. *BRAF* mutations are found in 30% to 60% of melanomas, and the kinase activating *BRAF* V600E mutation confers sensitivity to vemurafenib, a small molecule inhibitor.

The clinical utility of the *MGMT* methylation status as a biomarker for benefit from alkylating agent therapy in gliomas is still being evaluated and there is no consensus as to which procedure is most suitable for routine clinical testing. While most protocols measure the level of methylation accurately, presence of contaminating normal cells in every specimen makes it difficult to set up a consistent cut off point between low positive and negative test results. The extent of methylation required and the sets of CpGs that are crucial for complete silencing are still under investigation. Given the complexity of the biological relationship between promoter methylation and gene silencing and the difficulties to integrate these features into a test that is in addition complicated by presence of nontumoral tissue, there are unavoidable drawbacks for any technology attempting to predict loss of MGMT expression for potential benefit from alkylating agent therapy. Key to introducing tests for diagnostics is their careful prospective validation.

3.2. MGMT methylight assay validation - A one lab experience

Epigenetic silencing of the *MGMT* gene through promoter hypermethylation and resulting transcriptional inactivation is now routinely used as a prognostic and possibly predictive biomarker in evaluating treatment choices in patients diagnosed with glioma. Patients enrolling in clinical trials are also evaluated for the *MGMT* promoter methylation status. For that reason, a sensitive, clinically validated assay for detection of *MGMT* promoter methylation can be of great help in patient management.We previously developed a simplified *MGMT* MSP protocol [53] that utilized formalin fixed paraffin embedded specimens. This MSP protocol proved reliable with majority of glioma patients, however, result interpretation was sometimes challenging when evaluating specimens with few malignant cells and/or extensive necrosis, both of which gave faint bands on agarose gels.To further enhance our ability to accurately assess methylation status of the *MGMT* promoter region in glioma specimens, we investigated the use of real-time PCR technology as a way of enhancing assay sensitivity. Our ultimate goal was to develop a more sensitive detection method that would give reliable, semi-quantitative results, even with suboptimal specimens. Previous studies have shown sodium bisulfite conversion to be a reproducible method, with subsequent quantitative real-time PCR methylation assays having acceptable precision for clinical work [54].

The goal of this study was to evaluate the MethyLight protocol, as compared to the *MGMT*-MSP protocol, and appropriateness of the MethyLight protocol for use in *MGMT* promoter methylation detection in routine clinical testing of glioma cases.

3.3. Materials and methods

3.3.1. Tumor samples

Thirty archival brain resection cases were selected for the study: glioblastomamultiforme (18), oligodendroglioma (3), anaplastic oligodendroglioma (3), and astrocytoma (6). For all tumor samples, histology was reviewed to confirm diagnosis and select blocks with greatest tumor involvement. Microdissection was performed on all samples showing an estimated tumor cell content of less than 50% except in cases where infiltrative pattern of tumor growth made this step unreliable.

3.3.2. DNA extraction and bisulfite treatment

Genomic DNA was isolated from 2 to 3 twenty micrometer thick paraffin sections after confirmation of the histology. DNA from formalin fixed, paraffin embedded tissue was extracted using Puregene kit (Gentra Systems, Minneapolis, MN). *MGMT* promoter methylation status was assessed using a two step approach. The first step involved bisulfite conversion of isolated DNA (200-500 ng) which was done using EZ DNA Methylation Gold kit (Zymo Research, Orange, CA). The second step involved detection of methylated and unmethylated DNA sequences, and was done using the following methods: 1) Methylation specific PCR (MSP) and 2) Real-time PCR amplification (MethyLight).

3.3.3. *Methylation-specific PCR*

MGMT MSP amplification was performed as previously reported [53] with specific primers designed to distinguish methylated from unmethylated DNA. Methylated and unmethylated DNA sequences were detected on 2.5% agarose gels. Samples giving signals approximately equivalent to the positive methylated control were designated as methylated. Samples giving no signals with positive methylated control, but demonstrating presence of unmethylated DNA, similar to the negative control, were designated as unmethylated.

3.3.4. *Quantitative real-time PCR (MethyLight)*

Real-time PCR assays were set-up in parallel to measure *MGMT* methylation. Two sets of primers and probes designed specifically for bisulfite-converted DNAwere used [55]: a set for *MGMT* gene and a set for collagen 2A1 (COL2A1) to normalize for the amount of input DNA. The *MGMT* forward primer is 5′-GCG TTT CGA CGT TCG TAG GT-3′, the *MGMT* reverse primer is 5′-CAC TCT TCC GAA AAC GAA ACG-3′, and the *MGMT* probe is 6FAM-5′-CGC AAA CGA TAC GCA CCG CGA-3′BHQ1. COL2A1 forward primer is 5′-TCT AAC AAT TAT AAA CTC CAA CCA CCA A-3′, the COL2A1 reverse primer is 5′-GGG AAG ATG GGA TAG AAG GGA ATA T-3′, and the COL2A1 probe is 6FAM-5′-CCT TCA TTC TAA CCC AAT ACC TAT CCC ACC TCT AAA-3′BHQ1. We used Rotor Gene 3000 real-time PCR instrument (Qiagen, Germantown, MD, USA). The PCR conditions were as previously described [56, 57]. Briefly, PCR amplification was performed in 0.2 ml PCR tubes with a final reaction mixture of 25 μl consisting of 12.5 μl of TaqMan Universal Master mix without uracil DNA glycosylase (Applied Biosystems, Foster City, CA), 3 μl of respective forward and reverse primers (10 μM) for either *MGMT* or COL2A1, 1 μl of probe, 5 μl (about 50 ng) of bisulfite-modified DNA, and water. PCR conditions were as follows: 95ºC for 10 min, followed by 50 cycles at 95ºC for 15 s and 60ºC for 1 min.

3.3.5. *Assay controls*

For assay controls, methylated DNA and unmethylated DNA were purchased from Chemicon International, Temecula, CA, and used as positive and negative controls for methylated sequences. The control DNA was subjected to bisulfite treatment and PCR amplification in parallel with patient samples for every run. Controls without DNA were also performed for each set of reactions. Additionally, for the MethyLight protocol, collagen 2A1 (COL2A1) gene was used as the internal reference to assess the quality and quantity of input DNA.

3.3.6. *Results*

To determine the limit of detection of the MehtyLight protocol, bisulfite treated methylated control DNA was serially diluted into bisulfite treated unmethylated control DNA. DNA mixing study with methylated and unmethylated DNA showed good linearity. The limit of detection of the MethyLight assay was determined to be 1% of methylated DNA in the background of unmethylated DNA. The MSP protocol was shown to be slightly less sensitive, with the limit of detection of 5% of methylated DNA in unmethylated background [53].

Tube No.	% of Methylated DNA	% of Unmethylated DNA	Cycle Threshold (Ct)
1	**100**	**0**	**28.80**
2	**50**	**50**	**29.77**
3	**20**	**80**	**30.77**
4	**10**	**90**	**31.83**
5	**5**	**95**	**32.74**
6	**1**	**99**	**35.22**
7	**0**	**100**	**0**
8	**0**	**0**	**0**

Table 3. Cycle threshold values of serial dilution of methylated DNA into unmethylated control DNA

To evaluate run-to-run variations, we tested the reproducibility of the MethyLight assay by performing eight independent runs of the serially diluted methylated control in the negative control background. Acceptable reproducibility was demonstrated between runs.

Of the 30 tumor specimens in the study group, we were able to extract DNA of sufficient quantity and quality to allow us to determine *MGMT* promoter methylation status for all samples. There was a complete concordance in test results between the two methods for 25/30 cases (83%). Overall, methylation specific PCR (MSP) identified 16 (53%) specimens as positive (methylated *MGMT* promoter was present) and 14 (47%) of tumors as negative (having unmethylated*MGMT* promoter). The MethyLight protocol identified 15 specimens (50%) as positive for *MGMT* promoter methylation. Among the discordant cases, two samples tested negative by MSP and were low positive by MethyLight; low DNA recovery was observed for both of these samples, and the small amount of bisulfite treated DNA that was available for analysis might have contributed to the discordance in results. The other three discordant cases tested as weak positive with MSP and were negative by MethyLight; all three of these cases had significant amount of necrotic tissue, which complicated interpretation of the MSP results.

As regards assay controls, in the MSP protocol, *MGMT* promoter hypermethylation was always accompanied by amplification in the unmethylated reaction as well. This is to be expected since the original tissue sections contained a mixture of tumor and non-malignant tissue. The presence of unmethylated promoter served as an internal amplification control that confirmed that the quality and quantity of bisulfite treated DNA was acceptable for clinical testing. Only tumor samples that contained a clearly visible methylated signal, with or without an additional unmethylated signal, were interpreted as positive for the *MGMT* promoter methylation. All the samples that only amplified with unmethylated primers were interpreted as negative. COL2A1 internal control was used with the MethyLight protocol to assess the quality and quantity of DNA. All samples demonstrated positive signals with the COL2A1 PCR amplification.

In comparing the two quality control methods, we observed 100% concordance between the two systems, with both methods indicating that all samples in the study group contained sufficient amount of bisulfite converted DNA for clinical testing. The gel signals observed with unmethylated DNA as an indicator of DNA quantity with the MSP protocol, and the expression of COL2A1 as an internal control standard in the MethyLight protocol proved to be equivalent and reliable indicators of quality of input DNA.

This study reports an improvement on our previously published MSP protocol for the detection of *MGMT* promoter methylation in glioma specimens. MethyLight protocol, a real-time PCR based approach, was used in a number of application [54, 55-57]. In our laboratory, the MethyLight assay proved to be easy to perform, reproducible, and sensitive in detecting the amount of methylated DNA sequences in formalin fixed, paraffin embedded brain tumor specimens. Furthermore, with the use of the real-time PCR approach, we were able to eliminate post PCR processing that is integral to the MSP protocol.

Recently Ogino and colleagues [54] performed an in-depth investigation of critical parameters that influence the success of quantitative DNA methylation analysis after sodium bisulfite conversion of DNA samples from archived formalin-fixed paraffin-embedded tumor specimens, demonstrating the value of percentage of methylated reference (PMR) estimation. Our system, however, proved impractical for measurement of PMR.To obtain PMR measurement in their study, the investigators microdissected tumor tissue to obtain pure populations of tumor cells. Exclusion of normal tissue allowed for precise calculation of PMR values, and consequently quantitation of the amount of methylation in each tumor sample. This approach proved to be impractical for some of the samples in our study due to the pattern of growth of gliomas, particularly GBM tumors, which grow in an infiltrating pattern, with many benign cells surrounding a few infiltrating tumor cells. Consequently, sections of these tumors contain both malignant and normal cells, with no easy way of dissecting out a pure tumor population, unless one performs laser capture microdissection. Since our aim was to optimize a simple *MGMT* promoter methylation detection assay for routine clinical use, we continued our practice of histology review and preselecting tissue blocks with greatest amount of tumor involvement and smallest amount of necrosis prior to analysis. Using the entire tissue block section proved to be a practical approach for routine testing in our laboratory, even when microdissection was not possible. At 1% sensitivity, we were able to detect *MGMT* promoter methylation even when tumor cells were in minority, as assessed by review of histology.

While this study group consisted of a relatively small number of samples, we were able to develop a testing protocol using MethyLighttechnique, that proved to be reliable and reproducible in a clinical setting. When applying this method to clinical use, it is important that proper controls be included with every assay run.After bisulfite treatment of isolated DNA, patient samples are tested in duplicates for the evidence of *MGMT* promoter, and for the expression of COL2A1 internal control sequences to normalize for input DNA. Additionally, three different concentrations (100%, 10% and 1%) of methylated DNA in unmethylated background are run as reference standards. This approach allows clear distinction between positive and negative signals. The assay results are interpreted as positive or negative for *MGMT* promoter methylation. In terms of patient management, temozolomide is give to all patients, regardless of *MGMT* promoter methylation status. It has been established that strongly positive patients will respond to temozolomide, however it is less clear how low positive patients will respond. When very low positive results are reported for a glioma specimen, the amount of tumor involvement in that particular sample, as assessed by review of histology, can serve as an additional guide for the clinical care provider.

In summary, while both MSP and MethyLight detection methods proved acceptable for clinical testing, with 83% concordance between the two methods, the MethyLight method proved superior in several different areas. It allowed easier interpretation of low positive results, because there was a clear distinction between positive and negative signals. This real-time, quantitative approach also allowed for reduced turn around time and high throughput specimen processing, because post PCR gel analysis steps were eliminated. Finally, the MethyLight method appeared to be more sensitive, even though the significance of very low positive results is unknown. The limit of detection of the MethyLight assay was determined to be 1% of methylated DNA in the background of unmethylated DNA, compared to 5% with the MSP assay.

3.4. Regulation of molecular genomic testing

Molecular testing falls under high complexity testing and is highly regulated. In the United States two federal agencies, the Food and Drug Administration (FDA) and the Centers for Medicare and Medicaid Services (CMS) have jurisdiction over this type of testing. The laws and policies concerning the development and implementation of molecular tests continue to evolve. Medical tests are regulated by the Center for devices and Radiologic Health, a branch of FDA. Devices are divided into 3 classes based primarily on the risks associated with their intended use. Class I tests are low risk, usually of a simple design. Class II tests pose moderate risks, are evaluated by the FDA through review of a 510(k) premarket notification, and are cleared for marketing once they are found to be substantially equivalent to a legally marketed device that was previously cleared by the FDA. Class III tests are those associated with the highest clinical risk. Each Class III test is reviewed through application for premarket approval (PMA). A demonstration of safety and effectiveness is needed to gain FDA approval. The FDA approval/clearance process provides reasonable assurance of safety and effectiveness, and that the test will provide clinically significant results.

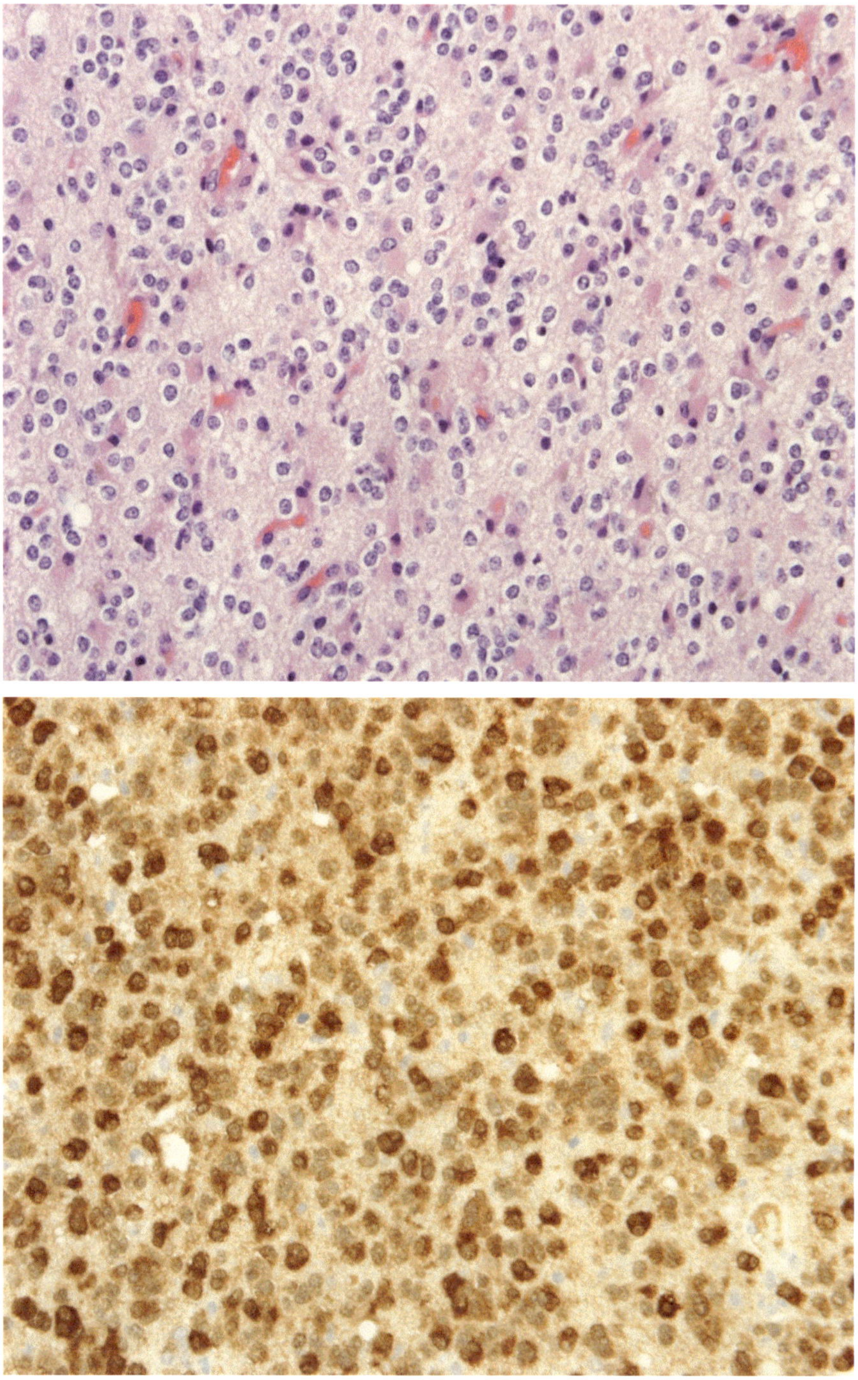

Figure 6. Oligodendroglioma, WHO grade II. (A) Sections show moderately cellular glial neoplastic proliferation. Tumor tissue tested positive for MGMT promoter methylation and 1p19q codeletion. (B) The IDH1 R132H is positive.

The rapid transition of new scientific knowledge to medical practice has led to development and use of diagnostic tests that are often called laboratory developed tests (LTDs). The FDA retains jurisdiction over this category of tests and until recently the oversight was basically directed towards critical reagents used to build these tests. With LTDs being used more widely in clinical decision making it is likely the FDA will develop clinical guidelines on Companion Diagnostics or molecular tests which directly impact the use of a pharmaceutical or biologic drug.

Clinical laboratories are governed through the Clinical Laboratory Improvement Amendment (CLIA) of 1988 administered by CMS. CLIA certification is a descriptor which is frequently associated with analytically valid assays performed in a clinical laboratory or a laboratory that has received a CLIA certification. CLIA certification requires that a laboratory adopt specific practices and perform prescribed measures of analytic validation while performing specific assays. Assays must be performed in CLIA certified laboratories if the results of the assays are going to be used to guide patient management. Key components of the regulation and oversight of CLIA accredited laboratories are inspections and proficiency tests. In most hospitals these are provided by the College of American Pathologists (CAP). CAP inspection guidelines essentially set the standards for overall biomarker laboratory operation, including assay validation, quality control, and quality assurance activities. The guidelines mandate regular proficiency testing for every clinical assay, and CAP runs an extensive program providing proficiency testing samples for all commonly used clinical assays.

4. Prognostic and predictive relevance of glioma biomarkers

Cancer-specific DNA methylation changes are hallmarks of human cancers, in which global hypomethylation is often seen concomitantly with hypermethylation of CpG islands. Promoter CpG island hypermethylation generally results in transcriptional silencing of the associated gene [58]. There have been several reports of promoter-associated CpG island hypermethylator phenotype in human GBM and other glioma subtypes [59-61]. Several studies have reported differences between primary and secondary GBMs with respect to epigenetic changes. Overall, secondary GBMs have a higher frequency of promoter methylation than primary GBMs [62]. Analysis of epigenetic changes from The Cancer Genome Atlas study [63] identified the existence of a proportion of GBM tumors with highly concordant DNA methylation of a subset of loci, indicative of a CpG island methylator phenotype (G-CIMP). G-CIMP positive samples were associated with secondary or recurrent (treated) tumors and tightly associated with *IDH*1 mutation. G-CIPM tumors also showed a relative lack of copy number variation commonly observed in GBM. Integration of the DNA methylation data with gene expression data showed that G-CIMP tumors represent a subset of proneural tumors. G-CIMP -positive tumors showed a favorable prognosis with GBMs as a whole and also with the proneural subset. These data suggest that G-CIMP-positive status may confer favorable outcome. When lower grade tumors were examined, nearly 10-fold more G-CIMP-positive gliomas were detected among grade II tumors as compared to grade IV GBMs. The study suggests that the improved survival of G-CIMP gliomas at all tumor grades might be due to certain molecular features within the G-CIMP gliomas that encourage a less aggressive tumor phenotype.

Low grade diffuse gliomas WHO grade II (diffuse astrocytoma, oligoastrocytoma, oligodendroglioma) are characterized by frequent *IDH*1/2 mutations (>80%) that occur at a very early stage. In addition, the majority of diffuse astrocytomas (about 60%) carry TP53 mutations, which constitute a prognostic marker for shorter survival. Limited data exists correlating *IDH*1/2 mutations with loss of heterozygosity (LOH) on chromosome arms 1p and 19q, methylation of the promoter region of DNA repair enzyme O-6-Methylguanine DNA methyl transferase (M-MGMT) rendering sensitivity to DNA alkylating agents, and epidermal growth factor receptor variant III (*EGFR*vIII), a constitutively active mutant form of *EGFR* frequently present in glioblastoma.

Diagnosis	GR	Micro dissected	IDH1 (+/total)	IDH2 (+/ total)	MGMT (+/total)	EGFRvIII (+/total)	LOH (+/total)
GBM	IV	5/20	0/20	0/20	10/20	3/20	nd
0	II	5/14	12/14	1/14	10/13	0/3	10/13
AO	III	0/2	2/2	0/2	1/2	0/1	1/1
A	II	2/6	2/6	0/6	3/6	0/4	0/2
AA	III	0/6	0/6	0/6	3/6	0/4	0/2
OA	II/III	3/8	8/8	0/8	6/7	0/4	2/8
AOA	III	1/6	1/6	0/6	3/5	0/3	3/3

Table 4. Biomarker distribution among different glioma types

High throughput profiling techniques in conjunction with sophisticated bioinformatics integrative tools are emerging to revolutionize our knowledge about the complexity of the disease. Development of novel array-based profiling techniques and next generation sequencing techniques has facilitated development of sophisticated tumor-specific genomic and transcriptional signatures. Integrative analysis of DNA copy number, gene expression and DNA methylation profiling indicate that molecular alterations may impact future treatment strategies. For example, as PIK3R1 encodes the regulatory protein p85a subunit, response to PI3K inhibitors may depend on whether the tumors bear mutations in this specific gene or not. Also, in predicting sensitivity and the development of resistance to temozolomide the Cancer Genome Atlas network added further support for a role of the DNA mismatch repair system. *MGMT* methylation in conjunction with temozolomide treatment may lead to a loss of mismatch repair function by introduction of mutations in mismatch repair genes [64, 65]. Thus patients who initially respond to front line therapy may evolve treatment resistance by developing a hypermutator phenotype. As a consequence, selective strategies targeting mismatch repair deficient cells might have to be used in combination with alkylating agent therapy to prevent or minimize resistance to temozolomide.

http://dx.doi.org/10.5772/52670

5. Conclusion

The list of clinically useful biomarkers in gliomas is expected to expand as novel markers are validated in large scale clinical trials [52]. *MGMT* promoter methylation is now routinely performed in many institutions. Alkylating agents cause cell death by forming cross-links between adjacent strands of DNA due to alkylation of the O^6 position of guanine. The cellular DNA repair protein O^6-methylguanine-DNA methyltransferase (*MGMT*) functions as a DNA repair enzyme that removes the mutagenic alkyl-adducts from the O^6-poasition of guanine and thereby causes resistance to alkylating drugs [66-68]. 1p/19q LOH has shown clinical utility, and is a part of guidelines for all oligodendroglioma and mixed tumor management. Some of the newer markers, such as *IDH*1/2 mutations and *EGFR*vIII mutations still need further evaluation, and are being used with increasing frequency to provide further definition of tumor stage and possibly subsequent behavior. Molecular laboratories are likely to evolve also, as clinical care providers continue to rely on genomic-type assays for guiding patient treatment.

Acknowledgements

The author gratefully acknowledges Lynda Szymanski, DO for her help with figures and Lisa Whiteley for help with data analysis.

Author details

Milena Cankovic

Address all correspondence to: mcankov1@hfhs.org

Division of Molecular Pathology and Genomic Medicine, Department of Pathology, Henry Ford Hospital, Detroit, Michigan, USA

References

[1] Louis DN, Ohgaki H, Wiestler OD, Cavanee WK (eds). WHO classification of tumors of the central nervous system. IARC, Lyon, 2007

[2] Hulleman E, Helin K. Molecular mechanisms in gliomagenesis. In: Adv Cancer Res 2005;94:1-21.

[3] Adamson C, Kanu OO, Mehta AI, Di C, Lin N, Mattox AK, Bigner DD. Glioblastoma-multiforme: A review of where we have been and where we are going. Expert OpinInvestig Drugs 2009;18:1061-1083.

[4] Furnari FB, Fenton T, Bachoo RM, Mukasa A, Stommel JM, Stegh A, Hahn WC, Ligon KL, Louis DN, Brennan C, et al. Malignant astrocyticglioma: Genetics, biology, and paths to treatment. Genes Dev 2007;21:2683-2710.

[5] Andesson U, Malmer B, Bergenheim AT, et al. Heterogeneity in the expression markers of drug resistance in brain tumors. ClinNeuropathol 2004;23:21-27.

[6] Nieder C, Adam M, Grosu AL. Combined modality treatment of glioblastomamultiforme: the role of Temozolomide. Rev on Recent Clin Trials 2006;1:43-51.

[7] Hegi ME, Diserens A-C, Gorlia T, et al. MGMT gene silencing and benefit from Temozolomide in glioblastomas. N Engl J Med 2005;352:997-1003.

[8] Stupp R, Dietrich P-Y, Kraljevic SO. Promising survival for patients with newly diagnosed glioblastomamultiforme treated with concomitant radiation plus Temozolomide followed by adjuvant Temozolomide. J ClinOncol 2002;20:1375-1382.

[9] Friedman HS, Kerby T, Calvert H. Temozolomide and treatment of malignant glioma. Clin Cancer Res 2000;6:2585-2597.

[10] Jenkins R. Gliomas. In: Leonard DGB (ed) Molecular Pathology in Clinical Practice. New York: Springer; 2007. p299-304.

[11] Riemenschneider MJ, Reifenberger G. Molecular neuropathology of gliomas. Int J Mol Sci 2009;10:184-212.

[12] Jaeckie KA, Eyre HJ, Townsend JJ, et al. Correlation of O^6methylguanine-DNA methyltransferase levels with survival of malignant astrocytoma patients treated with bischloroethylnitrosourea: A Southwest Oncology Group Study. J ClinOncol 1998;16:3310-3315.

[13] Hegi ME, Diserens A-C, Godard S, et al. Clinical trial substantiates the predictive value of O-6-methylguanine-DNA methyltransferase promoter methylation in glioblastoma patients treated with temozolomide. Clin Cancer Res 2004;10:1871-1874.

[14] Esteller M, Garcia-Foncillas J, Andion E, et al. Inactivation of the DNA-repair gene MGMT and the clinical response of gliomas to alkylating agents. N Engl J Med 2000;343:1350-1354.

[15] Brell M, Tortosa A, Verger E, et al. Prognostic significance of O^6-methylguanine-DNA methyltransferase determined by promoter hypermethylation and immunohistochemical expression in anaplastic gliomas. Cin Cancer Res 2005;11:5167-5174.

[16] Smith-Zagone MJ, Pulliam JF, Farkas DH. Molecular pathology methods. In: Leonard DGB (ed) Molecular Pathology in Clinical Practice. New York: Springer; 2007. p15-40.

[17] Sciuscio D, Diserens A-C, van Dommelen K, et al. Extent and patterns of MGMT promoter methylation in glioblastoma and respective glioblastoma-derived spheres. Clin Cancer Res 2011;17:255-266.

[18] Nagawachi T, Soejima H, Urano T, et al. Silencing effect of CpG island hypermethylation and histone modifications on O6-methylguanine-DNA methyltransferase (MGMT) gene expression in human cancer. Oncogene 2003;22:8835-8844.

[19] Stupp R, Hegi ME, Mason WP, et al. Effects of radiotherapy with concomitant and adjuvant temozolomide versus radiotherapy alone on survival in glioblastoma in a randomised phase III study: 5-year analysis of the EORTC-NCICtrial. Lancet Oncol 2009;10:459-466.

[20] Chen L, Lindeman NI. Glioblastoma multiforme. In:Schrijver I (ed) Diagnostic Molecular Pathology in Practice. Berlin;Springer;2011. p233-241.

[21] Herman JG, Baylin SB. Gene silencing in cancer in association with promoter hypermethylation. N Eng J Med 2003;349:2042-2054.

[22] Jones PA, Laird PW. Cancer epigenetics comes of age. Nat Genet 1999;21:163-167.

[23] Baylin SB, Herman JG. DNA hypermethylation in tumorigenesis: epigenetics joins genetics. Trends Genet 2000;16:168-174.

[24] Costello JE, Fruhwald MC, Smiraglia DJ, et al. Aberrant CpG-island methylation has nonrandom and tumour-type-specific patterns. Nat Genet 2000;24:132-138.

[25] Merlo A, Herman JG, Mao L, et al. 5′ CpG island methylation is associated with transcriptional silencing of the tumor suppressor p16/CDKN2/MTS1 in human cancers. Nat Med 1995;1:686-692.

[26] Herman JG, Jen J, Merlo A, et al. Hypermethylation-associated inactivation indicates a tumor suppressor role for p15 ^{INK4B}. Cancer Res 1996;56:722-727.

[27] Esteller M, Hamilton SR, Burger PC, et al. Inactivation of the DNA repair gene O-6-methylguanine-DNA methyltransferase by promoter hypermethylation is a common event in primary human neoplasia. Cancer Res 1999;59:793-797.

[28] Rein T, DePamphilis ML, Zorbas H. Identifying 5-methylcytosine and related modifications in DNA genomes. Nucleic Acids Res 1998;26:2255-2264.

[29] Langaee T, Ronaghi M. Genetic variation analysis by pyrosequencing. Mutat Res 2005;573:96-102.

[30] Metzger M. Emerging technologies in DNA sequencing. Genome Research 2005;15:1767-1776.

[31] Nygren AOH, Ameziane N, Duarte HMB, et al. Methylation-specific MLPA (MS-MLPA): simultaneous detection of CpG methylation and copy number changes of up to 40 sequences. Nucleic Acids Res 2005;33:e128.

[32] Jeuken JWM, Cornelissen SJB, Vriezen M, et al. MS-MLPA: an attractive alternative laboratory assay for robust, reliable, and semiquantitative detection of MGMT promoter hypermethylation in gliomas. Lab Invest 2007;87:1055-1065.

[33] Cairncross JG, Ueki K, Zlatescu MC, et al. Specific genetic predictors of chemotherapeutic response and survival in patients with anaplastic oligodendrogliomas. J Natl Cancer Inst 1998;90:1473-1479.

[34] Bourne TD, Schiff TD. Update on molecular findings, management and outcome in low-grade gliomas. Nat Rev Neurol 2010;6:695-701

[35] Ino Y, Betensky RA, Zlatescu MC, et al. Molecular subtypes of anaplastic oligodendroglioma: implications for patient management at diagnosis. Clin Cancer Res 2001;7:839-845

[36] Kaloshi G, Benouaich-Amiel A, Diakite F, et al. Temozolomide for low grade gliomas: predictive impact of 1p/19q loss on response and outcome. Neurology 2007;68:1831-1836

[37] Snuderl M, Hunt JL. Oligodendroglioma. In:Schrijver I (ed) Diagnostic Molecular Pathology in Practice. Berlin;Springer;2011. p227-232.

[38] Idbaih A, Kouwenhoven M, Jeuken J, et al. Chromosome 1p loss evaluation in anaplastic oligodendrogliomas. Neuropathology 2008;28:440-443

[39] Van den Bent M, Chinot OL, Cairnoss JG. Recent developments in the molecular characterization and treatment of oligodendroglial tumors. NeuroOncol 2003;5:128-138

[40] Smith JS, Alderete B, Minn Y, et al. Localization of common deletion regions on 1p and 19q in human gliomas and their association with histologic subtype. Oncogene 1999;18:4144-4152.

[41] Shinawi M, Cheung SW. The arary CGH and its clinical applications. Drug Discov Today 2008;13:760-770.

[42] Parsons DW, Jones S, Zhang X, et al. An integrated genomic analysis of human glioblastomamultiforme. Science 2008;321:1807-1812

[43] Houillier C, Wang X, Kaloshi G, et al. IDH1 or IDH2 mutations predict longer survival and response to temozolomide in low-grade gliomas. Neurology 2010;75:1560-1566

[44] Von Deimling A, Korshunov A, Hartmann C. The next generation of glioma biomarkers: MGMT methylation, BRAF fusions and IDH1 mutations. Brain Pathol 2011;21:74-87

[45] Dubbink HJ, Taal W, van Marion R, et al. IDH1 mutations in low grade astrocytomas predict survival but not response to temozolomide. Neurology 2009;73:1792-1795.

[46] Sanger F, Nicklen S, Coulson AR. DNA sequencing with chain terminating inhibitors. Proc natl. AcadSciUSA 1977;74:5463-5467.

[47] Capper D, Zentgraf H, Balss J, et al. Monoclonal antibody specific for IDH1 R132H mutation. ActaNeuropathol 2009;118:599-601.

[48] Heimberger A, Suki D, Yang D, et al. The natural history of EGFR and EGFRvIII on glioblastoma patients. Journal of Translational Medicine. 2005 (3):38.

[49] Nicholas M, Lukas R, Jafri N, et al. Epidermal Growth Factor Receptor – Medicated Signal Transduction in the Development and Therapy of Gliomas. Clinical Cancer Research. 2006; 12(24) 7261-7270.

[50] Yoshimito K, Dang J, Zhu S, et al. Development of a Real-Time RT-PCR Assay for Detecting EGFRvIII in Glioblastoma Samples. Clinical Cancer Research. 2008; 14(2): 488-493.

[51] McShane LM, Altman DG, Sauerbrei W, et al. Reporting recommendation for tumor marker prognostic studies (REMARK). J Natl Cancer Inst 2005;97:1180-1184

[52] Ohgaki H, Kleihues P. Genetic profile of astrocytic and oligodendroglialgliomas. Brain Tumor Pathol 2011;28:177-183.

[53] Febbo PG, Ladanyi M, Aldape KD, et al. NCCN Task Force Report: Evaluating the clinical utility of tumor markers in oncology. J Natl Cancer Netw 2011;9:S-1-S-32

[54] Cankovic M, Mikkelsen T, Rosenblum ML, Zarbo RJ. A simplified laboratory validated assay for MGMT MSP analysis of glioblastomamultiforme from formalin-fixed paraffin-embedded tissue. Laboratory Investigation 2007;87:392-397.

[55] Ogino S, Kawasaki T, Brahmandam M, et al. Precision and performance characteristics of bisulfite conversion and real-time PCR (MethyLight) for quantitative DNA methylation analysis. J MolDiagn 2006;8:209-217.

[56] Widschwendter M, Siegmund KD, Muller HM, et al. Association of breast cancer DNA methylation profiles with hormone receptor status and response to tamoxifen. Cancer Res 2004;64:3807-3813.

[57] Eads CA, Danenberg KD, Kawakami K, et al. MethyLight: a high-throughput assay to measure DNA methylation. Nucleic Acids Res 2000;28:e32.

[58] Shibata DM, Sato F, Mori Y, et al. Hypermethylation of HPP1 is associated with hMLH1 hypermethylation in gastric adenocarcinomas. Cancer Res 2002;62:5637-5640.

[59] Jones PA, Baylin SB. The epigenomics of cancer. Cell 2007;128:683-692.

[60] Kim TY, Zhong S, Fields CR, Kim JH, Robertson KD. Epigenomic profiling reveals novel and frequent targets of aberrant DNA methylation-mediated silencing in malignant glioma. Cancer Res 2006;66:7490-7501.

[61] Martinez R, Martin-Subero JI, Rohde V, Kirsch M, Alaminos M, et al. A microarray-based DNA methylation study of glioblastomamultiforme. Epigenetics 2009;4:255-264.

[62] Uhlmann K, Rohde K, Zeller C, Szymas J, et al. Distinct methylation profiles of glioma subtypes. Int J cancer 2003;106:52-59.

[63] Oghaki H, Kleihues P. Genetic pathways to primary and secondary glioblastoma. Am J Pathol 2007;170:1445-1453.

[64] Noushmehr H, Weisenberger DJ, Diefes K, et al. Identification of a CpG island methylator phenotype that defines a distinct subgroup of glioma. Cancer Cell 2010;17:510-522.

[65] Cahill DP, Levine KK, Betensky RA, et al. Loss of the mismatch repair protein MSH6 in human glioblastomas is associated with tumor progression during temozolomide treatment. Clin Cancer Res 2007;13:2038-2045.

[66] Hunter C, Smith R, Cahill DP, et al. A hypermutation phenotype and somatic MSH6 mutations in recurrent human malignant gliomas after alkylator therapy. Cancer Res 2006;66:3987-3991.

[67] Kaina B, Christmann M. DNA repair in resistance to alkylating anticancer drugs. Int J ClinPharmacolTher 2002;40:354-367.

[68] Gerson SL. MGMT: its role in cancer etiology and cancer therapeutics. Nat Rev Cancer 2004;4:296-307.

[69] Esteller M, Herman JG. Generating mutations but providing chemosensitivity: the role of O^6-methylguanine DNA methyltransferase in human cancer. Oncogene 2004;23:1-8.

Chapter 16

Telomeres and Brain Tumors

Domenico La Torre, Giovanni Raffa,
Chiara Tomasello, M'Hammed Aguennouz and
Antonino Germanò

Additional information is available at the end of the chapter

http://dx.doi.org/10.5772/52426

1. Introduction

Brain tumors are a large and heterogeneous group of neoplasms affecting the central nervous system that, despite the progress of the modern medicine, still represent a great challenge for physicians all over the world. The annual global age-standardized incidence of primary malignant brain tumors is ~3.7 per 100,000 for males and 2.6 per 100,000 for females. Rates appear to be higher in more developed countries (males 5.8, and females 4.1 per 100,000) than in less developed countries (males 3.0 and females 2.1 per 100,000). Conversely, the incidence of both primary malignant and non-malignant brain tumors is about 10 - 14 cases per 100,000/ year all over the world, with white males having the highest rate. Males also generally have higher rates of primary malignant brain tumors while females have higher rates of non-malignant tumors, primarily meningiomas. Worldwide age-standardized mortality for primary malignant brain tumors is ~2.8 for male and 2.0 for females per 100,000. Mortality rates differ significantly by histology and age. For example, glioblastoma multiforme (GBM) has a 5-year survival rate of 3.3%, low grade gliomas, such as pilocytic astrocytomas, oligodendrogliomas, and ependymomas have 5-year survival rates of over 70%, while anaplastic astrocytoma, malignant gliomas and lymphomas have 5-year survival rates less than 40% [1].

Due to these dramatic epidemiological data, in the past decades we assisted to the birth of an intensifying interest in understanding the causes of brain tumors among the scientific community. Despite notable advances achieved during recent years in both surgical and chemo/ radiotherapeutic approaches, an improved survival has not been clearly documented, especially for primary malignant brain tumors. This is partially due to the tumors' intrinsic clinical and molecular heterogeneity. As a matter of fact, choice of initial treatment, prediction of survival, stratification of patients, prediction and monitoring of response to therapy, still represent some of the greatest challenges in the management of patients affected by brain tumors. In these settings, different studies have been performed to better understand the pathophysiology of cerebral neoplasms, with the aim to identify new molecular prognostic markers and therapeutic targets. However, until now, molecular biomarkers that effectively predict response to therapy and/or survival outcomes in brain tumors are limited. Consequently, there is a strong need to develop novel and independent markers of prognosis for these neoplasms. One of the cellular structure candidate to accomplish this role is represented by telomeres.

Telomeres consist of long tandem arrays of TTAGGG repeats, bound by proteins, placed at the end of linear chromosomes, which are involved in several essential biological functions [2, 3]. These non-coding telomeric repeats represent a buffer zone preventing the adjacent coding region of the genome from erosion. In normal human cells, the telomeres decreases by some 5-20 repeats with every cell division [4]. Therefore telomere shortening limits the number of times a cell can divide.[5] Hence, they can be considered the mitotic clock by which cells count their divisions and regulate the onset of replicative senescence in somatic cells [6-8]. The alteration of telomere length homeostasis affects telomere structure and leads to genomic instability by generating chromosome end-to end fusion and chromosomal abnormalities [9]. It has been demonstrated that telomeres shortening could initiate successive events, such as aberrant fusions or recombination of the end of chromosomes, genomic instability, loss of cell growth control, and finally cancer development [10, 11]. Hence, cells exhibiting critical telomeres shortening and genomic instability present an increased capacity of dicentric chromosomes formation and susceptibility to oncogenic transformation [5, 12, 13]. Several studies showed the presence of an hypervariability of telomere length in different human solid tumors, including brain tumors, suggesting for telomeres and proteins involved in the modulation of their length a possible clinical role as diagnostic/prognostic marker or therapeutic target for cancer treatment.

2. Telomeres

Human telomeres are regions of 4-15 kilobases of repetitive hexameric (TTAGGG)n guanine-rich DNA sequences at the ends of each chromosome [14]. They end with a single-stranded 3'-overhang that folds back and invades its complementary strand to form a T-loop [15]. Formation of this structure is presumed to involve the insertion of the 3′-telomeric overhang into duplex telomeric DNA, its hybridization with the cytosine-rich strand, and dislodgment of the guanine-rich strand into a displacement loop (D-loop) [16]. It has been demonstrated that T-loops are especially well-adapted to shield the ends of chromosomes from DNA repair and DNA damage-sensing mechanisms [15, 17]. Moreover, a complex of telomere-specific proteins, named shelterin complex, binds and caps telomeres, further preventing chromosomal ends from being recognized as DNA double strand breaks (DSB) by the DNA damage response (DDR) machinery [18, 19]. As the lagging strands of telomeres are incapable of being fully replicated during each round of cell division, telomeres undergo progressive shortening during normal cellular proliferation. Eventually, they become so short that they trigger the DDR, causing cell crisis [4, 18, 20]. This normally results in replicative senescence and even-

http://dx.doi.org/10.5772/52426

tually checkpoint-driven cell death and apoptosis, defining cellular lifespan and safeguarding an organism against unlimited cellular proliferation and cancer [19, 21, 22].

Shelterin complex proteins interact selectively with telomeric DNA and localize to telomeres. In its most abundant form, the complex is composed of six core components: TRF1, TRF2, POT1, TIN2, TPP1 and RAP1[16]. TRF1 and TRF2 (Telomeric Repeat Factors 1 and 2) recognize duplex telomeric DNA whereas POT1 (Protection of Telomere 1) associates with the single-strand telomeric DNA present at the 3′-overhang [23, 24]. The scaffolding subunit TIN2 (TRF1-interacting nuclear protein 2) binds simultaneously to TRF1, TRF2 and TPP1, whereas TPP1 (previously known as TINT 1 [25]) connects POT1 with TIN2 [25-31]. A sixth component, RAP1 (Repressor Activator Protein 1), is a TRF2-associated factor [32]. Via protein–protein interactions, these DNA binding factors bring a number of other proteins to telomeres, where they localize to form a variety of complexes [33, 34], playing a key role in telomere capping and length regulation (see Figure 1).

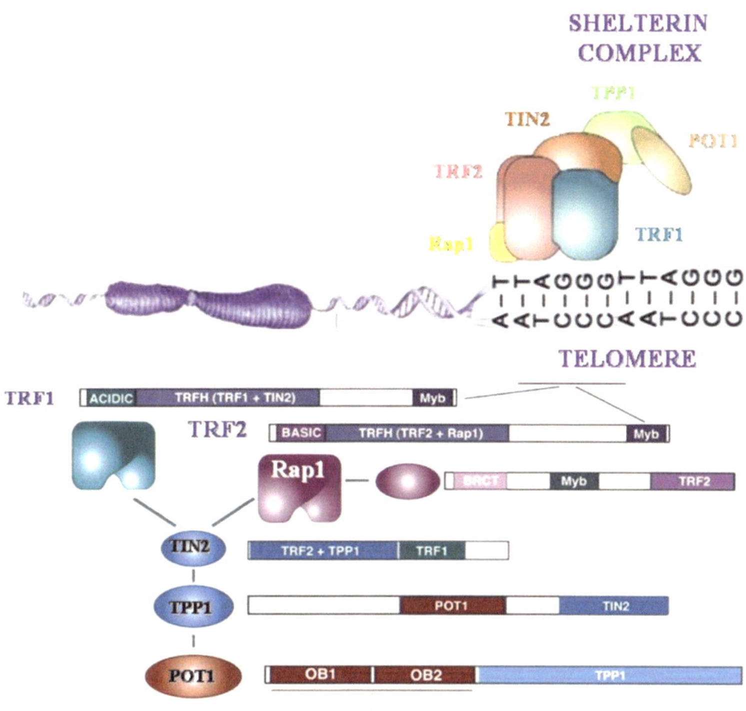

Figure 1. Schematic representation of the six subunits of the Shelterin complex on the telomeric DNA and of their molecular structure, including domains, protein interactions and DNA binding sites.

In addition to this 6-member complex, Shelterin may also be present in the form of sub-complexes that lack either TRF1 or TRF2/RAP1[30, 34-41]. While the importance of these different sub-complexes remains unclear, the particular function of each of the three DNA binding subunits (TRF1, TRF2 and POT1) is well-understood.

TRF1 has a key role in the modulation of telomere length. Its ADP-ribosylation, allow telomerase to bind telomeres and start their elongation.

TRF2 serves to block recognition of telomeres as double-strand DNA breaks. Loss of TRF2 function leads to the activation of the ATM kinase (Ataxia telangiectasia mutated kinase), formation of telomere dysfunction-induced foci (TIFs), and induction of either senescence or apoptosis [21, 36, 42-45]. Moreover, in cells lacking functional checkpoints, telomeres devoid of TRF2 serve as substrates for the NHEJ (non-homologous end-joining) repair mechanism and give rise to interchromosomal fusions [41, 46]. TRF2 also appears to protect telomeres, at least in part, through its ability to promote T-loop formation and maintenance [15, 17].

POT1 serves to hide the 3′-telomeric overhang from telomerase and from DNA damage sensing mechanisms. Hence, the loss of POT1 leads to the activation of the ATR kinase (ATM and Rad3-related kinase), formation of TIFs, and induction of either apoptosis or cell cycle arrest [38, 42, 47, 48]. In cells that lack functional checkpoints, POT1 dysfunction leads to a loss of telomerase regulation that results in longer telomeres [31, 39].

Therefore, through the interaction with the shelterin complex proteins, telomeres protect chromosomes from recombination, end-to-end fusion, and recognition as damaged DNA, providing a means for complete replication of chromosomes.

In summary, telomeres serve as a molecular clock that controls the replicative capacity of human cells and their entry into senescence, but they also contribute to the functional organization of chromosomes within the nucleus and participate in the regulation of gene expression [49, 50].

2.1. Telomere length modulation

During a process of DNA synthesis and cell division, telomeres shorten as a result of the incomplete replication of linear chromosomes. This progressive shortening represent the so-called 'end-replication problem'.

As previously described, in order to prevent degradation by exonucleases or processing as damaged DNA, the telomere 3′ single-strand overhang folds back into the D-loop of duplex telomeric DNA to form a protective 'T-loop', which is reinforced with TRF2 and other telomeric DNA-binding proteins that constitute the shelterin complex [51]. These proteins have a fundamental role in the modulation of telomere length, allowing telomeres elongation or conversely promoting their attrition.

In human cells, several pathways regulating telomeres length have been identified.

The most important mechanism is represented by telomerase, a highly specialized ribonuclear reverse transcriptase enzyme that catalyzes extension of 5′-ends of the lagging DNA strand by adding TTAGGG repeats onto the telomeres using its intrinsic RNA as a template for reverse transcription [52]. Two major subunits of the human telomerase core complex have been identified, named h-TERC and h-TERT. The former serves as a template for telomeres elongation; instead, the latter subunit (h-TERT) contains a reverse transcriptase domain that catalyzes this reaction [53] (see Figure 2).

http://dx.doi.org/10.5772/52426

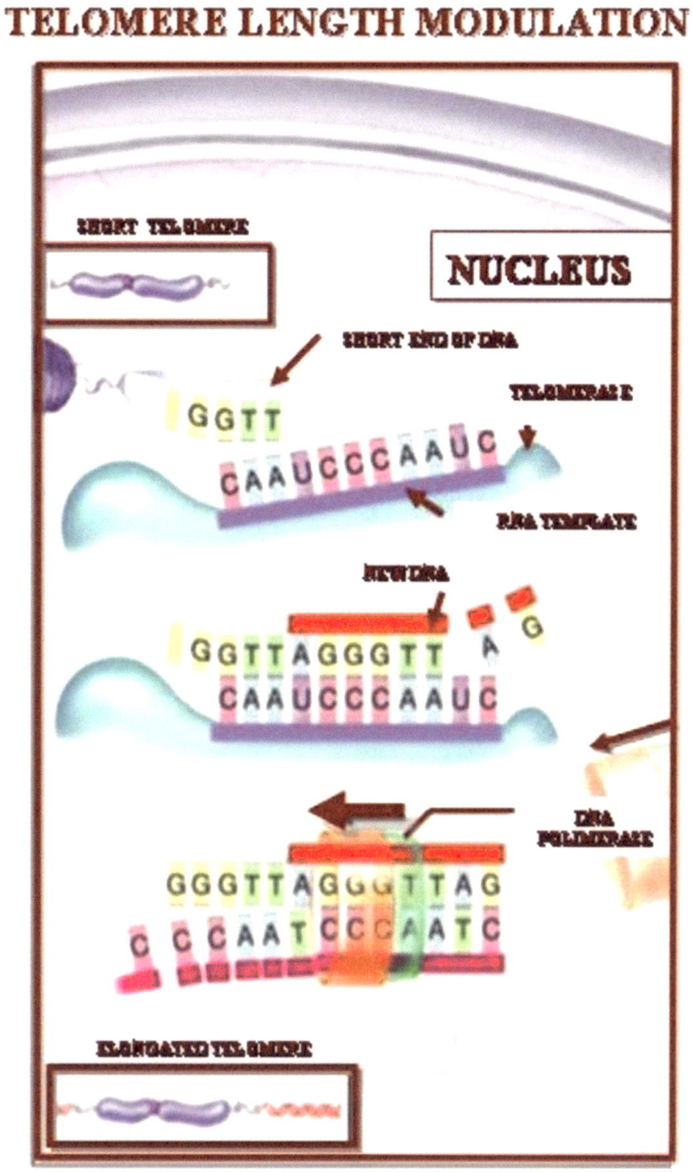

Figure 2. Schematic representation of telomere elongation by telomerase

However, the length and structure of telomeres are also controlled by a variety of proteins, working exclusively at the telomere or contemporarily participating in DNA repair process. Collectively, these telomeric proteins may function to protect telomere integrity and function, to connect the DNA damage/repair network with the controls of cellular senescence, to monitor telomere homeostasis and modify the access of telomerase to telomeres. Two major proteins are the TRF1 and TRF 2 that are localized at telomeres [54]. These proteins play key roles in the maintenance of telomere function and structure modifying telomerase activity [41, 55, 56]. Moreover, a recent evidence shows that TRF1 interacts with other telomere-binding molecules and is integrated into the functional telomere structure [57]. TRF1 accepts adenosine diphosphate (ADP)-ribosylation catalyzed by the tankyrase-poli-ADP-ribose polymerase (TANKs-PARP) complex. The ADP-ribosylation of TRF1 reduces its ability to bind telomeric DNA, allowing telomerase to elongate telomeres and extending the cellular life span [58-60].

In most somatic cells telomerase is produced at very low levels. In contrast, many malignant cells are able to upregulate this enzyme and extend their survival through continuous telomeric elongation [61].

The vast majority of tumor cells use telomerase as preferred mechanism for telomere maintenance, whereas only 10-15% of all cancer lose the functional activity of telomerase and use the telomerase-independent Alternative Lengthening of Telomeres pathway (ALT) that operates via DNA repair and recombination processes [22].

ALT was first deduced in human cell lines from the fact that some telomerase-deficient lines were able to be maintained in culture for many hundreds of population doubling times [62]. Later phenotypic studies revealed that, unlike telomerase-positive cells, ALT-dependent cells almost always contain heterogeneous telomere length distribution and form ALT-associated promyelocytic leukemia (PML) bodies or APBs. [63, 64] These phenotypes are either undetectable or have very low levels of activity in normal somatic cells. [22]

Several characteristic features are associated with ALT activity [65]. First, telomere length distribution is highly heterogeneous and ranges from less than 3 kb to more than 50 kb [66]. In contrast, in human telomerase-positive cells all telomeres typically have a similar length of around 10 kb. Second, ALT-positive cells have been described to contain several classes of extrachromosomal telomeric repeats (ECTRs) in the nucleus. ECTRs comprise double- and single-stranded circular molecules, linear telomeric DNA, and t-complex molecules that consist of high molecular weight DNA with highly branched structures [67-70]. These DNA fragments might be products of t-loop resolution by recombination enzymes. The function of ECTRs in the telomere lengthening process is unknown but the amount of partially single-stranded telomeric $(CCCTAA)_n$ DNA circles (C-circles) appears to correlate with ALT activity [71]. Third, the occurrence of telomere sister chromatid exchanges (T-SCE) is generally increased in ALT cells [72, 73]. Fourth, in ALT cells promyelocytic leukemia nuclear bodies (PML-NBs) associate with some telomeres [64, 74]. These complexes are called ALT-associated PML-NBs (APBs) [64, 65].

Which type of telomere maintenance mechanism is active seems to depend on the origin of the tumor. ALT is rarely found in carcinomas but frequently activated in tumors of mesenchymal and neuroepithelial origin like osteosarcomas, liposarcomas or astrocytomas [75, 76].

Therefore, at least two mechanisms of telomere maintenance, telomerase activity and the recombination-based ALT, may be more or less prevalent in different tissues undergoing tumour formation, leading to the aforementioned features [77, 78]. The activation of such a mechanisms causes the alteration of telomere length that is reflected by a hypervariability of telomere length already observed in different human solid tumors [79-81], and also in brain tumors [82-87]. Hence, analysis of telomere length variations and of length modulation mechanisms may provide promising information for their potential role as prognostic marker or therapeutic target in cancer.

3. Telomere in aging and disease

Aging can be defined as the progressive decline of tissue function that eventually results in mortality [88]. Aging is a natural occurring process and not a disease state. While aging is inevitable for all humans, the speed of age-related functional deterioration varies considerably amongst individuals. Why some individuals reach frailty earlier than others is not understood and genetic factors as well as environmental exposures are believed to modulate the senescence process. Currently, aging is viewed as a generalized process occurring in all organ systems in a parallel fashion [88]. However, recent studies point towards a much higher degree of complexity in the aging process and accumulating data support the notion that diseases incurred during life may accelerate the aging of certain organ systems [89].

Telomeres shorten as we age. Consequently, telomere length has been postulated as a marker of "genetic age" (mitotic clock), as a fundamental explanation for the aging process, and has been marketed as a simple predictor of longevity. Telomere length indeed reflects the cell's past proliferative history and future propensity to apoptosis, senescence, and transformation. However, cellular aging is not equivalent to organ or organismal aging. Studies in humans have attempted to relate short telomeres to longevity. In a provocative initial publication from the University of Utah, individuals around 60 years of age who had the longest telomeres lived longer than did subjects with the shortest telomeres, but the most associated cause of death in the latter group was, inexplicably, infection, and those with shorter telomeres did not have a higher rate of cancer deaths [90]. Heart disease as the cause of death was also more common in subjects with the shortest telomeres. Subsequent studies have produced conflicting findings. The Cardiovascular Health Study of subjects over 65 years of age found that individuals in the shortest quartile for telomere length were 60% more likely to die than those in the longest quartile [91]. Causes of death related to short telomeres were infectious. Two twin studies at older age also correlated shorter telomeres with poorer survival [92, 93]. Finally, a cohort study that looked at participants at time zero and after 10 years found that death within 10 years was significantly more common in those with shorter telomeres [94]. In contrast, these associations have not been confirmed in other studies of older subjects. Njajou and collegues reported that telomere length failed to predict survival, but correlated with years of healthy life [95]. In a Danish study of people aged 73 to 101 years, telomeres correlated with life expectancy in simple univariate analysis but, when corrected for age, did not predict longevity [96]. In Dutch men with a mean age of 78 years, telomere length eroded with aging but failed to correlate with mortality [97]. In a Finnish investigation, telomere length did not predict overall mortality [98]. Finally, in an analysis from California, short telomere length predicted death from cardiovascular disease in women but not in men, where the rate of shortening predicted mortality rather than length itself [99]. Collectively, data on association between telomere length and aging are quite inhomogeneous and contradictory, whereas data on the role of telomere length in human disease are more consistent.

Telomere dysfunction and telomere length alterations have been reported as responsible of various human pathologies, ranging from neurodegenerative to inherited genetic diseases. In the last decade, several studies elucidated telomere's role in the pathophysiology of different diseases at a molecular level. For this reason, measuring of telomeres in peripheral mononuclear cells or in whole blood samples has been applied to patients with a multitude of disease states [100].

Dyskeratosis congenital (DC), is a rare inherited bone marrow failure disease, and can be considered the classic "telomere disease". The inherited defect in X-linked dyskeratosis congenital was identified in a gene named DKC1 [101]. DKC1 encodes dyskerin, a protein that binds to the RNA component of telomerase and stabilizes the telomerase complex. Inheritance is X-linked recessive, autosomal dominant, or autosomal recessive. In addition to the diagnostic triad of nail dystrophy, lacey reticular pigmentation, and oral leukoplakia, patients with DC are at very high risk of bone marrow failure (BMF), cancer, pulmonary and liver disease, and multiple other medical problems [102, 103]. Several studies demonstrated that patients with dyskeratosis congenita have accelerated telomere shortening and that telomere length measurement by flow fluorescence *in situ* hybridization in peripheral blood lymphocytes is an important diagnostic test for DC: in particular, age-adjusted values provide a quantitative measure of disease severity, with shortest telomeres associated to severe variants of DC [104, 105].

Much attention has been given to individuals with atherosclerotic disease and, as a common rule, telomeric length of peripheral mononuclear cells seems to be a strong predictor for disease progression. In particular, leukocyte telomere length is associated with measures of subclinical atherosclerosis [106] and with HDL cholesterol levels [107]. Moreover, cellular aging reflected by shorter leukocyte telomere length is a predictor for advanced atherosclerosis and cardiovascular disease risk [108]. Patients with myocardial infarction have shorter telomeres as compared to controls [109], and reduced leukocyte telomere length has been linked to increased coronary artery calcium [110] and reduction in left ventricular mass.[111] Shortened telomeres have been observed also in white blood cells of patients affected by diabetes type I and II,[112-114] neurodegenerative disease including dementia and Alzheimer disease [115-119], ischemic stroke [120]. All these results suggest an important role of telomere and of its length modulation mechanisms in the pathophysiology of several common diseases, often age-related, encouraging new researches to improve the knowledge about telomere biology and to translate these new informations in the clinical practice for a better patient's management in terms of diagnosis, treatment and prognostic stratification.

4. Telomeres and cancer

Functional telomeres protect chromosome ends from recombination and fusion, and are therefore essential for maintenance of chromosomal stability [3, 121, 122]. The alteration of telomere length homeostasis affects telomere structure and leads to genomic instability by generating chromosome end-to-end fusion and chromosomal abnormalities [9]. It has been demonstrated that telomeres shortening could initiate successive events, such as aberrant fusion or recombination of the end of chromosomes, genomic instability, loss of cell growth control, and finally cancer development [10, 11]. Cells exhibiting critical telomeres shortening and genomic instability thus present an increased capacity of dicentric chromosomes formation and susceptibility to oncogenic transformation [5, 12, 13].

The phenomenon of telomeres alteration during carcinogenesis and cancer progression is well known and established at the molecular level [123-125]. Several studies demonstrated the presence of telomere length alterations in different human solid tumors, such as prostate, breast, colorectal, head and neck cancer [81]. These alterations are widely variable, resulting in both telomere attrition and elongation as compared to adjacent normal tissues. In the majority of cases, telomere length seems to be reduced in human tumors [126-131], even if it tends to increase along with malignancy of tumors [79, 132, 133].

In particular, telomere dysfunction has been extensively studied in the most common solid tumors. These studies demonstrated telomere length modification in different histologies as compared to normal tissue due to the alteration of telomere length modulation mechanisms [81]. This differences have been widely analysed in order to identify new cancer biomarkers, to investigate the eventual correlation with patient's prognosis and to discover new targeted molecular therapies.

In breast cancer, multiple studies have showed that telomere shortening is associated with increased risk and poor outcome, and can thus be used as a prognostic factor to predict the course of disease. The first report describing the use of telomere length as a possible prognostic marker in breast cancer was published by Odagiri and collegues [130]. In this study, telomere length analysis was performed in a cohort of 41 patients diagnosed with breast cancer and showed that telomere length was significantly reduced in tumor tissues (8.1 ± 0.6 kb) as compared to that of the adjacent normal breast tissues (9.7 ± 0.5 kb) in 18 of 22 patients ($p > 0.05$). Subsequent studies confirmed the potential role of telomere length as clinical biomarker in breast cancer, including Fordyce et al. [127] who reported measurements of telomere length in 2 independent sets of breast tumors containing a total of 140 samples. This study showed that telomere alterations include both telomere attrition and elongation. In fact, only 50% of all tumors had telomere values in the normal range. Moreover, in this study telomere length was associated with tumor size ($p = 0.02$), TNM stage ($p = 0.004$), 5-year overall survival ($p = 0.0001$) and 5-year disease-free survival ($p = 0.0004$) and, in particular, reduced telomere length was associated with nodal involvement ($p < 0.0001$).

Recent investigations concerning prostate cancer suggest that reduced telomere length is associated with poor clinical outcome and markers of disease progression [126, 128]. The first reported study was performed by Donaldson and colleagues in 1999 and represented a retrospective investigation of the relationship between clinical outcomes in patients with organ-confined prostate adenocarcinoma and telomere length [128]. In this archival case-controlled study, association analysis for telomere length and survival and telomere length and biochemical recurrence indicated by PSA levels of > 2.5ng/ml, revealed that reduced telomere length correlated with death ($p < 0.0001$) and disease recurrence ($p < 0.0001$), even if there was no statistical association with patients' ages at diagnosis, nodal statuses, pathological grades or Gleason sum scores. This finding was recently confirmed in a larger retrospective population-based study comprising 77 men who underwent prostatectomy between 1982 and 1995 [126]. In this cohort, telomere length was a predictor of time to recurrence when adjusted for age at diagnosis, Gleason sum score and pelvic node involvement.

Although relatively rare, researches on the role of telomeres in lung cancer showed that telomerase expression and activity can be considered important contributors to the malignant phenotype in lung epithelial cells, and have been proposed to be of potential prognostic value [134]. Conversely, reports on the use of telomere length to predict lung cancer progression are scarce. Shirotani et al. investigated the relationship between telomere length and various characteristics of tumor cells in 46 lung cancer specimens, comprising 40 primary and 6 metastatic lesions [135]. In partial accordance with recent studies in breast and prostate cancers [126, 127], the authors observed both elongation (2 cases) and reduction of telomere length (13 cases) in the 16 small cell carcinomas of the sample set. The 2 cases with telomere elongation were associated with a poor prognosis. Similarly, in the adenocarcinoma samples of this study, both telomere reduction and elongation were observed, but a clear association with patients prognosis was not reported. Hirashima et al. evaluated the prognostic significance of telomere length alterations in cancer and normal lung tissues obtained from 72 patients with histologically confirmed pathological stage I-IIIA non-small cell lung cancer (NSCLC) [136]. In this study, the 25 patients (34.7%) with alterations in telomere length, elongation or attrition, had significantly shorter survival durations than those of the others.

The use of telomeres as prognostic factors in colorectal carcinoma has been suggested in several studies performed by the groups led by Siewert and coworkers[132, 137] and by Iniesta and collegues [133]. It is interesting that these studies showed an opposite relationship as compared to studies in other cancer types [126-129, 131], with longer telomeres associated with poor prognosis. This difference may be explained considering the different regulation of telomerase expression in colorectal epithelial cells. Normal colorectal epithelium, in fact, has been showed to contain cells of possible stem cell origin that are telomerase-positive and presumably counteract telomere attrition due to physiologically high cell proliferation rates, and total cell loss due to physiological shedding in this specialized cell compartment [138]. Consequently, it is possible that the existing high telomerase activity may affect cells undergoing tumor initiation and results in elongated telomeres in cells of colorectal cancer.

Studies indicating the prognostic potential of telomeres have also been reported for head and neck cancer. Patel et al. studied telomere alterations in tumor and adjacent normal tissues in 110 patients with head and neck cancer (squamous cell carcinomas of the oral cavity, larynx and pharynx) and 40 patients with precancerous and benign conditions (leukoplakia, submucous fibrosis, erythroplakia, hemangioma) [79]. Telomere lengths in this sample set were significantly lower in malignant tissues as compared with the tumor adjacent normal tissues. In addition, 2-year disease-free survival analysis showed that patients with longer telomeres in malignant tissues had poor disease-free survival. These findings are in agreement with that reported for colorectal carcinoma and lung [132, 133, 135, 137], and in contrast to other cancer histologies [126-129]. A possible explanation for these interesting discrepancies in head and neck cancer is the fact that telomerase activity was observed in over half of the adjacent normal tissues. As before discussed for colorectal carcinoma, altered regulation of telomerase expression in cells undergoing transformation may explain the elongated telomeres in the tumors.

Collectively, these findings suggest that hypervariability of telomere length in various human solid tumors probably reflects the differential regulation of telomerase expression in cancer cells and depends on the different stages of carcinogenesis and tumor progression. Therefore, analysis of telomere length may have a clinical relevance as a prognostic marker in human solid tumors, whereas analysis of the mechanisms of length modulation, such as telomerase and ALT, can suggest new molecular target for advanced therapeutic strategies.

5. Telomeres and brain tumors

Brain tumors research is being performed worldwide at a remarkable pace, with some of the more recent promising studies focused on identification of aberrant genetic events and signalling pathways, tumor stem cell identification and characterization, modulation of tumor immunological responses, combination therapies, and understanding of the rare long-term survivors. Identification of additional indicators will enable better patients' stratification and individualization of treatment is needed to more accurately determine patient's prognosis and to identify novel therapeutic approaches that can optimize patient's outcome. A growing body of knowledge suggests a potential role of telomere length measurement in different tumors. Nevertheless, even if its clinical use is not completely established, a number of studies demonstrated that it can be helpful to patients stratification, to provide useful information about patient's prognosis and, in some case, to suggest new therapeutic strategies in cancer.

Although not entirely consistent in the type of telomere alteration, i.e., attrition vs. elongation, and unclear on the underlying mechanisms, multiple studies have showed that telomere dysfunctions are associated with parameters of clinical outcome in patients with brain tumors. A possible explanation for these interesting discrepancies in brain tumors is the fact that different expression and/or altered regulation of telomerase expression in tumor cells may reflects the underlying biology of telomere maintenance and its dysfunction over time. In telomerase positive tumor cells, telomere length is balanced by telomere shortening due to cell division and telomere elongation by telomerase. Therefore, telomere length is maintained by telomerase activity that can be influenced in different ways and by various factors. This mechanism keeps tumour cells proliferating and growing by the stabilization of their telomeres which is essential to maintain the unlimited dividing potential and to escape from 'crisis' [49, 123, 139]. As well as in almost all malignant tumors, World Health Organization (WHO) high grade brain tumors are associated to higher telomerase activity than benign tumors, such as schwannomas, meningiomas [140] or normal brain tissue [141]. Increased telomerase expression has been also associated with higher proliferative index, tumor grading, age, vascular and endothelial proliferation [142], poor outcome [83, 143, 144], and it increases with malignancy from low-grade to high-grade brain tumors [83, 145].

Therefore, understanding the context and mechanisms by which telomeres length contribute to cancer development is the next logical research step and may represent an interesting research field in order to elucidate brain tumors biology. Moving toward the study of molecular mechanisms controlling telomere length, included telomerase and ALT, will not only provide insight into the complex etiology of brain tumors but also promises to provide novel targets for cancer therapy.

In these settings, several studies have been performed to analyze telomere biology in brain tumors, with the aim to better understand the patophysiology of these tumors for improving prognosis of patients affected by such terrible neoplasms.

5.1. Astrocytic gliomas

Astrocytic tumors represent about the 23% of primary brain and CNS tumours and, in particular, astrocytomas and glioblastomas (GBMs) account for 76% of all gliomas. The incidence of such tumours tends to increase with age, although some histological variants are more frequent in specific age ranges. For example, pilocytic astrocytomas affect exclusively childhood, being the most common brain tumor between 5 and 14 years old. Conversely, the incidence of glioblastomas increases with age, with the highest rates in the 75 to 84 years old. The prognosis can be different according to histology. For low grade astrocytomas (grade I and II), prognosis is usually good and a gross total surgical excision alone represents a sufficient therapeutic strategy. Conversely, for high grade astrocytomas (i.e. glioblastomas WHO IV), although a multimodal therapeutic strategy consisting of radical surgical removal, chemotherapy and radiotherapy, prognosis remains poor. For example, five–year survival rates are 94% for pilocytic astrocytomas but are less than 5% for glioblastomas. Survival generally decreases with older age at diagnosis. Children and young adults have better survival for most histologies [146].

Several studies focused on astrocytomas showed an association between telomerase activity and reduced telomeres length in high grade tumors. Liu et al. analyzed telomere length in a series of astrocytic tumors. Telomere length measurement was performed using a telomere specific restriction enzyme and Southern blot analysis. The authors observed a progressive shortening of the telomere restriction fragments (TRFs) in astrocytomas from WHO grade I to IV as compared to TRFs of normal brain tissue, with no significant differences between primary and recurrent GBMs [87]. These findings support the hypothesis that telomere shortening is one of the important genetic events during transformation of astrocytomas and progression to higher grades.

Subsequent studies were focused on the analysis of the relationship between telomere length and telomerase activity, suggesting new interesting hypothesis about telomere maintenance mechanisms during the neoplastic transformation and progression of astrocytic tumors. In 1997, Morii and colleagues, analysed telomere length and telomerase activity in a series of 20 gliomas (WHO grade I to IV), including 1 pilocytic astrocytomas, 7 oligoastrocytomas, 1 anaplastic astrocytoma (AA) and 11 GBMs. In their series, telomerase-positive samples had a mean TRF length of <10 kb, whereas telomerase-negative samples all had long heterogeneous TRFs which exhibited an increased signal peak from 10 to 20 kb. The authors concluded that telomerase-negative gliomas had longer TRFs compared with telomerase positive ones, suggesting that, in addition to the telomerase-dependent mechanism, an alternative telomerase-independent mechanism (ALT) for telomere maintenance may be present in human gliomas [86]. Hiraga et al, in 1998, performed the most complete analysis of telomere length in human brain tumors, comparing TRFs length and telomerase activity in 160 neuroepithelial and non-neuroepithelial brain tumors. Among grade I-IV astrocytomas, the authors compared telomere length between telomerase-positive and telomerase-negative samples vs normal brain tissue (NBT). TRFs were shorter in tumors with telomerase activity than telomerase-negative samples and NBT samples. Specifically, the detection rates of telomerase activity were widely different for different histopathological entities. Telomerase activity was detected in none of pilocytic astrocytomas, in 20.0% (3 of 15) of grade II astrocytomas, 40% (6 of 15) of anaplastic astrocytomas and 72.3% (34 of 47) of glioblastomas, suggesting that telomerase activity tend to increase with the malignancy of astrocytic tumors. In particular, all pilocytic astrocytomas (3 of 3) were telomerase negative and showed longer TRFs as compared to normal brain tissue. TRFs in grade II astrocytomas and anaplastic astrocytomas with telomerase activity were shorter as compared to the same tumors without telomerase activity. Lastly, 80% of the progression GBMs exhibited reduced mean TRF length (7.747 kb) compared with NBT and origin tumors, and telomerase was reactivated in 100% (10 of 10) of cases. In summary, the mean TRF length of tumors with telomerase activity was significantly shorter than that of tumors with undetectable telomerase activity for each tumor entity [139].

These results suggest that telomerase activity strongly correlates with malignancy and potential progression of the astrocytic tumors, being often associated with reduced telomere length.

These findings were confirmed by Le et collegues, in 1998 [83]. The authors performed an analysis of telomere length and telomerase activity in a series of 69 grade I-IV gliomas. From the analysis of all series, the authors concluded that telomerase activity is present in most glioma samples (72%), but that the frequency of such activity increases with malignancy, being higher in high grade gliomas (HGGs) than in low grade gliomas (LGGs), and is often associated with telomeres shortening. This can be explained with the relative low replicative rate of LGG tumor cells. When the proliferative activity increases, such as during the progression to HGGs, the increased mitotic activity causes a progressive telomeres shortening. In this condition, the activation of telomerase activity represents the only way to escape from cell crisis and apoptosis. This can explain the presence of high telomerase activity and reduced TRFs only in a small percentage of LGGs that probably presents a more aggressive behavior than the telomerase negative LGGs with normal or elongated telomeres. This demonstrates an increasing telomerase activity with the more malignancy of gliomas samples, underlying the role of telomerase and TRFs length as marker of malignancy.

Similar findings were found by Maes and collegues in 2007 [145]. They conducted a study focusing on the relationship between telomerase activity and telomere length in a series of 53 intracranial tumors, including 2 low grade astrocytomas, 1 anaplastic astrocytomas, and 11 GBMs. Again, in this study the authors demonstrated that telomere length was reduced in high-grade tumours, whereas it was compatible or elongated as compared to normal brain tissues in low-grade astrocytomas, suggesting that telomerase activity with shortened telomeres correlates with the aggressive growth of high-grade gliomas.

Harada and colleagues [147] analyzed possible differences of telomerase activity and telomere length among primary and secondary GBMs. Summarizing their findings, TRFs were always shorter than NBT samples, but not statistically significant differences between primary and secondary GBMs were found. Interestingly, although the latter presented significantly higher levels of telomerase activity and hTERT expression than the former, telomere length was anyway shorter than normal brain tissue. The authors explained this apparent discrepancy suggesting that telomerase activation occurs late in carcinogenesis, when the high replication rate of tumor cells already caused telomeres shortening. At this point, activation of telomerase represents the principal mechanism to escape from apoptosis and cell death. Conversely, in primary GBMs, shorter telomere length can be explained by a reduced telomerase activity that might have less influence on carcinogenesis and, hence, other unknown factors might facilitate their cellular immortality.

Although the vast majority of the researches have been performed focusing their attention to telomere length and telomerase expression in astrocytic gliomas, recently several studies showed an increasing interest also to the analysis of the relation between ALT mechanism, telomere length and patients prognosis.

The presence of elongated telomeres and of an alternative mechanism of telomere length maintenance (ALT) was demonstrated to be associated to a better prognosis in patients affected by GBMs by Hakin-Smith et al. in 2003 [148]. Their work represents the first report describing the relationship among ALT pattern, telomere length, and prognosis in human GBMs. In this study, the authors analyzed telomerase activity and telomere lengths in 77 GBM patients. ALT phenotype patients had a median survival of 542 days compared with 247 days in those without the ALT phenotype. Moreover, ALT phenotype was associated with elongated telomeres, benign biology and better prognosis. Therefore, the presence of ALT could be a positive prognostic marker in glioblastoma multiforme.

The first study that analyzed the ALT prevalence among different grades of astrocytic tumors was performed by Henson and coworkers in 2005. In their study, the authors analyzed the prevalence of ALT phenotype and telomerase activity in a series of 40 astrocytomas, composed by 7 WHO grade II-III astrocytomas and 33 GBMs. This study showed for the first time that the prevalence of ALT associated to elongated telomeres is significantly higher in grade II to III astrocytomas as compared to GBMs.

On the basis of Henson's results, in 2010 Slatter and collegues conducted a study focusing on the analysis of ALT prevalence in a series of 48 astrocytic tumors from grade I to IV. In agreement with previous studies by Hakin-Smith and Henson [148, 149], ALT phenotype was more frequent in low grade astrocityc tumors, whereas telomerase activity was prevalent in the higher grades.

Collectively, these studies demonstrated that telomerase activity correlates with malignancy of astrocytic tumors, being higher with the increasing WHO grading [83, 86, 87, 139, 145, 147, 150]. Therefore, telomerase activity and reduced telomeres should be considered a potential biomarker of aggressive behaviour of these neoplasms. Conversely, low grade astrocytomas are usually telomerase-negative and have compatible or elongated telomeres as compared to normal brain tissue [83, 86, 139, 145, 149]. In these tumors, the only telomere length maintenance mechanism is represented by ALT [149, 150]. Henson et al [149] and Slatter and collegues [150] documented that ALT phenotype is associated to elongated telomeres and it is more frequent in low grade astrocityc tumors as compared to GBMs. Moreover, Hakin-Smith and collegues [148] demonstrated that, despite the ALT phenotype associated to elongated telomeres is rarely documented in GBMs, when present it is associated to a longer survival, suggesting its possible role as a positive prognostic markers in GBMs. These findings can be explained considering the biological role of telomeres. In normal tissues as in neoplastic cells, telomeres undergo progressive shortening during each cell replication. When telomeres are critically shortened, the cell cannot preserve anymore its own chromosomic ends and goes toward cell crisis and subsequent apoptosis. Therefore, telomeres represent the biologic clock of cells and constitute one of the most important structure that can preserve cells from senescence. This is the reason why tumor cells need a robust telomere maintenance mechanism to allow an high replicative activity, escaping from cell death. It is well known that high grade brain tumors are malignant neoplasms with an high replicative activity. Consequently, they need a mechanism of telomere maintenance that allows cell division avoiding excessive telomere shortening that can determine cell death. Telomerase seems to accomplish this role with success, especially in high grade tumors. This can be the explanation of the higher telomerase activity found in brain tumors with the increasing of WHO grading. Hence, the highest levels of telomerase expression are found in GBMs. Conversely, low grade astrocytic tumor have a slow replication rate and thus they does not need telomerase. According to the aforementioned studies, in these tumors the slow growing rate is accompanied by a sluggish cell division rate. This can be the reason why the most part of the studies in the literature documents elongated telomeres in low grade tumors. In these neoplasms, the main telomere length maintenance mechanism is represented by ALT. Being specific of benign or slightly aggressive tumors, ALT and elongated telomere are associated to a better survival [149, 150] even if these features are found in a low percentage of high grade brain tumors, such as GBMs [148]. When low grade tumors progress to higher grade, the increasing replicative activity causes a progressive telomere shortening. In this condition, the only way to escape from cell death is the activation of telomerase activity. This is typically observed in progression GBMs [139].

In summary, high telomerase activity and reduced telomere seem to be features of high grade astrocytic tumors, whereas elongated telomeres and ALT phenotype are specific of low grade ones and, therefore, correlates with a better prognosis.

Different studies have also been performed to analyze the role of the Shelterin proteins in the pathophysiology of several neoplasms, including brain tumors. Telomere-specific DNA-binding proteins, such as TRF1, have been put forward as additional candidates for the role of molecules modifying telomerase activity, and they have been suggested to play key roles in the maintenance of telomere function [41, 55, 56]. It has been demonstrated that overexpression of TRF1 inhibits telomere elongation in telomerase-positive cells [151], resulting in gradual and progressive telomeres shortening to the "mortality stages," the proliferative barriers that lead to a non-dividing state and cell death [24, 151, 152]. The mutation or deletion of TRF1 can result in telomere elongation and extend cell survival [151]. Overexpression of a dominant negative TRF1, which removes endogenous TRF1 from telomeres, results in telomere lengthening in telomerase-positive cells [151] [153]. Therefore, the expression of TRF1 is considered a physiological homeostatic mechanism that controls the proliferative potential of normal cells by inhibiting the activity of telomerase [151].

It has been demonstrated that TRF1 is expressed in astroglial brain tumors of different grades, whereas it is not expressed in normal brain tissue. Such expression decreases from low-grade through high grade astrocytomas [123]. This finding may suggest that the loss of TRF1 expression capability, being the result of down- regulation of TRF1 expression in malignant gliomas cells, may play a role in the cell immortalization of astroglial brain tumors.

Furthermore, according to the role of telomerase in the elongation of telomeres in high grade astrocytic tumors, several studies suggested its possible role as molecular target for new therapeutic strategies. Marian et al demonstrated that the telomerase antagonist Imetelstat efficiently targets glioblastoma tumor-initiating cells leading to a decreased proliferation and tumor growth [154]. Gurung and collegues showed that Thymoquinone induces telomere attrition, DNA damage, cell cycle arrest and apoptosis in the glioblastoma cells by inhibiting the activity of telomerase [155]. Lin et al documented that Butylidenephthalide (BP) inhibits proliferation and induces senescence in human glioblastomas by downregulating hTERT expression and consequently telomerase activity [156]. From this perspective, telomerase represent a promising target for new specific therapeutic approaches for the personalized treatment of telomerase-positive high grade astrocytic tumors.

5.2. Ependymomas, oligodendrogliomas and mixed tumors

Ependymomas are tumors that arise from ependymal cells lining the cerebral ventricles and the central canal of the spinal cord. They represent the 5-6% of intracranial gliomas (69% occur in children) and 60% of spinal cord gliomas (96% occur in adult) [157]. In pediatrics they are usually intracranial (the most common localization is the posterior fossa), whereas in adults they tend to be spinal. The treatment of choice is the radical surgical excission followed by radiotherapy (XRT), whereas the role of chemotherapy is very limited. The operative mortality is 5-8%, the 5 year survival is 20-30% in pediatrics and 80% in adults [158, 159].

Data on telomeric alterations in adult and pediatric intracranial ependymomas are slightly inhomogeneous. In 2008 Ridely et al. performed an analysis of telomere length in a series of 21 primary and recurrent pediatric intracranial ependimomas from 7 patients (6 primary tumors and 15 recurrences) [84]. Telomerase activity was detected in 19 tumors (86%), and particularly it was evident in 11 of 14 primary tumors and in all recurrent tumors. Mean telomere length ranged from 7.3 to 16.7 kb, with telomere maintenance observed in five of seven patients (71%). Of these five cases, four showed telomere lengthening and one had compatible TRFs in relapsed tumors as compared to the primary tumor. Conversely, telomere shortening occurred in two of seven recurrent cases (29%).

The authors concluded that variable TRFs length and evidence for telomerase-mediated telomere maintenance were present in the majority of pediatric ependymoma recurrent cases (71%), whereas TRFs shortening was evident in a minority (29%). These results implicate telomerasemediated telomere maintenance as a key mechanism facilitating tumor progression in pediatric ependymoma.

This was demonstrated by the fact that all recurrent tumors analyzed were telomerase positive, although telomere length was reduced only in small percentage of cases.

In the same year, Tabori et al evaluated TRFs length in a series of 26 pediatric intracranial ependymomas (grade II and III), analyzing an eventual correlation with patients' prognosis [85]. Telomerase activity was detected in 73% of tumor samples but TRFs length was widely variable (mean 6.5 kb,range 3.6–9.1 kb). Based on these findings, although ependymomas rely predominantly on telomerase activity to maintain their telomere length, the authors concluded that there was no correlation between telomere length and telomerase expression or survival. Although it seems to emerge that the majority of intracranial ependymomas (especially in children) shows telomerase activity, telomere length appears to be widely variable. Therefore, there is a lack of a firm correlation of telomere length with telomerase expression that do not allows to get definitive conclusions about their possible role as prognostic marker in these neoplasms. It is more probable that these findings reflect an high molecular variability of intracranial ependymomas.

Oligodendrogliomas arise from oligodendroglia cells. They represent 25-33% of glial tumors [160, 161] and have an incidence peak at 40 years, with a smaller earlier peak in childhood between 6-12 years [162]. They show a slight preference for male, with a male-female ratio of 3:2. In 90% of cases they are supratentorial. Surgery is the treatment of choice; chemotherapy is recommended, whereas XRT is suggested only for anaplastic variants [163]. The median survival for surgically treated lesions is 35 months [164], although the ten-year survival is about 10-30% [165]. According to Nurnberg [82] and Hiraga [139], oligodendrogliomas seem to have compatible or longer telomeres than normal brain tissues and detectable telomerase activity. The lack of reduced telomeres in telomerase positive tumor samples can be considered a marker of the less aggressive behavior of such tumors.

Different results have been reported for oligoastrocytomas, that show shorter telomeres than normal brain tissue associated to high telomerase activity [86]. This pattern is more frequent in the anaplastic variant, confirming the role of telomerase activity associated to reduced telomeres as markers of aggressive behavior in these neoplasms as in astrocytic gliomas[139].

5.3. Meningiomas

Meningiomas are extra-axial, usually benign tumors with a slow growing rate that arise from arachnoid cells. They account for 34% of all primary brain and CNS tumors [146]. The incidence peak is at 45 years with a male-female ratio of 1:2,2. About 1.5% occur in childhood and adolescence between 10-20-yeras age [166]. Surgery is the treatment of choice for symptomatic meningiomas and the five-year survival is 91.3% [167].

Benign mengiomas (WHO grade I) show a variable telomere length [82, 139, 168], sometimes slightly shorter than normal meningeal tissue [145], whereas atypical and anaplastic meningiomas show telomerase activity associated with a significant telomere length shortening [169]. This can be explained considering that the slow growth of benign meningiomas and the absence of telomerase activity cause an equally slow shortening of telomeres, whereas the higher replicative capacity of atypical and especially of malignant meningiomas determines a more evident reduction of telomere length. In these settings, the activation of telomerase activity can give to the cell the capacity to escape from senescence and, consequently, an high proliferative strength. Therefore detectable telomerase activity and shortened telomere length suggest that the tumor contains a cell population with the capacity for unlimited proliferation.

These results indicate that telomere shortening together with telomerase activity may be a critical step in pathogenesis of atypical and malignant meningiomas and may correlate with their malignant behavior. Indeed, as previously discussed for astrocytic tumors, the association of telomerase activity with reduced telomeres length may be considered a marker of an aggressive behavior also in meingiomas, being more frequent in atypical and malignant meningiomas.

5.4. Schwannomas

Schwannomas are benign, usually encapsulated, peripheral nerve sheath tumor composed of neoplastic Schwann cells that can have an intracranial or spinal localization. They account for about 8-10% of intracranial and 25-30% of spinal tumors. The peak of incidence is between the 4th and 6th decades [146]. The vast majority of intracranial Schwannomas develops from vestibular nerve. Tumors of trigeminal or facial nerve are far less common. Management includes many options: surgery, wait and see strategy for little or no growth tumors, radiation therapy alone or in conjunction with surgery, chemotherapy, radiosurgery [170].

Schwannomas usually show reduced telomeres, benign pathological features, low proliferative indices and a lack of telomerase activity [169, 171]. These peculiarities allows such tumors to have a benign clinical course. Conversely, rarely they can assume an aggressive behaviour that is characterized by malignant pathological features and high replicative potential that are usually associated to elongated telomeres. This can be explained considering that long telomeres allow tumor cells to maintain an high proliferative capacity without the need of telomerase activity. When the length of the telomere is long enough for proliferation, the telomerase activity subsides.

For these reasons, telomeres elongation, even in absence of telomerase activity, can be considered a marker of aggressive clinicopathological behaviour in schwannomas [169, 171].

5.5. Primitive Neuroectodermal Tumors (PNETS)

Primary neuroectodermal tumors (PNETs), also called embryonal tumors, represent 1 % of all primary central nervous system (CNS) tumors. They are frequent especially in children, representing the most frequent brain and CNS tumor in the range between 0 and 4 years old [146].

They are highly malignant lesions and can disseminate via CSF spontaneously or iatrogenically [172]. Extraneural metastases can also occur. Radical surgical excision is the treatment of choice. XRT is indicated following surgical removal, but it should be avoided at all if possible before 3 years of age to avoid intellectual impairment and growth retardation. Overall survival rate for PNETs is substantially poor with an expected 3 year progression free survival of approximately 50% for localized supratentorial PNETs [173].

PNETs usually show telomerase activity even if there is not a clear association with telomere length. Despite Hiraga [139] and Rahman [174] reported reduced telomeres in the most part of tumor samples, data from Didiano [175] document a wide variability of telomeres length. Interestingly, Rahman reported shorter telomere length in PNETs cells than GBMs, suggesting an higher replicative activity in the former as compared to the latter. These results underline and explain the aggressive behaviour of neuroectodermal tumors. The same author, reported a minority of cases with elongated telomeres and undetectable telomerase activity, suggesting ALT as alternative mechanism of telomere maintenance in these tumors [174].

In summary, telomerase activity can be considered a marker of PNETs and can explain the malignancy of these tumors, although there is not an evident correlation with telomere length. Moreover, in a little percentage of cases without telomerase activity, the aggressive behaviour of PNETs is due to ALT and is associated to elongated telomeres, that allow tumour cells to actively replicate [175].

5.6. Pituitary adenomas

Pituitary adenomas are usually benign tumors that arise from anterior pituitary cells (adenohypophysis). They represent about 13% of primary brain and CNS tumors with an incidence peak on 3th and 4th decades of life [146]. Treatment of pituitary adenomas include medical treatment (dopamine agonists, somatostatin, etc), surgery (transcranial or transsphenoidal approach) or XRT (in case of recurrence that cannot be surgically removed or treated medically).

Their usually benign behaviour can be explained with the lack of telomerase activity, although telomere length is slightly reduced as compared to normal brain tissue [139]. Sometimes they can recur or, rarely, they can progress to pituitary adenocarcinomas. As demonstrated by Harada and colleagues, during progression to carcinoma, the replicative activity of tumor cells causes a progressive shortening of telomeres and the reactivation of telomerase [176]. Therefore, also in pituitary adenomas, telomerase activity and reduced telomere length can be considered marker of aggressive behaviour and can be used to predict the progression to carcinomas.

5.7. Primary Central Nervous System Lymphomas (PCNSLs)

Primary central nervous system lymphomas (PCNSL) also known as primary brain lymphomas are a primary intracranial tumors appearing mostly in patients with severe immunosoppression (typically patients with AIDS). They represent the 0.5-1.2% of intracranial tumours and less than 1 % of extranodal non-Hodgkin lymphomas (NHL), although in the last years there was a progressive increase of incidence also in immunocompetent patients. They affect all age groups, but are most commonly diagnosed in people who are over 50 years of age. Histologically they are a form of extranodal, high-grade non-Hodgkin lymphoma. Most PCNSLs (about 90%) are diffuse large B-cell lymphomas (DLBCLs); the remaining 10% are poorly characterized low-grade lymphomas, Burkitt lymphomas, and T-cell lymphomas [177]. PCNSLs originate inside the CNS and typically remain confined, rarely spreading outside the nervous system. Although the origin cells are lymphocytes, PCNSLs can be assimilated to brain tumors for their intracranial localization and relationship with brain parenchyma and brain blood barrier that gives PCNSLs the same therapeutic challenges (i.e. in terms of drug delivery through the blood brain barrier) of the other brain tumors.

Data from the literature demonstrate that in PCNSLs have variable telomere length, usually reduced as compared with normal brain tissue, and show high telomerase activity [139, 178].

Harada et al demonstrated a statistically significant correlation between telomerase activity and the survival period of patients with PCNSL. In particular, patients with high telomerase activity had poor prognosis and short survival, regardless of telomere length [178].

These findings suggest that telomerase activity represents a common features in PCNSLs and can be considered by itself a marker for predicting a poor prognosis, regardless of telomeres length, the age at onset and the KPS score before the initial treatment. Nevertheless, telomeres are usually shortened in these tumors and this can explain the aggressive behavior of such tumors, even if the association with patients' survival has not been demonstrated.

5.8. Other intracranial tumors

Only few studies have been performed focusing on the analysis of telomere length and telomerase activity among less common non-neuroepithelial tumors, such as hemangioblastomas, hemangioperycitomas and germ cell tumors.

Hemangioblastomas are benign tumors that usually show normal telomere length and undetectable telomerase activity. Nevertheless, the rare cases of hemangioblastomas with aggressive behavior show shorter telomeres than normal brain tumors and are telomerase-positive [139].

Conversely, malignant non-neuroepithelial tumors such as hemangioperycitomas and germ cell tumors, usually show high telomerase activity associated to an important shortening of telomere length [139].

This suggest that, also for these rare non-neuroepithelial brain tumors, telomerase activity associated to reduced telomere length can be considered a marker of malignancy.

6. Conclusions

There is a desperate need for developing innovative diagnostic tools and therapies for brain tumors.

According to their role in the regulation of cell replication and senescence, telomeres and telomeric proteins represent a new interesting research field to better understand the alterations responsible of carcinogenesis and malignant progression of human brain tumors. In these settings, elucidation of telomeres biology represents the new frontier of cancer research. Although a lot of studies have already been focused on this promising field, further studies should be performed to better understand the pathways involved in the telomeres length maintenance and, consequently, in the process of carcinogenesis and malignant progression of human brain tumors, in order to discover new diagnostic/prognostic tools or new therapeutic strategies for improving prognosis of patients affected by these terrible neoplasms.

Acknowledgements

The study was financed by COFIN 2008 prot. 2008979M8K-001 by Italian Ministry of University and Research

Author details

Domenico La Torre[1*], Giovanni Raffa[1], Chiara Tomasello[2], M'Hammed Aguennouz[1] and Antonino Germanò[1]

*Address all correspondence to: dlatorre@unime.it

1 Department of Neurosciences, University of Messina, Messina, Italy

2 Department of Medical Oncology, University of Messina School of Medicine, Messina, Italy

References

[1] Bondy, M. L, Scheurer, M. E, Malmer, B, Barnholtz-sloan, J. S, & Davis, F. G. Il'yasova D, et al. Brain tumor epidemiology: consensus from the Brain Tumor Epidemiology Consortium. Cancer (2008). Suppl) , 1953-68.

[2] Blackburn, E. H. Structure and function of telomeres. Nature (1991). , 350(6319), 569-73.

[3] Wright, W. E, & Shay, J. W. Time, telomeres and tumours: is cellular senescence more than an anticancer mechanism? Trends in cell biology (1995). , 5(8), 293-7.

[4] Harley, C. B. Telomere loss: mitotic clock or genetic time bomb? Mutation research (1991).

[5] Rudolph, K. L, Chang, S, Lee, H. W, Blasco, M, Gottlieb, G. J, Greider, C, et al. Longevity, stress response, and cancer in aging telomerase-deficient mice. Cell (1999). , 96(5), 701-12.

[6] Harley, C. B, Futcher, A. B, & Greider, C. W. Telomeres shorten during ageing of human fibroblasts. Nature (1990). , 345(6274), 458-60.

[7] Shay, J. W, Wright, W. E, & Werbin, H. Defining the molecular mechanisms of human cell immortalization. Biochimica et biophysica acta (1991). , 1072(1), 1-7.

[8] Counter, C. M, & Avilion, A. A. LeFeuvre CE, Stewart NG, Greider CW, Harley CB, et al. Telomere shortening associated with chromosome instability is arrested in immortal cells which express telomerase activity. The EMBO journal (1992). , 11(5), 1921-9.

[9] De Lange, T. How telomeres solve the end-protection problem. Science (2009). , 326(5955), 948-52.

[10] Wright, W. E, & Shay, J. W. Telomere biology in aging and cancer. Journal of the American Geriatrics Society (2005). Suppl) S, 292-4.

[11] Hastie, N. D, Dempster, M, Dunlop, M. G, Thompson, A. M, Green, D. K, & Allshire, R. C. Telomere reduction in human colorectal carcinoma and with ageing. Nature (1990). , 346(6287), 866-8.

[12] Maser, R. S, & Depinho, R. A. Connecting chromosomes, crisis, and cancer. Science (2002). , 297(5581), 565-9.

[13] Chin, L, Artandi, S. E, Shen, Q, Tam, A, Lee, S. L, Gottlieb, G. J, et al. deficiency rescues the adverse effects of telomere loss and cooperates with telomere dysfunction to accelerate carcinogenesis. Cell (1999). , 53.

[14] Moyzis, R. K, Buckingham, J. M, Cram, L. S, Dani, M, Deaven, L. L, Jones, M. D, et al. A highly conserved repetitive DNA sequence, (TTAGGG)n, present at the telomeres of human chromosomes. Proceedings of the National Academy of Sciences of the United States of America (1988). , 85(18), 6622-6.

[15] Griffith, J. D, Comeau, L, Rosenfield, S, Stansel, R. M, Bianchi, A, Moss, H, et al. Mammalian telomeres end in a large duplex loop. Cell (1999). , 97(4), 503-14.

[16] Choi, K. H, Farrell, A. S, Lakamp, A. S, & Ouellette, M. M. Characterization of the DNA binding specificity of Shelterin complexes. Nucleic acids research (2011). , 39(21), 9206-23.

[17] De Lange, T. T-l. o. o. p. s. and the origin of telomeres. Nature reviews Molecular cell biology (2004). , 5(4), 323-9.

[18] Vaziri, H, & Benchimol, S. From telomere loss to induction and activation of a DNA-damage pathway at senescence: the telomere loss/DNA damage model of cell aging. Experimental gerontology (1996). , 53.

[19] Shay, J. W, & Wright, W. E. Telomerase activity in human cancer. Current opinion in oncology (1996). , 8(1), 66-71.

[20] Vaziri, H, Dragowska, W, Allsopp, R. C, Thomas, T. E, Harley, C. B, & Lansdorp, P. M. Evidence for a mitotic clock in human hematopoietic stem cells: loss of telomeric DNA with age. Proceedings of the National Academy of Sciences of the United States of America (1994). , 91(21), 9857-60.

[21] d'Adda di Fagagna F, Reaper PM, Clay-Farrace L, Fiegler H, Carr P, Von Zglinicki T, et al. A DNA damage checkpoint response in telomere-initiated senescence. Nature 2003;426(6963) 194-8.

[22] Durant, S. T. Telomerase-independent paths to immortality in predictable cancer subtypes. Journal of Cancer (2012). , 367-82.

[23] Baumann, P, & Cech, T. R. Pot1, the putative telomere end-binding protein in fission yeast and humans. Science (2001). , 292(5519), 1171-5.

[24] Broccoli, D, Smogorzewska, A, Chong, L, & De Lange, T. Human telomeres contain two distinct Myb-related proteins, TRF1 and TRF2. Nature genetics (1997). , 17(2), 231-5.

[25] Houghtaling, B. R, Cuttonaro, L, Chang, W, & Smith, S. A dynamic molecular link between the telomere length regulator TRF1 and the chromosome end protector TRF2. Current biology : CB (2004). , 14(18), 1621-31.

[26] Connor, O, Safari, M. S, Xin, A, Liu, H, & Songyang, D. Z. A critical role for TPP1 and TIN2 interaction in high-order telomeric complex assembly. Proceedings of the National Academy of Sciences of the United States of America (2006). , 103(32), 11874-9.

[27] Kim, S. H, Beausejour, C, Davalos, A. R, Kaminker, P, Heo, S. J, & Campisi, J. TIN2 mediates functions of TRF2 at human telomeres. The Journal of biological chemistry (2004). , 279(42), 43799-804.

[28] Kim, S. H, Kaminker, P, & Campisi, J. TIN2, a new regulator of telomere length in human cells. Nature genetics (1999). , 23(4), 405-12.

[29] Liu, D, Safari, A, Connor, O, Chan, M. S, Laegeler, D. W, & Qin, A. J, et al. PTOP interacts with POT1 and regulates its localization to telomeres. Nature cell biology (2004). , 6(7), 673-80.

[30] Ye, J. Z, Donigian, J. R, Van Overbeek, M, Loayza, D, Luo, Y, Krutchinsky, A. N, et al. TIN2 binds TRF1 and TRF2 simultaneously and stabilizes the TRF2 complex on telomeres. The Journal of biological chemistry (2004). , 279(45), 47264-71.

[31] Ye, J. Z, Hockemeyer, D, Krutchinsky, A. N, Loayza, D, Hooper, S. M, Chait, B. T, et al. POT1-interacting protein PIP1: a telomere length regulator that recruits POT1 to the TIN2/TRF1 complex. Genes & development (2004). , 18(14), 1649-54.

[32] Li, B, Oestreich, S, & De Lange, T. Identification of human Rap1: implications for telomere evolution. Cell (2000). , 101(5), 471-83.

[33] De Lange, T. Protection of mammalian telomeres. Oncogene (2002). , 21(4), 532-40.

[34] Palm, W, & De Lange, T. How shelterin protects mammalian telomeres. Annual review of genetics (2008). , 42301-34.

[35] Liu, D, Connor, O, Qin, M. S, Songyang, J, & Telosome, Z. a mammalian telomere-associated complex formed by multiple telomeric proteins. The Journal of biological chemistry (2004). , 279(49), 51338-42.

[36] Celli, G. B, & De Lange, T. DNA processing is not required for ATM-mediated telomere damage response after TRF2 deletion. Nature cell biology (2005). , 7(7), 712-8.

[37] Celli, G. B, Denchi, E. L, & De Lange, T. Ku70 stimulates fusion of dysfunctional telomeres yet protects chromosome ends from homologous recombination. Nature cell biology (2006). , 8(8), 885-90.

[38] Hockemeyer, D, Palm, W, Else, T, Daniels, J. P, Takai, K. K, Ye, J. Z, et al. Telomere protection by mammalian Pot1 requires interaction with Tpp1. Nature structural & molecular biology (2007). , 14(8), 754-61.

[39] Loayza, D, & De Lange, T. POT1 as a terminal transducer of TRF1 telomere length control. Nature (2003). , 423(6943), 1013-8.

[40] Takai, K. K, Hooper, S, Blackwood, S, Gandhi, R, & De Lange, T. In vivo stoichiometry of shelterin components. The Journal of biological chemistry (2010). , 285(2), 1457-67.

[41] Van Steensel, B, Smogorzewska, A, & De Lange, T. TRF2 protects human telomeres from end-to-end fusions. Cell (1998). , 92(3), 401-13.

[42] Denchi, E. L, & De Lange, T. Protection of telomeres through independent control of ATM and ATR by TRF2 and POT1. Nature (2007). , 448(7157), 1068-71.

[43] Karlseder, J, Broccoli, D, Dai, Y, Hardy, S, & De Lange, T. p. and ATM-dependent apoptosis induced by telomeres lacking TRF2. Science (1999). , 283(5406), 1321-5.

[44] Smogorzewska, A, & De Lange, T. Different telomere damage signaling pathways in human and mouse cells. The EMBO journal (2002). , 21(16), 4338-48.

[45] Takai, H, Smogorzewska, A, & De Lange, T. DNA damage foci at dysfunctional telomeres. Current biology : CB (2003). , 13(17), 1549-56.

[46] Konishi, A, & De Lange, T. Cell cycle control of telomere protection and NHEJ revealed by a ts mutation in the DNA-binding domain of TRF2. Genes & development (2008). , 22(9), 1221-30.

[47] Veldman, T, Etheridge, K. T, & Counter, C. M. Loss of hPot1 function leads to telomere instability and a cut-like phenotype. Current biology : CB (2004). , 14(24), 2264-70.

[48] Yang, Q, Zheng, Y. L, & Harris, C. C. POT1 and TRF2 cooperate to maintain telomeric integrity. Molecular and cellular biology (2005). , 25(3), 1070-80.

[49] Aragona, M, Maisano, R, Panetta, S, Giudice, A, & Morelli, M. La Torre I, et al. Telomere length maintenance in aging and carcinogenesis. International journal of oncology (2000). , 17(5), 981-9.

[50] Cong, Y. S, Wright, W. E, & Shay, J. W. Human telomerase and its regulation. Microbiology and molecular biology reviews : MMBR (2002). table of contents., 66(3), 407-25.

[51] De Lange, T. Shelterin: the protein complex that shapes and safeguards human telomeres. Genes & development (2005). , 19(18), 2100-10.

[52] Greider, C. W, & Blackburn, E. H. Identification of a specific telomere terminal transferase activity in Tetrahymena extracts. Cell (1985). Pt 1) 405-13.

[53] Counter, C. M, Hahn, W. C, Wei, W, Caddle, S. D, Beijersbergen, R. L, Lansdorp, P. M, et al. Dissociation among in vitro telomerase activity, telomere maintenance, and cellular immortalization. Proceedings of the National Academy of Sciences of the United States of America (1998). , 95(25), 14723-8.

[54] Zhong, Z, Shiue, L, Kaplan, S, & De Lange, T. A mammalian factor that binds telomeric TTAGGG repeats in vitro. Molecular and cellular biology (1992). , 12(11), 4834-43.

[55] Ancelin, K, Brunori, M, Bauwens, S, Koering, C. E, Brun, C, Ricoul, M, et al. Targeting assay to study the cis functions of human telomeric proteins: evidence for inhibition of telomerase by TRF1 and for activation of telomere degradation by TRF2. Molecular and cellular biology (2002). , 22(10), 3474-87.

[56] Nakanishi, K, Kawai, T, Kumaki, F, Hiroi, S, Mukai, M, Ikeda, E, et al. Expression of mRNAs for telomeric repeat binding factor (TRF)-1 and TRF2 in atypical adenomatous hyperplasia and adenocarcinoma of the lung. Clinical cancer research : an official journal of the American Association for Cancer Research (2003). , 9(3), 1105-11.

[57] Iwano, T, Tachibana, M, Reth, M, & Shinkai, Y. Importance of TRF1 for functional telomere structure. The Journal of biological chemistry (2004). , 279(2), 1442-8.

[58] d'Adda di Fagagna F, Hande MP, Tong WM, Lansdorp PM, Wang ZQ, Jackson SP. Functions of poly(ADP-ribose) polymerase in controlling telomere length and chromosomal stability. Nature genetics 1999;23(1) 76-80.

[59] Pennisi, E. A possible new partner for telomerase. Science (1998).

[60] Smith, S, Giriat, I, Schmitt, A, & De Lange, T. Tankyrase, a poly(ADP-ribose) polymerase at human telomeres. Science (1998). , 282(5393), 1484-7.

[61] Donate, L. E, & Blasco, M. A. Telomeres in cancer and ageing. Philosophical transactions of the Royal Society of London Series B, Biological sciences (2011). , 366(1561), 76-84.

[62] Bryan, T. M, Englezou, A, Gupta, J, Bacchetti, S, & Reddel, R. R. Telomere elongation in immortal human cells without detectable telomerase activity. The EMBO journal (1995). , 14(17), 4240-8.

[63] Reddel, R. R, Bryan, T. M, Colgin, L. M, Perrem, K. T, & Yeager, T. R. Alternative lengthening of telomeres in human cells. Radiation research (2001). Pt 2) 194-200.

[64] Yeager, T. R, Neumann, A. A, Englezou, A, Huschtscha, L. I, Noble, J. R, & Reddel, R. R. Telomerase-negative immortalized human cells contain a novel type of promyelocytic leukemia (PML) body. Cancer research (1999). , 59(17), 4175-9.

[65] Chung, I, Osterwald, S, Deeg, K. I, & Rippe, K. PML body meets telomere: The beginning of an ALTernate ending? Nucleus (2012).

[66] Henson, J. D, Neumann, A. A, Yeager, T. R, & Reddel, R. R. Alternative lengthening of telomeres in mammalian cells. Oncogene (2002). , 21(4), 598-610.

[67] Cesare, A. J, & Griffith, J. D. Telomeric DNA in ALT cells is characterized by free telomeric circles and heterogeneous t-loops. Molecular and cellular biology (2004). , 24(22), 9948-57.

[68] Ogino, H, Nakabayashi, K, Suzuki, M, Takahashi, E, Fujii, M, Suzuki, T, et al. Release of telomeric DNA from chromosomes in immortal human cells lacking telomerase activity. Biochemical and biophysical research communications (1998). , 248(2), 223-7.

[69] Tokutake, Y, Matsumoto, T, Watanabe, T, Maeda, S, Tahara, H, Sakamoto, S, et al. Extra-chromosomal telomere repeat DNA in telomerase-negative immortalized cell lines. Biochemical and biophysical research communications (1998). , 247(3), 765-72.

[70] Cesare, A. J, & Reddel, R. R. Alternative lengthening of telomeres: models, mechanisms and implications. Nature reviews Genetics (2010). , 11(5), 319-30.

[71] Henson, J. D, Cao, Y, Huschtscha, L. I, Chang, A. C, Au, A. Y, Pickett, H. A, et al. DNA C-circles are specific and quantifiable markers of alternative-lengthening-of-telomeres activity. Nature biotechnology (2009). , 27(12), 1181-5.

[72] Bechter, O. E, Zou, Y, Walker, W, Wright, W. E, & Shay, J. W. Telomeric recombination in mismatch repair deficient human colon cancer cells after telomerase inhibition. Cancer research (2004). , 64(10), 3444-51.

[73] Londono-vallejo, J. A, Sarkissian, H, Cazes, L, Bacchetti, S, & Reddel, R. R. Alternative lengthening of telomeres is characterized by high rates of telomeric exchange. Cancer research (2004). , 64(7), 2324-7.

[74] Lang, M, Jegou, T, Chung, I, Richter, K, Munch, S, Udvarhelyi, A, et al. Three-dimensional organization of promyelocytic leukemia nuclear bodies. Journal of cell science (2010). Pt 3) 392-400.

[75] Johnson, J. E, & Broccoli, D. Telomere maintenance in sarcomas. Current opinion in oncology (2007). , 19(4), 377-82.

[76] Heaphy, C. M, Subhawong, A. P, Hong, S. M, Goggins, M. G, Montgomery, E. A, Gabrielson, E, et al. Prevalence of the alternative lengthening of telomeres telomere maintenance mechanism in human cancer subtypes. The American journal of pathology (2011). , 179(4), 1608-15.

[77] Neumann, A. A, & Reddel, R. R. Telomere maintenance and cancer-- look, no telomerase. Nature reviews Cancer (2002). , 2(11), 879-84.

[78] Kim, N. W, Piatyszek, M. A, Prowse, K. R, Harley, C. B, West, M. D, Ho, P. L, et al. Specific association of human telomerase activity with immortal cells and cancer. Science (1994). , 266(5193), 2011-5.

[79] Patel, M. M, Parekh, L. J, Jha, F. P, Sainger, R. N, Patel, J. B, Patel, D. D, et al. Clinical usefulness of telomerase activation and telomere length in head and neck cancer. Head & neck (2002). , 24(12), 1060-7.

[80] Yokota, T, Suda, T, Igarashi, M, Kuroiwa, T, Waguri, N, Kawai, H, et al. Telomere length variation and maintenance in hepatocarcinogenesis. Cancer (2003). , 98(1), 110-8.

[81] Bisoffi, M, Heaphy, C. M, & Griffith, J. K. Telomeres: prognostic markers for solid tumors. International journal of cancer Journal international du cancer (2006). , 119(10), 2255-60.

[82] Nurnberg, P, Thiel, G, Weber, F, & Epplen, J. T. Changes of telomere lengths in human intracranial tumours. Human genetics (1993). , 91(2), 190-2.

[83] Le, S, Zhu, J. J, Anthony, D. C, Greider, C. W, & Black, P. M. Telomerase activity in human gliomas. Neurosurgery (1998). discussion 4-5., 42(5), 1120-4.

[84] Ridley, L, Rahman, R, Brundler, M. A, Ellison, D, Lowe, J, Robson, K, et al. Multifactorial analysis of predictors of outcome in pediatric intracranial ependymoma. Neuro-oncology (2008). , 10(5), 675-89.

[85] Tabori, U, Vukovic, B, Zielenska, M, Hawkins, C, Braude, I, Rutka, J, et al. The role of telomere maintenance in the spontaneous growth arrest of pediatric low-grade gliomas. Neoplasia (2006). , 8(2), 136-42.

[86] Morii, K, Tanaka, R, Onda, K, Tsumanuma, I, & Yoshimura, J. Expression of telomerase RNA, telomerase activity, and telomere length in human gliomas. Biochemical and biophysical research communications (1997). , 239(3), 830-4.

[87] Liu, J, Li, H, & Luo, Y. Analysis of telomere restriction fragments in human astrocytomas and glioblastomas]. Zhonghua yi xue za zhi (1996). , 76(8), 588-90.

[88] Aubert, G, & Lansdorp, P. M. Telomeres and aging. Physiological reviews (2008). , 88(2), 557-79.

[89] Hohensinner, P. J, Goronzy, J. J, & Weyand, C. M. Telomere dysfunction, autoimmunity and aging. Aging and disease (2011). , 2(6), 524-37.

[90] Cawthon, R. M, Smith, K. R, Brien, O, Sivatchenko, E, & Kerber, A. RA. Association between telomere length in blood and mortality in people aged 60 years or older. Lancet (2003). , 361(9355), 393-5.

[91] Fitzpatrick, A. L, Kronmal, R. A, Kimura, M, Gardner, J. P, Psaty, B. M, Jenny, N. S, et al. Leukocyte telomere length and mortality in the Cardiovascular Health Study. The journals of gerontology Series A, Biological sciences and medical sciences (2011). , 66(4), 421-9.

[92] Bakaysa, S. L, Mucci, L. A, Slagboom, P. E, Boomsma, D. I, Mcclearn, G. E, Johansson, B, et al. Telomere length predicts survival independent of genetic influences. Aging cell (2007). , 6(6), 769-74.

[93] Kimura, M, Hjelmborg, J. V, Gardner, J. P, Bathum, L, Brimacombe, M, Lu, X, et al. Telomere length and mortality: a study of leukocytes in elderly Danish twins. American journal of epidemiology (2008). , 167(7), 799-806.

[94] Ehrlenbach, S, Willeit, P, Kiechl, S, Willeit, J, Reindl, M, Schanda, K, et al. Influences on the reduction of relative telomere length over 10 years in the population-based Bruneck Study: introduction of a well-controlled high-throughput assay. International journal of epidemiology (2009). , 38(6), 1725-34.

[95] Njajou, O. T, Hsueh, W. C, Blackburn, E. H, Newman, A. B, Wu, S. H, Li, R, et al. Association between telomere length, specific causes of death, and years of healthy life in health, aging, and body composition, a population-based cohort study. The journals of gerontology Series A, Biological sciences and medical sciences (2009). , 64(8), 860-4.

[96] Bischoff, C, Petersen, H. C, Graakjaer, J, Andersen-ranberg, K, Vaupel, J. W, Bohr, V. A, et al. No association between telomere length and survival among the elderly and oldest old. Epidemiology (2006). , 17(2), 190-4.

[97] Houben, J. M, Giltay, E. J, Rius-ottenheim, N, Hageman, G. J, & Kromhout, D. Telomere length and mortality in elderly men: the Zutphen Elderly Study. The journals of gerontology Series A, Biological sciences and medical sciences (2011). , 66(1), 38-44.

[98] Strandberg, T. E, Saijonmaa, O, Tilvis, R. S, Pitkala, K. H, Strandberg, A. Y, Miettinen, T. A, et al. Association of telomere length in older men with mortality and midlife body mass index and smoking. The journals of gerontology Series A, Biological sciences and medical sciences (2011). , 66(7), 815-20.

[99] Epel, E. S, Merkin, S. S, Cawthon, R, Blackburn, E. H, Adler, N. E, Pletcher, M. J, et al. The rate of leukocyte telomere shortening predicts mortality from cardiovascular disease in elderly men. Aging (2009). , 1(1), 81-8.

[100] Calado, R, & Young, N. Telomeres in disease. F1000 medicine reports (2012).

[101] Heiss, N. S, Knight, S. W, Vulliamy, T. J, Klauck, S. M, Wiemann, S, Mason, P. J, et al. X-linked dyskeratosis congenita is caused by mutations in a highly conserved gene with putative nucleolar functions. Nature genetics (1998). , 19(1), 32-8.

[102] Dokal, I. Dyskeratosis congenita in all its forms. British journal of haematology (2000). , 110(4), 768-79.

[103] Savage, S. A, & Alter, B. P. Dyskeratosis congenita. Hematology/oncology clinics of North America (2009). , 23(2), 215-31.

[104] Alter, B. P, Rosenberg, P. S, Giri, N, Baerlocher, G. M, Lansdorp, P. M, & Savage, S. A. Telomere length is associated with disease severity and declines with age in dyskeratosis congenita. Haematologica (2012). , 97(3), 353-9.

[105] Alter, B. P, Baerlocher, G. M, Savage, S. A, Chanock, S. J, Weksler, B. B, Willner, J. P, et al. Very short telomere length by flow fluorescence in situ hybridization identifies patients with dyskeratosis congenita. Blood (2007). , 110(5), 1439-47.

[106] Panayiotou, A. G, Nicolaides, A. N, Griffin, M, Tyllis, T, Georgiou, N, Bond, D, et al. Leukocyte telomere length is associated with measures of subclinical atherosclerosis. Atherosclerosis (2010). , 211(1), 176-81.

[107] Chen, W, Gardner, J. P, Kimura, M, Brimacombe, M, Cao, X, Srinivasan, S. R, et al. Leukocyte telomere length is associated with HDL cholesterol levels: The Bogalusa heart study. Atherosclerosis (2009). , 205(2), 620-5.

[108] Willeit, P, Willeit, J, Brandstatter, A, Ehrlenbach, S, Mayr, A, Gasperi, A, et al. Cellular aging reflected by leukocyte telomere length predicts advanced atherosclerosis and cardiovascular disease risk. Arteriosclerosis, thrombosis, and vascular biology (2010). , 30(8), 1649-56.

[109] Maubaret, C. G, Salpea, K. D, Jain, A, Cooper, J. A, Hamsten, A, Sanders, J, et al. Telomeres are shorter in myocardial infarction patients compared to healthy subjects: correlation with environmental risk factors. J Mol Med (Berl) (2010). , 88(8), 785-94.

[110] Diaz, V. A, & Mainous, A. G. rd, Everett CJ, Schoepf UJ, Codd V, Samani NJ. Effect of healthy lifestyle behaviors on the association between leukocyte telomere length and coronary artery calcium. The American journal of cardiology (2010). , 106(5), 659-63.

[111] Kuznetsova, T, Codd, V, Brouilette, S, Thijs, L, Gonzalez, A, Jin, Y, et al. Association between left ventricular mass and telomere length in a population study. American journal of epidemiology (2010). , 172(4), 440-50.

[112] Jeanclos, E, Krolewski, A, Skurnick, J, Kimura, M, Aviv, H, Warram, J. H, et al. Shortened telomere length in white blood cells of patients with IDDM. Diabetes (1998). , 47(3), 482-6.

[113] Sampson, M. J, Winterbone, M. S, Hughes, J. C, Dozio, N, & Hughes, D. A. Monocyte telomere shortening and oxidative DNA damage in type 2 diabetes. Diabetes care (2006). , 29(2), 283-9.

[114] Tentolouris, N, Nzietchueng, R, Cattan, V, Poitevin, G, Lacolley, P, Papazafiropoulou, A, et al. White blood cells telomere length is shorter in males with type 2 diabetes and microalbuminuria. Diabetes care (2007). , 30(11), 2909-15.

[115] Honig, L. S, Schupf, N, Lee, J. H, Tang, M. X, & Mayeux, R. Shorter telomeres are associated with mortality in those with APOE epsilon4 and dementia. Annals of neurology (2006). , 60(2), 181-7.

[116] Von Zglinicki, T, Serra, V, Lorenz, M, Saretzki, G, Lenzen-grossimlighaus, R, Gessner, R, et al. Short telomeres in patients with vascular dementia: an indicator of low antioxidative capacity and a possible risk factor? Laboratory investigation; a journal of technical methods and pathology (2000). , 80(11), 1739-47.

[117] Hochstrasser, T, Marksteiner, J, & Humpel, C. Telomere length is age-dependent and reduced in monocytes of Alzheimer patients. Experimental gerontology (2012). , 47(2), 160-3.

[118] Panossian, L. A, Porter, V. R, Valenzuela, H. F, Zhu, X, Reback, E, Masterman, D, et al. Telomere shortening in T cells correlates with Alzheimer's disease status. Neurobiology of aging (2003). , 24(1), 77-84.

[119] Thomas, P, & Fenech, N. J O. C. M. Telomere length in white blood cells, buccal cells and brain tissue and its variation with ageing and Alzheimer's disease. Mechanisms of ageing and development (2008). , 129(4), 183-90.

[120] Ding, H, Chen, C, Shaffer, J. R, Liu, L, Xu, Y, Wang, X, et al. Telomere length and risk of stroke in Chinese. Stroke; a journal of cerebral circulation (2012). , 43(3), 658-63.

[121] Blackburn, E. H. Telomere states and cell fates. Nature (2000). , 408(6808), 53-6.

[122] Blackburn, E. H. Switching and signaling at the telomere. Cell (2001). , 106(6), 661-73.

[123] La Torre Dde Divitiis O, Conti A, Angileri FF, Cardali S, Aguennouz M, et al. Expression of telomeric repeat binding factor-1 in astroglial brain tumors. Neurosurgery (2005). , 56(4), 802-10.

[124] Callen, E, & Surralles, J. Telomere dysfunction in genome instability syndromes. Mutation research (2004). , 567(1), 85-104.

[125] Lundblad, V. Genome instability: McClintock revisited. Current biology : CB (2001). R, 957-60.

[126] Fordyce, C. A, Heaphy, C. M, Joste, N. E, Smith, A. Y, Hunt, W. C, & Griffith, J. K. Association between cancer-free survival and telomere DNA content in prostate tumors. The Journal of urology (2005). , 173(2), 610-4.

[127] Fordyce, C. A, Heaphy, C. M, Bisoffi, M, Wyaco, J. L, Joste, N. E, Mangalik, A, et al. Telomere content correlates with stage and prognosis in breast cancer. Breast cancer research and treatment (2006). , 99(2), 193-202.

[128] Donaldson, L, Fordyce, C, Gilliland, F, Smith, A, Feddersen, R, Joste, N, et al. Association between outcome and telomere DNA content in prostate cancer. The Journal of urology (1999). , 162(5), 1788-92.

[129] Griffith, J. K, Bryant, J. E, Fordyce, C. A, Gilliland, F. D, Joste, N. E, & Moyzis, R. K. Reduced telomere DNA content is correlated with genomic instability and metastasis in invasive human breast carcinoma. Breast cancer research and treatment (1999). , 54(1), 59-64.

[130] Odagiri, E, Kanada, N, Jibiki, K, Demura, R, Aikawa, E, & Demura, H. Reduction of telomeric length and c-erbB-2 gene amplification in human breast cancer, fibroadenoma, and gynecomastia. Relationship to histologic grade and clinical parameters. Cancer (1994). , 73(12), 2978-84.

[131] Hiyama, E, Hiyama, K, Yokoyama, T, Ichikawa, T, & Matsuura, Y. Length of telomeric repeats in neuroblastoma: correlation with prognosis and other biological characteristics. Japanese journal of cancer research : Gann (1992). , 83(2), 159-64.

[132] Gertler, R, Rosenberg, R, Stricker, D, Friederichs, J, Hoos, A, Werner, M, et al. Telomere length and human telomerase reverse transcriptase expression as markers for progression and prognosis of colorectal carcinoma. Journal of clinical oncology : official journal of the American Society of Clinical Oncology (2004). , 22(10), 1807-14.

[133] Garcia-aranda, C, De Juan, C, Diaz-lopez, A, Sanchez-pernaute, A, Torres, A. J, Diaz-rubio, E, et al. Correlations of telomere length, telomerase activity, and telomeric-repeat binding factor 1 expression in colorectal carcinoma. Cancer (2006). , 106(3), 541-51.

[134] Chen, K. Y, Lee, L. N, Yu, C. J, Lee, Y. C, Kuo, S. H, & Yang, P. C. Elevation of telomerase activity positively correlates to poor prognosis of patients with non-small cell lung cancer. Cancer letters (2006). , 240(1), 148-56.

[135] Shirotani, Y, Hiyama, K, Ishioka, S, Inyaku, K, Awaya, Y, Yonehara, S, et al. Alteration in length of telomeric repeats in lung cancer. Lung Cancer (1994).

[136] (Hirashima T, Komiya T, Nitta T, Takada Y, Kobayashi M, Masuda N, et al. Prognostic significance of telomeric repeat length alterations in pathological stage I-IIIA non-small cell lung cancer. Anticancer research 2000;20(3B) 2181-7). 2181-7.

[137] Rosenberg, R, Gertler, R, Stricker, D, Lassmann, S, Werner, M, Nekarda, H, et al. Telomere length and hTERT expression in patients with colorectal carcinoma. Recent

results in cancer research Fortschritte der Krebsforschung Progres dans les recherches sur le cancer (2003). , 162177-81.

[138] Kolquist, K. A, Ellisen, L. W, Counter, C. M, Meyerson, M, Tan, L. K, Weinberg, R. A, et al. Expression of TERT in early premalignant lesions and a subset of cells in normal tissues. Nature genetics (1998). , 19(2), 182-6.

[139] Hiraga, S, Ohnishi, T, Izumoto, S, Miyahara, E, Kanemura, Y, Matsumura, H, et al. Telomerase activity and alterations in telomere length in human brain tumors. Cancer research (1998). , 58(10), 2117-25.

[140] Sano, T, Asai, A, Mishima, K, Fujimaki, T, & Kirino, T. Telomerase activity in 144 brain tumours. British journal of cancer (1998). , 77(10), 1633-7.

[141] Weil, R. J, Wu, Y. Y, Vortmeyer, A. O, Moon, Y. W, Delgado, R. M, Fuller, B. G, et al. Telomerase activity in microdissected human gliomas. Modern pathology : an official journal of the United States and Canadian Academy of Pathology, Inc (1999). , 12(1), 41-6.

[142] Kleinschmidt-DeMasters BKHashizumi TL, Sze CI, Lillehei KO, Shroyer AL, Shroyer KR. Telomerase expression shows differences across multiple regions of oligodendroglioma versus high grade astrocytomas but shows correlation with Mib-1 labelling. Journal of clinical pathology (1998). , 51(4), 284-93.

[143] Kanauchi, H, Wada, N, Ginzinger, D. G, Yu, M, Wong, M. G, Clark, O. H, et al. Diagnostic and prognostic value of fas and telomeric-repeat binding factor-1 genes in adrenal tumors. The Journal of clinical endocrinology and metabolism (2003). , 88(8), 3690-3.

[144] Maitra, A, Yashima, K, Rathi, A, Timmons, C. F, Rogers, B. B, Shay, J. W, et al. The RNA component of telomerase as a marker of biologic potential and clinical outcome in childhood neuroblastic tumors. Cancer (1999). , 85(3), 741-9.

[145] Maes, L, Van Neste, L, Van Damme, K, Kalala, J. P, De Ridder, L, Bekaert, S, et al. Relation between telomerase activity, hTERT and telomere length for intracranial tumours. Oncology reports (2007). , 18(6), 1571-6.

[146] CBTRUSCBTRUS Statistical Report: Primary Brain and Central Nervous System Tumors Diagnosed in the United States in Central Brain Tumor Registry of the United States, Hinsdale, IL 2011., 2004-2007.

[147] Harada, K, Kurisu, K, Tahara, H, Tahara, E, & Ide, T. Telomerase activity in primary and secondary glioblastomas multiforme as a novel molecular tumor marker. Journal of neurosurgery (2000). , 93(4), 618-25.

[148] Hakin-smith, V, Jellinek, D. A, Levy, D, Carroll, T, Teo, M, Timperley, W. R, et al. Alternative lengthening of telomeres and survival in patients with glioblastoma multiforme. Lancet (2003). , 361(9360), 836-8.

[149] Henson, J. D, Hannay, J. A, Mccarthy, S. W, Royds, J. A, Yeager, T. R, Robinson, R. A, et al. A robust assay for alternative lengthening of telomeres in tumors shows the significance of alternative lengthening of telomeres in sarcomas and astrocytomas. Clinical cancer research : an official journal of the American Association for Cancer Research (2005). , 11(1), 217-25.

[150] Slatter, T, Gifford-garner, J, Wiles, A, Tan, X, & Chen, Y. J. MacFarlane M, et al. Pilocytic astrocytomas have telomere-associated promyelocytic leukemia bodies without alternatively lengthened telomeres. The American journal of pathology (2010). , 177(6), 2694-700.

[151] Smogorzewska, A, Van Steensel, B, Bianchi, A, Oelmann, S, Schaefer, M. R, Schnapp, G, et al. Control of human telomere length by TRF1 and TRF2. Molecular and cellular biology (2000). , 20(5), 1659-68.

[152] Van Steensel, B, & De Lange, T. Control of telomere length by the human telomeric protein TRF1. Nature (1997). , 385(6618), 740-3.

[153] Karlseder, J, Smogorzewska, A, & De Lange, T. Senescence induced by altered telomere state, not telomere loss. Science (2002). , 295(5564), 2446-9.

[154] Marian, C. O, Cho, S. K, Mcellin, B. M, Maher, E. A, Hatanpaa, K. J, Madden, C. J, et al. The telomerase antagonist, imetelstat, efficiently targets glioblastoma tumor-initiating cells leading to decreased proliferation and tumor growth. Clinical cancer research : an official journal of the American Association for Cancer Research (2010). , 16(1), 154-63.

[155] Gurung, R. L, Lim, S. N, Khaw, A. K, Soon, J. F, & Shenoy, K. Mohamed Ali S, et al. Thymoquinone induces telomere shortening, DNA damage and apoptosis in human glioblastoma cells. PloS one (2010). e12124.

[156] Lin, P. C, Lin, S. Z, Chen, Y. L, Chang, J. S, Ho, L. I, Liu, P. Y, et al. Butylidenephthalide suppresses human telomerase reverse transcriptase (TERT) in human glioblastomas. Annals of surgical oncology (2011). , 18(12), 3514-27.

[157] Mork, S. J, & Loken, A. C. Ependymoma: a follow-up study of 101 cases. Cancer (1977). , 40(2), 907-15.

[158] Duffner, P. K, Cohen, M. E, & Freeman, A. I. Pediatric brain tumors: an overview. CA: a cancer journal for clinicians (1985). , 35(5), 287-301.

[159] Sutton, L. N, Goldwein, J, Perilongo, G, Lang, B, Schut, L, Rorke, L, et al. Prognostic factors in childhood ependymomas. Pediatric neurosurgery (1990). , 16(2), 57-65.

[160] Coons, S. W, Johnson, P. C, Scheithauer, B. W, Yates, A. J, & Pearl, D. K. Improving diagnostic accuracy and interobserver concordance in the classification and grading of primary gliomas. Cancer (1997). , 79(7), 1381-93.

[161] Daumas-duport, C, Varlet, P, Tucker, M. L, Beuvon, F, Cervera, P, & Chodkiewicz, J. P. Oligodendrogliomas. Part I: Patterns of growth, histological diagnosis, clinical and

imaging correlations: a study of 153 cases. Journal of neuro-oncology (1997). , 34(1), 37-59.

[162] Chin, H. W, Hazel, J. J, Kim, T. H, Webster, J. H, & Oligodendrogliomas, I. A clinical study of cerebral oligodendrogliomas. Cancer (1980). , 45(6), 1458-66.

[163] Fortin, D, Cairncross, G. J, & Hammond, R. R. Oligodendroglioma: an appraisal of recent data pertaining to diagnosis and treatment. Neurosurgery (1999). discussion 191., 45(6), 1279-91.

[164] Mork, S. J, Lindegaard, K. F, Halvorsen, T. B, Lehmann, E. H, Solgaard, T, Hatlevoll, R, et al. Oligodendroglioma: incidence and biological behavior in a defined population. Journal of neurosurgery (1985). , 63(6), 881-9.

[165] Wallner, K. E, Gonzales, M, & Sheline, G. E. Treatment of oligodendrogliomas with or without postoperative irradiation. Journal of neurosurgery (1988). , 68(5), 684-8.

[166] Youmans, J. R. Neurological Surgery. 3rd ed. Philadelphia: W.B.Saunders; (1990).

[167] Mahaley, M. S. Jr., Mettlin C, Natarajan N, Laws ER, Jr., Peace BB. National survey of patterns of care for brain-tumor patients. Journal of neurosurgery (1989). , 71(6), 826-36.

[168] Chen, H. J, Liang, C. L, Lu, K, Lin, J. W, & Cho, C. L. Implication of telomerase activity and alternations of telomere length in the histologic characteristics of intracranial meningiomas. Cancer (2000). , 89(10), 2092-8.

[169] Chen, H. J, Cho, C. L, Liang, C. L, Chen, L, Chang, H. W, Lu, K, et al. Differential telomerase expression and telomere length in primary intracranial tumors. Chang Gung medical journal (2001). , 24(6), 352-60.

[170] Plotkin, S. R, Stemmer-rachamimov, A. O, & Barker, F. G. nd, Halpin C, Padera TP, Tyrrell A, et al. Hearing improvement after bevacizumab in patients with neurofibromatosis type 2. The New England journal of medicine (2009). , 361(4), 358-67.

[171] Chen, H. J, Cho, C. L, Liang, C. L, Lu, K, & Lin, J. W. Implication of telomere length as a proliferation-associated marker in schwannomas. Journal of surgical oncology (2002). discussion, 81(2), 93-100.

[172] Tomita, T, & Mclone, D. G. Spontaneous seeding of medulloblastoma: results of cerebrospinal fluid cytology and arachnoid biopsy from the cisterna magna. Neurosurgery (1983). , 12(3), 265-7.

[173] Reddy, A. T, Janss, A. J, Phillips, P. C, Weiss, H. L, & Packer, R. J. Outcome for children with supratentorial primitive neuroectodermal tumors treated with surgery, radiation, and chemotherapy. Cancer (2000). , 88(9), 2189-93.

[174] Rahman, R, Osteso-ibanez, T, Hirst, R. A, Levesley, J, Kilday, J. P, Quinn, S, et al. Histone deacetylase inhibition attenuates cell growth with associated telomerase inhibi-

tion in high-grade childhood brain tumor cells. Molecular cancer therapeutics (2010). , 9(9), 2568-81.

[175] Didiano, D, Shalaby, T, Lang, D, & Grotzer, M. A. Telomere maintenance in childhood primitive neuroectodermal brain tumors. Neuro-oncology (2004). , 6(1), 1-8.

[176] Harada, K, Arita, K, Kurisu, K, & Tahara, H. Telomerase activity and the expression of telomerase components in pituitary adenoma with malignant transformation. Surgical neurology (2000). , 53(3), 267-74.

[177] Miller, D. C, Hochberg, F. H, Harris, N. L, Gruber, M. L, Louis, D. N, & Cohen, H. Pathology with clinical correlations of primary central nervous system non-Hodgkin's lymphoma. The Massachusetts General Hospital experience (1958). Cancer 1994;, 74(4), 1383-97.

[178] Harada, K, Kurisu, K, Arita, K, Sadatomo, T, Tahara, H, Tahara, E, et al. Telomerase activity in central nervous system malignant lymphoma. Cancer (1999). , 86(6), 1050-5.

Chapter 17

Chromosomal Analysis: Clinical Applicability to Brain Cancers

Fabio P. Estumano da Silva and
Edivaldo H. C. de Oliveira

Additional information is available at the end of the chapter

http://dx.doi.org/10.5772/52354

1. Introduction

Cytogenetics is the branch of genetics that studies the cell activity focusing mainly on the chromosome structure, organization and function, isolated or as the whole karyotype, in order to understand aspects of cell biology, evolution or implicated diseases. The behavior of DNA and genes is greatly constrained by the fact that they are incorporated into chromosomes. The DNA is associated with proteins that control and catalyze the processes of transcription and replication. Gene expression is controlled by modifications in histones and by chromatin remodeling complexes. It can also be influenced by the position of the gene in the chromosome. Hence, errors in chromosome behavior are an important cause of ill-health. The presence of chromosomal abnormalities is usual in cancer, and specific chromosome abnormality may often be one of the first events in the development of cancer [1]. The importance of cytogenetic analysis in oncology is demonstrated by the number of researches made on this area since the discovery of the Philadelphia chromosome, a 9/22 translocation, which is seen in chronic myelogenous leukemia (CML) patients [2]. The focus of these studies is the relation between specific chromosome alterations to prognosis, drug resistance and diagnosis for some tumors entities. Moreover, DNA repair problems and others genomic stability pathways defects may lead to genome-wide genetic instability, which can drive further cancer progression [3]. Although chromosome rearrangements are mainly used as markers in hematologic cancers, these alterations have been increasingly studied in solid tumors (90% of all human malignancies), showing that chromosomal numerical/structural aberrations are common in this kind of neoplasia.

Brain cancers are very diverse solid tumors that demonstrate a wide range of complex karyotypes. The chromosomal features of each tumor can provide information that helps in clinical decisions, stratifying it in low and high risk in complementation to the grading aspects usually considered to the central nervous system (CNS) cancers [4]. On this chapter we will consider the implications of the presence of some chromosome mutations for specifics brain tumors. How can these specific alterations help in risk stratification? How these aberrations influence on the choice of treatment? What these rearranged chromosomes indicate about recurrence, metastasis, overall survival or resistance? Obviously, chromosomal mutations have many implications to the cell behavior, affecting the gene dosage by a deletion or amplification, or driving the formation of chimerical transcripts because of chromosomal translocations, etc. Each chromosomal rearrangement has an effect in gene expression or global metabolic equilibrium of the cells. The variety of chromosomal rearrangements is great, involving numerical and structural, and also including very specific types found mainly in cancer, such as double minutes (DMs) and homogeneously staining regions (HSRs), which correspond to gene amplifications (Figure 1).

The importance of chromosomal studies in brain tumors is highlighted by the fact that the most recent World Health Organization's (WHO) book of the CNS neoplasm classification [4] has improved the knowledge about the tumors entities with molecular and cytogenetic markers that, together with the histopathology features, helps in identifying, stratifying or understanding the behavior of tumors.

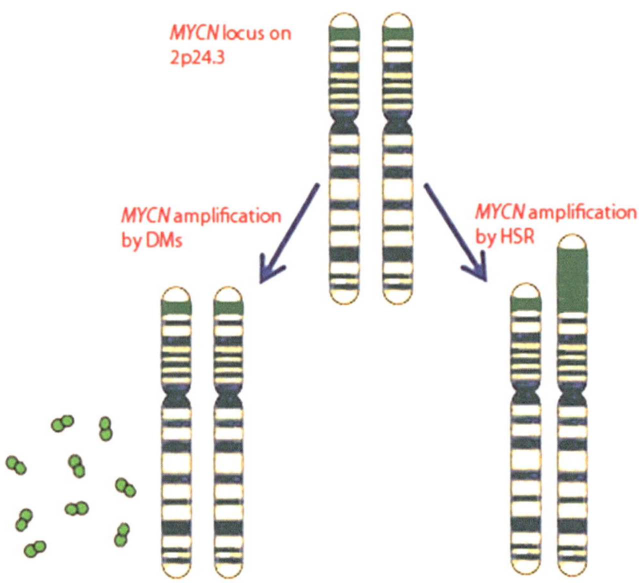

Figure 1. Amplification represents one of the major molecular pathways through which the oncogenic potential of proto-oncogenes is activated during tumorigenesis. In the example, *MYCN* (a MYC family gene) on 2p24.3 is showed amplified by two different mechanisms: extra-chromosomal amplifications (double minutes – DM), and intrachromosomal amplifications (Homogeneously Staining Region (HSR).

http://dx.doi.org/10.5772/52354

2. Cytogenetics and cancer

The idea that chromosomal rearrangements might be causally involved in early stages of carcinogenesis is not new. The first reports hypothesizing that karyotypic aberrations, typical of tumor cells, may possibly be involved in the transformation of normal cells into malignant ones was published more than a century ago by Theodor Boveri [5] in 1914. Although limited by the poor techniques and the restricted knowledge of cell biology, those early findings allowed him to formulate what is now known as the somatic mutation theory of cancer, which still holds the central stage of cancer research [6]. Because cancer cells usually exhibit abnormal karyotypes, a number of questions have emerged: are these abnormal chromosomes a cause or a consequence of tumorigenesis? Can a single gene mutation drive the neoplastic transformation? One assumption is correct: Some cytogenetic alterations have demonstrated that they are directly linked to tumor formation, progression or metastases, as they are found since the very beginning of tumorigenesis. The observation that some genes affected by chromosomal rearrangements were involved in critical stages in cell growth, development, or survival has focused the interest on how these rearrangements alter the function of target genes. These studies have led to a better understanding of origin of chromosomal alterations and their role in cancer development.

It is widely accepted that the process of tumorigenesis is initiated by an acquired mutation that confers a selective advantage on a dividing cell. This mutated cell will be exposed to new mutations and each new mutation will be passible of a new round of Darwinian selection [7]. The cell genome is far from stable, with intrinsic errors in replication, checkpoint, repair, apoptosis, chromosome segregation, recombination, etc. Some of these mutations can guide to chromosomal instability (CIN) and consequently to higher tendency to cancer formation [8], a situation well illustrated in patients with repair process mutation syndromes, such as *Xeroderma Pigmentosum* and Fanconi anemia, which are associated with an increased risk of cancer.

Albertson and coworkers [9] affirmed that the importance of chromosomal aberrations to tumor development varies substantially between tumors. While there are some tumors with marked chromosome rearrangements, others may evolve by mechanisms that result in little chromosomal change. The difference resides on tumor initiation or the manner in which genome instability is formed. In the same way, the ratio of chromosome rearrangement is accompanied by the malignant stage evolution of a neoplasm, and those pre-malignant tumors show few chromosomal aberrations, which are substantially increased on the malignant ones, supporting a role in chromosomal aberration acquisition in tumor progression. An important advance in the study of chromosomal rearrangements, especially aneuploidy, was the discovery that many cancer cell lines exhibit CIN, a phenotype in which cell division is accompanied by an abnormally high rate of chromosome loss and gain. Thus, CIN can be considered as one form of genomic instability, along with elevated rates of mutation, errors in DNA repair and somatic hyperrecombination [10, 11].

Many studies have also focused on the elucidation of the differential response to treatment of cancers from the same histological classification. Because resistance for multiple drugs cannot be explained solely in the light of gene mutation, Duesberg and coworkers [12] developed a theory in which they affirm that the dynamic evolution of karyotypes in cancers cells can be responsible for resistance acquisition to most drugs utilized on treatments of cancers. This karyotype evolution is derived by rounds of chromosome mutations facilitated by CIN, followed by Darwinian selection which increases oncogenic functions in cells. It can explain the rapid evolution of a tumor to gain resistance to drugs administrated on the chemotherapy transforming itself autocatalytically. The natural selection drives the constitution of some chromosome mutation to give a selective advantage to cell not only in growth but also in resistance to drugs and other features of the cancer environment. It is not surprising that the presence of chromosomal abnormalities in malignancies has been pivotal in the discovery of targeted therapy against cancer cells, or in discriminating patients sensitive or insensitive to traditional or new therapies [8]. Today we can say that chromosome abnormalities can be used as markers in many different types of malignancy in the cases when it is observed that specific rearrangements are found in tumors with a certain behavior or grade. In many different kinds of tumors, the presence of a specific chromosomal abnormality has improved the quality of the diagnosis, allowing a clearer definition of the prognosis and permitting the definition of new targets on cancer therapy.

The origin and progression of cancer always were unsolved questions to majority of tumor types. Li and coworkers [13] accompanied the chromosomal alterations in human cell lineages for many generations after transformation by SV40 aneuploidogenics genes. They proposed a theory in which cancer-causing karyotypes represent chromosomal equilibria between destabilizing aneuploidy and stabilizing selection for oncogenic function. Furthermore, they concluded that karyotypes are more likely to initiate and maintain cancers than specific gene mutations (Figure 2). One of the great questions concerns the quasi-stable karyotype observed in different passages of a long time cultured cell lineage or between different samples of the same tumor type versus de CIN observed on cancer cells. The answer comes from the Darwinian selection to give oncogenic function to cell, much like new species. Thus, this tumor karyotype increases and maintains the CIN and can form nonneoplastic and nonviable karyotypic compositions which will be eliminated (Figure 2: B, C and D); however, it can evolve to a karyotype that provides new capability to cells such as drug-resistance or metastasis (Figure 2: C, D and E). So, they defined two steps to cancer initiation: 1) the chromosomal instability initiation by carcinogens that generate random aneuploidy and 2) the karyotype Darwinian selection to give oncogenic function, that emerge from unstable randomly aneuploid karyotypes. In our opinion, Li's theory of cancer-causing karyotypes is very concise and is supported by different studies. Routine cancer cell culture experience demonstrates easily that tumor samples show different karyotypic compositions, with clonal structural or numerical chromosomal abnormalities, which are examples of CIN with the so called selection for oncogenic function. In complementation, oncogenic chromosomal compositions can be maintained quasi-stable in distant passages of a cancer cell culture.

The recognition of the importance of cytogenetic science to cancer surveillance has accompanied the technological development of microscopy, computer image acquisition's software and fluorochrome applications. Although chromosome-banding is still the gold standard for all routine techniques of clinical and tumor cytogenetics, the technical restrictions of this methodology are well known. Only changes that affect the normal pattern such as size variations or position in a chromosomal band or the chromosome itself can be detected, and the origin of additional material or gain/loss of small amounts in a structurally altered chromosome often remains questionable. To overcome such limitations, fluorescence *in situ* hybridization (FISH) approaches were introduced into cytogenetics. FISH is a technique based on the probe-sample hybrid formation labeled with a detectable fluorescent dye. It is a reliable technique that has made a revolution to chromosome mutation detection. Many other techniques have derived from FISH: Interphase FISH, chromosome region specific FISH (telomere, centromere, etc.), multicolor FISH, SKY, Multiplex-FISH, CGH, array-CGH, microarray-CGH, FISH banding, etc. In general, these techniques are very informative and can be utilized in complementation to those classical clinical histopathology diagnostic procedures.

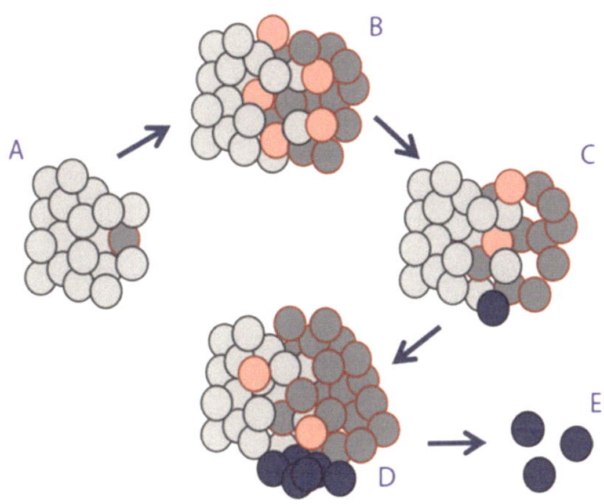

Figure 2. Li's theory of cancer-causing karyotypes. (A) Cells with CIN (gray cells) generate karyotypes with oncogenic functions (dark gray cell). (B) Cells with oncogenic functions will develop and grow forming nonneoplastic and nonviable cells (pink cells), which will be continually generated and eliminated (C and D). However, some karyotypes evolve to more aggressive behavior, like metastatic or drug-resistance cells (blue cells) which can migrate to others sites (C, D and E).

Some of these techniques, such as SKY, M-FISH or CGH-based methodologies (Figure 3), are able to show all chromosomal alterations of a sample in a single experiment, each respecting its limitation, of course. SKY and M-FISH (Figure 3A) can differently dye every chromosome pair in a metaphase spread of a tumor sample, using five different fluorochromes in 24 distinct combinations (22 autosomes, X and Y). These techniques allow the definition of the origin of each chromosome segment involved in rearrangement, but cannot indicate microdeletions or the gain/loss of specific loci. The CGH-based methodologies (Figure 3B) use only two different fluorochromes, for cancer and negative control, showing all losses, gains and amplifications in a tumor sample. These technological advances had led to an exponential increase on the number of patients cytogenetically analyzed. After decades of cancer genome and karyotype analysis, is estimated that 14% (about 3000) of the human genes are involved on cancer formation and progression [8], and the quantity of chromosome alterations involved is equally large. Therefore, some web tools were created to permit a faster search of these genic and chromosomal mutations on cancer for specific entities, as for example the "Mitelman Catalog of chromosomal alterations" [14].

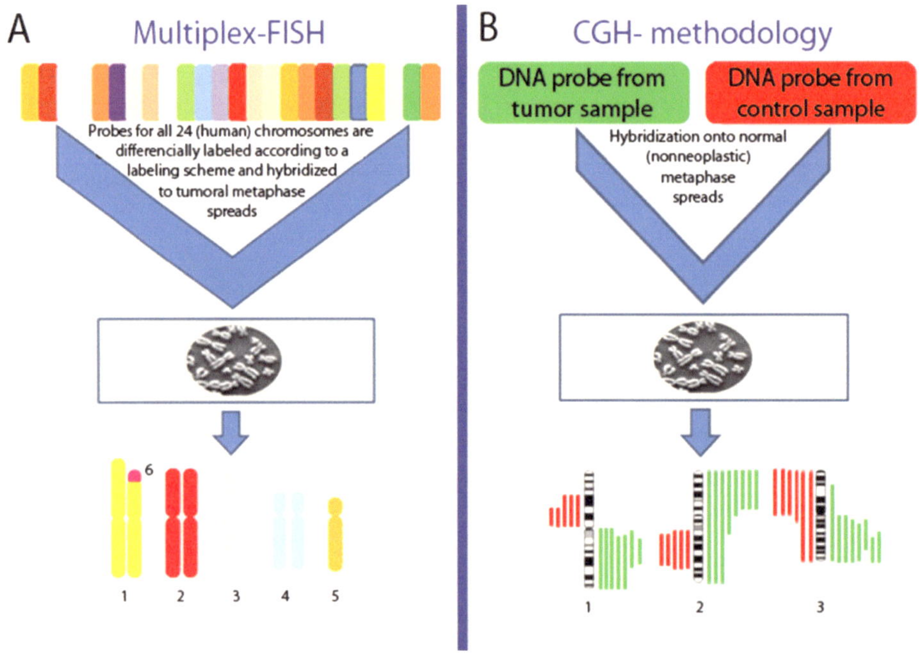

Figure 3. Whole-genome analysis of a tumor cell can be obtained by (A) M-FISH, SKY or (B) CGH methodologies. (A) SKY or M-FISH utilizes a pool with 24 differently labeled chromosomes with a combination of five distinct fluorochromes to show all chromosomal rearrangements in a metaphase, including structural and numerical rearrangements and markers chromosome. (B) CGH utilizes two different DNA probes, from tumor and from a control nonneoplastic sample, to hybridize onto a spread metaphase, or more recently in a slide array, to demonstrate DNA loss, gain or amplification in the tumor sample.

Further down we will list some of the new and well established correlations between brain tumors entities clinical behavior and some specific chromosome abnormalities. Some of the imbalances were correlated with particular pathways or genic imbalances, others have no well-established correlation with a specific gene function disturbance or cell pathways modifications, although are systematically found in some brain tumor types.

3. Brain tumors

Brain tumors are the second most common type of cancer in children and are associated with poor survival both in infants and adults, representing, therefore, a heavy burden for the patients and their relatives [15]. These tumors can be devastating because they are difficult to treat, and frequently cause mental impairment or death. The incidence of brain tumors has increased during the past three decades for all age and gender groups as a result of imaging with computed tomography (CT) and magnetic resonance imaging (MRI), lymphomas secondary to HIV/AIDS, and changes in coding and classification [16]. With the exception of meningiomas and pituitary adenomas, women are less likely than men to be diagnosed with a brain tumor, particularly glioblastoma multiforme and anaplastic astrocytoma, as well as medulloblastomas. The lifetime risk of contracting a primary malignant brain tumor is 0.52% for women and 0.67% for men. Similarly, the chance of dying from a malignant brain tumor is 0.40% for women and 0.49% for men. There have been growing amount of studies dedicated to detecting chromosomal imbalances and intercellular genomic variations both in benign and malign brain tumors. Currently, it is suggested that almost all the chromosomes are involved in aberrations associated with brain tumorigenesis [17]. Moreover, some specifics chromosome structures can differentiate the tumor grades, in accordance to WHO classification, simply by determining its proliferative potential, it is the case of Nucleolar Organizer Region (NOR), which can be analyzed by AgNOR to discriminate benign and malignant brain tumors [18]. Nevertheless, there are a number of chromosomal regions that are recurrently rearranged in brain tumors.

In order to illustrate the importance of cytogenetic studies and the relation of some recurrent rearrangements and tumor behavior/classification, we are going to describe the most common chromosomal rearrangements in some brain tumors.

4. Gliomas

The most common malignant primary brain tumors are gliomas, corresponding to more than 70% of the total primary brain tumors. They include a variety of malignant grades and histological tumor types. Gliomas can be classified in Astrocytic tumors, oligodendrogliomas and Ependymal tumors in accordance with the WHO classification of the tumors [4]. The most common gliomas are astrocytic tumors in which the most malignant entity is the glioblastoma (WHO grade IV). Gliomas are characterized as non-curable tumors. Today histopathology is still the gold standard for diagnosis and grading of gliomas tumors. However some markers have emerged and have important applications to their classification and prognosis.

4.1. Astrocytic tumors

The Astrocytic tumors are very diverse and represent the largest and most common group of brain tumors. The Astrocytomas, Anaplastic Astrocytomas and the secondary Glioblastomas (GBMs) are examples of tumors that show linear progression from benign to malignant neoplasms [4]. This progression is driven by some specific genetic events including chromosomal mutations. The most common cytogenetic observation is an increased complexity of the karyotype, both structural and numerically, concurrent with the progression in malignancy. Amplifications of *EGFR* locus on 7p12 and *PTEN* mutations on 10q23.3 are the best known genetic markers that distinguish the *de novo* GBM from GBM that has a progression from a low grade astrocytic tumor, which is frequently associated with *TP53* and *IDH1* gene mutations [19-21]. Trisomy of 7 and monosomy of 10 as well as frequent gains of 12p, 19q, and 20q differ primary from secondary glioblastomas [22]. Despite of these cytogenetic differences, primary or secondary glioblastomas can be assigned to a common set of functional pathways [23].

EGFR-mediated signaling is up regulated in about 30% of malignant gliomas and 60% of GBM [24-26]. In GBM the overexpression generally is driven by *EGFR* gene amplification [27, 28]. Several contradictory studies have been made in prognostic value determination of *EGFR* amplification [29]. Erlotinib and gefitinib are two drugs that target the *EGFR* amplification/ overexpression positive patients. These drugs presented unclear results up to date, with different researches demonstrating contradictory results. However, a recent study showed that co-expression of *PTEN* and *EGFRvIII* (a mutant form of *EGFR* molecules that constitutively activates the EGFR-phosphoinositide 3-kinase pathway) was associated with an increased sensitivity to erlotinib, whereas tumors without *PTEN* expression did not respond to erlotinib [30]. In another study, glioblastoma patients treated with these drugs did not show major response or survival improvement [31, 32]. On the other hand, a mixed result was obtained by the combined use of erlotinib with temozolomide and radiotherapy [33, 34]: a group with no overall benefit that did not help to identify a subgroup of tumors that might respond to therapy [33], and other group suggested that this regime might be useful for patients with tumors with *MGMT* promoter methylation and intact *PTEN* [34]. There is no consensus about use of these drugs in gliomas and glioblastomas patients to date, but new drugs and new molecularly targeted drugs reached clinical trials [35].

A more informative scenery is obtained by the simultaneous analyses of *EGFR* gene amplification and *EGFRvIII* in gliomas. An estimative of 50-60% of the amplified *EGFR* patients presents the *EGFRvIII* mutation. This condition is considered both diagnostic and prognostically informative, indicating a high grade malignancy. It is suggested that anaplastic or low-grade gliomas with this combination are more malignant than indicated by their histopathology and an unfavorable impact on the prognosis has been described for these patients [36]. To high grade gliomas, like primary glioblastomas, the *EGFR* amplification/ *EGFRvIII* poor prognosis is less obvious [37] but some studies have reported a poor prognosis association [38-41].

In glioblastomas, *EGFR* amplification mostly occurs as double-minutes (DM), which are small fragments of extra-chromosomal DNA. FISH assessment of this amplification is an accessible technique to be made in conventional pathology laboratories, which can be made in interphasic nuclei of a paraffin-embeded section [42, 43]. Quantitative PCR or reverse transcriptase PCR can be used to detect *EGFR* amplification as well [44]. Immunohistochemistry is used, but its value is less clear [45].

Some alterations in astrocytomas can indicate an increased risk of dying, independently of its histological grade, such as the presence of +7q and -10q chromosomal alterations detected by the CGH analysis of astrocytomas [46]. Misra and coworkers [47] identified three groups in GBM patients: those with both 7 gain and 10 loss, some with 10 loss without gain of 7 and the group without these two alterations. In clinical evaluation, the patients with 7 gain and 10 loss showed typical characteristic of GBM short-term survivors. In contrast, patients who had none of these alterations showed characteristics of typical and long-term survivors. In this research it was showed that *EGFR* is amplified on 7 gain 10 loss group of primary GBM. In a review using interphase-based FISH to chromosomes 7 and 10, it was found that 75% of the astrocytomas grade II and 100% of the grade III and IV exhibited cells with polysomy of chromosome 7 and that 75% of the grades II and III or 100% of the GBM samples showed cells with loss of chromosome 10 [20].

A gene expression profile (GEP) in a series of gliomas was associated with the cytogenetic of the glioblastomas and with the histopathology of gliomas [48]. When low-grades versus high-grades gliomas were compared, divergent profiles both cytogenetic and GEP were exhibited. High grades gliomas demonstrated higher intratumoral cytogenetic heterogeneity (demonstrated by a higher number of cell clones). The authors correlated this with the genomic instability or with the ancestral tumor cell clone chromosomal alterations in which karyotype composition led to an increased CIN. According to this study, three distinct glioblastomas GEP groups were formed: GEP1 with *EGFR* amplification, GEP2 with isolated trisomy 7 and GEP3 demonstrating more complex karyotype. All these three groups were formed after analysis of ancestral tumor cell clone and further cytogenetic evolution of the tumor cells of GEP1, GEP2 and GEP3 glioblastomas were related with 7 gain, 9p and 10q deletions, suggesting a simultaneous occurrence of *EGFR* activation (normal or mutant variants) and loss of both *Ink4A/Arf* and *PTEN* tumor suppressor genes.

4.2. Oligodendroglial tumors

Oligodendroglial tumors are diffusely infiltrating, well differentiated gliomas, typically located in cerebral hemispheres in adults, composed of neoplastic cells morphologically resembling oligodendroglia [4]. In oligodendrogliomas (WHO grade II) 80-90% are correlated to simultaneous deletion of 1p and 19q, whereas more malignant tumors demonstrate lower frequencies of this same alteration. The anaplastic oligodendrogliomas (WHO grade III) present 1p/19q co-deletions in approximately 50-60%, oligoastrocytomas in 30-50%, anaplastic oligoastrocytomas in 20-30%, and diffuse astrocytic gliomas in less than 10%, including glioblastomas. Currently, loss of 1p and 19q is the genetic hallmark of oligodendroglial tumors [4, 49]. Theses deletions were firstly associated with PVC (Procarbazine, CCNU and vincristine) sensitivity, demonstrating a favorable outcome in contrast with patients who don't show these chromosomal deletions, simultaneously [50]. Nowadays, this substantially improved survival times was correlated with others drugs (like temozolomide) or procedures (like radiotherapy) sensitivity, suggesting that 1p/19q co-deletion is an indicator of tumor vulnerability to a broad range of therapeutic options than as a specific predictor of chemosensitivity [35].

Interestingly, although the 1p and 19q regions have been extensively mapped, no tumorigenic gene was implicated. Another observation is that 1p/19q co-deletion tumors generally present a classical histology [51-53] and is correlated with *IDH1* and *IDH2* mutations [54]. On the other hand, *TP53* mutation, 10q deletions and *EGFR* amplifications were inversely correlated with 1p/19q co-deletion tumors [53]. Another association is obtained from tumor location: when anaplastic oligodendrogliomas and low grade oligodendrogliomas occur in the frontal, parietal, and occipital lobes, they are generally related to 1p/19q co-deletions [55-57]. In glioblastomas 1p/19q co-deletion is uncommon, however, when it is detected, the results observed are opposite, predicting shortened survival [52]. Thus, this cytogenetic marker denotes a clinically distinct tumor, with progression, prognosis, and treatment responses that are different of others gliomas. Therefore detection of 1p/19q alterations in oligodendrogliomas has become a useful and common test procedure [35]. FISH is the most reliable procedure to detect this marker in the laboratories, which can be substituted by array CGH in the next future when this technique may become less expensive.

By contrast, when the short arm of chromosome 1 is deleted alone, which is a rare cytogenetic finding in gliomas, it is associated with a poorer prognosis. On the other hand, in glioblastomas, primary or secondary, loss of heterozygosity (LOH) of 1p (other rare observation) is associated with longer survival [50]. In contrast, the oligodendroglial tumors are associated with poorer outcome when 8q gains are observed [20].

4.3. Pediatric gliomas

Pilocytic astrocytomas commonly present a characteristic *BRAF* proto-oncogene activation at 7q34, mainly by gene fusion or duplication, which is infrequent in diffusely infiltrating astrocytic gliomas [58-61]. Therefore, difficult diferential diagnosis between pilocytic astrocytoma and low-grade diffuse astrocytoma could be improved by the detection of *BRAF* activation. *BRAF* is target of a new therapy that inhibits the MAPK pathway, as showed in a case report [62]. The detection of *BRAF* fusion can be made by specific FISH probes or by specialized RT-PCR assays.

5. CNS Embryonal tumors

Embryonal tumors of the CNS form by far the largest group of malignant brain tumors in childhood. They are characterized by a mass of cells that begins its growth in the embryonic tissue in the brain. Despite the progress in the knowledge of these tumors, few studies were translated on clinical improvement. The WHO classification divides embryonal tumors into three entities: Medulloblastomas, CNS Primitive Neuroectodermal tumors (PNETs) and Atypical teratoid/rhabdoid tumor (AT/RT) [4].

5.1. Medulloblastomas

Medulloblastomas (MBs) are the most frequent embryonal tumors and the most frequent CNS tumor in childhood. They affect the cerebellum and are defined as grade IV in the WHO classification. Histopathological classification differentiates five distinct medulloblastoma variants: the classic MB, desmoplastic/nodular MB, MB with extensive nodularity, anaplastic MB and large cell MB [4].

In a recent comprehension made by [63], MB comprises four distinct molecular subgroups: WNT, SHH, group C and group D. This subgroup classification was made in accordance with its GEP of important genes in medulloblastoma disease. The authors also created an immunohistochemistry (an easier methodology to install on the conventional histopathology laboratories) four-antibody approach to discriminate the medulloblastoma patients into the four distinct molecular variants. Children patients classified as group C demonstrate a marked reduction in survival regardless of it metastatic stage. After a recent discussion about the classification of MB in the light of its transcriptome, involving researchers of different laboratories and countries, these subgroup were renamed, to WNT, SHH, Group 3 and Group 4 [64].

Analyzing the somatic copy number aberrations (SCNA) of the MB, Northcott and coworkers [65] concluded that SCNA in MB are common and are predominantly subgroup-enriched. Only the WNT subgroup demonstrated no significant deletions and a small subset of focal gains, which were found in a proportional frequency in non-WNT tumors, concluding that there are no frequent, targetable SCNA on this subgroup. SHH tumors, however, exhibit multiple focal SCNAs restricted/enriched on this group and have important clinical implications [65]. Group 3 and Group 4, which were generically named because less is known about its biology [64], presented important SCNAs restricted/enriched on them. *MYC* amplification (Figure 4A) mutually with *OTX2* oncogene demonstrated that are largely restricted to Group 3, and were extremely prognostic. Furthermore, TGF-β signaling is the unique restricted pathway involved in group 3 tumors, which may indicating a new therapy for Group 3 patients that present a dismal prognosis. In group 4 MB patients, the NF-kB pathway could represent a rational therapeutic target, because *NFKBIA* (14q13) and *USP4* (3p21.3), regulators of NF-kB, were consistently deleted on this group [65]

The most frequent chromosomal abnormality in MB is the isochromosome 17q (i17q), found in approximately 30%-50% of patients [66, 67]. The i17q structure consists of two centromeres, two very centromeric "17p" region that are fused together, mainly in the Smith-Magenis region, and two copies of 17 long arm. It was observed in increased levels of recurrent meduloblastomas compared with the initials ones, suggesting a role in progression of medulloblastomas [68]. But, although there are well-known tumor suppressor genes and oncogenes on chromosome 17, the tumor suppressor genes on the 17p or the oncogenes in the 17q directly involved on MB disease were not yet identified, however the tumor growth advantage may occur by haploinsufficiency for genes on 17p and an increased expression of genes on 17q driven by the copy number alterations. For this reason, 17q gain, 17p loss or both represent the same biological effect of an i17q (Figure 4C), which is an alteration commonly seen in MB patients [63, 68, 69]. The presence of this abnormality was the unique chromosomal alteration that occurs at a high frequency in [63] and was significantly prominent in Group D (Group 4) molecular subgroup of MBs (65.7%). The others chromosomal alterations were seen at a low frequency [63]. The monossomy 6 in the same study and others was detected exclusively in WNT tumors [63, 70-73], while the 9q loss was detected only in SHH tumors [72]. These and others chromosomal markers presents on the four molecular subgroups will be shown in Table 1.

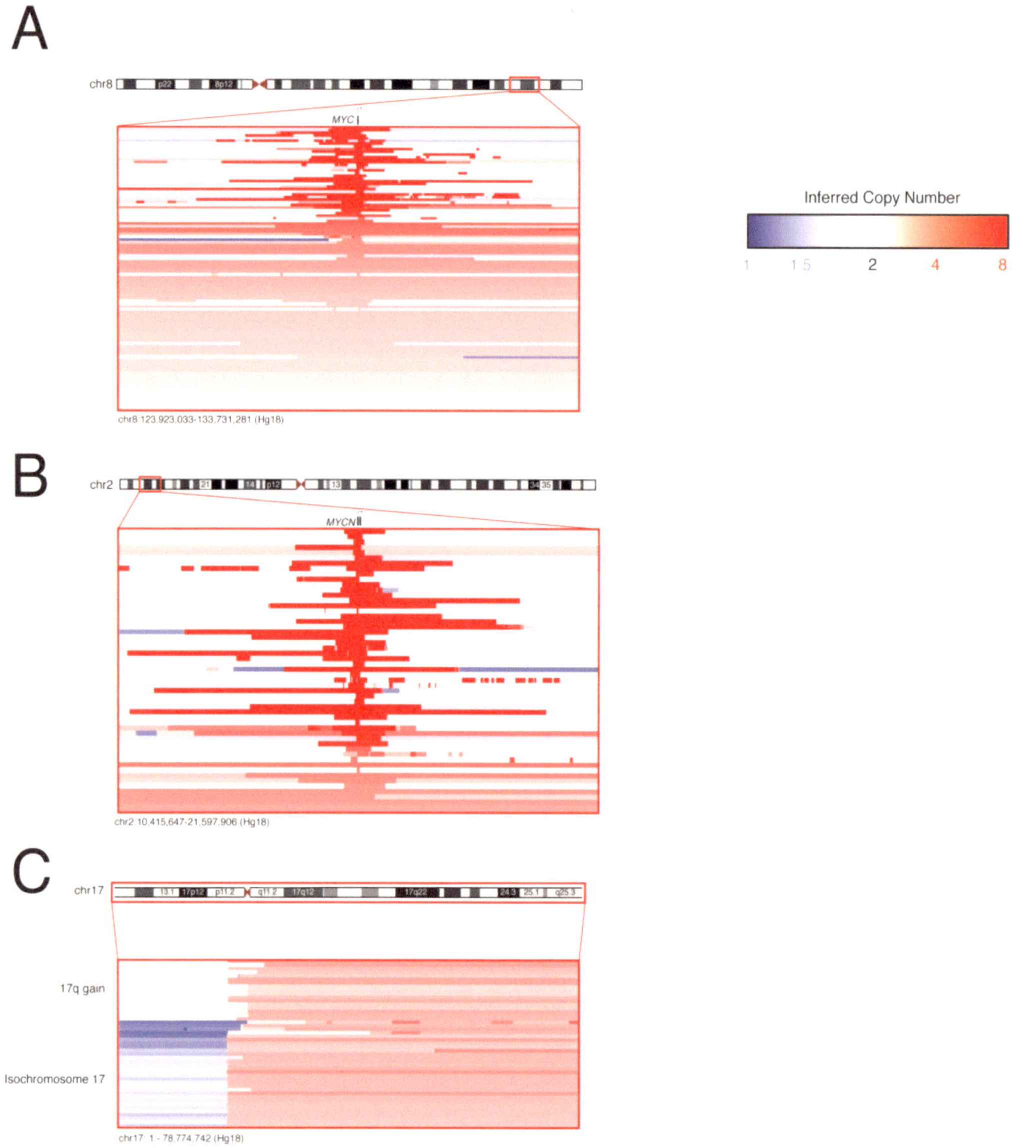

Figure 4. Somatic Copy Number Aberrations (SCNA) in medulloblastomas involving chromosomes (A) 8, (B) 2 and (C) 17. The colors represent the inferred copy number for each chromosome locus, in which red spectrum represent gains/amplification and blue spectrum represent loss/deletions, normal SCNA is represented in white. (A) Chromosome 8 SCNA exhibiting amplification on the *MYC* locus on 8q24.21. (B) Chromosome 2 SCNA showing amplification on *MYCN* locus on 2p24.3. (C) Chromosome 17 SCNA demonstrating 17q gain and both 17p loss and 17q gain (representing i17q). Courtesy of Dubuc AM, Taylor MD, Northcott PA and Shih D. See [65] for details.

The investigation of *MYC* and *MYCN* locus provided consistent prognostic information to medulloblastoma patients [66, 74-79], and can be accessed by FISH or CGH experiments (Figure 4A and 4B), being related mutated in up to 10% of medulloblastomas. *MYC* amplification is associated with poor prognosis and with the large cell/anaplastic medulloblastoma variants, but histologically aggressive cases diagnosed, like large cell/anaplastic MB without amplification of *MYC*, were not significantly associated with worse outcome [68]. *MYCN* amplification (Figure 4B) is associated with poor prognosis and correlated with large cell/ anaplastic variants, but is clinically more heterogeneous than *MYC*. The MYC family was considered in Northcott molecular stratification of MBs [63, 65], and *MYC* amplification on 8q24 (Figure 4A) was detected exclusively on Group C (Group 3) patients. MYCN was demonstrated amplified (Figure 4B) both in SHH and Group D (Group 4) MB patients [63, 65].

	Losses	Gains	Others
WNT	-	-	Monossomy 6
SHH	9q, 10q, 14	2, 3q, 9p, 20q, 21q	
Group C	5q, 8p, 10q, 11p, 16q	1q, 17q, 18	i17q,
Group D	X, 8p, 8q, 11p	17q, 18	i17q,

Table 1. Significant chromosomal abnormalities observed on the four distinct molecular variants of the Northcott study.

For adult Medulloblastomas, different genetic and cytogenetic changes were observed in relation to pediatric ones, with profiles of chromosomal abnormalities greatly differing from childhood. *CDK6* amplification, 17q gain and 10q loss were strongly associated with shortened survival. The WNT signaling pathway activation does not demonstrate the excellent prognosis seen in pediatrics MB [80].

5.2. Atypical teratoid/rhabdoid tumor

Atypical teratoid/rhabdoid tumors (AT/RT) are very malignant embryonal neoplasms (WHO grade IV) that occur in very young children [4]. Very constant alterations in *SMARCB1* locus on 22q11 were published. These alterations can be detected like deletions, loss of heterozygosity (LOH) or gene mutation in all the exons of this gene. SMARCB1 protein immunohistochemistry search has demonstrated great utility in diagnosis of AT/RT or in determinate patients with poor therapy response and aggressive clinical course, even in the absence of AT/ RT cell [81, 82]. When combined FISH, genomic sequencing, MLPA and SNP-based oligonucleotide arrays were used to diagnosis AT/RT in 36 patients, all demonstrated biallelic alteration in *SMARCB1* locus [83]. The molecular diagnostic became yet more important when it is possible to determinate adult carriers, to genetic counseling finalities.

5.3. Ependymoblastomas

Ependymoblastoma and ETANTR (Embryonal Tumor with Abundant Neuropil and True Rosettes) are rare and very aggressive Primitive Neuroectodermal Tumors (PNETs) characterized by the presence of multilayred rosette [4]. They were recently associated with focal amplification of 19q13.42 that contains a cluster of mi-RNA-coding gene. This amplification was seen in virtually all the embryonal brain tumor with true multilayered rosettes [84-86]. These results indicate that they may represent a single biological entity that can be diagnosed by the detection of 19q13.42 amplification. The term Embryonal Tumor with Multilayered Rosettes (ETMR) was proposed to designate these entities that apparently affect only children and have a very poor prognosis.

6. Ependymal tumors

Ependymomas form a group of heterogeneous tumors anywhere along the craniospinal axis that can occur in adult or childhood. They can originate from the radial glial cells [87, 88] which originate the ependymal cells during normal cellular development. The WHO classification [4] designates ependymal tumors in different histology entities, as hereafter: Subependymomas and myxopapillary ependymomas (WHO grade I); Classic ependymomas (WHO grade II); anaplastic ependymomas (WHO grade III). The classic ependymoma was subdivided in four variant cellular, papillary, clear cell and tanycytic [89]. For these tumors the WHO grading was the most powerful prognostic factor in adult population. In the same way, the tumor location has been demonstrated as having potential prognostic value, with those in the supratentorial regions demonstrating poor prognosis and with higher risk of recurrence.

The chromosomal abnormalities reflect the heterogeneity of topology and age of Ependymomas. A study made by Korshunov and coworkers [90] has presented a comprehensive work that subdivides the ependymomas in three groups:

a. Group 1: five years of Overall survival of 100% - tumors with gain of chromosomes 9, 15q, or 18, or loss of chromosome 6, without 1q gain or *CDKN2A* deletion.

b. Group 2: five years of Overall survival of 78% - tumors balanced for chromosome 1q, 6, 9, 15q, and 18, without a homozygous deletion of *CDKN2A*.

c. Group 3: five years of Overall survival of 32% - tumors with 1q gain or homozygous deletions of *CDKN2A*.

Group 1 demonstrates an excellent response to standard therapy protocols, demonstrating an excellent prognosis. Group 3 demonstrates a propensity to generate metastasis and generally show an aggressive clinical behavior, having its chromosomal composition associated with a poor prognosis. Another possibility for this group is the association of 1q21.1-32.1 gain correlated with an increased propensity to recurrence.

Some chromosome alterations remain unclear between the groups. The 6q23 loss in group 1 can be correlated with a decreased progression-free survival, while 6q25.3 loss in anaplastic ependymomas has been correlated with an improved overall survival. The 9q gain in pediatric group 1 patients was correlated with a frequent recurrence.

Yang and coworkers [91] conclude that diagnosis based only in the light of histologic procedures may be insufficient to assign an appropriate risk stratification strategy. In our opinion the enlargement of cytogenetic analysis could generate a map of chromosomal alterations on ependymomas that would help in creating a personalized treatment for these tumors and indicate targets to avoid growth, recurrence or metastasis.

7. Meningiomas

Meningiomas are the second most common tumor of the CNS in adults. They are classified as benign, atypical or anaplastic corresponding to 80%, 15-20% and 1-3%, respectively, and stratified in grades I, II and III, respectively [92]. Even the grade I meningiomas, with a favorable prognosis under the classical treatment with surgical resection, radiation and chemotherapy, presents an aggressive remaining group which needs molecular or cytogenetic markers to distinct its diagnosis and treatment.

The karyotypes of meningiomas show diversity among the WHO grades. The WHO grade I benign meningiomas rarely exhibit chromosomal aberrations beyond 22q losses. More complex karyotype compositions are seen in higher grade meningiomas with more aggressive behavior. The losses are common to 1p, 10q, 14q and less frequent on 6q and 18q in Atypical and Anaplastic meningiomas. Higher grade meningiomas are characterized by gains on 1q, 9q, 12q, 15q, 17q and 20q. Anaplastic meningiomas have demonstrated losses on 9p with amplification on 17q23 in a higher frequency. Alterations on chromosome 1 always represent important alterations on CNS tumors. In meningioma losses on 1p can be related as a strong indicator of recurrence: only 4.3% of the meningiomas with recurrence are seen with an intact 1p. The presence of deletions of 1p can be related to a strong propensity to recur. LOH on 1p, 10q and 9p are also associated with recurrence propensity. At the same way, 9p losses are associated with anaplastic meningiomas (grade III) with *p14ARF* (encoding p14), *CDKN2B/p15ARF* (encoding p15), and *CDKN2A/p16INKa* (encoding p16) tumor suppressor genes losses. The most important is the *CDKN2A* impairment causing poorer outcome when compared to patients with intact *CDKN2A* genes. Losses in 14q also are found in meningiomas, and are associated with a worse prognosis. 14q deletions serve as a powerful and reliable prognostic factor indicating tumor recurrence [93].

8. Others brain tumors

Less well understood involvement of chromosome abnormalities are reported for some infrequent tumors of the CNS. The low frequency can explain the low number of cytogenetic studies, but the involvement of a multigroup work to understand them could provide a solution to compile these patients. However, some works have made a suggestive involvement of specific chromosomal alterations in the genesis, development, aggressiveness or response to therapies. For these, a brief description will be made here.

An example is the Olfactory Neuroblastoma (also named Esthesioneuroblastoma), that originate from the olfactory epithelium, that form a group of neoplasm less studied at the cytogenetic point of view, but the first comprehensive study has suggested that the prevalence of 3q deletion demonstrates that it can be adopted as an early genetic event in Esthesioneuroblastoma and the involvement of deletion on chromosomes 5, 6q, 7q, 11p/q, 15q21 as well as gains of 1p32-34, 1q12, and 2p22-24 can be associated with a metastatic phenotype and a worse prognosis [94].

Rickert and coworkers [95] in a study applying CGH in choroid plexus papillomas and choroid plexus carcinomas made the follow correlation: patients with choroid plexus carcinomas were associated to have a significantly longer survival when +9p and -10q alterations were present.

9. Brain metastases

Brain metastases are tumors that originate outside the CNS and secondarily spread to the CNS via the haematogenous route (metastasis) or by direct invasion from adjacent tissues [4]. Metastatic tumors form a heterogeneous group, in which primary site can be from any location in body. But the frequencies of tumors that metastasize to brain are non-random, because there is an organ tropism to each tumor. However, brain metastases can occur in up to 40% of the cancer patients and represent a major cause of mortality and morbidity in cancer patients; some authors indicate that there are under notification of brain metastases [96]. The most commons primary sites that metastasize to brain are the lung, breast and melanoma with frequencies of 40-50%, 15-25% and 5-20%, respectively. However, melanoma will be not considered here since the *BRAF* gene mutation, it the main molecular marker, can't be detected by cytogenetic procedures.

A consensus is that up to date the role of current chemotherapy with cytotoxic drugs is limited to palliation, and the efficacy depends on the chemosensitivity of the primary tumor [97]. A new possibility is to create a therapy that prevents brain metastasis; it will be possible when targeted therapies to known molecular pathways to brain colonization become clear. This possibility could become a common strategy to those tumors that frequently form brain metastases.

On established brain metastases the therapy mainly consists on the use of whole brain radiation therapy (WBRT). Less frequently targeted agents, either alone or in combination with WBRT, have been investigated in newly diagnosed brain metastases [98].

A correlation can be made to Non-small Cell Lung Cancer (NSCLC). NSCLC patients show activating epidermal growth factor receptor (*EGFR*) mutations in 10-25% of the cases, with the highest prevalence in never-smoking women from East Asia, in up to 55%. Erlotinib and gefitinib, *EGFR* tyrosine kinase inhibitors, have been demonstrated to be useful in patients with brain metastases from NSCLC [99-106]. Nevertheless, Brain metastasis from NSCLC patients with mutant *EGFR* confronted with those wild type *EGFR* have demonstrated an improved overall survival, when receiving *EGFR* inhibitors [107]. Another molecular marker in NSCLC patient, a FISH detectable rearrangement in 2p23 in 4% of patients, the ALK rearrangement can be treated with crizotinib (a specific ALK inhibitor) demonstrating objective response or stabilization of the malignancy [108]. A speculation about a brain barrier to crizotinib agent could permit a poorer penetration into the brain leading to a lower efficacy, but no data about any treatment with crizotinib to brain metastasis exist to date [109].

The most informative molecular marker on brain metastases of breast cancer came from *HER2*. Breast tumors positive for *HER2*, triple negative lacking expression of HER2, estrogen and progesterone receptors, or the basal-like subtype form the high risk group that can metastasize to brain. The *HER2* breast cancer patients represent 25% of overall population, and have the highest risk of brain metastases development, especially if estrogen/progesterone negative [110]. A recent work analyzed alterations on chromosome 17 in metastatic brain tumors from breast cancers using a dual color experiment with CEP17 and *TP53* locus specific probe. The result was a high incidence of chromosome 17p deletion in these neoplasms, suggesting a role of 17p loss in the metastatic capability acquisition for breast tumor cells [111].

When breast cancer patients are treated with trastuzumab, a monoclonal antibody that target *HER2*, 25-40% tend to present brain metastasis [112-116], which can increase when compared with trastuzumab-no treated patients [117]. An explanation is that trastuzumab efficiently controls the systemic disease spread [118], associated with a *HER2* propensity to brain colonization [119, 120] and with the trastuzumab decreases penetration through the blood-brain barrier [118]. Recent works have demonstrated that a higher penetrance of trastuzumab into the brain, which could be provided by lesion in blood-brain barrier or increased vascular permeability driven by tumor activity or by radiation therapy, have revealed an improved prognosis to *HER2*-positive patients with brain metastases [116, 121-124].

The *HER2* gene, a member of *EGFR* gene family, is located on 17q21.1 and the amplification can be detected by a FISH experiment. HER2 protein overexpression can be detected by an immunohistochemistry method. Both, FISH or immunohistochemistry, can be made in paraffin-embedded tissues. The higher cost and longer time required to cell scoring in FISH experiments make the immunohistochemistry the most utilized procedure in laboratories, but FISH was demonstrated as more efficient and accurate scoring systems to determine *HER2* amplification than immunohistochemistry [125, 126]. More recently, a study aimed to determine a relationship between HER2 protein expression level or *HER2* gene amplification ratio (by FISH with a *HER2* gene probe and CEP17 probe in a dual color experiment) correlated with the time to brain metastases formation in *HER2*+ advanced breast cancer patients. It showed that HER2 protein expression level detection demonstrated a more sensitive method to determinate the time to brain metastases, shown a shorter time to brain metastases in higher level of HER2 protein expression [127].

10. Conclusions

After analyzing all these cumulative information, one can conclude that chromosomal analysis of brain tumors can strongly improve the clinical diagnostic and prognostic in clinical practice and the knowledge about the biology of brain tumors. This information has helped in the choice of the best therapy in widely studied tumor types, and could help even more. Also, the great number of chromosome abnormalities associated to specific tumor entities improves the search for target genes or cell pathways that direct or indirect act in tumorigenesis or tumor progression. On the other hand, if Li's theory [13] is true and the tumors are generated by aneuploidogenics carcinogens or mutations, targeted preventions to avoid aneuploidy/aneuploidy cells or a methodology that enhances genomic stability/cell defense mechanisms against cells with CIN could provide an effective approach.

Similarly, it is clear that some chromosomal alterations are more important to a wide range of brain tumor, participating in the genesis, progression, metastases and others hallmarks of cancer than to a specific entity. Alterations on chromosome 1, 7, 8, 10, 17 and 22 appear to be important to a variety of tumors of the brain. 1q gain is an example of alteration that leads to a worse prognosis, correlated with tumor recurrence or progression. At the same way, 17q gains and 17p losses almost always represent a poor prognosis. The presence of important tumor suppressor genes or oncogenes in these loci can explain its higher participation on the evolution of tumors cells to achieve the malignancy. Gain of chromosome 7q could be related with *EGFR* amplification, which is implicated with a large number of brain tumors entities. Likewise 17q gain could be related to *HER2* amplification, or 17p losses could be associated with the selective advantage of *TP53* pathways inactivation.

Obviously, as molecular markers, locus amplifications/deletions, structural abnormal chromosomes or aneuploidies are important genetic mutations that confer to tumors different clinical and biological behavior. These markers can be applied in clinical routine to determine prognostic, a better diagnostic or indicate alternative chemotherapy to brain tumor patient treatment.

Nomenclature

AT/RT	Atypical Teratoid/Rhabdoid Tumors
BRAF	v-raf murine sarcoma viral oncogene homolog B1
CDK6	cyclin-dependent kinase 6
CDKN2A	cyclin-dependent kinase inhibitor 2A
CDKN2A/p16INKa	cyclin-dependent kinase inhibitor 2A (encoding p16)
CDKN2B/p15ARF	cyclin-dependent kinase inhibitor 2B (encoding p15)
CGH	Comparative Genomic Hybridization
CIN	Chromosomal Instability
CML	Chronic Myelogenous Leukemia
CNS	Central Nervous System
DM	Double-minutes
EGFR	Epidermal Growth Factor Receptor
ETANTR	Embryonal Tumors with Abundant Neuropil and True Rosettes

http://dx.doi.org/10.5772/52354

ETMR	Embryonal Tumors with Multilayered Rosettes
FISH	Fluorescence in situ Hybridization
GBM	Glioblastomas
GEP	Gene Expression Profile
HER2	v-erb-b2 erythroblastic leukemia viral oncogene homolog 2, neuro/glioblastoma derived oncogene homolog
HSR	Homogeneously Staining Region
IDH1	isocitrate dehydrogenase 1
IDH2	isocitrate dehydrogenase 2
Ink4A/Arf	cyclin-dependent kinase inhibitor 2A
LOH	Loss of Heterozygosity
MB	Medulloblastoma
M-FISH	Multiplex-FISH
MGMT	O-6-methylguanine-DNA methyltransferase
MYC	v-myc myelocytomatosis viral oncogene homolog
MYCN	v-myc myelocytomatosis viral related oncogene, neuroblastoma derived
NF-kB	Nuclear Factor kappa B
NFKBIA	nuclear factor of kappa light polypeptide gene enhancer in B-cells inhibitor, alpha
NSCLC	Non-small Cell Lung Cancer
OTX2	orthodenticle homeobox 2
P14ARF	cyclin-dependent kinase inhibitor 2A (encoding p14)
PCR	Polymerase Chain Reaction
PNET	Primitive Neuroectodermal Tumors
PTEN	phosphatase and tensin homolog
SCNA	Somatic Copy Number Aberrations
SHH	Sonic Hedgehog
SKY	Spectral Karyotyping
SMARCB1	SWI/SNF related, matrix associated, actin dependent regulator of chromatin, subfamily b, member 1.
TGF-β	transforming growth factor, beta
TP53	tumor protein p53
USP4	ubiquitin specific peptidase 4
WBRT	Whole Brain Radiation Therapy
WHO	World Health Organization

Acknowledgements

We would like to thank Programa de Pós-graduação em Genética e Biologia Molecular, Instituto Federal do Pará and Instituto Evandro Chagas for supporting and motivation. We are grateful to Adriene Costa and Lorena da Silva for text and reference formatting. The authors are in debt to Dr. Adrian M. Dubuc, Dr. Michael D. Taylor, Dr. Paul A. Northcott and Dr. David Shih for the important contributions.

Author details

Fabio P. Estumano da Silva[1] and Edivaldo H. C. de Oliveira[2]

1 Instituto Federal do Pará, Tucuruí, PA, Brazil / Programa de Pós-graduação em Genética e Biologia Molecular, ICB, Universidade Federal do Pará, Belém, PA, Brazil

2 SAMAM-Instituto Evandro Chagas, Ananindeua, PA, Brazil / ICEN, Universidade Federal do Pará, Belém, PA, Brazil

References

[1] Sumner AT. Chromosomes: organization and function. North Berwick: Blackwell Publishing; 2003.

[2] Nowell PC, Hungerford DA. Chromosome studies on normal and leukemic human leukocytes. Journal of the National Cancer Institute 1960; 25: 85-109.

[3] Baak JP, Path FR, Hermsen MA, Meijer G, Schmidt J, Janssen EA. Genomics and proteomics in cancer. European Journal of Cancer 2003; 39(9):1199-215.

[4] Louis DN, Ohgaki H, Wiestler OD, Cavanee WK, editors. Who classification of tumours of the central nervous system. Lyon, France: IARC Press; 2007.

[5] Boveri T. Zur Frage der Entstehung maligner tumoren. Jena: Gustav Fisher; 1914.

[6] Bonassi S, Znaor A, Norppa H, Hagmar L. Chromosomal aberrations and risk of cancer in humans: an epidemiologic perspective. Cytogenetic and Genome Research 2004; 104(1-4):376-82.

[7] Gisselsson D. Chromosomal instability in cancer: causes and consequences. Atlas of genetics and cytogenetics in oncology and haematology 2001; 5(3): 237-244.

[8] Bernheim A. Cytogenomics of cancers: From chromosome to sequence. Molecular Oncology 2010; doi:10.1016/j.molonc.2010.06.003.

[9] Albertson DG, Collins C, McCormick F, Gray JW. Chromosome aberrations in solid tumors. Nature Genetics 2003; 34(4): 369-376.

[10] Lengauer C, Kinzler KW, Vogelstein B. Genetic instabilities in human Cancers. Nature 1998; 396:643-49.

[11] Draviam VM, Xic S, Sorger PK. Chromosome segregation and genomic stability. Current Opinion in Genetics and Development. 2004; 14(2):120-5.

[12] Duesberg P, Li R, Sachs R, Fabarius A, Upender MB, Hehlmann R. Cancer drug resistance: The central role of the Karyotype 2007; 10: 51-58.

[13] Li L, McCormack AA, Nicholson JM, Fabarius A, Hehlmann R, Sachs RK, Duesberg PH. Cancer-causing karyotype: chromosomal equilibria between destabilizing aneuploidy and stabilizing selection for oncogenic function. Cancer Genetics and Cytogenetics 2009; 188: 1-25.

[14] Mitelman F, Johansson B and Mertens F, Editors. Mitelman Database of Chromosome Aberrations and Gene Fusions in Cancer. http://cgap.nci.nih.gov/Chromosomes/Mitelman. (accessed 16 July 2012).

[15] Jemal A, Siegel R, Ward E, Hao Y, Xu J, Murray T, Thun MJ. Cancer statistics 2008. CA: a cancer Journal for Clinicians 2008; 58:71-96.

[16] Jukich PJ, McCarthy BJ, Surawicz TS, Freels S, Davis FG. Trends in incidence of primary brain tumors in the United States, 1985-1994. Neuro-Oncololy 2001; 3(3):141-51.

[17] Iourov IY, Vorsanova SG, Yurov YB. Molecular cytogenetics and cytogenomics of brain diseases. Current Genomics 2008; 9(7):452-65.

[18] Quintana LG, da Silva FP, Pieczarka JC, Nagamachi CY, Anselmo NP, de Oliveira EH. Correlation between argyrophilic nucleolar organizer region staining and brain tumor classification and grading. Cancer Investigation 2010; 28(5):459-64.

[19] Kleihues P, Ohgaki H. Primary and Secondary glioblastomas: from concept to clinical diagnosis. Neuro-Oncology 1999; 1: 44-51.

[20] Bayani J, Pandita A, Squire JA. Molecular cytogenetic analysis in the study of brain tumors: findings and applications. Neurosurgical Focus 2005; 19(5): 1-36.

[21] Ohgaki H, Kleihues P. Genetic pathways to primary and secondary glioblastoma. The American journal of pathology 2007; 170: 1445-1453.

[22] Toedt G, Barbus S, Wolter M, Felsberg J, Tews B, Blond F, Sabel MC, Hoffman S, Becker N, Hartmann C, Ohgaki H, von Deimling A, Wiestler OD, Hahn M, Lichter P, Reifenberger G, Radlwimmer B. Molecular signatures classify astrocytic gliomas by IDH1 mutation status. International Journal of cancer 2010; 28(5): 1095-1103.

[23] Cancer Genome Atlas Research Network. Comprehensive genomic characterization defines human glioblastoma genes and core pathways. Nature 2008; 455:1061-1068. doi:10.1038/nature07385.

[24] Humphrey PA, Wong AJ, Vogelstein B, Friedman HS, Werner MH, Bigner DD, Bigner SH. Amplification and expression of the epidermal growth factor receptor gene in human gliomaxenografts. Cancer Research 1988; 48: 2231-38.

[25] Agosti RM, Leuthold M, Gullick WJ, Yasargil MG, Wiestler OD. Expression of the epidermal growth factor receptor in astrocytic tumours is specifically associated with glioblastoma and Histopathology 1992; 420: 321-25.

[26] Omuro AM, Faivre S, Raymond E. Lessons learned in the development of targeted therapy for malignant gliomas. Molecular Cancer Therapeutics 2007; 6: 1909-19.

[27] Bigner SH, Humphrey PA, Wong AJ, Vogelstein B, Mark J, Friedman HS, Bigner DD. Characterization of the epidermal growth factor receptor in human glioma cell lines and xenografts. Cancer Research 1990; 50: 1909-19.

[28] McLendon RE, Turner K, Rich J. Second messenger systems in human gliomas. Archives Pathology and Laboratory Medicine 2007; 131: 1585-90.

[29] Heimberger AB, Suki D, Yang D, Shi W, Aldape K. The natural history of EGFRvIII in glioblastoma patients. Journal of Translational Medicine 2005; 3: 287-90.

[30] Mellinghoff IK, Wang MY, Vivanco I, Haas-Kogan DA, Zhu S, Dia EQ, Lu KV, Yoshimoto K, Huang JH, Chute DJ, Riggs BL, Horvath S, Liau M, Cavenee WK, Rao PN, Beroukhim R, Pec TC, Lee JC, Sellers WR, Stokoe D, Prados M, Cloughesy TF, Sawyers CL, Mischel PS. Molecular determinants of the response of glioblastomas to EGFR kinase inhibitors. New England Journal of Medicine 2005; 353: 2012-24.

[31] Rich JN, Reardon DA, Peery T, Dowell JM, Quinn JA, Penne KL, Wikstrand CJ, Van Duyn LB, Dancey JE, McLendon RE, Kao JC, Stenzel TT, Ahmed Rasheed BK, Tourt-Uhlig SE, Herndon JE 2nd, Vredenburgh JJ, Sampson JH, Friedman AH, Bigner DD, Friedman HS. Phase II trial of gefitinib in recurrent glioblastoma. Journalof Clinical Oncology 2004; 22: 133-42.

[32] Kesari S, Ramakrishna N, Sauvageot C, Stiles CD, Wen PY. Targeted molecular therapy of malignant gliomas. Current Neurology and Neuroscience Reports 2005; 5: 186-97.

[33] Brown PD, Krishnan S, Sarkaria JN, Wu W, Jaeckle KA, Uhm JH, Geoffroy FJ, Arusell R, Kitange G, Jenkins RB, Kugler JW, Morton RF, Rowland KM Jr., Mischel P, Yong WH, Scheithauer BW, Schiff D, Giannini C, Buckner JC, Soori GS, Dakhil SR, Fitch TR, Windschitl HE, Flynn PJ, Anderson DM, Nair S, Nikcevich DA, Wender DB, Stella PJ, Jillella AP. Phase I/II trial of erlotinib and temozolomide with radiation therapy in the treatment of newly diagnosed glioblastoma multiforme: North Central Cancer Treatment Group Study N0177. Journal of Clinical Oncology 2008; 26: 5603-09.

[34] Prados MD, Chang SM, Butowski N, DeBoer R, Parvataneni R, Carline H, Kabuubi P, Ayers-Ringler J, Rabbitt J, Page M, Fedoroff A, Sneed PK, Berger MS, McDermott MW, Parsa AT, Vandenberg S, James CD, Lamborn KR, Stokoe D, Haas-Kogan DA. Phase II study of erlotinib plus termozolomide during and after radiation therapy in patients with newly diagnosed glioblastoma multiforme or gliosarcoma. Journal of Clinical Oncology 2009; 27: 579-84.

[35] Jansen M, Yip S, Louis DN. Molecular pathology in adult gliomas: diagnostic, prognostic, and predictive markers. Lancet Neurology 2010; 9(7): 717-26.

[36] Riemenschneider, MJ, Jeuken, JWM, Wesseling, P, Reifenberger. Molecular diagnostics of gliomas: state of the art. Acta Neuropathologica 2010; 120: 567-584.

[37] Weller, M, Felsberg, J, Hartmann, C, Berger, H, Steinbach, JP, Schramm, J, Westphal, M, Schackert, G, Simon, M, Tonn, JC, Heese, O, Krex, D, Nikkhah, G, Pietsch, T, Wiestler, O, Reifenberger, G, von Deimling, A, Loeffler, M, . Molecular predictors of progression- free and overall survival in patients with newly diagnosed glioblastoma: a prospective translational study of the German Glioma Network. Journal of Clinical Oncology 2009; 27: 5743-5750.

[38] Shinojima N, Tada K, Shiraishi S, Kamiryo T, Kochi M, Nakamura H, Makino K, Saya H, Hirano H, Kuratsu J, Oka K, Ishimaru Y, Ushio Y. Prognostic value of epidermal growth factor receptor in patients with glioblastoma multiforme. Cancer Research 2003; 63:6962–6970.

[39] Dehais C, Laigle- Donadey F, Marie Y, Kujas M, Lejeune J, Benouaich-Amiel A, Pedretti M, Polivka M, Xuan KH, Thillet J, Delattre JY, Sanson M. Prognostic stratification of patients with anaplastic gliomas according to genetic profile . Cancer 2006; 107: 1891-1897.

[40] Pelloski CE, Ballman KV, Furth AF, Zhang L, Lin E, Sulman EP, Bhat K, McDonald JM, Yung WK, Colman H, Woo SY, Heimberger AB, Suki D, Prados MD, Chang SM, Barker FG 2nd, Buckner JC, James CD, Aldape K. Epidermal growth factor receptor variant III status defines clinically distinct subtypes of glioblastoma. Journal f Clinical Oncology 2007; 25: 2288-94.

[41] Murat A, Migliavacca E, Gorlia T, Lambiv WL, Shay T, Hamou MF, de Tribolet N, Regli L, Wick W, Kouwenhoven MC, Hainfellner JA, Heppner FL, Dietrich PY, Zimmer Y, Cairncross JG, Janzer RC, Domany E, Delorenzi M, Stupp R, Hegi ME. Stem cell-related "self- renewal" signature and high epidermal growth factor receptor expression associated with resistance to concomitant chemoradiotherapy in glioblastoma. Journal of Clinical Oncology 2008; 26:3015-3024.

[42] Okada Y, Hurwitz EE, Esposito JM, Brower MA, Nutt CL, Louis DN. Selection Pressures of TP53 mutation and microenvironmental location influence epidermal growth factor receptor gene amplification in human glioblastomas. Cancer Research 2003; 63: 413-16.

[43] Aldape KD, Ballman K, Furth A, Buckner JC, Giannini C, Burger PC, Scheithauer BW, Jenkins RB, James CD. Immunohistochemical detection of EGFRvIII in high malignancy grade astrocytomas and evaluation of prognostic significance. Journal of Neuropathology E Experimental Neurology 2004; 63: 700-07.

[44] Arjona D, Bello MJ, Alonso ME, Aminoso C, Isla A, de Campos JM, Sarasa JL, Gutierrez M, Villalobo A, Rey JA. Molecular analysis of the EGFR gene in astrocytic gliomas: mRNA expression, quantitative-PCR analysis of non-homogeneous gene amplification and DNA sequence alterations. Neuropathology and Applied Neurobiology 2005; 31: 384-94.

[45] Kersting C, Packeisen J, Leidinger B, Brandt B, von Wasielewski R, Winkelmann W, van Diest PJ, Gosheger G, Buerger H. Pitfalls in immunohistochemical assessment of EGFR expression in soft tissue sarcomas. Journal of Clinical Pathology 2006; 59: 585-90.

[46] Wiltshire RN, Herndon JE II, Lloyd A, Friedman HS, Bigner DD, Sandra HB, McLendon RE. Comparative genomic hybridization analysis of astrocytomas: Prognostic and diagnostic implications. Journal of Molecular Diagnostics 2004; 6(3)166-179.

[47] Misra A, Pellarin M, Nigro J, Smirnov I, Moore D, Lamborn KR, Pinkel D, Albertson DG, Feuerstein BG. Array comparative genomic hybridization identifies genetic subgroups in grade 4 human astrocytoma. Clinical Cancer Research 2005; 11:2907–2918.

[48] Viltal AL, Tabernero MD, Castrillo A, Rebelo O, Tão H, Gomes F, Nieto AB, Oliveira CR, Lopes MC, Orfao A. Gene expression profiles of human glioblastomas are associated with both tumor cytogenetics and histopathology. Neuro-Oncology 2010; 12(9): 991-1003.

[49] Jeuken JW, von Deimling A, Wesseling P. Molecular pathogenesis of oligodendroglial tumors. Journal Neuro-oncology 2004; 70: 161–181.

[50] Ohgaki H, Kleihues P. Genetic alterations and signaling pathways in the evolution of gliomas. Cancer Science 2009; 100(12): 2235-2241.

[51] Smith JS, Alderete B, Minn Y, Borell TJ, Perry A, Mohapatra G, Hosek SM, Kimmel D, O'Fallon J, Yates A, Feuerstein BG, Burger PC, Scheithauer BW, Jenkins RB. Localization of common deletion regions on 1p and 19q in human gliomas and their association with histological subtype. Oncogene 1999;18(28):4144-52.

[52] Smith JS, Perry A, Borell TJ, Lee HK, O'Fallon J, Hosek SM, Kimmel D, Yates A, Burger PC, Scheithauer BW, Jenkins RB. Alterations of chromosome arms 1p and 19q as predictors of survival in oligodendrogliomas, astrocytomas, and mixed oligoastrocytomas. Journal Clinical Oncology 2000; 18: 636–45.

[53] Nutt CL. Molecular genetics of oligodendrogliomas: a model for improved clinical management in the field of neurooncology. Neurosurgical Focus 2005; 19: E2.

[54] Yan H, Parsons DW, Jin G, McLendon PR, Rasheed BA, Yuan W, Kos I, Batinic-Haberle I, Jones S, Riggins GJ, Friedman H, Friedman A, Reardon D, Herndon J, Kinzler

KW, Velculescu VE, Vogelstein B, Bigner DD. IDH1 and IDH2 mutations in gliomas. The New England Journal of Medicine 2009; 360: 765–73.

[55] Zlatescu MC, TehraniYazdi A, Sasaki H, Megyesi JF, Betensky RA, Louis DN, Cairncross JG. Tumor location and growth pattern correlate with genetic signature in oligodendroglial neoplasms. Cancer Research 2001; 61(18):6713-5.

[56] Laigle-Donadey F, Martin-Duverneuil N, Lejeune J, Crinière E, Capelle L, Duffau H, Cornu P, Broët P, Kujas M, Mokhtari K, Carpentier A, Sanson M, Hoang-Xuan K, Thillet J, Delattre JY. Correlations between molecular profile and radiologic pattern in oligodendroglial tumors. Neurology 2004; 63(12):2360-2.

[57] Kouwenhoven MC, Gorlia T, Kros JM, Ibdaih A, Brandes AA, Bromberg JE, Mokhtari K, van Duinen SG, Teepen JL, Wesseling P, Vandenbos F, Grisold W, Sipos L, Mirimanoff R, Vecht CJ, Allgeier A, Lacombe D, van den Bent MJ. Molecular analysis of anaplastic oligodendroglial tumors in a prospective randomized study: A report from EORTC study 26951. Neuro-Oncology 2009; 11(6):737-46.

[58] Bar EE, Lin A, Tihan T, Burger PC, Eberhart CG. Frequent gains at chromosome 7q34 involving BRAF in pilocytic astrocytoma. Journal of Neuropathology Experimental Neurology 2008; 67:878–887.

[59] Jones DT, Kocialkowski S, Liu L, Pearson DM, Backlund LM, Ichimura K, Collins VP. Tandem duplication producing a novel oncogenic BRAF fusion gene defines the majority of pilocytic astrocytomas. Cancer Research 2008; 68:8673–8677.

[60] Pfister S, Janzarik WG, Remke M, Ernst A, Werft W, Becker N, Toedt G, Wittmann A, Kratz C, Olbrich H, Ahmadi R, Thieme B, Joos S, Radlwimmer B, Kulozik A, Pietsch T, Herold-Mende C, Gnekow A, Reifenberger G, Korshunov A, Scheurlen W, Omran H, Lichter P. BRAF gene duplication constitutes a mechanism of MAPK pathway activation in low-grade astrocytomas. The Journal of Clinical Investigation 2008; 118:1739–1749.

[61] Jones DT, Kocialkowski S, Liu L, Pearson DM, Ichimura K, Collins VP. Oncogenic RAF1 rearrangement and a novel BRAF mutation as alternatives to KIAA1549:BRAF fusion in activating the MAPK pathway in pilocytic astrocytoma. Oncogene 2009; 28:2119–2123.

[62] Rokes CA, Remke M, Guha-Thakurta N, Witt O, Korshunov A, Pfister S, Wolff JE. Sorafenib plus valproic acid for infant spinal glioblastoma. Journal of Pediatric Hematology Oncology 2010; 32(6): 511-4.

[63] Northcott PA, Korshunov A, Witt H, Hielscher T, Eberhart CG, Mack S, Bouffet E, Clifford SC, Hawkins CE, French P, Rutka JT, Pfister S, Taylor MD. Medulloblastoma comprises four distinct molecular variants. Journal of Clinical Oncology 2011; 29(11): 1408-1414.

[64] Taylor MD, Northcott PA, Korshunov A, Remke M, Cho YJ, Clifford SC, Eberhart CG, Parsons DW, Rutkowski S, Gajjar A, Ellison DW, Lichter P, Gilbertson RJ, Pom-

eroy SL, Kool M, Pfister SM. Molecular subgroups of medulloblastoma: the current consensus. Acta Neuropathologica 2012; 123(4):465-72. doi: 10.1007/s00401-011-0922-z.

[65] Northcott PA, Shih DJ, Peacock J, Garzia L, Morrissy AS, Zichner T, Stütz AM, Korshunov A, Reimand J, Schumacher SE, Beroukhim R, Ellison DW, Marshall CR, Lionel AC, Mack S, Dubuc A, Yao Y, Ramaswamy V, Luu B, Rolider A, Cavalli FM, Wang X, Remke M, Wu X, Chiu RY, Chu A, Chuah E, Corbett RD, Hoad GR, Jackman SD, Li Y, Lo A, Mungall KL, Nip KM, Qian JQ, Raymond AG, Thiessen NT, Varhol RJ, Birol I, Moore RA, Mungall AJ, Holt R, Kawauchi D, Roussel MF, Kool M, Jones DT, Witt H, Fernandez-L A, Kenney AM, Wechsler-Reya RJ, Dirks P, Aviv T, Grajkowska WA, Perek-Polnik M, Haberler CC, Delattre O, Reynaud SS, Doz FF, Pernet-Fattet SS, Cho BK, Kim SK, Wang KC, Scheurlen W, Eberhart CG, Fèvre-Montange M, Jouvet A, Pollack IF, Fan X, Muraszko KM, Gillespie GY, Di Rocco C, Massimi L, Michiels EM, Kloosterhof NK, French PJ, Kros JM, Olson JM, Ellenbogen RG, Zitterbart K, Kren L, Thompson RC, Cooper MK, Lach B, McLendon RE, Bigner DD, Fontebasso A, Albrecht S, Jabado N, Lindsey JC, Bailey S, Gupta N, Weiss WA, Bognár L, Klekner A, Van Meter TE, Kumabe T, Tominaga T, Elbabaa SK, Leonard JR, Rubin JB, Liau LM, Van Meir EG, Fouladi M, Nakamura H, Cinalli G, Garami M, Hauser P, Saad AG, Iolascon A, Jung S, Carlotti CG, Vibhakar R, Ra YS, Robinson S, Zollo M, Faria CC, Chan JA, Levy ML, Sorensen PH, Meyerson M, Pomeroy SL, Cho YJ, Bader GD, Tabori U, Hawkins CE, Bouffet E, Scherer SW, Rutka JT, Malkin D, Clifford SC, Jones SJ, Korbel JO, Pfister SM, Marra MA, Taylor MD. Subgroup-specific structural variation across 1,000 medulloblastoma genomes. Nature 2012; 488(7409):49-56. doi:10.1038/nature11327

[66] Pfister S, Remke M, Benner A, Mendrzyk F, Toedt G, Felsberg J, Wittmann A, Devens F, Gerber NU, Joos S, Kulozik A, Reifenberger G, Rutkowski S, Wiestler OD, Radlwimmer B, Scheurlen W, Lichter P, Korshunov A. Outcome prediction in pediatric medulloblastoma based on DNA copy-number aberrations of chromosomes 6q and 17q and the MYC and MYCN loci. Journal of Clinical Oncology 2009; 27:1627-1636.

[67] Northcott PA, Nakahara Y, Wu X, Feuk L, Ellison DW, Croul S, Mack S, Kongkham PN, Peacock J, Dubuc A, Ra YS, Zilberberg K, McLeod J, Scherer SW, Sunil Rao J, Eberhart CG, Grajkowska W, Gillespie Y, Lach B, Grundy R, Pollack IF, Hamilton RL, Van Meter T, Carlotti CG, Boop F, Bigner D, Gilbertson RJ, Rutka JT, Taylor MD. Multiple recurrent genetic events converge on control of histone lysine methylation in medulloblastoma. Nature Genetics 2009; 41:465-472.

[68] Pfister SM, Korshunov A, Kool M, Hasselblatt M, Eberhart C, Taylor MD. Molecular diagnostics of CNS embryonal tumors. Acta Neuropathologica 2010; 120: 553-566.

[69] da Silva FE, Cordeiro AB, Nagamachi CY, Pieczarka JC, Rens W, Weise A, Liehr T, Mkrtchyan H, Anselmo NP, de Oliveira EH. A case of aggressive medulloblastoma with multiple recurrent chromosomal alterations. Cancer Genetics and Cytogenetics 2010; 196(2):198-200.

[70] Clifford SC, Lusher ME, Lindsey, Langdon JA, Gilbertson RJ, Straughton D, Ellison DW. Wnt/Wingless pathway activation and chromosome 6 loss characterize a distinct molecular sub-group of medulloblastomas associated with a favorable prognosis. Cell Cycle 2006; 5:2666-2670.

[71] Thompson MC, Fuller C, Hogg TL, Dalton J, Finkelstein D, Lau CC, Chintagumpala M, Adesina A, Ashley DM, Kellie SJ, Taylor MD, Curran T, Gajjar A, Gilbertson RJ. Genomics identifies medulloblastoma subgroups that are enriched for specific genetic alterations. Journal of Clinical Oncology 2006; 24:1924-1931.

[72] Kool M, Koster J, Bunt J, Lakeman A, van Sluis P, Troost D, Meeteren N, Caron HN, Cloos J, Mršić A, Ylstra B, Grajkowska W, Hartmann W, Pietsch T, Ellison D, Clifford SC, Versteeg R. Integrated genomics identifies five medulloblastoma subtypes with distinct genetic profiles, pathway signatures and clinicopathological features. PLoS One 2008; 3:e3088.

[73] Northcott PA, Fernandez LA, Hagan JP, Ellison DW, Grajkowska W, Gillespie Y, Grundy R, Van Meter T, Rutka JT, Croce CM, Kenney AM, Taylor MD. The miR-17/92 polycistron is up-regulated in sonic hedgehog-driven medulloblastomas and induced by N-myc in sonic hedgehog-treated cerebellar neural precursors. Cancer Research 2009; 69:3249-3255.

[74] Scheurlen WG, Schwabe GC, Joos S, Mollenhauer J, Sorensen N, Kuhl J. Molecular analysis of childhood primitive neuroectodermal tumors defines markers associated with poor outcome. Journal of Clinical Oncology 1998; 16:2478–2485.

[75] Aldosari N, Bigner SH, Burger PC, Becker L, Kepner JL, Friedman HS, McLendon RE. MYCC and MYCN oncogene amplification in medulloblastoma. A fluorescence in situ hybridization study on paraffin sections from the Children's Oncology Group. Archives of Pathology & Laboratory Medicine 2002; 126:540–544.

[76] Eberhart CG, Kratz JE, Schuster A, Goldthwaite P, Cohen KJ, Perlman EJ, Burger PC. Comparative genomic hybridization detects an increased number of chromosomal alterations in large cell/anaplastic medulloblastomas. Brain Pathology 2002; 12:36–44.

[77] Lamont JM, McManamy CS, Pearson AD, Clifford SC, Ellison DW. Combined histopathological and molecular cytogenetic stratification of medulloblastoma patients. Clinical Cancer Research 2004; 10:5482–5493.

[78] Takei H, Nguyen Y, Mehta V, Chintagumpala M, Dauser RC, Adesina AM. Low-level copy gain versus amplification of myc oncogenes in medulloblastoma: utility in predicting prognosis and survival. Laboratory investigation. Journal Neurosurgery Pediatrics 2009; 3:61–65

[79] Brown HG, Kepner JL, Perlman EJ, Friedman HS, Strother DR, Duffner PK, Kun LE, Goldthwaite PT, Burger PC. "Large cell/anaplastic" medulloblastomas: a Pediatric Oncology Group Study. Journal Neuropathology & Experimental Neurology 2010; 59:857–865.

[80] Korshunov A, Remke M, Werft W, Benner A, Ryzhova M, Witt H, Sturm D, Wittmann A, Scho°ttler A, Felsberg J, Reifenberger G, Rutkowski S, Scheurlen W, Kulozik A, von Deimling A, Lichter P, Pfister S. Adult and pediatric medulloblastomas are genetically distinct and require different algorithms for molecular risk stratification. Journal of Clinical Oncoogyl 2010; 28:3054–3060.

[81] Haberler C, Laggner U, Slavc I, Czech T, Ambros IM, Ambros PF, Budka H, Hainfellner JA. Immunohistochemical analysis of INI1 protein in malignant pediatric CNS tumors: lack of INI1 in atypical teratoid/rhabdoid tumors and in a fraction of primitive neuroectodermal tumors without rhabdoid phenotype. The American Journal of Surgical Pathology 2006; 30:1462–1468.

[82] Bourdeaut F, Freneaux P, Thuille B, Lellouch-Tubiana A, Nicolas A, Couturier J, Pierron G, Sainte-Rose C, Bergeron C, Bouvier R, Rialland X, Laurence V, Michon J, Sastre-Garau X, Delattre O. hSNF5/INI1-deficient tumours and rhabdoid tumours are convergent but not fully overlapping entities. The Journal of Pathology 2007; 211:323–330.

[83] Jackson EM, Sievert AJ, Gai X, Hakonarson H, Judkins AR, Tooke L, Perin JC, Xie H, Shaikh TH, Biegel JA. Genomic analysis using high-density single nucleotide polymorphism- based oligonucleotide arrays and multiplex ligationdependent probe amplification provides a comprehensive analysis of INI1/SMARCB1 in malignant rhabdoid tumors. Clinical Cancer Research 2009; 15:1923–1930

[84] Li M, Lee KF, Lu Y, Clarke I, Shih D, Eberhart C, Collins VP, Van Meter T, Picard D, Zhou L, Boutros PC, Modena P, Liang M-L, Scherer SW, Bouffet E, Rutka JT, Pomeroy SL, Lau CC, Taylor MD, Gajjar A, Dirks PB, Hawkins CE, Huang A. Frequent amplification of a chr19q13.41 microRNA polycistron in aggressive primitive neuroectodermal brain tumors. Cancer Cell 2009; 16:533–546.

[85] Pfister S, Remke M, Castoldi M, Bai A, Muckenthaler M, Kulozik A, von Deimling A, Pscherer A, Lichter P, Korshunov A. Novel genomic amplification targeting the microRNA cluster at 19q13.42 in a pediatric embryonal tumor with abundant neuropil and true rosettes. Acta Neuropathology 2009; 117:457–464.

[86] Korshunov A, Remke M, Gessi M, Ryzhova M, Witt H, Tobias V, Buccoliero A, Gardiman M, Bonnin J, Scheithauer B, Kulozik A, Witt O, Mork S, von Deimling A, Giangaspero F, Rosenblum M, Pietsch T, Lichter P, Pfister S. Focal genomic amplification at 19q13.42 comprises a diagnostic marker for embryonal tumors with ependymoblastic rosettes. Acta Neuropathology 2010; 120:253–260.

[87] Hadjipanayis CG, Van Meir EG. Brain cancer propagating cells: biology, genetics and targeted therapies. Trends in Molecular Medicine 2009; 15:519–30.

[88] Andreiuolo F, Puget S, Peyre M, Dantas-Barbosa C, Boddaert N, Philippe C, Mauguen A, Grill J, Varlet P. Neuronal differentiation distinguishes supratentorial and infratentorial childhood ependymomas. Neuro- Oncology 2010; 12:1126–34.

[89] Hasselblatt M. Ependymal tumors. Recent Results in Cancer Research. 2009; 171:51-66.

[90] Korshunov A, Witt H, Hielscher T, Benner A, Remke M, Ryzhova M, Milde T, Bender S, Wittmann A, Schöttler A, Kulozik AE, Witt O, von Deimling A, Lichter P, Pfister S. Molecular staging of intracranial ependymoma in children and adults. Journal of Clinical Oncology. 2010; 28(19):3182-90.

[91] Yang I, Nagasawa DT, Kim W, Spasic M, Trang A, Lu DC, Martin NA. Chromosomal anomalies and prognostic markers for intracranial and spinal ependymomas. Journal of Clinical Neuroscience 2012; 19(6):779-85.

[92] Choy W, Kim W, Nagasawa D, Stramotas S, Yew A, Gopen Q, Parsa AT, Yang I. The molecular genetics and tumor pathogenesis of meningiomas and the future directions of meningioma treatments. Neurosurgical Focus 2011; 30(5):E6.

[93] Yew A, Trang A, Nagasawa DT, Spasic M, Choy W, Garcia HM, Yang I. Chromosomal alterations, prognostic factors, and targeted molecular therapies for malignant meningiomas. Journal of Clinical Neuroscience 2012. [Epub ahead of print] doi: http://dx.doi.org/10.1016/j.jocn.2012.02.007

[94] Bockmühl U, You X, Pacyna-Gengelbach M, Arps H, Draf W, Petersen I. CGH pattern of esthesioneuroblastoma and their metastases. Brain Pathology 2004; 14(2): 158-63.

[95] Rickert CH, Wiestler OD, Paulus W. Chromosomal imbalances in choroid plexus tumors. The American Journal of Pathology 2002; 160(3):1105-13.

[96] Nayak L, Lee EQ, Wen PY. Epidemiology of brain metastases. Current Oncology Reports 2012; 14(1): 48–54.

[97] Soffietti R, Rudà R, Trevisan E. Brain metastases: current management and new developments. Current Opinion in Oncology 2008; 20:676–684.

[98] Soffietti R, Trevisan E, Ruda R. Targeted therapy in brain metastasis. Current Opinion in Oncology 2012, 24:000–000.

[99] Chiu CH, Tsai CM, Chen YM, Chiang SC, Liou JL, Perng RP. Gefitinib is active in patients with brain metastases from non-small cell lung cancer and response is related to skin toxicity. Lung Cancer 2005; 47(1):129-38.

[100] Lai CS, Boshoff C, Falzon M, Lee SM. Complete response to erlotinib treatment in brain metastases from recurrent NSCLC. Thorax 2006; 61(1):91.

[101] Fekrazad MH, Ravindranathan M, Jones DV Jr. Response of intracranial metastases to erlotinib therapy. Journal of Clinical Oncology 2007; 25(31):5024-6.

[102] Popat S, Hughes S, Papadopoulos P, Wilkins A, Moore S, Priest K, Meehan L, Norton A, O'Brien M. Recurrent responses to non-small cell lung cancer brain metastases with erlotinib. Lung Cancer 2007; 56(1):135-7.

[103] Wu C, Li YL, Wang ZM, Li Z, Zhang TX, Wei Z. Gefitinib as palliative therapy for lung adenocarcinoma metastatic to the brain. Lung Cancer 2007; 57(3):359-64.

[104] Altavilla G, Arrigo C, Santarpia MC, Galletti G, Picone G, Marabello G, Tomasello C, Pitini VV. Erlotinib therapy in a patient with non-small-cell lung cancer and brain metastases. Journal of Neurooncology 2008; 90(1):31-3.

[105] Porta R, Sánchez-Torres JM, Paz-Ares L, Massutí B, Reguart N, Mayo C, Lianes P, Queralt C, Guillem V, Salinas P, Catot S, Isla D, Pradas A, Gúrpide A, de Castro J, Polo E, Puig T, Tarón M, Colomer R, Rosell R. Brain metastases from lung cancer responding to erlotinib: the importance of EGFR mutation. The European Respiratory Journal 2011; 37(3):624-31.

[106] Bai H, Han B. The effectiveness of erlotinib against brain metastases in nonsmall-cell lung cancer patients. American Journal of Clinical Oncology 2012; (Epub ahead of print).

[107] Eichler AF, Kahle KT, Wang DL, Joshi VA, Willers H, Engelman JA, Lynch TJ, Sequist LV. EGFR mutation status and survival after diagnosis of brain metastasis in nonsmall cell lung cancer. Neuro-Oncology 2010; 12:1193–1199.

[108] Kwak EL, Bang YJ, Camidge DR, Shaw AT, Solomon B, Maki RG, Ou S-HI, Dezube BJ, Jänne PA, Costa DB, Varella-Garcia M, Kim W-H, Lynch TJ, Fidias P, Stubbs H, Engelman JA, Sequist LV, Tan W, Gandhi L, Mino-Kenudson M, Wei GC, Shreeve SM, Ratain MJ, Settleman J, Christensen JG, Haber DA, Wilner K, Salgia R, Shapiro GI, Clark JW, Iafrate AJ. Anaplastic lymphoma kinase inhibition in nonsmall-cell lung cancer. The New England Journal of Medicine 2010; 363:1693–1703.

[109] Costa DB, Kobayashi S, Pandya SS, Yeo W-L, Shen Z, Tan W, Wilner KD. CSF concentration of the anaplastic lymphoma kinase inhibitor crizotinib. Journal of Clinical Oncology 2011; 29:443–e445.

[110] Kennecke H, Yerushalmi R, Woods R, Cheang MCU, Voduc D, Speers CH, Nielsen TO, Gelmon K. Metastatic behavior of breast cancer subtypes. Journal of Clinical Oncology 2010; 28:3271–3277.

[111] Vasconcelos DS, Da Silva FPE, Quintana LG, Anselmo NP, Othman MAK, Liehr T, De Oliveira EHC. Numerical aberrations of chromosome 17 and TP53 in brain metastases derived from breast cancer. Genetics and Molecular Research 2012; in press.

[112] Stemmler HJ, Kahlert S, Siekiera W, Untch M, Heinrich B, Heinemann V. Characteristics of patients with brain metastases receiving trastuzumab for HER2 overexpressing metastatic breast cancer. Breast 2006; 15(2):219-25.

[113] Yau T, Swanton C, Chua S, Sue A, Walsh G, Rostom A, Johnston SR, O'Brien ME, Smith IE. Incidence, pattern and timing of brain metastases among patients with advanced breast cancer treated with trastuzumab. Acta Oncologica 2006; 45(2):196-201.

[114] Lin NU, Winer EP. Brain metastases: the HER2 paradigm. Clinical Cancer Research 2007; 13(6):1648-55.

[115] Leyland-Jones B. Human epidermal growth factor receptor 2-positive breast cancer and central nervous system metastases. Journal of Clinical Oncology 2009; 27(31): 5278-86.

[116] Brufsky AM, Mayer M, Rugo HS, Kaufman PA, Tan-Chiu E, Tripathy D, Tudor IC, Wang LI, Brammer MG, Shing M, Yood MU, Yardley DA. Central nervous system metastases in patients with HER2-positive metastatic breast cancer: incidence, treatment, and survival in patients from registHER. Clinical Cancer Research 2011; 17:4834–4843.

[117] Yin W, Jiang Y, Shen Z, Shao Z, Lu J. Trastuzumab in the adjuvant treatment of HER2- positive early breast cancer patients: a meta-analysis of published randomized controlled trials. PLoS One 2011; 6:e21030.

[118] Stemmler HJ, Schmitt M, Willems A, Bernhard H, Harbeck N, Heinemann V. Ratio of trastuzumab levels in serum and cerebrospinal fluid is altered in HER2-positive breast cancer patients with brain metastases and impairment of blood–brain barrier. Anticancer Drugs 2007; 18:23–28.

[119] Pestalozzi BC, Zahrieh D, Price KN, Holmberg SB, Lindtner J, Collins J, Crivellari D, Fey MF, Murray E, Pagani O, Simoncini E, Castiglione-Gertsch M, Gelber RD, Coates AS, Goldhirsch A. Identifying breast cancer patients at risk for Central Nervous System (CNS) metastases in trials of the International Breast Cancer Study Group (IBCSG). Annals of Oncology 2006; 17:935–944.

[120] Palmieri D, Bronder JL, Herring JM, Yoneda T, Weil RJ, Stark AM, Kurek R, Vega-Valle E, Feigenbaum L, Halverson D, Vortmeyer AO, Steinberg AM, Aldape K, Steeg PS. Her-2 overexpression increases the metastatic outgrowth of breast cancer cells in the brain. Cancer Research 2007; 67:4190–4198.

[121] Lin NU, Carey LA, Liu MC, Younger J, Come SE, Ewend M, Harris GJ, Bullitt E, Van den Abbeele AD, Henson JW, Li X, Gelman R, Burstein HJ, Kasparian E,Kirsch DG, Crawford A, Hochberg F, Winer EP. Phase II trial of lapatinib for brain metastases in patients with human epidermal growth factor receptor 2-positive breast cancer. Journal of Clinical Oncology 2008; 26:1993–1999.

[122] Dawood S, Gonzalez-Angulo AM, Albarracin C, Yu TK, Hortobagyi GN, Buchholz TA, Woodward WA. Prognostic factors of survival in the trastuzumab era among women with breast cancer and brain metastases who receive whole brain radiotherapy: a single-institution review. Cancer 2010; 116:3084–3092.

[123] Le Scodan R, Jouanneau L, Massard C, Gutierrez M, Kirova Y, Cherel P, Gachet J, Labib A, Mouret-Fourme El. Brain metastases from breast cancer: prognostic significance of HER-2 overexpression, effect of trastuzumab and cause of death. BioMed Central Cancer 2011; 11:395.

[124] Xu Z, Marko NF, Chao ST, Angelov L, Vogelbaum MA, Suh JH, Barnett GH, Weil RJ. Relationship between HER2 status and prognosis in women with brain metastases from breast cancer. International Journal of Radiation Oncology Biology Physics 2012; 82:e739–e747.

[125] Pauletti G, Dandekar S, Rong H, Ramos L, Peng HJ, Seshadri R, Slamon DJ. Assessment of Methods for Tissue-Based Detection of the HER-2/neu Alteration in Human Breast Cancer: A Direct Comparison of Fluorescence In Situ Hybridization and Immunohistochemistry. Journal of Clinical Oncology 2000; 18(21): 3651-3664.

[126] Ellis CM, Dyson MJ, Stephenson TJ, Maltby EL. HER2 amplification status in breast cancer: a comparison between immunohistochemical staining and fluorescence in situ hybridisation using manual and automated quantitative image analysis scoring techniques. Journal of Clinical Pathology 2005; 58:710–714.

[127] Duchnowska R, Biernat W, Szostakiewicz B, Sperinde J, Piette F, Haddad M, Paquet A, Lie Y, Czartoryska-Arłukowicz B, Wysocki P, Jankowski T, Radecka B, Foszczynska-Kłoda M, Litwiniuk M, Debska S, Weidler J, Huang W, Buyse M, Bates M, Jassem J. Correlation between quantitative HER-2 protein expression and risk for brain metastases in HER-2+ advanced breast cancer patients receiving trastuzumab-containing therapy. The Oncologist 2012; 17(1):26-35.

Section 7

Brainstem Gliomas

Chapter 18

Brainstem Gliomas

Zhiping Zhou and Mark M. Souweidane

Additional information is available at the end of the chapter

http://dx.doi.org/10.5772/53887

1. Introduction

Brainstem gliomas are a heterogeneous group of tumors occurring in the brainstem and cervicomedullary junction. They occur more often in children than in adults. Brainstem tumors, according to data prior to early 1980s, represent 10-20% of all central nervous system neoplasms in the pediatric population [1-3]. Approximately 90% of brainstem tumors are gliomas in origin [4].

Diffuse intrinsic pontine glioma (DIPG) is the most common type representing approximately 80% of brainstem gliomas [5, 6]. They have a dismal prognosis with a median survival of only a year. Their natural history is often compared to but worse than that of supratentorial glioblastoma seen primarily in the adult population. Nondiffuse brainstem gliomas, including focal, dorsal exophytic and cervicomedullary gliomas, are encountered less often and have a better prognosis. However, if untreated, they could also lead to progressive brainstem dysfunction and ultimately death.

2. Epidemiology

True incidence studies of brainstem gliomas are lacking. According to the Central Brain Tumor Registry of the United States, there were 400-450 cases of brainstem gliomas in children per year in the U.S. during 2004-2008, representing 10.7% of primary central nervous system tumors [7]. This number is higher than those previously estimated for the period between 1970s-1990s [8]. The increase is thought primarily to be a result of increased detection by the use of magnetic resonance imaging (MRI) and better data reporting as opposed to a true increase in the incidence of these tumors.

The most common age at diagnosis for DIPG is 5-9 years old with a median of 6.5 years, but cases have been seen in all age groups from infants to adults [5, 9]. Nondiffuse brainstem gliomas have roughly the same age distribution.

Neurofibromatosis type 1 (NF1) patients have higher incidence of brainstem gliomas. These tumors, whether diffuse or nondiffuse, appear to have a more benign course compared with tumors from patients without NF1 [10].

There does not appear to be a sex predilection in any of the brainstem tumor subgroups [5, 9]. Because of the low incidence and lack of diagnosis in less developed countries, there is not sufficient data to determine if there is a geographic propensity. No specific risk factors, either environmental or infectious, have been described to be related to the incidence of brainstem gliomas.

3. Classification

Brainstem gliomas are classified based on their location, focality and growth patterns. Classification systems were created using the current form of imaging available. Brainstem gliomas can be broadly categorized as diffuse intrinsic pontin glioma (DIPG) and nondiffuse brainstem gliomas. Nondiffuse brainstem gliomas can be further classified into three groups: focal gliomas (tectal and other locations), dorsal exophytic gliomas and cervicomedullary gliomas.

DIPG accounts for approximately 80% of brainstem gliomas in children [5, 6]. Surgical resection is not possible due to the location and infiltrative nature of the tumor. The standard of care for DIPG is radiation therapy. They have a median survival of about 10-12 months [6].

Focal gliomas account for about 5% of brainstem gliomas in children. They may be located anywhere within the brainstem but are typically not in the ventral pons. Most focal gliomas occur in the midbrain, especially the tectum of the midbrain. Focal gliomas in other areas of the brainstem, such as medulla, are less often seen. As a result, some discussions about focal gliomas may focus on tectal gliomas. Focal gliomas have well defined margins. They usually have an indolent course, and depending on location, are often amenable to surgical resection. The majority of tectal glioma patients have non-communicating hydrocephalus at initial presentation due to compression of cerebral aqueduct. Focal gliomas have a good prognosis [11].

Dorsal exophytic gliomas account for 10-15% of brainstem gliomas in children. They present insidiously with a long history of nonspecific headache and vomiting. They are amenable to surgical resection. These tumors have a good outcome after surgical resection [12].

Cervicomedullary gliomas account for 5-10% of brainstem gliomas in childrens. They arise from the lower medulla or the upper cervical spinal cord. They are amenable to surgical resection. Long-term tumor control can be achieved in most patients with surgical resection alone [13, 14].

http://dx.doi.org/10.5772/53887

4. Pathology and pathophysiology

Brainstem gliomas are typically astrocytomas. Focal, dorsal exophytic and cervicomedullary gliomas are usually pilocytic astrocytoma (WHO grade I) and fibrillary astrocytoma (WHO grade II). Other low-grade gliomas with indolent growth such as ganglioglioma are also seen. DIPGs are typically anaplastic astrocytoma (WHO grade III) and glioblastoma multiforme (WHO grade IV). Growth of low-grade gliomas typically respect fiber tracts and pial borders. In contrast, high-grade gliomas grow and expand without respecting anatomic boundaries of these surrounding tissues.

70-90% of DIPGs are anaplastic astrocytoma (WHO grade III) and glioblastoma multiforme (WHO grade IV) if biopsied before radiation therapy is given [15-17]. The remainders are mainly fibrillary astrocytoma (WHO grade II). At a later stage, invasion of adjacent levels of the brainstem and cerebellar peduncles is common. At autopsy, the vast majority of DIPGs are high-grade and more than 50% have disseminated within the neuraxis [18].

Most focal gliomas are low-grade [11, 19]. Low-grade gliomas seen in this subgroup include pilocytic astrocytoma, fibrillary astrocytoma and ganglioglioma. Most tectal gliomas cause hydrocephalus at an early stage due to its compression on the cerebral aqueduct.

Dorsal exophytic gliomas arise from subependymal glial tissue. Over 90% of these tumors are pilocytic astrocytomas [20] that grow along the path of least resistance. As a result, most of the tumor extends into the fourth ventricle rather than infiltrating the brainstem ventrally. Tumors that extend laterally and/or ventrally into the brainstem are usually more aggressive and of higher grade on pathological examination.

Cervicomedullary gliomas arise from either the lower medulla or upper cervical spinal cord. Most of them are low-grade astrocytomas, but gangliogliomas and ependymomas are also seen [14, 21]. Tumors with epicenters in the upper cervical cord grow dorsally into the cisterna magna. Those with epicenters in the lower medulla grow centrifugally as focal nodules.

5. Molecular genetics

Partially because of the low incidence of brainstem gliomas, their molecular genetics is less studied compared with some more common primary central nervous system tumors. However, there are some significant advances in the last a few years concerning both DIPG and focal brainstem gliomas.

DIPGs are genetically complex and distinct from both adult and pediatric supratentorial high-grade gliomas (HGG). Recent evidence points to platelet-derived growth factor (PDGF) and its receptors (PDGFR) as among the major driving forces of tumorigenesis in the majority of cases [22-26]. Another type of growth factor receptors involved in DIPG is epidermal growth factor receptor (EGFR). Expression of EGFR was reported in the majority of high grade and less than 20% of low grade DIPG by immunohistochemistry staining [27]. The same study also reported that 25% of grade III and 50% of grade IV tumors had EGFR gene amplification. Recent data show that strong EGFR immunohistochemistry staining was seen in about 27% cases [23], lower than in the earlier report, and that amplification rate of the EGFR gene is also much lower (about 7-9%) [23, 25]. Unlike the case in pediatric supratentorial HGG, CDKN2A deletion is non-existent in DIPG [25, 28] and amplification of CDK4 and CDK6 only occurs at a low rate [25]. Approximately 50% of DIPG had p53 mutation [29, 30] and three groups reported loss of a region of 17p containing the p53 gene in 31%, 57% and 64% cases, respectively [23, 28, 31]. In approximately 50% of DIPG patients, allelic loss of a region of 10q where PTEN is located was observed [31-33].

There have been fewer molecular genetics studies of nondiffuse brainstem gliomas. Recently it was reported that BRAF gene duplication and mutation are often observed in pediatric pilocytic astrocytomas and fibrillary astrocytomas, including those located in the brainstem [34-36].

6. Clinical presentation

The clinical behavior and presentation of brainstem gliomas are highly variable, depending on the anatomic location and growth pattern of the tumor, age of the patient and certain other factors. Symptom evolution reflects aggressiveness of the tumor. Low-grade tumors typically present with an insidious course over several months of gradual symptom progression. By comparison, a shorter and more abrupt onset of symptoms is indicative of higher-grade tumors.

Nondiffuse gliomas are often low-grade lesions with expectedly slow growth. Symptoms are insidious in onset and may not be readily appreciated. Careful history taking, including comparison to photographs, may be necessary to evaluate subtle changes associated with cranial nerve dysfunction in these slow-growing tumors. DIPGs, in comparison, typically present with a short prodrome of symptoms (usually 1-2 months or shorter) [9].

In brainstem gliomas, the pattern of symptoms reflects the extent of the tumor. Diffusely growing tumors are associated with multiple and bilateral cranial neuropathies, long tract signs and ataxia. Hydrocephalus in these tumors is uncommon at initial presentation. Nondiffuse gliomas often present with isolated cranial neuropathies, signs and symptoms of increased intracranial pressure, and ataxia. Rarely, hemiparesis may be part of the clinical presentation.

Brainstem glioma patients can have a combination of the following at presentation.

Cranial neuropathies are common in most tumors of the brainstem. Simultaneous involvement of multiple cranial nerves is more frequently encountered with diffuse lesions. Focal lesions, in contrast, are often associated with more limited cranial nerve involvement. Upper brainstem involvement is often associated with oculomotor deficits, and lesions of the lower

http://dx.doi.org/10.5772/53887

brainstem are frequently found to have lower cranial nerve involvement resulting in changes in voice, dysphagia and/or aspiration pneumonias.

Long tract signs, including motor dysfunction and hyperreflexia, are most often associated with diffusely growing tumors or focal tumors of the cervicomedullary junction. Long tract signs are often conspicuously absent with dorsal exophytic gliomas [12].

In brainstem glioma patients, ataxia can be a result of loss of proprioceptive sensation, CN VIII involvement and/or invasion of cerebellar peduncles by the tumor. Ataxia is frequently seen in DIPG patients.

Obstructive hydrocephalus is usually the first sign seen in focal tectal gliomas as a result of the tumor compressing cerebral aqueduct. Hydrocephalus and its associated signs and symptoms are also often seen in dorsal exophytic gliomas which grow dorsally into the fourth ventricle resulting in the obstruction of normal cerebrospinal fluid (CSF) flow.

Failure to thrive is commonly encountered in infants with tumors of the cervicomedullary junction due to lower cranial nerve dysfunction resulting in swallowing difficulties.

6.1. Diffuse intrinsic pontine gliomas

DIPG patients usually have an acute onset and present with a history of rapid deterioration of 1-2 months or even shorter. Physical examination reveals classic brainstem signs: cranial nerve deficits, long tract signs and ataxia, or combinations of the three. At least two of the triad need to be present along with MRI evidence to establish the diagnosis of DIPG.

Bilateral and multiple cranial nerve involvement is frequent in DIPG. Abducens (CN VI) palsy is the most frequent cranial neuropathy at presentation [5]. Facial palsy is also frequently seen at initial presentation. Involvement of CN VIII causes deadness and contributes to ataxia. Lower cranial nerve involvement causes aspiration, and difficulty in speech, swallowing and maintaining normal head positions.

These children often present with severe limb weakness and hyperreflexia, resulting in their difficulty to walk and sometimes even to sit. Long tract involvement also causes loss of tactile, nociceptive and proprioceptive sensations, causing numbness and contributing to ataxia.

In DIPG patients, both CN VIII involvement and loss of proprioceptive sensation contribute to ataxia. Invasion of cerebellar peduncles is also common in DIPG, which is another factor contributing to ataxia.

DIPG patients may also have other symptoms including headache, nausea and vomiting etc. indicating increased intracranial pressure from edema or hydrocephalus. Approximately 10% of DIPG patients have hydrocephalus at initial presentation [5].

6.2. Focal gliomas

Focal gliomas can occur anywhere in the brainstem, but usually not in the vental pons. Their clinical presentations depend on the location.

Focal tectal gliomas have an insidious clinical course and often compress on cerebral aqueduct to cause a non-communicating hydrocephalus [11, 37]. As a result the initial presentation is usually those signs reflecting increased intracranial pressure: headache, vomiting, diplopia and papilledema.

Focal gliomas in the midbrain tegmentum and the medulla are usually larger than tectal gliomas and presents with cranial nerve dysfunction, long tract signs and ataxia [11, 38].

6.3. Dorsal exophytic gliomas

Dorsal exophytic gliomas grow into the fourth ventricle and typically present with signs and symptoms of increased intracranial pressure including headache, nausea and/or vomiting, lethargy, downward gaze preference, changes in vision and cranial nerve palsies (including abducens palsy). Infants with these tumors may present primarily with failure to thrive. Long tract signs are rare with these tumors [12].

6.4. Cervicomedullary gliomas

Cervicomedullary gliomas usually have an indolent course because the majority of these tumors are slow growing low-grade lesions. Two presenting syndromes have been described based on the epicenter of these tumors [39]. Medullary syndrome often presents as a failure to thrive secondary to nausea, vomiting or dysphagia. Also seen with this syndrome are sleep apnea, dysarthria and recurrent upper respiratory tract infections. Cervical cord syndrome presents with chronic neck pain and/or progressive myelopathy with spasticity and weakness. Hydrocephalus is unusual in cervicomedullary gliomas.

7. Imaging studies

Diagnosis of brainstem gliomas is based on clinical presentations and imaging studies. MRI is the imaging method of choice because of its high resolution and ability to differentiate the natures of lesions (tumor vs. inflammation etc.), which is especially important in the diagnosis of DIPG. MRI enables identification of important anatomic features and localization of tumors with multi-planar views. It allows a precise evaluation of the growth pattern and accurate preoperative diagnosis in most cases. Both T1- and T2-weighted axial and sagittal sequences should be obtained for the basic studies. Other useful sequences include fluid attenuated inversion recovery (FLAIR), diffusion tensor imaging (DTI), gradient echo (GRE) and susceptibility weighted imaging (SWI). DTI tractography may be useful in evaluating the relationship between the tumor and white matter tracts [40], which can be a part of the preoperative planning for nondiffuse brainstem gliomas.

7.1. Diffuse intrinsic pontine gliomas

DIPGs are diagnosed with clinical presentation and magnetic resonance imaging. Since the publication of the Children's Cancer Group (CCG) report in 1993 [41], when a brainstem tumor presents with typical symptoms and radiological appearance, it is usually considered that these findings are diagnostic and a biopsy is rarely performed. If, however, the clinical or radiological presentation is not typical, where brainstem encephalitis or an inflammatory process of the pons cannot be ruled out, a stereotactic biopsy would be needed before initiating radiation therapy and/or chemotherapy.

DIPGs infiltrate widely. MRI scans show infiltrative expansion of the pons that is typically hypointense on T1-weighted, hyperintense on T2-weighted and FLAIR images, and has no significant dorsal exophytic component. Involvement of adjacent levels of the brainstem and/or cerebellar peduncles is common. Envelopment of the basilar artery is commonly present in DIPG showing the tumor growing ventrally outside of the boundary of the brainstem. Contrast enhancement with gadolinium is variable, with no enhancement being common [42]. Enhancement, if present, is usually patchy, without known prognostic significance. Neuraxis dissemination of DIPG can be seen on MRI in more than 50% of patients during progression [18]. In some cases the tumor may show atypical features including prominent enhancement and/or hypointense T2-weighted/FLAIR signals.

Magnetic resonance spectroscopy (MRS) is helpful in differential diagnosis when the tumor shows atypical features. Increased Cho/NAA (choline/N-acetyl aspartate) and Cho/Cr (choline/creatine) ratios in DIPG are useful in differentiating it from brainstem encephalitis, demyelination and other inflammatory processes when clinical and MRI presentations are atypical [43, 44]. However, the differentiating power of MRS is limited in NF1-associated DIPG [43].

7.2. Focal gliomas

Before the availability of computed tomography (CT) and MRI for the diagnosis of intracranial lesions, focal tectal gliomas could only be found in autopsy evaluations. In the 1950s, when CSF diversion procedures were not as universally successful as of today, Kernohan and Sayre stated that tectal gliomas were "in all probability the smallest tumors in the human body that lead to the death of the patient [45]."

Focal gliomas show as focal lesions on MRI. Focal tectal gliomas are usually isointense on MRI and show as thickened tectal plate. Tectal gliomas rarely enhance with gadolinium [11, 37]. Central calcification may be noted rarely [46]. Hydrocephalus is seen in the vast majority of tectal gliomas, causing symptoms for which the patients are seeking medical attention.

Focal gliomas in other areas of the brainstem are usually hypointense on T1-weighted and hyperintense on T2-weighted images. The margins are well defined in focal tegmentum and medullary gliomas, and most are more or less round or spherical. They are frequently cystic with an intense rim enhancement after intravenous contrast agent administration. Most midbrain focal gliomas show upward extension to the thalamus and downward extension to the pons.

7.3. Dorsal exophytic gliomas

Dorsal exophytic gliomas typically erupt through the pia/ependyma early in their growth, so imaging will show that the bulk of tumor outside of the brainstem. Imaging of patients suspected of dorsal exophytic gliomas should include MRI studies with and without intravenous gadolinium of the brain to differentiate this type of tumor from tumors in the fourth ventricle such as primitive neuroectodermal tumors (PNETs). On MRI, dorsal exophytic gliomas appear as a dorsal exophytic expansion into the fourth ventricle or below the cerebellum. They usually show as sharply demarcated hypointense signals on T1-weighted and hyperintense on T2-weighted images. Bright homogeneous contrast enhancement and hydrocephalus are common MRI findings [20].

7.4. Cervicomedullary gliomas

Imaging of patients suspected cervicomedullary gliomas should include MRI studies with and without intravenous gadolinium of the brain and cervical spine to determine the extent of tumor growth and involvement.

Cervicomedullary gliomas arise from either the lower medulla or upper cervical spinal cord. Growth pattern of the tumor will give some hints as to their epicenters and what structures are being placed at risk by tumor growth. Tumors with epicenters in the upper cervical cord will have their rostral growth blocked by the decussating fibers of the sensory and motor pathways. Instead, the tumor curves dorsally to grow into the cisterna magna at the cervicomedullary junction. Tumors with epicenters in the lower medulla grow centrifugally as focal nodules pushing the surrounding fibers to their side [21].

Cervicomedullary gliomas appear as solid masses within the above-described areas. They are hypointense on T1-weighted and hyperintense on T2-weighted images. They typically enhance homogeneously upon gadolinium injection.

8. Diagnosis and differential diagnosis

Diagnosis of brainstem gliomas is based on clinical presentations and imaging studies and needs to address the location and nature of the lesion.

It is expected that the patient's clinical course, examination and imaging studies be in agreement. With nondiffuse brainstem gliomas this congruence often prompts surgical intervention (resection and/or relief of hydrocephalus), particularly for those located at the cervicomedullary junction or dorsal exophytic in growth.

Incongruence between presentation and clinical studies suggests the need for biopsy prior to definitive treatment. In cases with disagreement between the imaging findings and clinical course (i.e. rapidly progressive course with imaging consistent with a focal or low-grade lesion), frozen sections should be obtained at the time of surgery prior to progressing to an aggressive resection. These instances may be representative of a more malignant tumor in which case the potential for iatrogenic injury during resection outweighs the potential benefit of an extensive resection.

Differential diagnosis includes other tumors in the brainstem and adjacent regions and lesions of other natures. Other tumors include lymphoma, metastatic tumors, germinoma and nongerminomatous germ cell tumors, PNET, hemangioblastoma, lipoma, acoustic neuroma, etc. Some of these tumors typically arise from nearby regions and may encroach into the brainstem, e.g., primary intracranial germ cell tumors usually occur in the pineal region and can invade the brainstem. The majority of nongerminomatous germ cell tumors can be differentiated by testing for secreted markers in the blood such as α-fetoprotein and β-human chorionic growth hormone. PNET occurring in the brainstem, even though relatively rare, can appear similar to DIPG or nondiffuse brainstem gliomas. Because of the difference in treatment options from those for brainstem gliomas, it should be carefully differentiated when suspected. Lesions of other natures include infectious, autoimmune, other inflammatory, vascular and metabolic lesions etc.

The role of biopsy in the diagnosis of DIPG remains intensely debated [47, 48]. Before the wide adoption of MRI in the diagnosis of brainstem gliomas, biopsy was performed to confirm diagnosis and provide information on prognosis. However, biopsy has been only performed infrequently since mid-1990s. Of note is that since the Children's Cancer Group (CCG) report in 1993 [41], MRI has superseded biopsy as the main method of diagnosing DIPG. As better methods to characterize tumors become available and more molecularly targeted therapies have become available or are under development in recent years, there are increasing calls to perform biopsy more frequently in clinically diagnosed DIPGs. Brainstem biopsy is safe with low morbidity and mortality rates [49-51]. Survey showed that parents of children with DIPG are generally amenable to biopsy, even if the results may not benefit the patient [52]. Various focus groups have been holding discussions on criteria of recommending biopsy. Some investigational protocols of DIPG have included biopsy and molecular characterization as mandatory components in stratifying subjects for experimental therapy.

9. Treatment

Treatment of brainstem gliomas includes management of pain, bulbar symptoms and motor impairment, relief of hydrocephalus and general support. Brainstem glioma patients should be cared for by a multidisciplinary team including neurosurgeons, non-surgical specialists and other therapists.

Surgical intervention is indicated for certain nondiffuse brainstem gliomas. Tectal gliomas are usually indolent and present with hydrocephalus. Hydrocephalus is relieved by endoscopic third ventriculostomy (ETV) or ventricular shunt placement. Early resection of tectal gliomas is controversial. Dorsal exophytic gliomas are the most amenable to surgical resection in brainstem gliomas. The goal is to remove the exophytic component, and when safe, followed by debulking of the intrinsic component. Surgical resection is typically recommended early for cervicomedullary gliomas. Subtotal resection can be safely performed in most cases.

Adjuvant therapy for brainstem gliomas depends on the tumor location, pathological diagnosis and extent of previous surgical resection. Radiation therapy is the standard of care for DIPG, but it is not recommended as an early treatment for nondiffuse brainstem gliomas if pathology shows a low-grade glioma. It is usually used in patients with high-grade pathology, upon clinical and imaging evidence of progression, or late in the disease course [5, 38]. Stereotactic radiosurgery is also used in nondiffuse brainstem gliomas. Chemotherapy has limited use in the management of brainstem gliomas. It is mainly used for high-grade pathology or at late stage of the disease.

9.1. Diffuse intrinsic pontine glioma

Surgical resection of DIPG is not safe because of its location and infiltrative nature. Biopsy is not indicated for patients with typical clinical presentation and MRI findings. Hydrocephalus, if present, should be treated with either an ETV or a shunt. A histological confirmation might be needed if imaging or clinical history is not typical for a DIPG, or if an investigational protocol requests it.

The standard of care for DIPG is involved field external beam radiation therapy, typically delivered at 1.8Gy/fraction for 30-33 fractions in the North America. Significant clinical improvement occurs in 85% of patients receiving radiation therapy, but the improvement is usually transient, lasting only 3-4 months, before progressive decline in clinical status returns [6].

Various chemotherapeutic regimens have been studied either alone or in combination with radiation therapy. However, up to date, no chemotherapeutic agent, either alone or in combination, or in conjunction with radiation therapy, has altered the natural history of DIPG. Many patients are enrolled in clinical trials of new agents or previously used agents in previously untested combinations.

9.2. Focal gliomas

Most tectal gliomas in children have indolent growth with few symptoms except those caused by hydrocephalus. Early resection of focal tectal gliomas is controversial and infrequently done. Often, these tumors are managed by relief of hydrocephalus, followed by clinical observation and periodic MRI scans [53, 54]. Treatment of the hydrocephalus typically includes ETV to restore CSF flow. Shunting is an alternative or can be considered for patients who fail ETV. Surgical resection may be considered on rare occasions.

Focal gliomas in other areas of the brainstem, including tegmentum and medulla, are usually indicated for surgical resection. Tissue diagnosis before radical resection is indicated for lesions with atypical clinical and imaging findings. For those patients initially put on observation, when tumor progression is observed, biopsy or sometimes radical resection is indicated. Transventricular endoscopic biopsy may be performed with or without CSF diversion

http://dx.doi.org/10.5772/53887

when the tumor is adjacent to a ventricle's walls [55]. Stereotactic biopsies may be considered for lesions that cannot be approached with endoscopy where accurate histological diagnosis is warranted but more aggressive surgical resection is deemed unsafe. Surgical resection of focal, well-circumscribed lesions provides not only a tissue diagnosis but also a prolonged event-free survival in many cases.

Conventional radiation therapy has demonstrated limited efficacy in patients with focal gliomas. Tumors with high-grade features should be treated with radiation therapy after recovery from surgery or when surgery is not indicated, while low-grade tumors may be observed and treated only if there is subsequent tumor progression [5, 38]. Implantation of iodine-129 (I-129) or iodine-125 (I-125) seeds has been used in some patients with acceptable tumor control. I-125 is an alternative to resection, external beam radiation therapy and chemotherapy in children with progressively symptomatic low-grade gliomas in deep and eloquent areas where high postoperative morbidity would be expected with open surgery [56]. Stereotactic radiosurgery has been used as an alternative means for managing focal brainstem gliomas [57]. Its use has been reported in patients with progressive tumor growth or worsening neurological deficits.

The role of chemotherapy has not been well evaluated for focal brainstem gliomas. In general, for tumors that total or subtotal resection has been performed on and subsequently progress, chemotherapy may be considered with or without radiation therapy. In children younger than 3 years old, chemotherapy may be used alone in attempts to delay the need for radiation therapy.

9.3. Dorsal exophytic gliomas

Dorsal exophytic gliomas are the group most amenable to surgical resection among brainstem gliomas and total or near total resection alone usually results in a good prognosis [12, 20]. Long-term event-free survival is expected when these tumors are simply shaven down to the level of the floor of the fourth ventricle. They should not be aggressively "chased" into the brainstem. In patients with findings consistent with an obstructive hydrocephalus who have not previously undergone a CSF diversion procedure (e.g. ETV or shunting), placement of an external ventricular drain may be considered. Tumor specimens should be sent early for frozen sections. A high-grade lesion is an indication to halt the surgery, as there is no proven long-term benefit to debulking aggressive lesions. Resection of the tumor takes place primarily within the fourth ventricle on the extra-axial part. In instances where there is a large intramedullary component to the tumor or if it is felt that damage to the functional tissues of the brainstem would be unavoidable, subtotal resection should be attempted. Some have advocated that resection carried to the level of the floor of the fourth ventricle confers a sufficient balance between disease control and preservation of neurological function by minimizing the risk of injuring functional brainstem tissues.

Radiation therapy is used for inoperable tumors or recurrent disease not amenable to re-resection [5, 38]. Treatment primarily consists of conventional external beam radiation therapy with 30-33 daily fractions of 1.8Gy/fraction [58-60]. The use of stereotactic radiation therapy and radiosurgery has also been examined in small cohorts. Chemotherapy has no proven efficacy in the treatment of dorsal exophytic gliomas [61].

9.4. Cervicomedullary gliomas

Cervicomedullary gliomas are treated in a fashion similar to that of an intramedullary spinal cord glioma or a focal glioma of the medulla depending on the location of the epicenter. Specimens should be sent early for frozen sections. Identification of a high-grade lesion is an indication to halt the surgery, as there is no proven long-term benefit to debulking aggressive lesions. Surgical resection should begin with internal debulking from the center to periphery.

As the majority of these tumors are low grade, surgery is typically the initial treatment modality. Radiation therapy should be reserved for advanced or recurrent diseases not amenable to surgical resection [5, 38]. Treatment primarily consists of conventional fractionated external beam radiation given at 1.8Gy/fraction for 30-33 fractions [58-60]. The use of stereotactic radiation therapy and radiosurgery has also been examined in small cohorts. Although a number of trials have examined the efficacy of chemotherapy in the treatment of DIPG, no role has been defined for its use in the treatment of cervicomedullary tumors [61].

10. Outcomes

The outcome of brainstem gliomas depends on the location and pathological grade of the tumor. Focal, dorsal exophytic and cervicomedullary gliomas typically have a fairly good prognosis. In contrast, the median survival of DIPG patients is only about one year despite numerous investigational therapies. In both DIPG and nondiffuse brainstem gliomas, patients with neurofibromatosis, older age, and longer duration of symptoms before diagnosis are thought to have a more favorable outcome [10].

10.1. Diffuse intrinsic pontine gliomas

External beam radiation therapy transiently improves the neurological condition in 85% of DIPG patients, but the disease usually progresses within 3-4 months. No treatment has been shown to be effective at the time of progression. Clinical deterioration is usually fast once progression is detected. Median survival is 10-12 months. Only 10% of patients survive beyond two years after diagnosis [6]. Children under the age of 3 years, young adults over 18 and those with NF1 may have a better prognosis.

10.2. Focal gliomas

Lesions typical of tectal gliomas on imaging studies usually need treatment for hydrocephalus only and rarely progress over many years. Hydrocephalus can be well managed in tectal gliomas. ETV for tectal gliomas has a success rate exceeding 70% and as high as 90%. Focal gliomas in other areas of the brainstem, especially if the pathology is pilocytic astrosytoma, can be cured by gross total resection but long-term follow-up is necessary. One study noted a 4-year progression-free survival rate of 94% and an overall 4-year survival rate of 100% in 17 patients with focal midbrain gliomas, which included tectal gliomas [11]. Stereotactic radiosurgery may be an effective primary treatment or adjunct to open surgery for focal brainstem gliomas. After gamma knife radiosurgery, most patients improved or stabilized but some worsened [57].

10.3. Dorsal exophytic gliomas

Dorsal exophytic gliomas are amenable to surgical resection. Gross total or subtotal resection can be achieved in most cases. They have a good outcome after surgical resection. Among 18 patients who underwent surgery, 17 survived and only four showed evidence of radiological progression after a median follow-up of 113 months [12]. Subsequent progression may require re-resection or radiation therapy.

10.4. Cervicomedullary gliomas

Tumor control can be achieved by surgical resection in most patients with cervicomedullary gliomas. 5-year progression-free survival rate is 60% and overall 5-year survival rate about 90% after surgical resection alone [14].

11. Recent advances and future directions

Because of the dismal prognosis of DIPG and the lack of therapeutic efficacy of current chemotherapies, innovative approach is urgently needed for the disease. One promising drug delivery method that may improve the outcome of DIPG patients is convection-enhanced delivery (CED). Another recent advance is the molecular characterization of DIPG, which may provide guidance for developing new therapies.

11.1. Convection-enhanced delivery

The blood-brain barrier (BBB) presents a significant obstacle to achieving therapeutic concentrations of systemically delivered agents in brain tumors. Convection-enhanced delivery (CED) is a method of local delivery that bypasses the BBB [62]. CED is typically accomplished by inserting a small-bore cannula directly into a tumor followed by drug infusion through the cannula. Experimental studies have led to the recognition that CED can be characterized by several common features:

- Local drug concentration can exceed that achieved with systemic administration by several thousand times.
- Systemic exposure by efflux into the vasculature is minimal.
- Tissue penetration by CED is well beyond that achieved by other local delivery methods that rely on diffusion rather than bulk flow such as drug-impregnated polymers.

- Distribution is preferentially along white matter tracts, a pattern reminiscent of glioma cell invasion.
- CED can be used to deliver macromolecules such as monoclonal antibodies or recombinant toxins, which is not possible by systemic administration in the brain parenchyma or tumor.

It is hypothesized that CED is ideally suited for the treatment of DIPG based on several features particular to this disease such as the tumor's relative compact growth pattern, its tendency to migrate along white matter fibers, the rarity of tumor related cysts and the lack of cavitary changes from radiation therapy.

The safety of CED in the brainstem has been well established in rodents and non-human primates [63-71]. The tolerability of several therapeutic agents delivered using CED into the brainstem has also been investigated and most of them proven to be safe at high concentrations [72-78]. This approach has been safely used on a limited clinical basis.

Although it is clear that certain limitations exist in the application of CED for the treatment of DIPG, currently existing preclinical data are sufficient to guide the design of clinical studies. Decisions in the design of these studies include the selection of an appropriate agent or agents, surgical technique, parameters of infusion, timing of treatment and methods of assessing distribution, local concentration, safety and therapeutic efficacy. These questions, however, should not be a barrier for clinical implementation, but rather as goals for early phase clinical studies. Based on current preclinical data, CED may serve as the basis for a new approach in the treatment of DIPG.

11.2. Molecular characterization of diffuse intrinsic pontine gliomas

A promising advance that may aid the development of therapeutic agents for the treatment of DIPG is the recent molecular characterization of this tumor. Four groups independently discovered that platelet-derived growth factor (PDGF) and its receptors (PDGFR) are amplified or over-expressed in the majority of these tumors [22-26]. Another type of growth factor receptors involved in DIPG is epidermal growth factor receptor (EGFR). Expression of EGFR was reported in the majority of high grade and less than 20% of low grade DIPG by immunohistochemistry staining [27]. The same study also reported that 25% of grade III and 50% of grade IV tumors had EGFR gene amplification. Recent data show that strong EGFR immunohistochemistry staining was seen in about 27% cases [23], lower than in the earlier report, and that amplification rate of the EGFR gene is also much lower (about 7-9%) [23, 25]. Unlike the case in pediatric supratentorial HGG, CDKN2A deletion is non-existent in DIPG [25, 28] and amplification of CDK4 and CDK6 only occurs at a low rate [25]. Approximately 50% of DIPG had p53 mutation [29, 30] and three groups reported loss of a region of 17p containing the p53 gene in 31%, 57% and 64% cases, respectively [23, 28, 31]. In approximately 50% of DIPG patients, allelic loss of a region of 10q where PTEN is located was observed [31-33]. Like in adult malignant gliomas, the interleukin-13 receptor subtype IL-13Rα2 is highly expressed in DIPG [79].

Some of these genetic aberrations have been the basis for DIPG animal models that could be powerful tools for studying the disease, *e.g.*, Becher *et al.* designed a mouse model of DIPG based on PDGF overexpression [22]. Some of the molecular abnormalities have already been used as therapeutic targets. There are therapeutic monoclonal antibodies targeting PDGFR, namely IMC-3G3 (ImClone) and MEDI-575 (MedImmune), that need to be tested for efficacy in treating DIPG, preferably delivered through CED into the tumor since they are macromolecules unable to cross the BBB. There are numerous small molecule tyrosine kinase inhibitors with strong inhibitory effects on PDGFR and/or EGFR kinases, and inhibitors of downstream signaling molecules such as AKT and mTOR, that are undergoing clinical trials for the treatment of DIPG. There are also targeted recombinant toxins, e.g. IL13-PE38QQR, utilizing IL-13 as the targeting moiety to target tumor cells overexpressing IL-13 receptors. Even though biopsy of DIPG is far from being routine, when these molecularly targeted therapies come to clinical use, it would be ideal for the tumor to be pre-screened for specific targets of those agents.

12. Conclusion

Brainstem gliomas are a heterogeneous group of neoplasms with considerably diverse natural histories and prognoses. They are classified into four groups based on their location, focality and growth patterns. Diffuse intrinsic pontine gliomas (DIPG) account for approximately 80% of brainstem gliomas. The overwhelming majority of them is high grade. They are not resectable and the standard of care is involved field external beam radiation therapy. They have a dismal prognosis. The vast majority of focal, dorsal exophytic and cervicomedullary gliomas is low grade, often amenable to surgical resection and has a more favorable outcome.

Developing effective therapy for DIPG is so far frustrating as neither new schedules of radiation therapy nor chemotherapeutic regimens being studied have improved survival of these patients. As better molecular characterization methods become available, there are increasing calls to perform biopsy and tissue diagnosis in clinically diagnosed DIPGs. Recent molecular characterization of DIPG identified some genetic aberrations that could be used as effective therapeutic targets, including PDGF and PDGF receptors. There are both large and small molecule agents targeting these genetic aberrations that are either available or under development. However, most of these agents are unable to cross the blood-brain barrier (BBB) to reach the tumor. Convection-enhanced delivery (CED) is a drug delivery method to bypass the BBB. It has proven capability to deliver high local drug concentrations and the safety of its use in the brainstem has been established in small and large animals and a small number of patients. CED, combined with conventional chemotherapeutic drugs and novel targeted agents, has the potential to produce an effective treatment for DIPG.

Author details

Zhiping Zhou[1*] and Mark M. Souweidane[1,2]

*Address all correspondence to: zhz2004@med.cornell.edu

1 Department of Neurological Surgery, Weill Medical College of Cornell University, New York, NY, USA

2 Department of Neurosurgery, Memorial Sloan-Kettering Cancer Center, New York, NY, USA

References

[1] Panitch, H.S. and B.O. Berg, *Brain stem tumors of childhood and adolescence.* Am J Dis Child, 1970. 119(6): p. 465-72.

[2] Farwell, J.R., G.J. Dohrmann, and J.T. Flannery, *Central nervous system tumors in children.* Cancer, 1977. 40(6): p. 3123-32.

[3] Albright, A.L., R.A. Price, and A.N. Guthkelch, *Brain stem gliomas of children. A clinicopathological study.* Cancer, 1983. 52(12): p. 2313-9.

[4] Pierre-Kahn, A., et al., *Surgical management of brain-stem tumors in children: results and statistical analysis of 75 cases.* J Neurosurg, 1993. 79(6): p. 845-52.

[5] Freeman, C.R. and J.P. Farmer, *Pediatric brain stem gliomas: a review.* Int J Radiat Oncol Biol Phys, 1998. 40(2): p. 265-71.

[6] Hargrave, D., U. Bartels, and E. Bouffet, *Diffuse brainstem glioma in children: critical review of clinical trials.* Lancet Oncol, 2006. 7(3): p. 241-8.

[7] Central Brain Tumor Registry of the United States, *CBTRUS Statistical Report: Primary Brain and Central Nervous System Tumors Diagnosed in the United States in 2004-2008.* 2012.

[8] Smith, M.A., et al., *Trends in reported incidence of primary malignant brain tumors in children in the United States.* J Natl Cancer Inst, 1998. 90(17): p. 1269-77.

[9] Kaplan, A.M., et al., *Brainstem gliomas in children. A Children's Cancer Group review of 119 cases.* Pediatr Neurosurg, 1996. 24(4): p. 185-92.

[10] Ullrich, N.J., et al., *Brainstem lesions in neurofibromatosis type 1.* Neurosurgery, 2007. 61(4): p. 762-6; discussion 766-7.

[11] Robertson, P.L., et al., *Pediatric midbrain tumors: a benign subgroup of brainstem gliomas.* Pediatr Neurosurg, 1995. 22(2): p. 65-73.

[12] Pollack, I.F., et al., *The long-term outcome after surgical treatment of dorsally exophytic brain-stem gliomas.* J Neurosurg, 1993. 78(6): p. 859-63.

[13] Young Poussaint, T., et al., *Cervicomedullary astrocytomas of childhood: clinical and imaging follow-up.* Pediatr Radiol, 1999. 29(9): p. 662-8.

[14] Weiner, H.L., et al., *Intra-axial tumors of the cervicomedullary junction: surgical results and long-term outcome.* Pediatr Neurosurg, 1997. 27(1): p. 12-8.

[15] Wolff, J.E., et al., *Subpopulations of malignant gliomas in pediatric patients: analysis of the HIT-GBM database.* J Neurooncol, 2008. 87(2): p. 155-64.

[16] Wolff, J.E., et al., *Intensive chemotherapy improves survival in pediatric high-grade glioma after gross total resection: results of the HIT-GBM-C protocol.* Cancer, 2010. 116(3): p. 705-12.

[17] Cartmill, M. and J. Punt, *Diffuse brain stem glioma. A review of stereotactic biopsies.* Childs Nerv Syst, 1999. 15(5): p. 235-7; discussion 238.

[18] Sethi, R., et al., *Prospective neuraxis MRI surveillance reveals a high risk of leptomeningeal dissemination in diffuse intrinsic pontine glioma.* J Neurooncol, 2011. 102(1): p. 121-7.

[19] Hoffman, H.J., L. Becker, and M.A. Craven, *A clinically and pathologically distinct group of benign brain stem gliomas.* Neurosurgery, 1980. 7(3): p. 243-8.

[20] Khatib, Z.A., et al., *Predominance of pilocytic histology in dorsally exophytic brain stem tumors.* Pediatr Neurosurg, 1994. 20(1): p. 2-10.

[21] Epstein, F.J. and J.P. Farmer, *Brain-stem glioma growth patterns.* J Neurosurg, 1993. 78(3): p. 408-12.

[22] Becher, O.J., et al., *Preclinical evaluation of radiation and perifosine in a genetically and histologically accurate model of brainstem glioma.* Cancer Res, 2010. 70(6): p. 2548-57.

[23] Zarghooni, M., et al., *Whole-genome profiling of pediatric diffuse intrinsic pontine gliomas highlights platelet-derived growth factor receptor alpha and poly (ADP-ribose) polymerase as potential therapeutic targets.* J Clin Oncol, 2010. 28(8): p. 1337-44.

[24] Puget, S., et al., *Mesenchymal transition and PDGFRA amplification/mutation are key distinct oncogenic events in pediatric diffuse intrinsic pontine gliomas.* PLoS One, 2012. 7(2): p. e30313.

[25] Paugh, B.S., et al., *Genome-wide analyses identify recurrent amplifications of receptor tyrosine kinases and cell-cycle regulatory genes in diffuse intrinsic pontine glioma.* J Clin Oncol, 2011. 29(30): p. 3999-4006.

[26] Paugh, B.S., et al., *Integrated molecular genetic profiling of pediatric high-grade gliomas reveals key differences with the adult disease.* J Clin Oncol, 2010. 28(18): p. 3061-8.

[27] Gilbertson, R.J., et al., *ERBB1 is amplified and overexpressed in high-grade diffusely infiltrative pediatric brain stem glioma.* Clin Cancer Res, 2003. 9(10 Pt 1): p. 3620-4.

[28] Barrow, J., et al., *Homozygous loss of ADAM3A revealed by genome-wide analysis of pediatric high-grade glioma and diffuse intrinsic pontine gliomas.* Neuro Oncol, 2011. 13(2): p. 212-22.

[29] Badhe, P.B., P.P. Chauhan, and N.K. Mehta, *Brainstem gliomas--a clinicopathological study of 45 cases with p53 immunohistochemistry.* Indian J Cancer, 2004. 41(4): p. 170-4.

[30] Zhang, S., et al., *p53 gene mutations in pontine gliomas of juvenile onset.* Biochem Biophys Res Commun, 1993. 196(2): p. 851-7.

[31] Louis, D.N., et al., *Molecular genetics of pediatric brain stem gliomas. Application of PCR techniques to small and archival brain tumor specimens.* J Neuropathol Exp Neurol, 1993. 52(5): p. 507-15.

[32] Cheng, Y. and H. Wu, *[Recent advances on molecular biology of diffuse astrocytoma].* Zhonghua Bing Li Xue Za Zhi, 1999. 28(3): p. 165-8.

[33] Cheng, Y., et al., *Genetic alterations in pediatric high-grade astrocytomas.* Hum Pathol, 1999. 30(11): p. 1284-90.

[34] Pfister, S., et al., *BRAF gene duplication constitutes a mechanism of MAPK pathway activation in low-grade astrocytomas.* J Clin Invest, 2008. 118(5): p. 1739-49.

[35] Schindler, G., et al., *Analysis of BRAF V600E mutation in 1,320 nervous system tumors reveals high mutation frequencies in pleomorphic xanthoastrocytoma, ganglioglioma and extra-cerebellar pilocytic astrocytoma.* Acta Neuropathol, 2011. 121(3): p. 397-405.

[36] Horbinski, C., et al., *Association of molecular alterations, including BRAF, with biology and outcome in pilocytic astrocytomas.* Acta Neuropathol, 2010. 119(5): p. 641-9.

[37] Bowers, D.C., et al., *Tectal gliomas: natural history of an indolent lesion in pediatric patients.* Pediatr Neurosurg, 2000. 32(1): p. 24-9.

[38] Ueoka, D.I., et al., *Brainstem gliomas--retrospective analysis of 86 patients.* J Neurol Sci, 2009. 281(1-2): p. 20-3.

[39] Epstein, F. and J. Wisoff, *Intra-axial tumors of the cervicomedullary junction.* J Neurosurg, 1987. 67(4): p. 483-7.

[40] Helton, K.J., et al., *Diffusion tensor imaging of brainstem tumors: axonal degeneration of motor and sensory tracts.* J Neurosurg Pediatr, 2008. 1(4): p. 270-6.

[41] Albright, A.L., et al., *Magnetic resonance scans should replace biopsies for the diagnosis of diffuse brain stem gliomas: a report from the Children's Cancer Group.* Neurosurgery, 1993. 33(6): p. 1026-9; discussion 1029-30.

[42] Mauffrey, C., *Paediatric brainstem gliomas: prognostic factors and management.* J Clin Neurosci, 2006. 13(4): p. 431-7.

[43] Porto, L., et al., *Proton magnetic resonance spectroscopy in childhood brainstem lesions.* Childs Nerv Syst, 2007. 23(3): p. 305-14.

[44] Thakur, S.B., et al., *Longitudinal MR spectroscopic imaging of pediatric diffuse pontine tumors to assess tumor aggression and progression.* AJNR Am J Neuroradiol, 2006. 27(4): p. 806-9.

[45] Kernohan, G.W. and G.S. Sayre, *Tumors of the central nervous system*, in *Atlas of Tumor Pathology: Section X*1952, Armed Forces Institute of Pathology: Washington, DC.

[46] Daglioglu, E., O. Cataltepe, and N. Akalan, *Tectal gliomas in children: the implications for natural history and management strategy.* Pediatr Neurosurg, 2003. 38(5): p. 223-31.

[47] Leach, P.A., et al., *Diffuse brainstem gliomas in children: should we or shouldn't we biopsy?* Br J Neurosurg, 2008. 22(5): p. 619-24.

[48] Wilkinson, R. and J. Harris, *Moral and legal reasons for altruism in the case of brainstem biopsy in diffuse glioma.* Br J Neurosurg, 2008. 22(5): p. 617-8.

[49] Pincus, D.W., et al., *Brainstem stereotactic biopsy sampling in children.* J Neurosurg, 2006. 104(2 Suppl): p. 108-14.

[50] Pirotte, B.J., et al., *Results of positron emission tomography guidance and reassessment of the utility of and indications for stereotactic biopsy in children with infiltrative brainstem tumors.* J Neurosurg, 2007. 107(5 Suppl): p. 392-9.

[51] Roujeau, T., et al., *Stereotactic biopsy of diffuse pontine lesions in children.* J Neurosurg, 2007. 107(1 Suppl): p. 1-4.

[52] Bartels, U., et al., *Proceedings of the diffuse intrinsic pontine glioma (DIPG) Toronto Think Tank: advancing basic and translational research and cooperation in DIPG.* J Neurooncol, 2011. 105(1): p. 119-25.

[53] Walker, D.A., J.A. Punt, and M. Sokal, *Clinical management of brain stem glioma.* Arch Dis Child, 1999. 80(6): p. 558-64.

[54] Sandri, A., et al., *Diffuse and focal brain stem tumors in childhood: prognostic factors and surgical outcome. Experience in a single institution.* Childs Nerv Syst, 2006. 22(9): p. 1127-35.

[55] Ahn, E.S. and L. Goumnerova, *Endoscopic biopsy of brain tumors in children: diagnostic success and utility in guiding treatment strategies.* J Neurosurg Pediatr, 2010. 5(3): p. 255-62.

[56] Korinthenberg, R., et al., *Long-term results of brachytherapy with temporary iodine-125 seeds in children with low-grade gliomas.* Int J Radiat Oncol Biol Phys, 2011. 79(4): p. 1131-8.

[57] Yen, C.P., et al., *Gamma knife surgery for focal brainstem gliomas.* J Neurosurg, 2007. 106(1): p. 8-17.

[58] Schild, S.E., et al., *The results of radiotherapy for brainstem tumors.* J Neurooncol, 1998. 40(2): p. 171-7.

[59] Skowronska-Gardas, A., *Evaluation of radiotherapy for pediatric CNS tumors.* Expert Rev Neurother, 2003. 3(4): p. 491-500.

[60] Hoffman, K.E. and T.I. Yock, *Radiation therapy for pediatric central nervous system tumors.* J Child Neurol, 2009. 24(11): p. 1387-96.

[61] Allen, J.C. and J. Siffert, *Contemporary chemotherapy issues for children with brainstem gliomas.* Pediatr Neurosurg, 1996. 24(2): p. 98-102.

[62] Bobo, R.H., et al., *Convection-enhanced delivery of macromolecules in the brain.* Proc Natl Acad Sci U S A, 1994. 91(6): p. 2076-80.

[63] Sandberg, D.I., M.A. Edgar, and M.M. Souweidane, *Effect of hyperosmolar mannitol on convection-enhanced delivery into the rat brain stem.* J Neurooncol, 2002. 58(3): p. 187-92.

[64] Sandberg, D.I., M.A. Edgar, and M.M. Souweidane, *Convection-enhanced delivery into the rat brainstem.* J Neurosurg, 2002. 96(5): p. 885-91.

[65] Occhiogrosso, G., et al., *Prolonged convection-enhanced delivery into the rat brainstem.* Neurosurgery, 2003. 52(2): p. 388-93; discussion 393-4.

[66] Croteau, D., et al., *Real-time in vivo imaging of the convective distribution of a low-molecular-weight tracer.* J Neurosurg, 2005. 102(1): p. 90-7.

[67] Krauze, M.T., et al., *Safety of real-time convection-enhanced delivery of liposomes to primate brain: a long-term retrospective.* Exp Neurol, 2008. 210(2): p. 638-44.

[68] Laske, D.W., et al., *Chronic interstitial infusion of protein to primate brain: determination of drug distribution and clearance with single-photon emission computerized tomography imaging.* J Neurosurg, 1997. 87(4): p. 586-94.

[69] Lonser, R.R., et al., *Image-guided, direct convective delivery of glucocerebrosidase for neuronopathic Gaucher disease.* Neurology, 2007. 68(4): p. 254-61.

[70] Lonser, R.R., et al., *Successful and safe perfusion of the primate brainstem: in vivo magnetic resonance imaging of macromolecular distribution during infusion.* J Neurosurg, 2002. 97(4): p. 905-13.

[71] Nguyen, T.T., et al., *Convective distribution of macromolecules in the primate brain demonstrated using computerized tomography and magnetic resonance imaging.* J Neurosurg, 2003. 98(3): p. 584-90.

[72] Souweidane, M.M., et al., *Interstitial infusion of IL13-PE38QQR in the rat brain stem.* J Neurooncol, 2004. 67(3): p. 287-93.

[73] Souweidane, M.M., et al., *Interstitial infusion of carmustine in the rat brain stem with systemic administration of O6-benzylguanine.* J Neurooncol, 2004. 67(3): p. 319-26.

[74] Luther, N., et al., *Intraparenchymal and intratumoral interstitial infusion of anti-glioma monoclonal antibody 8H9.* Neurosurgery, 2008. 63(6): p. 1166-74; discussion 1174.

[75] Luther, N., et al., *Interstitial infusion of glioma-targeted recombinant immunotoxin 8H9scFv-PE38.* Mol Cancer Ther, 2010. 9(4): p. 1039-46.

[76] Murad, G.J., et al., *Real-time, image-guided, convection-enhanced delivery of interleukin 13 bound to pseudomonas exotoxin.* Clin Cancer Res, 2006. 12(10): p. 3145-51.

[77] Murad, G.J., et al., *Image-guided convection-enhanced delivery of gemcitabine to the brainstem.* J Neurosurg, 2007. 106(2): p. 351-6.

[78] Szerlip, N.J., et al., *Real-time imaging of convection-enhanced delivery of viruses and virus-sized particles.* J Neurosurg, 2007. 107(3): p. 560-7.

[79] Joshi, B.H., et al., *Identification of interleukin-13 receptor alpha2 chain overexpression in situ in high-grade diffusely infiltrative pediatric brainstem glioma.* Neuro Oncol, 2008. 10(3): p. 265-74.

Section 8

Chemotherapy

Chapter 19

Chemotherapeutic Agent for Glioma

Shinji Kohsaka and Shinya Tanaka

Additional information is available at the end of the chapter

http://dx.doi.org/10.5772/54353

1. Introduction

Glioma is the most common primary tumors of the central nervous system, accounting approximately for 30% of entire CNS tumors, and classified into four clinical grades as I to IV. The most aggressive and lethal tumors is glioblastoma multiforme (GBM) with median survival of only 14.6 months, mainly because of limited effects of conventional post-surgical chemotherapeutic agents and irradiation [1]. In this chapter, we summarize chemotherapeutic agents for glioma focusing on their mechanism of anti-tumor action and the acquisition of resistance to the agents.

2. Temozolomide

2.1. Mechanism of action

Temozolomide (TMZ) is an alkylating agent which is applied to the treatment of malignant glioma including GBM. TMZ induces DNA methylation of guanine at O^6 position (O6-MG; 6% of adducts formed), as well as 7-methylguanine (N7-MG; 70% of adducts formed), and 3-methyladenine (N3-MA; 9% of adducts formed) [2]. O6-MG incorrectly pairs with thymine and triggers the mismatch repair (MMR) system leading to double strand break of the genome that result in the arrest of cell cycle and induction of apoptosis. N7-MG and N3-MA are removed by the methylpurine glycosylase followed by AP endonuclease which are the first two enzymes in the base excision repair (BER) pathway. Efficient BER system functions and repairs DNA lesions in normal and tumor cells. 573 patients with newly diagnosed as GBM were randomly assigned to be treated by radiotherapy alone or by radiotherapy plus continuous daily medication of temozolomide [3]. At a median follow-up of 28 months, the median survival was 14.6 months with radiotherapy plus temozolomide and 12.1 months with radiotherapy alone. The unadjusted hazard ratio for death in the radiotherapy-plus-temozolomide group was 0.63 (95 percent confidence interval, 0.52 to 0.75; $P<0.001$ by the log-rank test). The two-year survival rate was 26.5 percent with radiotherapy plus temozolomide and 10.4 percent with radiotherapy alone.

2.2. MGMT – a key molecule for TMZ resistance

MGMT specifically removes the methyl/alkyl group from the O^6-position of guanine and restore the guanine to its normal form escaping from DNA strand breaks (Fig. 1). Thus, the expression of MGMT in tumors has a protective effect against alkylating agents-dependent cell death correlating between MGMT activity and TMZ resistance. MGMT expressing tumor cells exhibit 4- to 10-folds increase of resistance to TMZ, BCNU, and their related compounds [4]. MGMT-mediated repair is unique compared with other DNA repair pathways because : (a) it acts alone without relying on any other proteins or cofactors; (b) it transfers the alkyl group to an internal cysteine residue in the protein, acting as both a transferase and an acceptor of the alkyl-group; (c) it inactivates itself after receiving the alkyl-group from guanine, and thus, it is a suicidal protein; (d) it repairs in a stoichiometric fashion. As one molecule of MGMT removes one alkyl molecule, an excess of DNA adducts at the O^6-position could completely deplete MGMT. MGMT is ubiquitously expressed in normal human tissues [5] but is overexpressed in all types of human tumors, including colon cancer, glioma, lung cancer, breast cancer, leukemia, lymphomas, and myeloma. These properties make MGMT as an important drug resistance factor and an ideal target for suppression of drug resistance [2].

2.3. Regulation of MGMT

2.3.1. Promoter methylation

It is well known that MGMT expression levels vary widely in tumor cells [6; 7]. Hypermethylation of CpG islands within the promoter region is associated with epigenetic inactivation of the MGMT. In the EORTC trial with 206 GBM patients, MGMT promoter methylation was observed in 45% cases [8]. In cases with methylated MGMT promoter which means negative of MGMT expression, TMZ was effective as median survival was 21.7 months treated with TMZ and RT compared with 15.3 months with only RT ($P = 0.007$). A study of German Glioma Network (GGN) also showed that MGMT promoter methylation was associated with prolonged progression-free survival (PFS) and OS in patients receiving TMZ [9]. Several other studies have also shown predictive and prognostic significance of MGMT promoter methylation in GBM [10].

2.3.2. Transcriptional regulation

In the MGMT promoter region, there are several specific sequences for the binding of transcription factors including SP1, GRE, AP-1, and NF-κB, thus MGMT can be induced by glucocorticoids, cyclic AMP, protein kinase C activators, and NF-κB [11; 12; 13; 14]. p53 is also reported to suppress MGMT expression by directly binding to the MGMT or by suppressing the transcription factor of SP1 [15; 16]. In addition, MGMT expression can be induced by radiation or other forms of DNA damages [17]. However, physiological roles and regulation of MGMT induction is not elucidated.

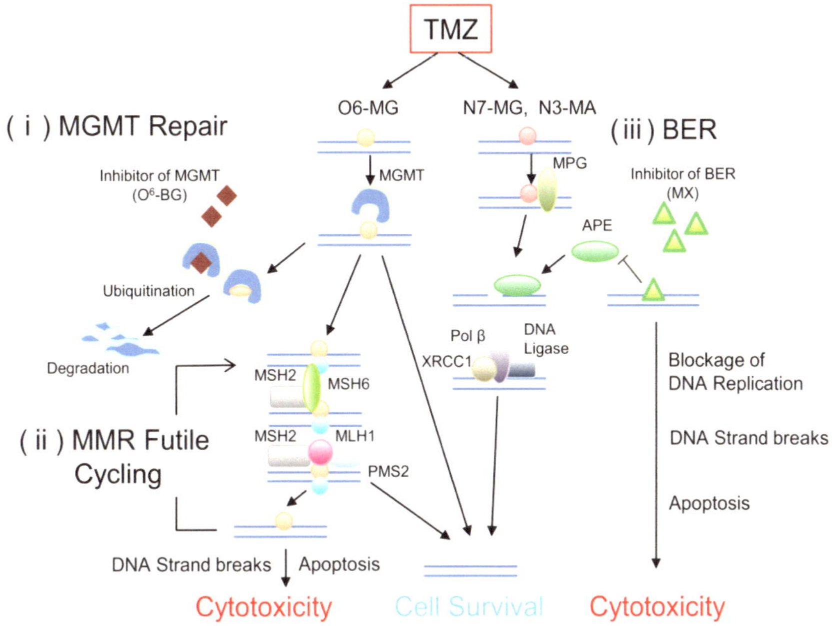

Figure 1. MGMT and other DNA repair mechanisms deal with DNA damage produced by the methylating therapeutic drug, temozolomide (TMZ), in human cells. TMZ and related drugs cause potentially cytotoxic DNA lesions such as O6-methylguanine (O6-MG, orange circle) and N7-methylguanine (N7-MG, brown circle). (i), MGMT (O6-MG DNA methyltransferase) removes the O6-alkylguanine DNA adduct through covalent transfer of the alkyl group to the conserved active-site cysteine and restores the guanine to normal. After receiving a methyl-group from O6-MG, MGMT is inactivated, and subject to ubiquitin-mediated degradation. A similar suicidal enzyme reaction occurs when MGMT transfers and accepts an alkyl-group from O6-benzylguanine (O6-BG), a therapeutic strategies. (ii), if an O6-MG DNA adduct escapes MGMT repair, it would form a base pair with thymine (blue circle) during DNA replication. The mismatched base pair of the persistent O6-MG with thymine is recognized by the mismatch repair pathway, resulting in futile cycles of repair leading to cell death. (iii), N7-MG DNA adducts (> 70% of total DNA adducts formed by TMZ) are efficiently repaired by the base excision repair (BER) pathway, and normally they contribute little to the cytotoxicity of TMZ. Methoxyamine binds to AP sites produced by methylpurine glycosylase (MPG), the first step in BER processing. Methoxyamine-bound AP sites are refractory to AP endonuclease (APE, green circle) cleavage, resulting in the blockage of the BER pathway. This leads to strand breaks, disrupted replication, and increased cytotoxicity of TMZ. Figure 1 is adapted from L. Liu et al. Clin Cancer Res. 2006;12(2):328-331.

2.3.3. Post-transcriptional regulation

MGMT protein was reported to be degraded *via* the ubiquitin proteolytic pathway [18]. According to the recent study, the correlation between MGMT promoter methylation and MGMT protein expression was poor (p = 0.27) [19]. *In silico* analysis predicted potential binding sites for several miRNAs within the 3'UTR of MGMT, suggesting a mechanism for post-transcriptional regulation of MGMT.

2.4. Candidate drugs for combination with TMZ

Strategies to potentiate the effecacy of TMZ by suppressing MGMT or BER pathway have been examined. Pseudosubstrates of MGMT such as O^6-benzylguanine were expected to suppress drug resistance by depleting MGMT [20; 21; 22]. However, clinical trials did not show significant restoration of TMZ sensitivity in patients with TMZ-resistant GBM [23]. IFN-β down-regulates the expression of MGMT and sensitizes resistant glioma to TMZ and phase II study has been started [15; 24].

We discovered post-transcriptional regulation of MGMT by signal transducer and activator of transcription-3 (STAT3) and demonstrated that STAT3 inhibitor or STAT3 knockdown potentiated TMZ efficacy in TMZ-resistant GBM cell lines [25] (Fig 2). Furthermore, immunohistochemical analysis of 44 malignant glioma specimens demonstrated significant positive correlation between expression levels of MGMT and phosphorylated STAT3 (pSTAT3) ($p<0.001$, $r=0.58$) (Fig 2). Therefore, STAT3 inhibitor might be one of the candidate reagents for combination therapy with TMZ for TMZ-resistant GBM patients.

2.5. Other molecules involving TMZ resistance

In spite of the correlation between promoter methylation of MGMT and temozolomide sensitivity, survival time of the patients who have methylated promoters of MGMT is still short and this suggests the involvement of other mechanism in TMZ resistance. Especially, key molecules of MMR, BER, and Fanconi anemia repair pathway such as MSH6 [26; 27], N-methyl purine DNA glycosylase (MPG) [28], DNA polymerase β (Polβ) [28], alkylpurine-DNA-N-glycosylase (APNG) [29] and FANCD1/BRCA2 [30] have been reported to affect to TMZ resistance. The unfolded protein response regulator GRP78/BiP was shown to act as a novel target for increased chemosensitivity in malignant gliomas [31]. Inhibition of Y-box binding protein-1 (YB-1) slows the increased growth of GBM and sensitizes to temozolomide independent of MGMT [32]. High levels of HOXA9/HOXA10 gene expression were associated with a shorter survival in pediatric high-grade glioma patient samples. [33]. Phosphatase and tensin homologue (PTEN) deficiency in GBM confers resistance to radiation and temozolomide that is reversed by the protease inhibitor nelfinavir [34].

Agent	Mechanism of Action	References
O^6-benzylguanine	pseudo-substrate of MGMT	Quinn JA, *et al.* J Clin Oncol. 27: 1262-1267, 2009.
Interferon-β	MGMT inhibition	Natsume A, *et al.* Cancer Res. 65: 7573-7579, 2005.
STAT3 inhibitor	MGMT inhibition	Kohsaka S, *et al.* Mol Cancer Ther. In press.
Levetiracetam	MGMT inhibition	Bobustuc GC, *et al.* NeuroOncol. 12:917-927, 2010.
PARP inhibitor(ABT888)	BER pathway inhibition	Palma JP , *et al.* Clin Cancer Res. 15:7277-7290, 2009.
Methoxyamine	BER pathway inhibition	Yan L, *et al.* Clin Cancer Res. 13:1532-1539, 2007.

Table 1. Candidate drugs for combiunation with TMZ. STAT3 indicates signal transducer and activator of transcription-3; PARP, poly(ADP-ribose) polymerase; BER, base excision repair.

http://dx.doi.org/10.5772/54353

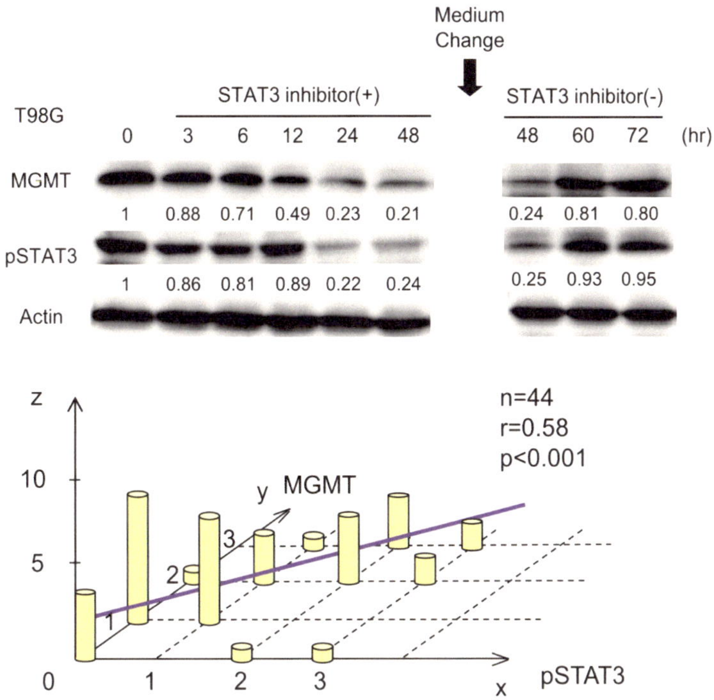

Figure 2. Correlation between expression levels of MGMT and phosphorylated STAT3. (A) Immunoblot analysis of MGMT in T98G treated with 200 mM of STAT3 inhibitor VI. Duration of the treatment is indicated at the top as 0 to 48hr. Medium change indicated removal of STAT3 inhibitor. The level of pSTAT3 was also evaluated (middle panel). Actin is shown as a loading control (bottom panel). (B) Correlation between pSTAT3 and MGMT in 44 cases of malignant glioma specimens. x and y axes indicate score of positivity of pSTAT3 and MGMT, respectively. z axis indicates the number of cases. n=44, correlation coefficient r=0.58, p<0.001. (A) Immunoblot analysis of MGMT in T98G treated with 200 mM of STAT3 inhibitor VI. Duration of the treatment is indicated at the top as 0 to 48hr. Medium change indicated removal of STAT3 inhibitor. The level of pSTAT3 was also evaluated (middle panel). Actin is shown as a loading control (bottom panel). (B) Correlation between pSTAT3 and MGMT in 44 cases of malignant glioma specimens. x and y axes indicate score of positivity of pSTAT3 and MGMT, respectively. z axis indicates the number of cases. n=44, correlation coefficient r=0.58, p<0.001.

3. Targeted molecular agents

3.1. Therapeutic targets in GBM

Identification of biological mechanisms contributing to GBM oncogenesis contributes to provide appropriate targeted therapies to improve patient outcomes. In a large-scale multidimensional analysis performed by the Cancer Genome Atlas involving, the most frequent gene amplifications were: epidermal growth factor receptor (EGFR) and platelet-derived growth factor receptor α (PDGFRα), 2 transmembrane receptors with tyrosine kinase activity; cyclin-dependent kinase 4 (CDK4), and murine double minute (MDM)2 and MDM4 which are suppressors for p53 [35]. The most frequent homozygous gene deletions were

CDKN2A, CDKN2B, and CDKN2C, which encode tumor suppressor proteins that suppress CDK4 and CDK6, phosphatase and tensin homolog (PTEN), a tumor suppressor that inhibits phosphatidylinositol-3 kinase (PI3K) signaling such as retinoblastoma (RB1), a cell-cycle inhibitor as PARK2, a regulator of dopaminergic cell death, and neurofibromin 1 (NF1), a negative regulator of the RAS signal transduction pathway. The most frequently mutated genes were p53, PTEN, NF1, EGFR, human epidermal growth factor receptor 2 (HER2), RB1, and PIK3R1 and PIK3CA-2 components/regulators of the PI3K signaling pathway. This study shows that several genes encoding proteins which are involved in signaling pathways of receptor tyrosine kinases/PI3K, and p53 and the cyclin/RB1, are considerably altered in GBM (Fig. 3). Another study has identified characteristic mutations in the active site of isocitrate dehydrogenase 1 (IDH1) in 12% of patients with GBM. IDH1 mutations occurred in a high proportion of young patients and in the majority of secondary GBM cases and were associated with increased OS (3.8 years), compared with wild-type IDH1 (1.1 years) [36]. This may be due to increased tumor sensitivity to chemotherapy, although a large controlled series in the German Glioma Network did not find any association between prolonged survival of patients with tumors with IDH1 mutations and administration of a specific therapy [9]. Mutation of the IDH1 active site prevents conversion of isocitrate to α-ketoglutarate but allows the mutated enzyme to catalyze the nicotinamide dinucleotide phosphate-dependent reduction of α-ketoglutarate to R(-)-2-hydroxyglutarate (2HG) [37]. Accumulated 2HG appears to act as an oncometabolite that contributes to glioma formation and malignant progression. This observation is supported by data from patients with inherited 2-hydroxyglutaric aciduria, in whom deficient 2HG dehydrogenase causes an accumulation of brain 2HG. These patients have an increased risk of developing brain tumors, possibly because of increased production of reactive oxygen species [38].

3.1.1. EGFR

EGFR is one of the most attractive therapeutic targets in GBM. Approximately 50% of GBM overexpress EGFR and 25% express a constitutively active mutated form of EGFR known as EGFRvIII, which has a large deletion in the extracellular domain and renders the receptor ligand independent for signaling [39]. Overexpression of EGFR is more common in primary tumors than in secondary GBM [40]. The deletion also renders a unique codon, which is not found in the wild-type receptor, thereby creating a tumor-specific epitope that can be exploited for therapeutic targeting. Increased EGFR signaling drives tumor cell proliferation, invasiveness, motility, angiogenesis, and inhibition of apoptosis.

3.1.1.1. Gefitinib, Erlotinib, Lapatinib and Cetuximab

Small-molecules of EGFR inhibitor such as gefitinib and erlotinib are well tolerated in patients with malignant gliomas, phase II trials have so far shown limited clinical benefit of erlotinib in patients with either recurrent or newly diagnosed GBM, either in combination regimens [41; 42; 43; 44] or as monotherapy [45]. Neither the EGFR/HER-2 inhibitor lapatinib [46], nor the monoclonal antibody against EGFR, cetuximab [47], have proven to be effective. Attempts to identify biomarkers to predict response to EGFR inhibitors have yielded

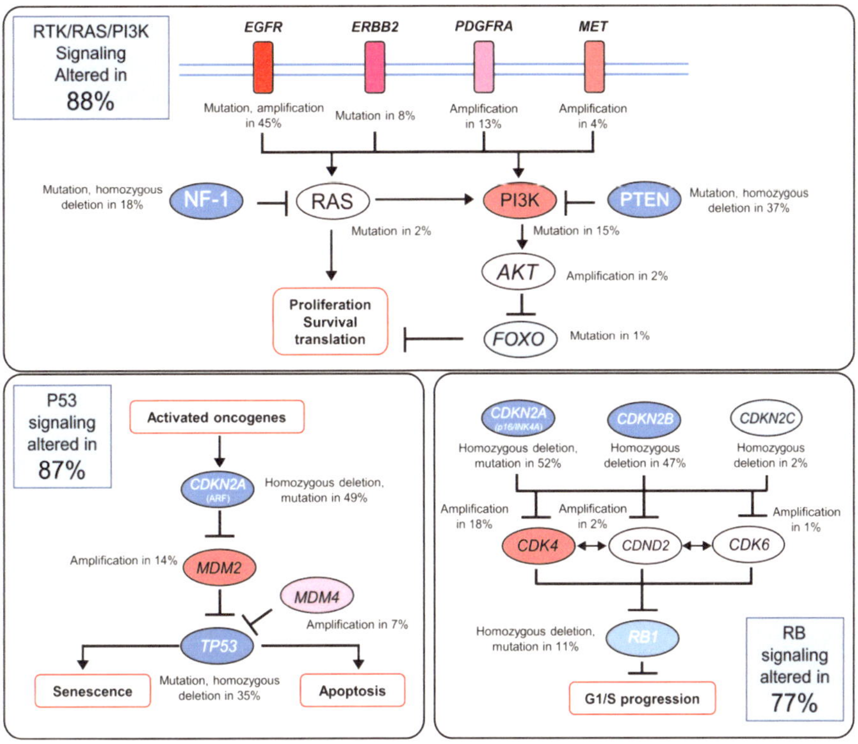

Figure 3. Genetic Alterations in Glioblastoma Occur Frequently in 3 Cellular Signaling Pathways. DNA alterations and copy number changes in the following signaling pathways are indicated in (a) receptor tyrosine kinase (RTK), RAS, and phosphoinositol-3-kinase (PI3K); (b) p53 tumor suppressor; and (c)retinoblastoma (Rb) tumor suppressor. Activating genetic alterations are shown in red. Genetic alterations that lead to a loss of function are indicated in blue. In each pathway, the altered components, the type of alteration, and the percentage of tumors carrying each alteration are shown. Blue boxes contain the total percentages of glioblastomas with alterations in at least 1 known component gene of the designated pathway. Figure 3 is adapted from The Cancer Genome Atlas Research Network. Comprehensive genomic characterization defines human glioblastoma genes and core pathways. Nature 2008;455(7216):1061–1068.

conflicting results. There is no convincing evidence of a correlation between the drug efficacy and the expression levels of EGFR in tumor tissue. In a phase I study, patients with gliomas expressing high levels of EGFR and low levels of activated AKT had better responses to erlotinib than did those with low EGFR expression and high levels of activated AKT [48]. Another study have shown significant correlation of therapeutic response of erlotinib and the presence of EGFR deletion mutant variant III [49]. However, not all studies confirmed these initial observations to predict the sensitivity to EGFR inhibitors [45].

3.1.2. PDGFR

PDGFR is a receptor tyrosine kinase with α and β isoforms. Overexpression of PDGFRα has been demonstrated in astrocytoma and GBM, indicating a potential role in tumor development [50]. Several PDGFR-targeting agents have been developed that may have therapeutic potential against tumors with elevated PDGFR expression.

3.1.2.1. *Sorafenib, Imatinib and Tandutinib*

Sorafenib is an orally available antiangiogenic agent that inhibits tumor cell growth and proliferation by blocking the action of intracellular and receptor kinases, including PDGFR, RAF kinase, VEGFR2, and c-KIT [51]. In human GBM cell lines, sorafenib inhibited proliferation synergistically in combination with bortezomib, a proteosome inhibitor [52], and rottlerin, an experimental inhibitor of protein kinase C [53]. A phase II trial found that first-line TMZ and radiotherapy followed by TMZ plus sorafenib was tolerated by patients with GBM, although preliminary efficacy data for this regimen (median PFS duration, 6 months; 12-month PFS rate, 16%) were similar to data for standard therapy.

Imatinib mesylate, a small-molecule inhibitor for PDGFR, ABL, and c-KIT, was reported to have significant antitumor activity both *in vitro* and *in vivo* as orthotopic glioma models (Kilic et al 2000). Especially, preclinical trials suggested that Imatinib have shows growth inhibition in a subpopulation of CXCL12-expressing GBM cells [54] and radiosensitizes them [55]. However, in phase II trials involving recurrent GBM, imatinib alone or combined with hydroxyurea had limited antitumor activity [56; 57; 58; 59; 60].

Tandutinib is an orally active inhibitor of PDGFR, FLT3, and c-KIT tyrosine kinase activity. Although no preclinical data was available for tandutinib in GBM, 2 early-phase trials are assessing tandutinib in recurrent/progressive GBM as monotherapy or combined with bevacizumab. As correlation between increased gene expression levels of PDGFR and preclinical data for therapeutic efficacy was reported, PDGFR may be a promising target for treating GBM. However, the available clinical data suggest otherwise. Trial data of combination regimens involving PDGFR inhibitors are awaited [61].

3.1.3. *VEGFR*

There are multiple reasons for adapting anti-angiogenic drugs to the treatment of malignant gliomas. Malignant glioma exhibits higher vascularization which is one of the pathological hallmarks of GBM. One of the difficulties of developing effective treatments for gliomas has been poor drug penetration through the blood-brain barrier. The dense network of angiogenic vessels in GBM typically display structural, functional, and biochemical abnormalities, including large endothelial cell fenestrae, deficient basement membrane, decreased pericytes and smooth muscle cells, haphazard interconnections with saccular blind-ended extensions, complex tortuosity, and dysregulated transport pathways [62; 63; 64; 65; 66; 67]. Therefore, by targeting the tumor vasculature, it is possible to bypass this dependence on drugs to pass the blood-brain barrier to reach their targets. Further, there is also both experimental [68] and clinical [69; 70] evidence that anti-angiogenic drugs can decrease vasogenic edema and patients' requirement for corticosteroids which contributes to morbidity in this population.

The VEGF family of growth factors and their respective receptors are the best characterized proangiogenic proteins in glioma. The VEGF family includes 6 secreted glycoproteins

(VEGF-A, VEGF-B, VEGF-C, VEGF-D, VEGF-E, and placenta growth factor [PlGF]). VEGF-A, the best characterized member, typically localizes adjacent to pseudopalisading necrosis in GBM [71], and the levels of VEGF-A is increased in higher grade of glioma [72; 73], and is associated with poor prognosis [74]. The VEGF receptor (VEGFR) family includes VEGFR-1 (Flt-1), VEGFR-2 (KDR), VEGFR-3, neuropilin-1 (NRP-1), and NRP-2, which exhibit different binding affinities of the VEGF homologs. VEGFR-1 and VEGFR-2 regulate angiogenesis, whereas VEGFR-3 regulates lymphangiogenesis. Vascular endothelial growth factor production and secretion by tumor cells is stimulated mainly by hypoxia, and malignant gliomas are rapidly growing and innately hypoxic tumors. More specifically, VEGF-A binds to VEGFR-2 expressed in blood vessels, which promotes endothelial cell migration and proliferation results in new blood vessel formation in a manner of paracrine signaling loop.

3.1.3.1. Bevacizumab

Bevacizumab, a recombinant humanized monoclonal antibody composed of human immunoglobulin G1 (IgG1; 93%) and murine VEGF-binding complementarity-determining regions (7%), binds all isoforms of VEGF with high affinity and specificity [75]. Despite initial reluctance to evaluate bevacizumab in patients with brain tumors owing to concerns of intracranial hemorrhage, a series of 29 patients with recurrent malignant glioma treated with bevacizumab and irinotecan showed no significant hemorrhage with remarkable tumor regression as radiographic response rate of 66% compared with ordinal chemotherapeutic reagents as rates of 9% [76; 77]. These results led rigorous prospective clinical trials of bevacizumab in recurrent malignant gliomas. The combination of bevacizumab and irinotecan was studied in single-arm phase 2 trials for recurrent malignant glioma (n = 33) and GBM (n = 35), showing response rates as 61% and 57%, and progression-free survival (PFS) at 6 months as 55% and 46% [78; 79], respectively. These results were compared with previous rates of PFS at 6 months as 9% to 15% for recurrent GBM and 17% to 31% for recurrent malignant gliomas [80]. A large phase 2 trial randomized 167 patients of recurrent GBM to analyze efficacy of combination of either bevacizumab or bevacizumab with irinotecan. This noncomparative randomized study showed radiographic response rates as 28% and 38%, and a PFS at 6 months of 43% and 50%, respectively [69]. In addition, patients treated with bevacizumab often exhibit less vasogenic edema and decreased corticosteroid dependence secondary to neutralization of VEGF, a known vascular permeability factor. Another phase 2 trial involved bevacizumab monotherapy in 48 heavily pretreated patients with recurrent GBM [70]. The radiographic response rate was 35%, and the PFS6 rate was 29%. Ongoing phase 3 studies are evaluating the combination of bevacizumab with temozolomide and radiotherapy. The results will be of great interest because of the uncertainty regarding the impact of bevacizumab on overall survival. Combinations of bevacizumab and other chemotherapeutics or targeted molecular drugs are also currently in clinical trials.

3.1.3.2. Aflibercept

VEGF Trap (aflibercept) sequesters all isoforms of VEGF-A and PDGF as a soluble, recombinant, decoy receptor, composed of the second Ig domain of VEGFR-1 and the third Ig domain of VEGFR-2 bound to the hinge region of the Fc portion of human IgG1 [81]. Single arm phase II study of aflibercept in recurrent malignant glioma was proceeded [82]. 42 patients with GBM and 16 patients with malignant glioma who had received concurrent radiation and temozolomide therapies, and adjuvant temozolomide were enrolled at first relapse. The 6-month progression-free survival rate was 7.7% for GBM cohort and 25% for patients with malignant glioma. Overall radiographic response rate was 24% (18% for GBM and 44% for malignant glioma). The median PFS was 24 weeks for patients with malignant glioma (95% CI, 5 to 31 weeks) and 12 weeks for patients with GBM (95% CI, 8 to 16 weeks). A total of 14 patients (25%) were removed from the study for toxicity, on average less than 2 months from treatment initiation. This study suggested Aflibercept monotherapy had moderate toxicity and minimal evidence of single-agent activity in unselected patients with recurrent malignant glioma.

3.1.3.3. Cediranib

Several inhibitors for VEGFR tyrosine kinase have shown significant antiangiogenic and antitumor activity in preclinical GBM models [83; 84; 85; 86; 87; 88], which may also enhance cytotoxic therapy [89; 90; 91]. In addition, several these agents are undergoing evaluation in phase I/II clinical trials, but only cediranib has advanced to phase III investigation. In an initial phase II study of single-agent cediranib (45 mg/d), 27% of patients with recurrent malignant glioma exhibited a radiographic response and a 6-month PFS was 26%. In addition, cediranib induced rapid normalization of tumor vasculature, including decreased diameter of microvessels and diminished permeability, which reversed after cediranib interruption. Adverse events including hypertension and fatigue were observed, and nearly half of the patients required a dose reduction or interruption of therapy because of its toxicity [92].

3.1.3.4. Mechanisms of resistance to antiangiogenic therapy

Although antiangiogenic therapies prolong PFS of GBM patients, further progression of disease is inevitable. Progression of tumors under antiangiogenic therapy cannot often be treated successfully thereafter, and most patients die of the disease within a few months. In the cediranib study, serum levels of the proangiogenic factors bFGF, stromal-derived factor 1 (SDF1), and soluble VEGFR2 increased at the time of failure [93]. The alternative proangiogenic pathways depends on these angiogenic factors may drive angiogenesis in the setting of VEGFR inhibition. Furthermore, for many gliomas, particularly malignant gliomas, there is often little evidence for vascular proliferation. As the individual infiltrating tumor cell tends to grow along normal cerebral vasculature, and thus there is no need for tumor-associated angiogenesis. Indeed, there is at least a theoretical concern that inhibition of angiogenesis in malignant glioma may prevent the formation bulky tumor but has little effect on sparsely infiltrative GBM cells results in little impact on OS of patients. Early clinical and radiographic observations of patients treated with bevacizumab suggest that this may be the case [94; 95]. Another concern is recent laboratory evidence that suggests that inhibition of VEGF may actually increase invasiveness of tumor cells [96]. The infiltrative tumor cells are often responsible for relapse leading to the death of patients.

Combination of antiangiogenic and anti-invasion therapy may delay disease progression. Studies of co-administration of cediranib (pan-VEGFR inhibitor) with cilengitide (integrin inhibitor) and bevacizumab (neutralizing VEGF antibody) with dasatinib (PDGFRβ inhibitor) are ongoing. Another potential mechanism of resistance to antiangiogenic therapies involves increased PDGF signaling. PDGF stabilizes neovasculature by recruiting pericytes and facilitating pericyte-endothelial cell interactions [97]. Preclinical data suggest that dual VEGFR/PDGFR inhibition potentiates antiangiogenic efficacy and reduces resistance to therapy [98], and this approach is currently being evaluated in clinical trials.

3.1.4. *c-MET*

Aberrant signaling by hepatocyte growth factor (HGF) and its receptor MET has been observed in various tumors including GBM, and potential involvement in tumorigenesis and metastasis has been reported [99]. Recently c-MET overexpression was detected in 18 (29%) of 62 GBM with shorter median survival durations than those of little or no expression of c-MET (median durations of survival, 11.7 vs 14.3 months) [100].

3.1.4.1. *AMG102 and PF02341066*

Inhibitors of HGF or c-MET have shown preclinical activity against GBM cell lines [99]. The anti-HGF antibody AMG102 enhanced TMZ-induced inhibition of growth of GBM cell line *in vitro* and *in vivo* as xenografts [101]. However, phase II trial suggests AMG 102 monotherapy did not significantly suppress tumor growth of recurrent GBM [102]. PF02341066, an orally available ATP-competitive inhibitor of c-MET inhibited growth and c-MET phosphorylation of GBM in preclinical studies [103]. This molecule is currently under clinical investigation in patients with advanced cancers.

3.1.5. *PI3K and related pathways*

PI3K plays a role in intracellular signaling pathways regulating in cell survival, growth, and proliferation. Activated PI3K is recruited to the cell membrane where it mediates signaling after activation of receptor tyrosine kinases. Downstream targets include AKT for cell proliferation and survival; glycogen synthase kinase-3 (GSK-3) for regulation of c-MYC; and mammalian target of rapamycin (mTOR) for regulation of protein synthesis and negative regulator of PI3K. In malignant glioma, PI3K/Akt/mTOR signaling is frequently activated because of the stimulation of receptor tyrosine kinases as EGFR, PDGFR, and mesenchymal-epithelial transition factor (MET), mutation of oncogenic PI3K subunits, and/or loss of PTEN tumor suppressor activity. Therefore inhibiting the PI3K pathway may have therapeutic potential.

3.1.5.1. *NVP-BEZ235 and Enzastaurin*

NVP-BEZ235, an orally available kinase inhibitor for PDK1, mTOR, and PI3K, induced G1 arrest of a GBM cell line *in vitro* and enhanced TMZ efficacy *in vivo* [104]. NVP-BEZ235 treatment is currently in phase I trials involving patients with solid tumors.

Enzastaurin, a PKC/PI3K/AKT inhibitor, suppressed proliferation and induced apoptosis *via* a caspase-dependent mechanism in GBM cells in vitro [105]. *In vivo* models showed that enzastaurin combined with radiotherapy synergistically reduced tumor volume, radiation-induced satellite tumor formation, upregulation of VEGF expression, neovascularization, and GSK-3β phosphorylation [106]. In phase II study of enzastaurin in patients with recurrent heavily pretreated GBM showed that objective radiographic responses occurred in 25% of patients [107]. The subsequent phase III trial comparing lomustine and enzastaurin at first or second recurrence was the first phase III trial to evaluate a targeted therapy for recurrent GBM. Enzastaurin was well tolerated and had a better hematologic toxicity profile but did not have superior efficacy compared with lomustine in patients with recurrent GBM [108].

3.1.6. SRC and SRC-Family kinases

SRC and SRC-Family Kinases (SFKs) are frequently activated in GBM [109] frequently due to their overexpression [110]. SRC and SFKs are promiscuous regulators of multiple signaling pathways for cell proliferation, adhesion, migration, and invasion, which are important processes in tumor invasion and metastasis.

3.1.6.1. Dasatinib

Dasatinib is a potent inhibitor of SRC and SFKs and has been approved for the treatment of certain types of leukemia on the basis of inactivation of BCR-ABL [111]. Dasatinib also inhibits c-KIT and PDGFR [112]. In GBM cells, dasatinib inhibited migration and induced autophagy, resulted in cell death which was enhanced by combination with TMZ [111; 113]. Dasatinib inhibited invasion, promoted tumor regression, induced apoptosis in EGFRvIII-expressing GBM, and enhanced the activity of anti-EGFR antibodies [111]. Trials of dasatinib are ongoing in GBM and several solid tumors. A phase I/II trial involving patients with newly diagnosed GBM is assessing dasatinib combined with radiotherapy and concomitant TMZ, followed by adjuvant dasatinib plus TMZ. Trials of dasatinib for treatment of recurrent GBM include a phase II trial of dasatinib monotherapy, a phase I trial of dasatinib in combination with erlotinib, and a randomized phase I/II trial of dasatinib in combination with CCNU that has started its phase I component with patients who have recurrent GBM.

3.1.7. Integrin

Integrin plays key roles regulating cell adhesion, migration, and invasion. In addition to a role for matrix-cell contact, integrin also activate intracellular signals including SRC-dependent pathway. In various tumors, integrin has an established role in metastasis and angiogenesis [114]. Therefore, targeting integrin function may have potential for treating GBM.

http://dx.doi.org/10.5772/54353

PRIMARY TARGET	AGENT	OTHER TARGETS	MECHANISM OF ACTION
EGFR	Gefitinib (ZD1839)		TKI
	Erlotinib (OSI-774)		TKI
	Lapatinib (GW-572016)	HER-2	TKI
	PF-00299804	HER-2, HER-4	TKI (irreversible)
	BIBW2992	HER-2, HER-4	TKI (irreversible)
	Cetuximab		Monoclonal antibody
	Nimotuzumab		Monoclonal antibody
EGFRvlll	CDX110		Vaccine
PDGFR-α	IMC3G3		Monoclonal antibody
PDGFR-β	Imatinib	BCR/Abl, c-Kit	TKI
	Dasatinib	Src, BCR/Abl, c-Kit, ephrin A2	TKI
	Tandutinib (MLN518)	Flt3, c-Kit	TKI
VEGF-A	Aflibercept (VEGF Trap)	VEGF-B, PlGF	Soluble decoy receptor
	Bevacizumab		Monoclonal antibody
VEGFR-2	Cediranib (AZD2171)	All VEGFR subtypes, PDGFR-β ,c-Kit	Adnectin
	CT-322	All VEGFR subtypes	TKI
	Pazopanib	All VEGFR subtypes, PDGFR-α And β, c-Kit	TKI
	Sorafenib	VEGFR-3, B-Raf, PDGFR-β , c-Kit, Ras, p38α	TKI
	Sunitinib	PDGFR-β, Flt3, c-Kit	TKI
	Vandetanib (ZD6474)	EGFR	TKI
c-Met	XL-184	VEGFR	TKI
HGF/SF	17-AAG		Monoclonal antibody
PI3K	XL765	mTOR	STKI
PKC	Enzastaurin (LY31761)		STKI
mTOR	Sirolimus (rapamycin)		mTOR inhibitor
	Everolimus (RAD001)		mTOR inhibitor
	Temsirolimus (CCI-779)		mTOR inhibitor
	Ridaforolimus (AP23573)		mTOR inhibitor
SRC	Dasatinib		TKI
Integrins	Cilengitide (EMD121974)		Synthetic RGD peptide
HDAC	Vorinostat (SAHA)		HDAC inhibitor
	Valproic acid		HDAC inhibitor
	LBH589		HDAC inhibitor

Table 2. Targeted molecular agents currently in clinical development for high-grade glioma TKI indicates tyrosine kinase inhibitor; SAHA, suberoylanilide hydroxamic acid; RGD, arginine-glycine-aspartate; STKI. serine-threnoine kinase inhibitor; PKC, protein kinase C.

3.1.7.1. *Cilengitide*

Cilengitide is a specific αV integrin inhibitor in clinical development. In a phase I/IIa trial, cilengitide combined with the current standard of therapy in patients with newly diagnosed GBM was well tolerated, with 6-month PFS as 69%. Methylation of promoter of O6-methylguanine-DNA methyltransferase (MGMT) predicts a higher likelihood of achieving 6-month PFS, as shown by increases in the durations of PFS and OS to 13.4 months and 23.2 months, respectively, compared with 3.4 and 13.1 months for patients without MGMT promoter methylation [115]. On the basis of these findings, a similar regimen is being compared with radiotherapy/TMZ alone in the phase III CENTRIC trial in patients with newly diagnosed GBM with hypermethylated MGMT promoter. In a phase IIa study of recurrent GBM, cilengitide monotherapy was well tolerated but was largely inactive (6-month PFS rate, 15%); long-term disease stabilization was seen in a small subset of patients: 10% were progression free for 12 months, and 5% were progression free for 24 months [116].

3.1.8. *Histone deacetylase inhibitor*

Histone deacetylases (HDACs) are involved in multiple processes to lead malignant phenotype of glioma including maintanance of stemness, angiogenesis, and resistance to DNA damage.

3.1.8.1. *Vorinostat*

Vorinostat is an orally available inhibitor of class I and II HDAC approved for advance cutaneous T cell lymphoma. In a phase II study of recurrent GBM, vorinostat monotherapy was well tolerated and had modest clinical activity (6-month PFS rate, 15.2%; median OS duration, 5.7 months) [117]. Vorinostat is currently being evaluated for use in newly diagnosed and recurrent GBM as a combination therapy.

4. Conclusion

Although TMZ prolonged the survival of GBM patients, GBM are still immortal disease with extremely poor prognosis because of acquisition of TMZ resistance. Therefore, other therapeutic agents which suppress MGMT expression or attenuate TMZ resistance are highly desired. As the efficacy of single agent of targeted molecular therapy seems to be limited, combination therapy should be evaluated since multi-pathway is involved in the chemoresistance in GBM. An 'tailor-made' selection of chemotherapeutic agents for each GBM patients based on molecular analysis is essential to obtain maximum efficacy of chemotherapeutic agents.

http://dx.doi.org/10.5772/54353

Author details

Shinji Kohsaka[1] and Shinya Tanaka[1,2]

*Address all correspondence to: tanaka@med.hokudai.ac.jp

1 Department of Cancer Pathology, Hokkaido University Graduate School of Medicine, Sapporo, Japan

2 Department of Translational Pathology, Hokkaido University Graduate School of Medicine, Sapporo, Japan

References

[1] E.G. Van Meir, C.G. Hadjipanayis, A.D. Norden, H.K. Shu, P.Y. Wen, J.J. Olson. Exciting new advances in neuro-oncology: the avenue to a cure for malignant glioma. CA Cancer J Clin. May-Jun 2010;60(3):166-193.

[2] L. Liu, S.L. Gerson. Targeted modulation of MGMT: clinical implications. Clin Cancer Res. Jan 15 2006;12(2):328-331.

[3] R. Stupp, W.P. Mason, M.J. van den Bent, et al. Radiotherapy plus concomitant and adjuvant temozolomide for glioblastoma. N Engl J Med. Mar 10 2005;352(10):987-996.

[4] S.C. Schold, Jr., T.P. Brent, E. von Hofe, et al. O6-alkylguanine-DNA alkyltransferase and sensitivity to procarbazine in human brain-tumor xenografts. J Neurosurg. Apr 1989;70(4):573-577.

[5] S.L. Gerson, J.E. Trey, K. Miller, N.A. Berger. Comparison of O6-alkylguanine-DNA alkyltransferase activity based on cellular DNA content in human, rat and mouse tissues. Carcinogenesis. May 1986;7(5):745-749.

[6] M. Citron, R. Decker, S. Chen, et al. O6-methylguanine-DNA methyltransferase in human normal and tumor tissue from brain, lung, and ovary. Cancer Res. Aug 15 1991;51(16):4131-4134.

[7] W.J. Washington, R.S. Foote, W.C. Dunn, W.M. Generoso, S. Mitra. Age-dependent modulation of tissue-specific repair activity for 3-methyladenine and O6-methylguanine in DNA in inbred mice. Mech Ageing Dev. Apr 1989;48(1):43-52.

[8] M.E. Hegi, A.C. Diserens, T. Gorlia, et al. MGMT gene silencing and benefit from temozolomide in glioblastoma. N Engl J Med. Mar 10 2005;352(10):997-1003.

[9] M. Weller, J. Felsberg, C. Hartmann, et al. Molecular predictors of progression-free and overall survival in patients with newly diagnosed glioblastoma: a prospective translational study of the German Glioma Network. J Clin Oncol. Dec 1 2009;27(34): 5743-5750.

[10] [10]P. Das, T. Puri, P. Jha, et al. A clinicopathological and molecular analysis of glioblastoma multiforme with long-term survival. J Clin Neurosci. Jan 2011;18(1):66-70.

[11] I. Lavon, D. Fuchs, D. Zrihan, et al. Novel mechanism whereby nuclear factor kappaB mediates DNA damage repair through regulation of O(6)-methylguanine-DNA-methyltransferase. Cancer Res. Sep 15 2007;67(18):8952-8959.

[12] A.E. Pegg. Repair of O(6)-alkylguanine by alkyltransferases. Mutat Res. Apr 2000;462(2-3):83-100.

[13] T. Grombacher, S. Mitra, B. Kaina. Induction of the alkyltransferase (MGMT) gene by DNA damaging agents and the glucocorticoid dexamethasone and comparison with the response of base excision repair genes. Carcinogenesis. Nov 1996;17(11): 2329-2336.

[14] T. Biswas, C.V. Ramana, G. Srinivasan, et al. Activation of human O6-methylguanine-DNA methyltransferase gene by glucocorticoid hormone. Oncogene. Jan 14 1999;18(2):525-532.

[15] A. Natsume, D. Ishii, T. Wakabayashi, et al. IFN-beta down-regulates the expression of DNA repair gene MGMT and sensitizes resistant glioma cells to temozolomide. Cancer Res. Sep 1 2005;65(17):7573-7579.

[16] D. Bocangel, S. Sengupta, S. Mitra, K.K. Bhakat. p53-Mediated down-regulation of the human DNA repair gene O6-methylguanine-DNA methyltransferase (MGMT) via interaction with Sp1 transcription factor. Anticancer Res. Oct 2009;29(10): 3741-3750.

[17] V. Vielhauer, M. Sarafoff, P. Gais, H.M. Rabes. Cell type-specific induction of O6-alkylguanine-DNA alkyltransferase mRNA expression in rat liver during regeneration, inflammation and preneoplasia. J Cancer Res Clin Oncol. Oct 2001;127(10):591-602.

[18] K.S. Srivenugopal, X.H. Yuan, H.S. Friedman, F. Ali-Osman. Ubiquitination-dependent proteolysis of O6-methylguanine-DNA methyltransferase in human and murine tumor cells following inactivation with O6-benzylguanine or 1,3-bis(2-chloroethyl)-1-nitrosourea. Biochemistry. Jan 30 1996;35(4):1328-1334.

[19] V. Ramakrishnan, D. Kushwaha, D.C. Koay, et al. Post-transcriptional regulation of O(6)-methylguanine-DNA methyltransferase MGMT in glioblastomas. Cancer Biomark. 2011;10(3-4):185-193.

[20] J.A. Quinn, A. Desjardins, J. Weingart, et al. Phase I trial of temozolomide plus O6-benzylguanine for patients with recurrent or progressive malignant glioma. J Clin Oncol. Oct 1 2005;23(28):7178-7187.

[21] M. Ranson, M.R. Middleton, J. Bridgewater, et al. Lomeguatrib, a potent inhibitor of O6-alkylguanine-DNA-alkyltransferase: phase I safety, pharmacodynamic, and pharmacokinetic trial and evaluation in combination with temozolomide in patients with advanced solid tumors. Clin Cancer Res. Mar 1 2006;12(5):1577-1584.

[22] O. Khan, M.R. Middleton. The therapeutic potential of O6-alkylguanine DNA alkyltransferase inhibitors. Expert Opin Investig Drugs. Oct 2007;16(10):1573-1584.

[23] J.A. Quinn, S.X. Jiang, D.A. Reardon, et al. Phase II trial of temozolomide plus o6-benzylguanine in adults with recurrent, temozolomide-resistant malignant glioma. J Clin Oncol. Mar 10 2009;27(8):1262-1267.

[24] A. Yoshino, A. Ogino, K. Yachi, et al. Effect of IFN-beta on human glioma cell lines with temozolomide resistance. Int J Oncol. Jul 2009;35(1):139-148.

[25] S. Kohsaka, L. Wang, K. Yachi, et al. STAT3 inhibition overcomes temozolomide resistance in glioblastoma by downregulating MGMT expression. Mol Cancer Ther. Jun 2012;11(6):1289-1299.

[26] D.P. Cahill, K.K. Levine, R.A. Betensky, et al. Loss of the mismatch repair protein MSH6 in human glioblastomas is associated with tumor progression during temozolomide treatment. Clin Cancer Res. Apr 1 2007;13(7):2038-2045.

[27] S. Yip, J. Miao, D.P. Cahill, et al. MSH6 mutations arise in glioblastomas during temozolomide therapy and mediate temozolomide resistance. Clin Cancer Res. Jul 15 2009;15(14):4622-4629.

[28] J.B. Tang, D. Svilar, R.N. Trivedi, et al. N-methylpurine DNA glycosylase and DNA polymerase beta modulate BER inhibitor potentiation of glioma cells to temozolomide. Neuro Oncol. May 2011;13(5):471-486.

[29] S. Agnihotri, A.S. Gajadhar, C. Ternamian, et al. Alkylpurine-DNA-N-glycosylase confers resistance to temozolomide in xenograft models of glioblastoma multiforme and is associated with poor survival in patients. J Clin Invest. Jan 3 2012;122(1): 253-266.

[30] N. Kondo, A. Takahashi, E. Mori, et al. FANCD1/BRCA2 plays predominant role in the repair of DNA damage induced by ACNU or TMZ. PLoS One. 2011;6(5):e19659.

[31] P. Pyrko, A.H. Schonthal, F.M. Hofman, T.C. Chen, A.S. Lee. The unfolded protein response regulator GRP78/BiP as a novel target for increasing chemosensitivity in malignant gliomas. Cancer Res. Oct 15 2007;67(20):9809-9816.

[32] Y. Gao, A. Fotovati, C. Lee, et al. Inhibition of Y-box binding protein-1 slows the growth of glioblastoma multiforme and sensitizes to temozolomide independent O6-methylguanine-DNA methyltransferase. Mol Cancer Ther. Dec 2009;8(12):3276-3284.

[33] N. Gaspar, L. Marshall, L. Perryman, et al. MGMT-independent temozolomide resistance in pediatric glioblastoma cells associated with a PI3-kinase-mediated HOX/stem cell gene signature. Cancer Res. Nov 15 2010;70(22):9243-9252.

[34] Z. Jiang, N. Pore, G.J. Cerniglia, et al. Phosphatase and tensin homologue deficiency in glioblastoma confers resistance to radiation and temozolomide that is reversed by the protease inhibitor nelfinavir. Cancer Res. May 1 2007;67(9):4467-4473.

[35] Comprehensive genomic characterization defines human glioblastoma genes and core pathways. Nature. Oct 23 2008;455(7216):1061-1068.

[36] D.W. Parsons, S. Jones, X. Zhang, et al. An integrated genomic analysis of human glioblastoma multiforme. Science. Sep 26 2008;321(5897):1807-1812.

[37] W. Xu, H. Yang, Y. Liu, et al. Oncometabolite 2-hydroxyglutarate is a competitive inhibitor of alpha-ketoglutarate-dependent dioxygenases. Cancer Cell. Jan 18 2011;19(1):17-30.

[38] L. Dang, D.W. White, S. Gross, et al. Cancer-associated IDH1 mutations produce 2-hydroxyglutarate. Nature. Dec 10 2009;462(7274):739-744.

[39] L. Frederick, X.Y. Wang, G. Eley, C.D. James. Diversity and frequency of epidermal growth factor receptor mutations in human glioblastomas. Cancer Res. Mar 1 2000;60(5):1383-1387.

[40] P. Kleihues, H. Ohgaki. Primary and secondary glioblastomas: from concept to clinical diagnosis. Neuro Oncol. Jan 1999;1(1):44-51.

[41] D.M. Peereboom, D.R. Shepard, M.S. Ahluwalia, et al. Phase II trial of erlotinib with temozolomide and radiation in patients with newly diagnosed glioblastoma multiforme. J Neurooncol. May 2010;98(1):93-99.

[42] M.D. Prados, S.M. Chang, N. Butowski, et al. Phase II study of erlotinib plus temozolomide during and after radiation therapy in patients with newly diagnosed glioblastoma multiforme or gliosarcoma. J Clin Oncol. Feb 1 2009;27(4):579-584.

[43] J.F. de Groot, M.R. Gilbert, K. Aldape, et al. Phase II study of carboplatin and erlotinib (Tarceva, OSI-774) in patients with recurrent glioblastoma. J Neurooncol. Oct 2008;90(1):89-97.

[44] D.A. Reardon, A. Desjardins, J.J. Vredenburgh, et al. Phase 2 trial of erlotinib plus sirolimus in adults with recurrent glioblastoma. J Neurooncol. Jan 2010;96(2):219-230.

[45] M.J. van den Bent, A.A. Brandes, R. Rampling, et al. Randomized phase II trial of erlotinib versus temozolomide or carmustine in recurrent glioblastoma: EORTC brain tumor group study 26034. J Clin Oncol. Mar 10 2009;27(8):1268-1274.

[46] B. Thiessen, C. Stewart, M. Tsao, et al. A phase I/II trial of GW572016 (lapatinib) in recurrent glioblastoma multiforme: clinical outcomes, pharmacokinetics and molecular correlation. Cancer Chemother Pharmacol. Jan 2010;65(2):353-361.

[47] B. Neyns, J. Sadones, E. Joosens, et al. Stratified phase II trial of cetuximab in patients with recurrent high-grade glioma. Ann Oncol. Sep 2009;20(9):1596-1603.

[48] D.A. Haas-Kogan, M.D. Prados, T. Tihan, et al. Epidermal growth factor receptor, protein kinase B/Akt, and glioma response to erlotinib. J Natl Cancer Inst. Jun 15 2005;97(12):880-887.

[49] I.K. Mellinghoff, M.Y. Wang, I. Vivanco, et al. Molecular determinants of the response of glioblastomas to EGFR kinase inhibitors. N Engl J Med. Nov 10 2005;353(19):2012-2024.

[50] T. Ozawa, C.W. Brennan, L. Wang, et al. PDGFRA gene rearrangements are frequent genetic events in PDGFRA-amplified glioblastomas. Genes Dev. Oct 1 2010;24(19): 2205-2218.

[51] S.M. Wilhelm, L. Adnane, P. Newell, A. Villanueva, J.M. Llovet, M. Lynch. Preclinical overview of sorafenib, a multikinase inhibitor that targets both Raf and VEGF and PDGF receptor tyrosine kinase signaling. Mol Cancer Ther. Oct 2008;7(10):3129-3140.

[52] C. Yu, B.B. Friday, J.P. Lai, et al. Cytotoxic synergy between the multikinase inhibitor sorafenib and the proteasome inhibitor bortezomib in vitro: induction of apoptosis through Akt and c-Jun NH2-terminal kinase pathways. Mol Cancer Ther. Sep 2006;5(9):2378-2387.

[53] E.P. Jane, D.R. Premkumar, I.F. Pollack. Coadministration of sorafenib with rottlerin potently inhibits cell proliferation and migration in human malignant glioma cells. J Pharmacol Exp Ther. Dec 2006;319(3):1070-1080.

[54] D. Hagerstrand, G. Hesselager, S. Achterberg, et al. Characterization of an imatinib-sensitive subset of high-grade human glioma cultures. Oncogene. Aug 10 2006;25(35):4913-4922.

[55] M. Holdhoff, K.A. Kreuzer, C. Appelt, et al. Imatinib mesylate radiosensitizes human glioblastoma cells through inhibition of platelet-derived growth factor receptor. Blood Cells Mol Dis. Mar-Apr 2005;34(2):181-185.

[56] A. Desjardins, J.A. Quinn, J.J. Vredenburgh, et al. Phase II study of imatinib mesylate and hydroxyurea for recurrent grade III malignant gliomas. J Neurooncol. May 2007;83(1):53-60.

[57] P.Y. Wen, W.K. Yung, K.R. Lamborn, et al. Phase I/II study of imatinib mesylate for recurrent malignant gliomas: North American Brain Tumor Consortium Study 99-08. Clin Cancer Res. Aug 15 2006;12(16):4899-4907.

[58] E. Raymond, A.A. Brandes, C. Dittrich, et al. Phase II study of imatinib in patients with recurrent gliomas of various histologies: a European Organisation for Research and Treatment of Cancer Brain Tumor Group Study. J Clin Oncol. Oct 1 2008;26(28): 4659-4665.

[59] D.A. Reardon, G. Dresemann, S. Taillibert, et al. Multicentre phase II studies evaluating imatinib plus hydroxyurea in patients with progressive glioblastoma. Br J Cancer. Dec 15 2009;101(12):1995-2004.

[60] G. Dresemann, M. Weller, M.A. Rosenthal, et al. Imatinib in combination with hydroxyurea versus hydroxyurea alone as oral therapy in patients with progressive pretreated glioblastoma resistant to standard dose temozolomide. J Neurooncol. Feb 2010;96(3):393-402.

[61] W. Wick, M. Weller, M. Weiler, T. Batchelor, A.W. Yung, M. Platten. Pathway inhibition: emerging molecular targets for treating glioblastoma. Neuro Oncol. Jun 2011;13(6):566-579.

[62] K.H. Plate, H.D. Mennel. Vascular morphology and angiogenesis in glial tumors. Exp Toxicol Pathol. May 1995;47(2-3):89-94.

[63] E. Bullitt, D.A. Reardon, J.K. Smith. A review of micro- and macrovascular analyses in the assessment of tumor-associated vasculature as visualized by MR. Neuroimage. 2007;37 Suppl 1:S116-119.

[64] S.K. Hobbs, W.L. Monsky, F. Yuan, et al. Regulation of transport pathways in tumor vessels: role of tumor type and microenvironment. Proc Natl Acad Sci U S A. Apr 14 1998;95(8):4607-4612.

[65] S. Morikawa, P. Baluk, T. Kaidoh, A. Haskell, R.K. Jain, D.M. McDonald. Abnormalities in pericytes on blood vessels and endothelial sprouts in tumors. Am J Pathol. Mar 2002;160(3):985-1000.

[66] P. Baluk, S. Morikawa, A. Haskell, M. Mancuso, D.M. McDonald. Abnormalities of basement membrane on blood vessels and endothelial sprouts in tumors. Am J Pathol. Nov 2003;163(5):1801-1815.

[67] T. Inai, M. Mancuso, H. Hashizume, et al. Inhibition of vascular endothelial growth factor (VEGF) signaling in cancer causes loss of endothelial fenestrations, regression of tumor vessels, and appearance of basement membrane ghosts. Am J Pathol. Jul 2004;165(1):35-52.

[68] W.S. Kamoun, C.D. Ley, C.T. Farrar, et al. Edema control by cediranib, a vascular endothelial growth factor receptor-targeted kinase inhibitor, prolongs survival despite persistent brain tumor growth in mice. J Clin Oncol. May 20 2009;27(15):2542-2552.

[69] H.S. Friedman, M.D. Prados, P.Y. Wen, et al. Bevacizumab alone and in combination with irinotecan in recurrent glioblastoma. J Clin Oncol. Oct 1 2009;27(28):4733-4740.

[70] T.N. Kreisl, L. Kim, K. Moore, et al. Phase II trial of single-agent bevacizumab followed by bevacizumab plus irinotecan at tumor progression in recurrent glioblastoma. J Clin Oncol. Feb 10 2009;27(5):740-745.

[71] D. Zagzag, H. Zhong, J.M. Scalzitti, E. Laughner, J.W. Simons, G.L. Semenza. Expression of hypoxia-inducible factor 1alpha in brain tumors: association with angiogenesis, invasion, and progression. Cancer. Jun 1 2000;88(11):2606-2618.

[72] N.O. Schmidt, M. Westphal, C. Hagel, et al. Levels of vascular endothelial growth factor, hepatocyte growth factor/scatter factor and basic fibroblast growth factor in human gliomas and their relation to angiogenesis. Int J Cancer. Feb 19 1999;84(1): 10-18.

[73] Y.H. Zhou, F. Tan, K.R. Hess, W.K. Yung. The expression of PAX6, PTEN, vascular endothelial growth factor, and epidermal growth factor receptor in gliomas: relationship to tumor grade and survival. Clin Cancer Res. Aug 15 2003;9(9):3369-3375.

[74] J.R. Flynn, L. Wang, D.L. Gillespie, et al. Hypoxia-regulated protein expression, patient characteristics, and preoperative imaging as predictors of survival in adults with glioblastoma multiforme. Cancer. Sep 1 2008;113(5):1032-1042.

[75] N. Ferrara, K.J. Hillan, H.P. Gerber, W. Novotny. Discovery and development of bevacizumab, an anti-VEGF antibody for treating cancer. Nat Rev Drug Discov. May 2004;3(5):391-400.

[76] E.T. Wong, K.R. Hess, M.J. Gleason, et al. Outcomes and prognostic factors in recurrent glioma patients enrolled onto phase II clinical trials. J Clin Oncol. Aug 1999;17(8):2572-2578.

[77] F.M. Iwamoto, H.A. Fine. Bevacizumab for malignant gliomas. Arch Neurol. Mar 2010;67(3):285-288.

[78] J.J. Vredenburgh, A. Desjardins, J.E. Herndon, 2nd, et al. Bevacizumab plus irinotecan in recurrent glioblastoma multiforme. J Clin Oncol. Oct 20 2007;25(30):4722-4729.

[79] A. Desjardins, D.A. Reardon, J.E. Herndon, 2nd, et al. Bevacizumab plus irinotecan in recurrent WHO grade 3 malignant gliomas. Clin Cancer Res. Nov 1 2008;14(21): 7068-7073.

[80] K.R. Lamborn, W.K. Yung, S.M. Chang, et al. Progression-free survival: an important end point in evaluating therapy for recurrent high-grade gliomas. Neuro Oncol. Apr 2008;10(2):162-170.

[81] J. Holash, S. Davis, N. Papadopoulos, et al. VEGF-Trap: a VEGF blocker with potent antitumor effects. Proc Natl Acad Sci U S A. Aug 20 2002;99(17):11393-11398.

[82] J.F. de Groot, K.R. Lamborn, S.M. Chang, et al. Phase II study of aflibercept in recurrent malignant glioma: a North American Brain Tumor Consortium study. J Clin Oncol. Jul 1 2011;29(19):2689-2695.

[83] S. de Bouard, P. Herlin, J.G. Christensen, et al. Antiangiogenic and anti-invasive effects of sunitinib on experimental human glioblastoma. Neuro Oncol. Oct 2007;9(4): 412-423.

[84] F. Hilberg, G.J. Roth, M. Krssak, et al. BIBF 1120: triple angiokinase inhibitor with sustained receptor blockade and good antitumor efficacy. Cancer Res. Jun 15 2008;68(12):4774-4782.

[85] J.N. Rich, S. Sathornsumetee, S.T. Keir, et al. ZD6474, a novel tyrosine kinase inhibitor of vascular endothelial growth factor receptor and epidermal growth factor receptor, inhibits tumor growth of multiple nervous system tumors. Clin Cancer Res. Nov 15 2005;11(22):8145-8157.

[86] J.J. Yiin, B. Hu, P.A. Schornack, et al. ZD6474, a multitargeted inhibitor for receptor tyrosine kinases, suppresses growth of gliomas expressing an epidermal growth factor receptor mutant, EGFRvIII, in the brain. Mol Cancer Ther. Apr 2010;9(4):929-941.

[87] F. Yang, C. Brown, R. Buettner, et al. Sorafenib induces growth arrest and apoptosis of human glioblastoma cells through the dephosphorylation of signal transducers and activators of transcription 3. Mol Cancer Ther. Apr 2010;9(4):953-962.

[88] Y. Zhang, F. Guessous, A. Kofman, D. Schiff, R. Abounader. XL-184, a MET, VEGFR-2 and RET kinase inhibitor for the treatment of thyroid cancer, glioblastoma multiforme and NSCLC. IDrugs. Feb 2010;13(2):112-121.

[89] A.J. Schueneman, E. Himmelfarb, L. Geng, et al. SU11248 maintenance therapy prevents tumor regrowth after fractionated irradiation of murine tumor models. Cancer Res. Jul 15 2003;63(14):4009-4016.

[90] V. Damiano, D. Melisi, C. Bianco, et al. Cooperative antitumor effect of multitargeted kinase inhibitor ZD6474 and ionizing radiation in glioblastoma. Clin Cancer Res. Aug 1 2005;11(15):5639-5644.

[91] Q. Zhou, P. Guo, J.M. Gallo. Impact of angiogenesis inhibition by sunitinib on tumor distribution of temozolomide. Clin Cancer Res. Mar 1 2008;14(5):1540-1549.

[92] T.T. Batchelor, D.G. Duda, E. di Tomaso, et al. Phase II study of cediranib, an oral pan-vascular endothelial growth factor receptor tyrosine kinase inhibitor, in patients with recurrent glioblastoma. J Clin Oncol. Jun 10 2010;28(17):2817-2823.

[93] T.T. Batchelor, A.G. Sorensen, E. di Tomaso, et al. AZD2171, a pan-VEGF receptor tyrosine kinase inhibitor, normalizes tumor vasculature and alleviates edema in glioblastoma patients. Cancer Cell. Jan 2007;11(1):83-95.

[94] F.M. Iwamoto, L.E. Abrey, K. Beal, et al. Patterns of relapse and prognosis after bevacizumab failure in recurrent glioblastoma. Neurology. Oct 13 2009;73(15):1200-1206.

[95] A.D. Norden, J. Drappatz, A. Muzikansky, et al. An exploratory survival analysis of anti-angiogenic therapy for recurrent malignant glioma. J Neurooncol. Apr 2009;92(2):149-155.

[96] M. Paez-Ribes, E. Allen, J. Hudock, et al. Antiangiogenic therapy elicits malignant progression of tumors to increased local invasion and distant metastasis. Cancer Cell. Mar 3 2009;15(3):220-231.

[97] P. Guo, B. Hu, W. Gu, et al. Platelet-derived growth factor-B enhances glioma angiogenesis by stimulating vascular endothelial growth factor expression in tumor endothelia and by promoting pericyte recruitment. Am J Pathol. Apr 2003;162(4): 1083-1093.

[98] R. Erber, A. Thurnher, A.D. Katsen, et al. Combined inhibition of VEGF and PDGF signaling enforces tumor vessel regression by interfering with pericyte-mediated endothelial cell survival mechanisms. FASEB J. Feb 2004;18(2):338-340.

[99] L. Toschi, P.A. Janne. Single-agent and combination therapeutic strategies to inhibit hepatocyte growth factor/MET signaling in cancer. Clin Cancer Res. Oct 1 2008;14(19):5941-5946.

[100] D.S. Kong, S.Y. Song, D.H. Kim, et al. Prognostic significance of c-Met expression in glioblastomas. Cancer. Jan 1 2009;115(1):140-148.

[101] H.T. Jun, J. Sun, K. Rex, et al. AMG 102, a fully human anti-hepatocyte growth factor/ scatter factor neutralizing antibody, enhances the efficacy of temozolomide or docetaxel in U-87 MG cells and xenografts. Clin Cancer Res. Nov 15 2007;13(22 Pt 1): 6735-6742.

[102] P.Y. Wen, D. Schiff, T.F. Cloughesy, et al. A phase II study evaluating the efficacy and safety of AMG 102 (rilotumumab) in patients with recurrent glioblastoma. Neuro Oncol. Apr 2011;13(4):437-446.

[103] S. Yamazaki, J. Skaptason, D. Romero, et al. Pharmacokinetic-pharmacodynamic modeling of biomarker response and tumor growth inhibition to an orally available cMet kinase inhibitor in human tumor xenograft mouse models. Drug Metab Dispos. Jul 2008;36(7):1267-1274.

[104] S.M. Maira, F. Stauffer, J. Brueggen, et al. Identification and characterization of NVP-BEZ235, a new orally available dual phosphatidylinositol 3-kinase/mammalian target of rapamycin inhibitor with potent in vivo antitumor activity. Mol Cancer Ther. Jul 2008;7(7):1851-1863.

[105] J. Rieger, D. Lemke, G. Maurer, et al. Enzastaurin-induced apoptosis in glioma cells is caspase-dependent and inhibited by BCL-XL. J Neurochem. Sep 2008;106(6): 2436-2448.

[106] G. Tabatabai, B. Frank, A. Wick, et al. Synergistic antiglioma activity of radiotherapy and enzastaurin. Ann Neurol. Feb 2007;61(2):153-161.

[107] T.N. Kreisl, S. Kotliarova, J.A. Butman, et al. A phase I/II trial of enzastaurin in patients with recurrent high-grade gliomas. Neuro Oncol. Feb 2010;12(2):181-189.

[108] W. Wick, V.K. Puduvalli, M.C. Chamberlain, et al. Phase III study of enzastaurin compared with lomustine in the treatment of recurrent intracranial glioblastoma. J Clin Oncol. Mar 1 2010;28(7):1168-1174.

[109] J. Du, P. Bernasconi, K.R. Clauser, et al. Bead-based profiling of tyrosine kinase phosphorylation identifies SRC as a potential target for glioblastoma therapy. Nat Biotechnol. Jan 2009;27(1):77-83.

[110] K.V. Lu, S. Zhu, A. Cvrljevic, et al. Fyn and SRC are effectors of oncogenic epidermal growth factor receptor signaling in glioblastoma patients. Cancer Res. Sep 1 2009;69(17):6889-6898.

[111] M. Brave, V. Goodman, E. Kaminskas, et al. Sprycel for chronic myeloid leukemia and Philadelphia chromosome-positive acute lymphoblastic leukemia resistant to or intolerant of imatinib mesylate. Clin Cancer Res. Jan 15 2008;14(2):352-359.

[112] L.J. Lombardo, F.Y. Lee, P. Chen, et al. Discovery of N-(2-chloro-6-methyl- phenyl)-2-(6-(4-(2-hydroxyethyl)- piperazin-1-yl)-2-methylpyrimidin-4- ylamino)thiazole-5-carboxamide (BMS-354825), a dual Src/Abl kinase inhibitor with potent antitumor activity in preclinical assays. J Med Chem. Dec 30 2004;47(27):6658-6661.

[113] V. Milano, Y. Piao, T. LaFortune, J. de Groot. Dasatinib-induced autophagy is enhanced in combination with temozolomide in glioma. Mol Cancer Ther. Feb 2009;8(2):394-406.

[114] J.S. Desgrosellier, D.A. Cheresh. Integrins in cancer: biological implications and therapeutic opportunities. Nat Rev Cancer. Jan 2010;10(1):9-22.

[115] R. Stupp, M.E. Hegi, B. Neyns, et al. Phase I/IIa study of cilengitide and temozolomide with concomitant radiotherapy followed by cilengitide and temozolomide maintenance therapy in patients with newly diagnosed glioblastoma. J Clin Oncol. Jun 1 2010;28(16):2712-2718.

[116] D.A. Reardon, K.L. Fink, T. Mikkelsen, et al. Randomized phase II study of cilengitide, an integrin-targeting arginine-glycine-aspartic acid peptide, in recurrent glioblastoma multiforme. J Clin Oncol. Dec 1 2008;26(34):5610-5617.

[117] E. Galanis, K.A. Jaeckle, M.J. Maurer, et al. Phase II trial of vorinostat in recurrent glioblastoma multiforme: a north central cancer treatment group study. J Clin Oncol. Apr 20 2009;27(12):2052-2058.

Chapter 20

Topoisomerase Therapy in the Treatment of Brain Tumors

George Theodore, Niramol Savaraj and Lynn Feun

Additional information is available at the end of the chapter

http://dx.doi.org/10.5772/53184

1. Introduction

The treatment of brain tumors remains a challenge for modern medicine and care. Therapy for these patients is often complicated by site accessibility and the risk of damage to surrounding tissue. The ability of chemotherapies to cross the blood brain barrier has also limited their use as compared with surgical resections and radiation therapy. (Groothuis, 2000) For these reasons, malignant gliomas of the central nervous system (CNS) have a poor prognosis. In fact, the majority of patients with high grade gliomas (glioblastomas) will die within the first couple of years after the diagnosis.(McLendon, 2003) The 5 year survival rate for these patients with glioblastoma is less than 4% with the majority of deaths in the first two years post-diagnosis. (Grossman, 2004; CBTRUS, 2012) This devastating impact has been the impetus behind much of the research that is ongoing into effective therapies to combat these tumors. Over the years many therapies have been studied, but in recent times the increased investigation into specific molecular pathways has led to targeting specific tumor expression patterns and cellular attributes. The enhanced understanding of cell division, including aspects of DNA replication are now being used to target tumor replication and treat many cancers from various tissues. In this fashion, tumors of the CNS should be more specifically targeted so that damage to the surrounding normal tissue is minimized.

2. Epidemiology

Even after treatment, the median survival after the primary diagnosis remains poor. Many multimodal treatment approaches are considered, but few patients have been reported to have long term survival greater than three years. In a recent study, analysis of 34,664 patients, diagnosed with GBM over the age of 20 from 1972-2008 in the Surveillance, Epidemiology, and End Results (SEER) NCI database, evaluated specific prognostic factors known to influence survival in these patients. (Thumma, 2012) This analysis included racial/ethnic characteristics in the description of specific subpopulations and found that Asian/Pacific Islanders had a better survival compared to the white population ($P<0.001$). Patients diagnosed with GBM during the years of 2000 to 2008 had a superior survival rate when compared with earlier decades ($P<0.001$). Statistically significant improvements in overall survival were also found for patients who received surgical resections, and adjuvant radiation treatment versus no radiation (P values <0.001). Young age was also found to be highly predictive of improved overall survival rates when separated into age groups as well as when studied as a continuous variable. (Thumma, 2012) Thus, there are subpopulations with varied genomic and environmental attributes that may affect survival of CNS tumors. Although these studies did not specifically identify the critical factors that dictate these differences, future studies may capitalize on differences that enhance efficacy.

Despite aggressive therapy for malignant gliomas, recurrence rate is quite high and the prognosis for most patients is extremely poor. The standard approach for high grade gliomas is radiation therapy combined with temozolomide. (Stupp, 2005) Temozolomide added to cranial radiation therapy improved Two year survival to 26.5% vs 10.4% to radiation therapy alone. Toxicity of temozolomide and radiation therapy was minimal. Despite the improved two-year survival with the addition of temozolomide to standard radiation therapy, the vast majority of patients progress and die of their disease. Thus, more effective drugs and approaches are definitely needed. Newer drugs being investigated include topoisomerase I inhibitors. This chapter will review topoisomerase I inhibitors in the treatment of malignant gliomas. Novel approaches using this class of compounds will also be discussed.

3. Current therapies

The DNA topoisomerases are a family of important enzymes involved in different stages of the cell cycle. They are essential nuclear enzymes important in DNA topology, repair, and replication by breaking and rejoining of the DNA double helix. The breakage that they induce in essence unwinds the DNA structure and releases the molecule from its wound configuration. In this configuration, DNA replication as well as transcription can occur in the cell nucleus. Two significant topoisomerase molecules are named topoisomerase I and topoisomerase II. Although these molecules are in the same family, they work in different steps to bind and cause the eventual unwinding of the helical DNA structure. Topoisomerase I is a monomeric protein that induces single stranded breaks in DNA, one strand at a time.(Redinbo, 1998) Topoisomerase II brings about double stranded breaks in DNA since it is a dimer in which each homologous monomer can cleave a strand of DNA.(Wang, 1996) These differences have lead to the development of specific inhibitors to these topoisomerase enzymes. Since these inhibitors actually damage DNA, they are sometimes referred to as poisons in the literature.

4. Topotecan

Topotecan (TPT) is an analogue of camptothecin, an FDA approved chemotherapy for many types of cancer.(Bookman, 1998; tenBukkel, 2004) TPT is water soluble, and inhibits an essential role of topoisomerase I, depleting it in tumor cells and resulting in DNA strand breaks that are not utilized or repaired.(Yamashita, 2007) Cells are then stopped in the G2 phase of the cell cycle, and the progression of replication does not occur eventually leading to programmed cell death through apoptotic processes. In subcutaneous xenograft models and in vitro, TPT therapy has shown significant activity against glioblastoma (GBM) which is the most common and malignant type of primary brain tumor.(Ciusani, 2005; Rapisarda, 2004) Topotecan treatment showed some efficacy in preclinical studies, and TPT was found to be distributed in the cerebrospinal fluid after systemic administration, leading to the initiation of clinical trials evaluating the efficacy of TPT monotherapy on patients with GBM. (Ciusani, 2005; Baker, 1996) Data from phase II clinical trials with TPT treatment of both newly diagnosed and recurrent GBM revealed modest tumor responses. It is proposed that the lack of efficacy in treatment may be due to rapid clearance of TPT from the CSF, and rapid inactivation in plasma. (Mi, 1995) Both of these processes provide a survival advantage to the tumors since drug concentrations may not be significant around the tumor site. In order to address this and other mechanisms, the approach to TPT therapy has changed from monotherapy to use in combination with different agents targeting alternate pathways.(MacDonald,1996; Blaney,1996; Reveiz,2012) These combinations may vary in the sequence of drug delivery or may be simultaneous depending on the protocol used.

Topotecan is being studied as a component of combination therapies in primary brain tumors as well as in the efficacy it may have in the treatment of brain metastases. In one recent large scale literature review, approximately 10% to 18% of patients presented with brain metastases (BM) at the time of initial diagnosis of small cell lung cancer (SCLC), and an additional 40% to 50% will develop brain metastases during the course of their disease. To evaluate the effectiveness and toxicity of systemic chemotherapy for the treatment of these types of brain metastases from SCLC, the large scale systematic literature review was conducted for publications up to July 2011.(Reveiz,2012) The literature searched included randomized controlled trials comparing systemic chemotherapy (single agent or combination chemotherapy) vs another chemotherapy regimen, palliative care, whole brain radiotherapy or any combination of these interventions for the treatment of brain metastases as the sole site of progression. (Reveiz,2012) After this extensive search, no significant differences for overall survival (OS) were reported from randomized controlled trials with whole brain radiation therapy, and no significant difference was found between those treated with topotecan and those not treated with topotecan. Hence the treatment efficacy was not established in that review. A second trial found that patients receiving teponoside plus whole brain radiotherapy had a higher complete response rate than those receiving only the topoisomerase inhibitor. Hence, available evidence is insufficient to judge the effectiveness and safety of chemotherapy for the treatment of brain metastasis from small cell lung cancer. This may depend on the characteristics of the primary tumor and the activated mechanisms of metastasis. Future research may better address the different combination therapies as well as monotherapies in head to head comparisons and trials in populations with primary tumors and metastatic tumors.

Liposomes are microscopic phospholipid particles with a bilayer membrane structure, and are used to encapsulate various anticancer drugs.(Allen, 2004; Drummond,1999,2005) Liposomes have been used to encapsulate TPT, while free TPT was found to be less active against subcutaneous xenografts of cancers than injection of nano-liposomal TPT.(Drummond, 2005;Tardi,2001) Liposomal encapsulation may improve the efficacy of TPT by increasing increasing drug circulatory half-life and by providing the appropriate pH to maintain drug activity.(Tardi, 2001;Burke, 1994) In either case, the effect may be an increased amount of active drug present at the tumor site. In orthotopic, intracranial xenograft models of GBM, nanoliposomal TPT demonstrated superior efficacy when administered directly into the tumor by convection-enhanced delivery (CED).(Tardi, 2001;Saito,2006) CED of nano-liposomal TPT increased TPT half-life in the brain vs free TPT, and conferred a highly significant survival advantage. In a recent study, systemically administered nano-liposomal TPT had enhanced efficacy in 3 orthotopic xenograft models of GBM.(Serwer,2011) Bioluminescence monitoring of tumor growth and therapeutic response, survival benefit to animal subjects, and immune-histochemical analysis of tumor apoptotic response to therapy were used to assess efficacy. Although these results were promising, data from clinical trials would be more significant and applicable to the demonstration of efficacy. Consistent with the inhibitor function, increased DNA strand breaks in TPT-treated tumors, and an increase in activated caspase-3 (marker of programmed cell death) were observed in this study.(Serwer,2011) Delivery of liposomal packaged TPT to tumors increased both of these molecular events, leading to cell death.

Nano-liposomal topotecan (nLS-TPT) has anti-tumor activity when administered directly to brain tumors by convection-enhanced delivery (CED).(Serwer,2011 poster) As a topoisomerase I inhibitor, topotecan (TPT) must be internalized in order to have a cytotoxic effect, hence increasing cellular internalization may increase the anti-tumor activity of nLS-TPT. Attaching an epidermal growth factor (EGFR)-specific antibody to the nLS-TPT surface increased EGFR-targeting. EGFR activation is considered a proliferative event leading to more cell replication. This receptor is commonly found on cell membranes in order to increase accessibility to ligand binding, hence the antibody used for targeting in this study may increase specific binding to cells that have increased expression of the receptor. Improved targeting rates of TPT-nLS internalization in vitro, and secondly nLS-TPT-EGFR offered superior efficacy compared to nLS-TPT in vivo.(Serwer,2011 poster) When coupled to the antibody, the internalization of the inhibitor was highly and significantly increased as was the rate of internalization of nLS-TPT-EGFR when compared to nLS-TPT in all cells that express EGFR. In vivo studies in both EGFR-expressing mouse models of glioblastoma models showed a substantial dose dependent benefit of nLS-TPT-EGFR treatment compared to nLS-TPT treatment.(Serwer, 2011 and poster) The use of nLS-TPT-EGFR against glioblastomas that overexpress EGFR increases targeting and improves internalization. This may ultimately increase survival by delaying tumor growth.

The prognosis for newly-diagnosed GBM remains poor, and one of the reasons for this is that GBM's have the highest levels of vascular endothelial growth factor (VEGF) and hypoxia inducing factor-1 alpha (HIF-1 alpha), an important regulator of VEGF. Topotecan therapy may play a role in this signalling pathway by inhibiting HIF-1 alpha in treated tumor cells, limiting tumor vascularization. (Vredenburgh, 2011) A phase II trial in newly diagnosed GBM added bevacizumab and topotecan to standard therapy. 80 newly diagnosed GBM patients received standard radiation therapy and temozolomide with bevacizumab at 10 mg/kg every 14 days was added a minimum of 4 weeks post-op. Two weeks after radiation therapy was completed, 12 monthly cycles of temozolomide, and oral topotecan were given for patients not on an enzyme inducing anti-epileptic drug.(Vredenburgh, 2011) The addition of bevacizumab to temozolomide and radiation followed by temozolomide, bevacizumab and oral topotecan was tolerable and safe. Six patients came off the study with recurrent grade IV thrombocytopenia, one each with grade 2 CNS hemorrhage, wound dehiscence requiring surgery and a GI perforation. Median PFS and OS were not reached at a median follow-up of 8 months but the 6 month EFS was 83%. Hence in this case, multifactorial combination therapies for DNA replication as well as vascularization may aid in treatment efficacy.

5. Irinotecan

Irinotecan is another water soluble topoisomerase inhibitor that is being used clinically for the treatment of tumors. (Hsiang, 1985) A recent prospective, phase II study evaluated the efficacy of irinotecan and bevacizumab in the treatment of recurrent glioblastoma multiforme (GBM). (Møller,2012) In the evaluation of 85 patients with different brain tumors, the investigators used response rate and progression free survival (PFS) in patients who received intravenous bevacizumab (10 mg/kg), and irinotecan (125/340 mg/m^2) every 14 days until progression. The median treatment that these patients received was four cycles. At 8 week intervals, the patients underwent MRI imaging and were evaluated based on the Macdonald response criteria. The following histologies were studied among the 85 patients: GBM (n = 32), glioma WHO gr. III (n = 33), glioma WHO gr. II (n = 12), others (n = 8). For glioblastoma, ORR (overall response rate) was 25%, with 59% achieving stable disease. The median PFS in this study was 5.2 months. Upon evaluating the other types of tumors, for grade III gliomas ORR was 21% and 45% had SD with a median PFS of 3.7 months. Objective responses were not found for any grade II gliomas in this study. (Møller,2012) Since the study included a non-glioma population, the investigators reported that they observed several long PFS times. Bevacizumab and irinotecan combination therapy was well tolerated and moderately efficacious in glioblastoma and glioma of WHO grade III with the majority of patients achieving some disease stabilization. (Møller, 2012) The current studies have evaluated irinotecan alone or in combination (ex:bevacizumab). (Table 1) Future studies should expand on these findings in larger cohorts since progression-free survival was prolonged in non-glioma patients.

6. Safety, adverse effects, and methods to minimize toxicity

Malignant gliomas are highly proliferative, resistant to therapy and often recurrent post radiation and chemotherapy. Lack of adequately tumoricidal concentrations of chemotherapeutic drugs in tumor cells may be be one of the primary causes of treatment failure in solid tumors. The blood-brain barrier (BBB) restricts the concentrations of chemotherapeutic drugs that may reach the tumor site. Methods that deliver drugs in a systemic fashion may increase toxicity and create off target site complications. Convection-enhanced delivery (CED) is a method that may provide drugs to the tumor in a more targeted fashion through the interstitial space.(Barker,1998; Bobo,1994) This approach results into more drug being delivered into tumors and surrounding brain through stereo-tactically placed catheters connected to pumps. (Barker,1998; Bobo,1994) By providing a continuous, low grade positive-pressure microinfusion that distributes drugs by bulk flow, CED may result in high local concentrations and reduce systemic toxicity. (Bruce,2011)

Topotecan, a topoisomerase I inhibitor, is cytotoxic to glioma cells and nontoxic to normal brain, and its levels are higher in glioma cells and tumor tissue than in normal brain. Topotecan is a natural-product drug with high molecular weight which allows it to minimally traverse the BBB from the brain to the systemic circulation. (Kaiser,2000;Bruce,2000;Borris,1998, Matsumoto, 1999) Now there is evidence that in colon tumors topotecan treatment results in the downregulation of hypoxia-inducible factor-1α (HIF1A) target genes along with an inhibition of HIF1A protein accumulation. (Guerin, 2012) Hence, topoisomerase I inhibitors may also influence the tumor environment by decreasing tumor angiogenesis leading to tumor size stabilization, although clinical trials of topotecan delivered intravenously had minimal effects on tumors. (Fridman,1999) In other studies, CED in rat in vivo models prolonged survival and had significant antitumor efficacy. (Kaiser,2000; Bruce,2000)

Recently, a prospective, dose-escalation phase Ib study of CED of topoisomerase-I was conducted in sixteen patients with recurrent malignant gliomas with a median age of 50 years. Ten patients had glioblastoma multiforme, and the other 6 had World Health Organization grade III glial tumors with an average enhancing volume of 16.1 cm^3. (Bruce,2011) Standard MRI/CT-guided stereotactic biopsy was used to histologically confirm the presence of recurrent malignant glioma. In this study, the investigators evaluated toxicity and quality of life (QOL) effects and confirmed antitumor activity radiographically. The change in contrast-enhancing volume of tumor on MRI was used to assess tumor response to treatment. Three response categories were used to characterize the tumors: early response; as a decrease in contrast-enhancing volume of >50% through the first 3 to 6 months after therapy, progressive disease; as increasing contrast-enhancing volume (>25%) at ≥1 month after therapy until surgical resection or death, and pseudoprogression; an increase in the contrast-enhancing volume of >50% followed by regression of enhancement and edema (changes had to be sustained for at least 4 weeks with patients on a stable or decreasing dose of steroids).(Bruce, 2011) The investigators noted significant antitumor activity in these tumors through radiographic changes, and treatment with CED topotecan prolonged overall survival. The maximum tolerated dose that can be used for phase II studies was determined in this trial. Drug-associated toxicity was minimal and topotecan convection-enhanced delivery had activity at concentrations that were nontoxic to normal brain. (Bruce,2011)

CED locally administered topotecan treatment was tested on a rat model of glioblastoma that is induced by intracerebral injection of PDGF (platelet-derived growth factor)-IRES (internal ribosome entry site) expressing retrovirus. (Lopez, 2011) Glial progenitor cells recruited to the tumor and the transformed tumor cells were analyzed by histopathology. Glial progenitor cells are proliferate within gliomas and contribute to the growth of the tumor. (Appolloni, 2009 OGDEN) This pro-growth process is influenced via PDGF signaling, another common proliferative pathway. (Assanah, 2006 Assanah, 2009) The transformed cell population was reduced about 10-fold and recruited progenitors by about 80-fold. A significant survival advantage was found in treated animals and this improved with greater treatment duration. (Lopez, 2011) In addition, the distribution of topotecan was traced with MRI of a tracer molecule and corresponded with regions of glial progenitor ablation. The decrease in progenitor recruitment was most likely due to the ablation of recruitable progenitor cells. These results showed that in a model of growth factor influenced gliomas, tumor cells and the induced progenitor cells are eradicated by topoisomerase inhibition based treatments. Hence, future characterization of tumors through these methods may enhance the efficacy of treatments in specific subpopulations. Topotecan administration by convection-enhanced delivery has significant antitumor activity at concentrations that are nontoxic to normal brain. The potential for use of this therapy as a generally effective treatment option for malignant gliomas will be tested in subsequent phase II and III trials. (Bruce, 2011)

Topoisomerase II (epipodophyllotoxin) has been implicated in the pathogenesis of treatment-related myelodysplastic syndrome/ treatment-related acute myelogenous leukemia (t-MDS/t-AML). (Baehring, 2012) Once patients develop these t-MDS/t-AML disorders they are treated with supportive care, including transfusion of blood products and administration of antibiotics; 5-azacytidine, decitabine, and lenalidomide are approved for the treatment of selected patients with MDS in the United States. Hence, some of the side effects of topoisomerase inhibition therapy for CNS tumors must be further investigated in additional head to head clinical studies with other monotherapies or combinations that may alleviate adverse effects. Additional ways to reduce or minimize toxicity include close monitoring of blood counts and limiting long term usage of the drug.

7. Emerging topoisomerase therapies and combinations

Genz-644282 is a new a non-camptothecin topoisomerase I inhibitor (Kurtzberg, 2011) in clinical development. Efficacy for this novel agent was tested and compared with the standard anticancer drugs; irinotecan, docetaxel, and dacarbazine in human tumor xenografts of colon cancer, renal cell carcinoma, non-small cell lung cancer, and melanoma. Genz-644282 had superior or equal antitumor activity than the standard drug comparators, although brain tumor models were not utilized. (Kurtzberg) Genz-644282 and its metabolites induce Top1 cleavage at similar, as well as unique genomic positions, compared with camptothecin which traps topoisomerase I (Top1)-DNA cleavage complexes. Protein-linked DNA breaks are induced by Genz-644282, and cleavage complexes persist longer after compound removal than camptothecin treatment. (Sooryakumar, 2011) The agent was tested against the pediatric preclinical testing program (PPTP) panel as well as *in vivo* using at its maximum tolerated dose (MTD) of 4 mg/kg (3 times per week × 2 schedule repeated at day 21).(Houghton, 2012) Testing was also conducted in model systems in order to determine a dose regulated response. Treatment exhibited potent cytotoxic activity in vitro models, and in vivo it induced and maintained complete responses in all 6 solid tumor models at MTD. At lower doses of 2 mg/kg it induced complete responses and maintained complete responses in tumor models relatively insensitive to Topotecan although responses were not observed at lower doses. A significant correlation was found between predictive response scores in baseline mRNA tumor gene expression profiles and the observed in vivo responses to Genz-644282. Future research on clinical activity in children impacted by CNS tumors will depend on tolerated drug exposures and safety profiles. (Houghton, 2012)

Topotecan has been studied in combination with other therapies that may increase treatment efficacy in brain tumors. In a recent study, the combination of nanoliposomal topotecan (nLs-TPT) and pegylated liposomal doxorubicin (PLD) was delivered with CED as treatment for malignant brain tumors. (Yamashita, 2007) Both drugs decreased proteins and enzymes with roles in cell replication in vitro, with some synergistic effects. Doxorubicin is also used to inhibit topoisomerase II, and although these studies used implantation of tumor cells in animals, the investigators conducted a survival study in which animals in the control group and the single agent groups had a median survival that was less than the median survival of the combination group. In this study combination therapy use two agents that were both encapsulated in liposomes. Furthermore, the use of CED was promoted as an enhanced drug delivery method, increasing drug availability at the brain tumor site and leading to tumor death.

New phase III randomized control trials incorporating the addition of bevacizumab for newly diagnosed GBM patients may be informative and increase treatment efficacy. (Vredenburg, 2011) In combination with the use of specific molecular biomarkers, data from these trials may clarify the role of anti-angiogenesis agents such as bevacizumab in combination therapy with topoisomerase inhibitors. The incorporation of molecular signatures elicited by therapies such as irinotecan will create a more descriptive situation of the tumor microenvironment, and lead to the elucidation of additional therapeutic targets. (Guerin, 2012)

Additional research into the use of low-dose etoposide (topoII inhibitor) with an oncolytic herpes simplex virus increased survival of mice-bearing intracranial human GSC–derived tumors. (Cheema) These results were found without adverse side effects, possibly leading to this as an effective combination strategy to treat resistant and recurrent GBM in the future. (Cheema)

In a recent study of both a neuroblastoma and astrocytoma cell line that were resistant to chemotherapy (eg. temozolomide) and radiation treatment, investigators found that a novel cytotoxic compound was toxic to these these cells but not to human primary astrocytes. This compound is an analog of thiobarbituric acid and is effective in subcutaneous and intracranial mouse tumor models with a good safety profile. (Lee, 2011) The mechanism of action of the lead compound has topoisomerase IIa inhibition activity but does not inhibit topoisomerase I activity. These types of studies may lead to the development of new agents that can overcome some of the tumor resistance mechanisms in temozolomide and radiation resistant astrocytomas.

8. Predictive biomarkers and tests

The development of molecular markers which predict response to chemotherapy is an important aspect of current neuro-oncology research. The studies and subsequent tests that may assess the status of these biomarkers are ongoing, but few molecules are being tested at this time. O 6-methylguanine-DNA methyltransferase MGMT promoter methylation is the only proved marker of glioblastoma. (Weller,2010) This DNA repair enzyme antagonizes the genotoxic effects of alkylating agents. The expression of MGMT in tumor cells is a marker for significant resistance to temozolomide therapy and other treatments. (Liu, 2006; Donson, 2007; Hegi, 2005) MGMT promoter methylation is the key mechanism of MGMT gene silencing and predicts a favorable outcome in patients with glioblastoma who are exposed to alkylating agent chemotherapy. (Weller,2010) The predictive or prognostic value of MGMT promoter methylation may differ depending on glioma subtypes, and the extent to which testing should be incorporated into routine clinical practice is still under investigation.

A recent study assessed the effect of topoisomerase expression on glioblastoma survival and the mechanisms involved. (Arivazhagan,2012) In an effort to correlate outcome with gene expression, the transcript levels of all isoforms of the topoisomerase family in all grades of diffuse astrocytoma were assessed in this prospective study of patients with glioblastoma treated by a uniform treatment procedure. Transcript levels of TOP2A, TOP2B, and TOP3A were up regulated significantly in GBM in comparison with lower grades of astrocytoma and normal brain samples. The mRNA levels of TOP2A correlated significantly with survival of the patients, and better prognosis in GBM patients. Temozolomide (Arivazhagan,2012) was also a TOP2A inhibitor, and TOP2A transcript levels determined the chemosensitivity of glioblastoma to temozolomide therapy. Very high levels of TOP2A were considered a good prognostic indicator in GBM patients receiving temozolomide chemotherapy. Methylation of the MGMT promoter was found to be the strongest predictor of outcome and benefit from temozolomide chemotherapy. (Stupp,2009) Analysis of progression free survival revealed an advantage solely for patients whose tumor had a methylated MGMT promoter and who were treated with temozolomide and radiotherapy. Hence, in this patient analysis relied on combination therapy was as opposed to monotherapy. These types of results may serve as the impetus for the identification of new genetic biomarkers for GBM and the development of therapies targeting new molecular targets.

9. Conclusions

The treatment of primary malignancies of the CNS continues to be a challenging problem since their treatment is complicated due to anatomical site and the intricacy of the blood brain barrier. Topoisomerase I (topo I) inhibitors, in addition to temozolomide and nitrosourea compounds, represent one promising one treatment option. While preclinical studies in glioma models were promising, clinical trials with topo I inhibitors with topotecan and CPT-11 showed only modest benefit in phase II clinical trials. Children with anaplastic astrocytoma or glioblastoma (Turner, 2002) appear to benefit more with higher response rates than adults with the same tumors. (Friedman,1999; Batchelor, 2004)

The combination of topo I inhibitors with drugs that block angiogenesis including VEGF appear promising, and further studies are needed in the establishment of efficacy, and the development of treatment strategy. However, serious toxicity such as CNS hemorrhage and leukoencephalopathy may occur with these agents. (Ozcan,2006) Further clinical trials are needed to better define the patients at risk for these major side effects.

Another future approach is combining topo I inhibitors together with targeted agents and antiangiogenesis drugs. For example, NF-κB activation in glioma cells may be induced by campothecins leading to inhibition of apoptosis in these cells. It has been shown that over-production of IL-1B can sustain NF-κB activation (Morandi,2006) and agents that inhibit NF-κB activation may increase the susceptibility of glioma cells y to apoptosis induced by campothecin. (Weaver,2003)

Other agents that may increase the efficacy of topo I drugs include the new chemotherapy drug, irofulven. (Woo,2005) PKC inhibitors in combination with CPT-11 have also shown promise in laboratory studies. (Chen TC, 2003) These studies demonstrated an increase in apoptosis and decrease in proliferation in glioma cell lines when exposed to both agents. A decrease in the antiapoptotic protein bcl-2 and an increase in the proapoptotic bax protein may be propagate this mechanism of apoptosis.

Other novel approaches include the use of agents to increase penetration of topotecan into glioma cells. (Carcaboso, 2010) It is possible that one mechanism of drug resistance to topotecan is increased pumping of drug out of the cell. It is known that topotecan is a substrate of the ATP-binding cassette (ABC) transporters P-glycoprotein and breast cancer resistance protein (BCRP/ABCG2). In mice it has been shown that the epidermal growth factor receptor tyrosine kinase inhibitor, Gefitinib, can increase intracellular drug penetration into glioma cells. Similar approaches in the treatment of brain tumors may increase drug availability to the tumor environment.

Immunotherapy for treatment of malignant gliomas has usually been unsuccessful. One new approach is to add topotecan to enhance immune clearance of gliomas. (Wei J,2009) Preclinical studies with the human glioma cell line U-87 using topotecan showed that the drug can upregulate functional Fas receptors and the resulting upregulated Fas expression can increase susceptibility to cytotoxic T cell killing. These findings will have to be substantiated through additional clinical studies and testing.

Another novel approach is to increase drug delivery across the blood brain barrier. Liposomes incorporating Tamoxifen and wheat germ agglutinin have improved the transport of topotecan across the blood brain barrier in brain tumor-bearing rats. (Du 2009) In these studies, improved survival may be related to the enhanced effect of Tamoxifen by inhibiting efflux of multidrug resistant proteins in the blood brain barrier and/or an enhanced effect by the wheat germ agglutinin via endocytosis in the blood brain barrier and in the brain tumor.

Another method to deliver more drug into brain tumors is by a convection-delivery system. This approach may be advantageous by potentially increasing drug delivery into the brain tumor while reducing systemic side effects. Regression of malignant gliomas by this convection-enhanced delivery system has been reported recently. (Bruce, 2011) Future phase II trials are being planned with this technique since the maximum tolerated dose has been established.

Finally, there are newer generations of topo I inhibitors being evaluated and several have entered into clinical trials in human patients. These newer topo I inhibitors include Diflomotecan, Karenitecin, Silatecan, PEG-camptothecin, Rubitecan, 9-aminocamptothecin, Exatecan mesylate, Lurtotecan, and Gimatecan. (Pommier, 2006) A phase II trial of Rubitecan in patients with glioblastoma showed disappointing results. (Raymond,2002) A phase I and pharmacokinetic study of Karenitecin in patients with recurrent malignant gliomas was recently reported. (Grossman, 2008)

Since the vast majority of patients with malignant gliomas die of their disease, it is clear that newer and more effective drugs are needed. There has been renewed interest in topoisomerase I inhibitors in brain tumors using innovative drug carriers or drug delivery systems. In addition, novel topoisomerase I inhibitors are promising and are currently being explored and investigated.

Investigator	n	Treatment	Response Rate	Ref.
Møller et al.	85	IV bevacizumab (10 mg/kg), irinotecan (125/340 mg/m^2) every 14d until progression	ORR (overall response rate) was 25%, with 59% achieving stable disease; median PFS of 5.2 months	Møller, 2012
Bruce et al.	16	Dose escalation of Ib study of CED of topotecan	Significant antitumor activity by radiographic changes, and treatment with prolonged OS	Bruce, 2011
Vredenburgh et al.	80	Add. bevacizumab to temozolomide and radiation followed by temozolomide, bevacizumab, topotecan	Median PFS and OS not reached at a median follow-up of 8 months but the 6 month EFS was 83%	Vredenburgh, 2011
Colavolpe et al.	25	After combined treatment with bevacizumab and itinotecandetermine the independent prognostic value of (FDG)-PET on PFS and OS of recurrent histologically proven high grade glioma, compared with other documented prognostic variables. Imaging was performed within 6 weeks of starting chemotherapy	Median PFS and OS were 4 months (range, 0.9-10.4 months) and 7.2 months (range, 1.2-41.7 months), respectively. At 6 months, PFS and OS rate were 16.0% and 72.0%. FDG uptake was the most powerful predictor of both PFS and OS	Colavolpe, 2012
Paldino et al.	15	Determine the prognostic significance of changes in parameters derived from diffusion tensor imaging (DTI) that occur in response to treatment with bevacizumab and	DTI detected a change in Apparent diffusion coefficient (ADC) within FLAIR signal abnormality (FSA). Patients with a change in ADC within FSA had significantly shorter	Paldino, 2012

Investigator	n	Treatment	Response Rate	Ref.
		irinotecan in patients with recurrent GM through serial 1.5 T MRI. Axial single-shot echo planar DTI was obtained on scans performed 3 days and 1 day prior to and 6 wks. after initiation of therapy.	overall survival (p=0.032) and progression free survival (p=0.046) than those with no change.	
Desjardins et al.	32	PII trial of combined protracted daily temozolomide 50 mg/m(2) and biweekly bevacizumab (10mg/kg) IV for patients with recurrent glioblastoma who had previously received radiation therapy and temozolomide. Underwent physical examination and brain MRI every 8 weeks.	6month PFS rate 18.8% (95% [CI], 7.6%-33.7%), median PFS 15.8 wks. Median OS of 37 wks.,6-m OS rate of 62.5% (95% CI, 43.5%-76.7%), 12-m OS rate of 31.3% (95% CI, 16.4%-47.3%). Patients progressed; locally (52%), diffuse pattern (38%), distant (10%). Regimen had some activity and was well tolerated but results obtained were inferior to those observed in studies of bevacizumab monotherapy and of combination with irinotecan. Patient population was more heterogeneous and pretreated more heavily than in previous studies.	Desjardins, 2012
Reardon et al.	40	Phase II, open, label, single arm trial on efficacy of carboplatin, irinotecan, and bevacizumab among bevacizumab-naïve, recurrent GBM patients. Patients received carboplatin (area under the plasma curve [AUC] 4 mg/ml-min) on day one, while bevacizumab (10 mg/kg) and irinotecan (340 mg/m(2) for patients on CYP3A-enzyme-inducing anti-epileptics [EIAEDs] and 125 mg/m(2) for patients not on EIAEDs) administered on days 1 and 14 of every 28-day cycle. Evaluated after each of the first 2 cycles and then after every other cycle. Treatment continued until progressive disease, unacceptable toxicity, non-compliance, or voluntary withdrawal.	All patients had progression after standard therapy, patients (40%) had a KPS of 90-100, while 68% were at first progression. PFS-6 rate was 46.5% (95% CI: 30.4, 61.0%) and median OS of 8.3 months [95% CI: 5.9, and 10.7 months]. Addition of carboplatin and irinotecan to bevacizumab significantly increases toxicity but does not improve anti-tumor activity to that achieved historically with single-agent bevacizumab among bevacizumab-naïve, recurrent GBM patients.	Reardon, 2012

Investigator	n	Treatment	Response Rate	Ref.
Reardon, et al.		Phase II, open, label, single arm trial on efficacy of carboplatin, irinotecan, and bevacizumab among recurrent glioblastoma (GBM) patients after prior progression on bevacizumab therapy. Received carboplatin (area under the plasma curve [AUC] 4 mg/ml-min) on day 1, bevacizumab (10 mg/kg) and irinotecan (340 mg/m(2) for patients on CYP3A enzyme-inducing anti-epileptics [EIAEDs] and 125 mg/m(2) for patients not on EIAEDs) were administered on days 1 and 14 of every 28-day cycle. Patients were evaluated after each of the first 2 cycles and then after every other cycle. Treatment continued until progressive disease, unacceptable toxicity, noncompliance, or voluntary withdrawal.	All patients had progression on at least 1 prior bevacizumab regimen and 56% enrolled after either 2nd or 3rd overall progression. Median OS was 5.8 months (95% [CI], 4.0-7.0 months) and PFS-6 rate was 16% (95% CI, 5.0%-32.5%). Carboplatin, irinotecan, and bevacizumab was associated with modest activity and adequate safety among these patients.	Reardon, 2011
Parekh et al.	8	Retrospectively reviewed the records of patients <21 yrs. of age with recurrent or progressive WHO grade 3-4 gliomas who were treated with bevacizumab containing regimens at institution between January 1/2006-9/2008.6 patients received irinotecan, temozolomide and bevacizumab, one patient received irinotecan and bevacizumab, and one patient received CCNU and bevacizumab.	3 patients had stable disease for 30-93 weeks, 5 patients progressed within 17 wks., median PFS was 15 weeks, 6-m PFS was 38%. Contrast enhancing disease responded or remained stable in 5/7 patients, and non-enhancing disease progressed in 3/4 patients. Bevacizumab was well tolerated when used in combination with conventional chemotherapy (irinotecan in most cases). PFS in cohort was much shorter and the response rate was inferior in this small cohort of patients when compared with published adult data, but bevacizumab regimens may have efficacy in a subset of pediatric patients with predominantly contrast-enhancing disease.	Parekh, 2011
Pope et al.	85	Evaluated patterns of tumor progression in patients with recurrent	79% treated with single-agent BEV and 70% of patients treated with	Pope, 2011

Investigator	n	Treatment	Response Rate	Ref.
		glioblastoma who were treated with bevacizumab (BEV) alone or in combination with irinotecan (CPT-11) while participating in the BRAIN study. Iindependent neuroradiologist reviewed MRI scans in patients who received BEV or BEV+CPT-11 while on BRAIN. 28% of patients who participated had nonlocal disease at baseline.	BEV+CPT-11 experienced disease progression while on BRAIN. Most patients did not have a change in radiographic pattern (i.e., "no shift") at the time of progression. 82% of BEV patients had no shift and BEV +CPT-11 patients (53%, $\chi(2)$ p = 0.0004), and a greater proportion of BEV+CPT-11 (39%) compared with BEV (16%) experienced local-to-diffuse tumor pattern at progression ($\chi(2)$ p = 0.002). Patients treated with BEV or BEV +CPT-11 who had local-to-local or local-to-diffuse progression patterns had similar efficacy outcomes, including objective response, PFS, and OS.	

Table 1. Recent studies of topoisomerase inhibitors as monotherapies or in combination with other chemotherapeutics for the treatment of brain tumors

Author details

George Theodore[1*], Niramol Savaraj[1,2*] and Lynn Feun[2,3]

1 Miami VA Medical Center, USA

2 University of Miami Miller School of Medicine, USA

3 Sylvester Comprehensive Cancer Center, USA

References

[1] Allen TM, Martin FJ. Advantages of liposomal delivery systems for anthracyclines. *Semin. Oncol.* 2004;31: 5–15.

[2] Appolloni I, Calzolari F, Tutucci E, Caviglia S, Terrile M, Corte G, et al. PDGF-B induces a homogeneous class of oligodendrogliomas from embryonic neural progenitors. *Int J Cancer* 2009;124:2251–9.

[3] Arivazhagan A, Kumar DM, Sagar V,et al. Higher topoisomerase 2 alpha gene transcript levels predict better prognosis in GBM patients receiving temozolomide chemotherapy: identification of temozolomide as a TOP2A inhibitor. *J Neurooncol.* 2012 Apr;107(2):289-97.

[4] Assanah M, Lochhead R, Ogden A, Bruce J, Goldman J, Canoll P. Glial progenitors in adult white matter are driven to form malignant gliomas by platelet-derived growth factor-expressing retroviruses. *J Neurosci.* 2006;26:6781–90.

[5] Assanah MC, Bruce JN, Suzuki SO, Chen A, Goldman JE, Canoll P. PDGF stimulates the massive expansion of glial progenitors in the neonatal forebrain. *Glia.* 2009;57:1835–47.

[6] Baehring JM, Peter W. Marks PW. Treatment-related myelodysplasia in patients with primary brain tumors. Neuro-Oncology. 2012;14(5)529–540.

[7] Baker SD, Heideman RL, Crom WR, et al. Cerebrospinal fluid pharmacokinetics and penetration of continuous infusion topotecan in children with central nervous system tumors. *Cancer Chemother Pharmacol.* 1996;37:195–202.

[8] Barker FG II, Chang SM, Gutin PH, et al. Survival and functional status after resection of recurrent glioblastoma multiforme. *Neurosurgery*. 1998;42(4):709-720.

[9] Batchelor *Neuro Oncol.* 2004; 24:21-27 , 2004)

[10] Blaney SM, Phillips PC, Packer RJ, et al. Phase II evaluation of topotecan for pediatric central nervous system tumors. *Cancer*. 1996;78(3):527–531.

[11] Bobo RH, Laske DW, Akbasak A, et al.Convection-enhanced delivery of macromolecules in the brain. *Proc Natl Acad Sci U S A*. 1994;91(6):2076-2080.

[12] Bookman MA, Malmstrom H, Bolis G, et al. Topotecan for the treatment of advanced epithelial ovarian cancer: an open-label phase II study in patients treated after prior chemotherapy that contained cisplatin or carboplatin and paclitaxel. *J Clin Oncol*. 1998;16: 3345–3352.

[13] Bruce JN, Falavigna A, Johnson JP, et al. Intracerebral clysis in a rat glioma model. *Neurosurgery*.2000;46(3):683-691.

[14] Bruce JN, Fine RL, Canoll P, et al. Regression of Recurrent malignant Gliomas With Convection-Enhanced Delivery of Topotecan *Neurosurgery*. 2011; 69:1272–1280.

[15] Burke TG, Gao X. Stabilization of topotecan in low pH liposomes composed of distearoylphosphatidylcholine. *J Pharm Sci*. 1994;83: 967–969.

[16] Burris HA III. Topotecan: incorporating It Into the treatment of solid tumors. *Oncologist*. 1998;3(1):1-3.

[17] Carcaboso AM, Elmeliegy MA, Shen J, et al. Tyrosine kinase inhibitor gefitinib enhances topotecan penetration of gliomas. *Cancer Res.* 2010;70(11):4499-508.

[18] CBTRUS Stat. Report: Primary brain tumors in the US, 1998-2002. http://www.cbtrusorg/reports//2005-2006/2006report.pdf. Assessed: May 1, 2012.

[19] Cheema TA, Kanai R, Kim GW, et al. Enhanced antitumor efficacy of low-dose etoposide with oncolytic Herpes Simplex Virus in human glioblastoma stem cell xenografts. *Clin Cancer Res.* 2011;17:7383-7393.

[20] Chen TC, Su S, Fry D, Liebes L. Combination therapy with irinotecan and protein kinase C inhibitors in malignant glioma. *Cancer.* 2003 May 1;97(9 Suppl):2363-73.

[21] Ciusani E, Croci D, Gelati M, et al. In vitro effects of topotecan and ionizing radiation on TRAIL/Apo2L-mediated apoptosis in malignant glioma. *J Neuro-Oncol.* 2005;71:19–25.

[22] Colavolpe C, Chinot O, Metellus P, et al. FDG-PET predicts survival in recurrent high-grade gliomas treated with bevacizumab and irinotecan. *Neuro Oncol.* 2012 May;14(5):649-57.

[23] Desjardins A, Reardon DA, Coan A, Marcello J, Herndon JE 2nd, Bailey L, Peters KB, Friedman HS, Vredenburgh JJ. Bevacizumab and daily temozolomide for recurrent glioblastoma. Cancer. 2012 Mar 1;118(5):1302-12.

[24] Donson AM, AddoYobo SO, Handler MH, et al. MGMT promoter methylation correlates with survival benefit and sensitivity to temozolomide in perdiatric glioblastoma. *Pediatr. Blood Cncer.* 2007;48:403-407.

[25] Drummond DC, Noble CO, Guo Z, et al. Development of a highly stable and targetable nanoliposomal formulation of topotecan. *J Control Release.* 2010;141(1):13–21.

[26] Drummond, DC, Meyer O, Hong K, et al. Optimizing liposomes for delivery of chemotherapeutic agents to solid tumors. *Pharmacol. Rev.* 1999;51:691–743.

[27] Drummond DC, Marx C, Guo Z, et al. Enhanced pharmacodynamics and antitumor properties of a histone deacetylase inhibitor encapsulated in liposomes or ErbB2-targeted immunoliposomes. *Clin. Cancer Res.* 2005;11:3392–3401.

[28] Du J, Lu WL, Ying X, et al. Dual-targeting topotecan liposomes modified with tamoxifen and wheat germ agglutinin significantly improve drug transport across the blood-brain barrier and survival of brain tumor-bearing animals. *Mol Pharm.* 2009 May-Jun;6(3):905-17.

[29] Friedman HS, Petros WP, Friedman AH, et al. Irinotecan therapy in adults with recurrent or progressive malignant glioma. *J Clin Oncol.* 1999;17(5):1516-25.

[30] Friedman HS, Kerby T, Fields S, et al. Topotecan treatment of adults with primary malignant glioma: the Brain Tumor Center at Duke. *Cancer.* 1999;85(5):1160-1165.

[31] Grossman SA, Carson KA, Phuphanich S, et al. Phase I and pharmacokinetic study of karenitecin in patients with recurrent malignant gliomas. *Neuro Oncol.* 2008;10(4): 608-16.

[32] Groothuis, DR. The blood-brain and blood-tumor barriers: A review of strategies for increasing drug delivery. *Neuro-Oncology* 2000;2: 45–59.

[33] Grossman SA, Batara JF. Current management of glioblastoma multiforme. *Semin. Oncol.* 2004;31:635-644.

[34] Guérin E, Raffelsberger W, Pencreach E. et al. In vivo topoisomerase I inhibition attenuates the expression of hypoxia-inducible factor 1 target genes and decreases tumor angiogenesis. *Mol. Med.* 2012;1 8 : 8 3 - 9 4.

[35] Gustavsson A, Svensson M, Jacobi F, et al in the CDBE2010 Study Group. Cost of disorders of the brain in Europe 2010. *Eur Neuropsychopharmacol*. 2011 Oct;21(10):718-79.

[36] Hegi ME, Diserens AC, Gorlia T. et al. MGMT gene silencing and benefit from temozolomide in glioblastoma. *N. Engl. J. Med.* 2005;352:997-1003.

[37] Houghton PJ, Lock R, Carol H, et al. Testing of the topoisomerase 1 inhibitor Genz-644282 by the pediatric preclinical testing program. *Pediatr Blood Cancer.* 2012;58(2):200-9.

[38] Hsiang YH, Hertzberg R, Hecht S, et al. Camptothecin induces protein-linked DNA breaks via mammalian DNA topoisomerase I. *J. Biol. Chem.* 1985;260:14873-878.

[39] Kurtzberg LS, Roth S, Krumbholz RGenz-644282, a novel non-camptothecin topoisomerase I inhibitor for cancer treatment. *Clin Cancer Res*. 2011 May 1;17(9):2777-87. Epub 2011 Mar 17.

[40] Kaiser MG, Parsa AT, Fine RL, et al. Tissue distribution and antitumor activity of topotecan delivered by intracerebral clysis in a rat glioma model. *Neurosurgery*. 2000;47(6):1391-1398.

[41] Lee SY, Slagle-Webb B, M. Sheehan JM, et al. Are topoisomerase inhibitors an alternative treatment option for therapy resistant brain tumors? NEU ONC 2011Abstract Number: ET-39.

[42] Liu L, Gerson SL. Targeted modulation of MGMT: clinical implications. *Clin. Cancer Res.* 2006;12:328-331.

[43] Lopez KA, Tannenbaum AM, Assanah MC, et al. Convection-enhanced delivery of topotecan into a PDGF-driven model of glioblastoma prolongs survival and ablates both tumor-initiating cells and recruited glial progenitors. *Cancer Res*. 2011:71(11); 3963–71.

[44] Macdonald D, Cairncross G, Stewart D, et al. Phase II study of topotecan in patients with recurrent malignant glioma. National Clinical Institute of Canada Clinical Trials Group. *Ann Oncol*. 1996;7(2):205–207.

[45] Matsumoto Y, Fujiwara T, Honjo Y, et al. Quantitative analysis of DNA topoisomerase I activity in human and rat glioma:characterization and mechanism of resistance to antitopoisomerase chemical,camptothecin-11. *J Surg Oncol*. 1993;53(2):97-103.

[46] McLendon RE, Halperin EC. Is the long-term survival of patients with intracranial glioblastoma multiforms overstated? *Cancer*. 2003;98:1745-1748.

[47] Mi Z, Malak H, Burke TG. Reduced albumin binding promotes the stability and activity of topotecan in human blood. *Biochemistry*. 1995;34(42):13722–13728.

[48] Møller S, Grunnet K, Hansen S, et al. A phase II trial with bevacizumab and irinotecan for patients with primary brain tumors and progression after standard therapy. *Acta Oncol*. 2012;51:797-804.

[49] Morandi E, Zingaretti C, Chiozzotto D, et al. A cDNA-microarray analysis of camptothecin resistance in glioblastoma cell lines. *Cancer Lett*. 2006;231(1):74-86.

[50] Mi Z, Malak H, Burke TG. Reduced albumin binding promotes the stability and activity of topotecan in human blood. *Biochemistry*. 1995;34(42):13722–13728.

[51] Macdonald D, Cairncross G, Stewart D, et al. Phase II study of topotecan in patients with recurrent malignant glioma. National Clinical Institute of Canada Clinical Trials Group. *Ann Oncol*. 1996;7(2):205–207.

[52] Ogden AT, Waziri AE, Lochhead RA, Fusco D, Lopez K, Ellis JA, et al. Identification of A2B5þCD133- tumor-initiating cells in adult human gliomas. *Neurosurgery*. 2008;62:505-15.

[53] Ozcan C, Wong SJ, Hari P. Reversible posterior leukoencephalopathy syndrome and bevacizumab. *N Engl J Med*. 2006;354(9):980-2; discussion 980-2.

[54] Paldino MJ, Desjardins A, Friedman HS, et al. A change in the apparent diffusion coefficient after treatment with bevacizumab is associated with decreased survival in patients with recurrent glioblastoma multiforme. *Br J Radiol*. 2012 Apr;85(1012):382-9.

[55] Parekh C, Jubran R, Erdreich-Epstein A, et al. Treatment of children with recurrent high grade gliomas with a bevacizumab containing regimen. *J Neurooncol*. 2011 Jul; 103(3):673-80.

[56] Pommier Y. Topoisomerase I inhibitors: camptothecins and beyond. *Nat Rev Cancer*. 2006;6(10):789-802.

[57] Pope WB, Xia Q, Paton VE, et al. Patterns of progression in patients with recurrent glioblastoma treated with bevacizumab. *Neurology*. 2011 Feb 1;76(5):432-7.

[58] Rapisarda A, Zalek J, Hollingshead M, et al. Schedule-dependent inhibition of hypoxia-inducible factor-1alpha protein accumulation, angiogenesis, and tumor growth by topotecan in U251-HRE glioblastoma xenografts. *Cancer Res*. 2004;64:6845–6848.

[59] Raymond E, Campone M, Stupp R, et al. Multicentre phase II and pharmacokinetic study of RFS2000 (9-nitro-camptothecin) administered orally 5 days a week in patients with glioblastoma multiforme. *Eur J Cancer*. 2002;38(10):1348-50.

[60] Reardon DA, Desjardins A, Peters KB, et al. Phase II study of carboplatin, irinotecan, and bevacizumab for bevacizumab naïve, recurrent glioblastoma. *J Neurooncol*. 2012 Mar;107(1):155-64. (ClinicalTrials.gov number NCT00953121).

[61] Reardon DA, Desjardins A, Peters KB, et al. Phase 2 study of carboplatin, irinotecan, and bevacizumab for recurrent glioblastoma after progression on bevacizumab therapy. *Cancer*. 2011 Dec 1;117(23):5351-8.

[62] Reveiz L, Rueda JR, Cardona AF. Chemotherapy for brain metastases from small cell lung cancer. Cochrane Database Syst Rev. 2012 Jun 13;6:CD007464.

[63] Redinbo MR, Stewart L, Kuhn P, et al. Crystal structures of human topoisomerase I in covalent and noncovalent complexes with DNA. *Science*. 1998;279:1504-1513.

[64] Saito R, Krauze MT, Noble CO, et al. Convection-enhanced delivery of Ls-TPT enables an effective continuous, low dose chemotherapy against malignant glioma xenograft model. *Neuro Oncol*. 2006;8(3):205–214.

[65] Serwer LP, Noble CO, Michaud K, et al. Investigation of intravenous delivery of nanoliposomal topotecan for activity against orthotopic glioblastoma xenografts. *Neuro-Oncology*. 2011;13(12):1288–1295.

[66] Serwer LP, Noble CO, Michaud K, et al. Increased efficacy of nanoliposomal topotecan via antibody-mediated EGFR-targeting . Abstract Number: ET-33 NEU ONC 2011

[67] Sooryakumar D, Dexheimer TS, Teicher BA, et al. Molecular and cellular pharmacology of the novel noncamptothecin topoisomerase I inhibitor Genz-644282. Mol Cancer Ther. 2011;10(8):1490-9.

[68] Stupp R, Mason WP, van den Bent MJ, et al. Radiotherapy plus concomitant and adjuvant temozolomide for glioblastoma. *N Engl J Med*. 2005;352(10):987-96.

[69] Stupp R, Hegi ME, Mason WP, et al. Effects of radiotherapy with concomitant and adjuvant temozolomide versus radiotherapy alone on survival in glioblastoma in a randomized phase III study: 5-year analysis of the EORTC-NCIC trial. *Lancet Oncol*. 2009 10:459–466.

[70] Tardi P, Choice E, Masin D, et al. Liposomal encapsulation of topotecan enhances anticancer efficacy in murine and human xenograft models. *Clin Cancer Res*. 2000;60: 3389–3393.

[71] Tardi P, Choice E, Masin D, Redelmeier T, Bally M, Madden TD. Liposomal encapsulation of topotecan enhances anticancer efficacy in murine and human xenograft models. *Clin Cancer Res*. 2001;60:3389–3393.

[72] Ten Bokkel HW, Lane SR, Ross GA, the International Topotecan Study Group. Long-term survival in a phase III, randomised study of topotecan vs paclitaxel in advanced epithelial ovarian carcinoma. *Ann Oncol*. 2004;15:100–103.

[73] Thumma SR, Fairbanks RK, Lamoreaux WT, et al. Effect of pretreatment clinical factors on overall survival in glioblastoma multiforme: a Surveillance Epidemiology and End Results (SEER) population analysis. *World J Surg Oncol.* 2012 May 3;10(1):75.

[74] Turner CD, Gururangan S, Eastwood J, et al. Phase II study of irinotecan (CPT-11) in children with high-risk malignant brain tumors: the Duke experience. *Neuro Oncol.* 2002;4(2):102-8.

[75] Vredenburgh JJ, Desjardins A, Reardon DA, et al. The addition of bevacizumab to temozolomide and radiation therapy followed by bevacizumab, temozolomide and oral topotecan for newly diagnosed glioblastoma multiforme (GBM) NEU ON 2011 Abstract Number: OT-19

[76] Wang JC. DNA Topoisomerases. *Annu. Rev. Biochem.* 1996;65:535-692.

[77] Weaver KD, Yeyeodu S, Cusack JC Jr, et al. Potentiation of chemotherapeutic agents following antagonism of nuclear factor kappa B in human gliomas. J Neurooncol. 2003;61(3):187-96.

[78] Weller M, Stupp R, Reifenberger G. MGMT promoter methylation in malignant gliomas: ready for personalized medicine? *Nature Reviews Neurology.* 2010;(6):39-51.

[79] Woo MH, Peterson JK, Billups C, et al. Enhanced antitumor activity of irofulven in combination with irinotecan in pediatric solid tumor xenograft models. *Cancer Chemother Pharmacol.* 2005;55(5):411-9.

[80] Wei J, DeAngulo G, Sun W, et al. Topotecan enhances immune clearance of gliomas. *Cancer Immunol Immunother.* 2009;58(2):259-70.

[81] Yamashita Y, Krauze MT, et al. Convection-enhanced delivery of a topoisomerase I inhibitor (nanoliposomal topotecan) and a topoisomerase II inhibitor (pegylated liposomal doxorubicin) in intracranial brain tumor xenografts. *Neuro Oncol.* 2007;9:20–28

Section 9

Central Nervous System Lymphoma

Chapter 21

Primary Central Nervous System Lymphoma – Recent Advance on Clinical Research

Ryuya Yamanaka

Additional information is available at the end of the chapter

http://dx.doi.org/10.5772/52757

1. Introduction

A primary central nervous system lymphoma (PCNSL) is an extranodal form of non-Hodgkin's lymphoma arising in the craniospinal axis. For many years, PCNSLs were reported to represent 3–5% of all primary central nervous system (CNS) tumors [1]. However, PCNSL appears to be increasing in incidence [2-4]. PCNSL age-adjusted incidence (0.15 to 0.48, a 3-fold increase) outpaced that of systemic lymphoma (14.1 to 18.5, a 33% increase) for the same registries over the same time periods [2]. The increase is evident in all age groups and in both genders [2]. The tumor manifestation is often diffuse and multifocal, and most frequently affects the supratentorial brain parenchyma. The absence of systemic lymphadenopathies and other extracranial localizations of disease should be confirmed. Most PCNSLs belong to the diffuse large B-cell lymphomas (DLBCLs), but differ from systemic DLBCLs by their less favorable prognosis. The systemic use of high-dose methotrexate (HD-MTX)-based chemotherapy with radiation therapy for newly diagnosed PCNSL has improved the median overall survival (OS) from 20 to 36 months [5-8]. However, more intense efforts are required to improve the outcome of the patients and to identify novel therapeutic strategies. In this article, we will review the recent developments of basic and clinical research on PCNSL.

2. Clinical characteristics

PCNSL has been described at all ages, but usually arise in the fifty to sixty years, with a male to female ratio of 1.5 [9]. The symptoms are focal neurological deficits, mental disturbance and increased intracranial pressure. The characteristics of radiographic findings of

PCNSL are homogenous contrast enhancement on MRI with gadolinium at least 15 mm in contact with the subarachnoid space [10], periventricular lesions involving the corpus callosum, basal ganglia, or thalamus. The eye is involved in about 20% of patients [11]. Leptomeningeal involvement is seen in about 18% [12]. The tumor is single in 60% of patients and multiple in the remainder [10]. Diffusion-weighted MRI (DW-MRI) and proton-MR-spectroscopy (1H-MRS) usually reveal a uniformly pathologic pattern of metabolite concentrations [10]. The absence of systemic lymphadenopathies and other extracranial localizations of disease should be confirmed. Corticosteroids can temporaly cause regression of the tumor in 40-85% of patients [13]. Diagnosis requires histologic conformation. Molecular analysis of the rearrangement of immunoglobulin heavy chain genes by means of polymerase chain reaction (PCR) and Southern blotting may be acceptable [14]. Most PCNSLs belongs to diffuse large B cell and phenotypically express pan-B-cell markers such as CD19, CD20, CD22 and CD79a. The majority of PCNSL express BCL-6, a marker of GCB (germinal center B-cell-like) cells, and MUM1, a marker of late GCB cells.

3. Treatment

PCNSL is sensitive to radiation therapy, however patients treated with radiotherapy alone had 5-year over all survivals of 3-4%, more than 80% patients relapsed within 10-14 months [15]. Standard radiotherapy for patients consists of 40 Gy to whole brain with an additional boost of 10-20 Gy on the tumor bed [16]. Shibamoto et al. [17] reported the recent improved results of radiation monotherapy, 5-year survival was 25% for patients 63 years old or younger, and 9.8% for those older than 63 years. Since total irradiation dose is an important predictor of delayed neurotoxicity, a decrease in the incidence of this complication should be expected if the total irradiation dose is reduced. Several studies have demonstrated that HD-MTX, with or without other chemotherapeutic agents, yielded high response rates with 33-45 months over all survival. These results are better than the results of radiotherapy alone. HD-MTX is widely recognized as the single most effective chemotherapeutic agent for PCNSL [18-23]. MTX is usually administered at high doses with various schedules. Recently, randomized trials for PCNSLs are reported. Ferreri et al. [6] assessed the effect of adding high-dose cytarabine to methotrexate in patients with newly diagnosed PCNSL in randomised phase 2 trial. Seventy-nine patients with PCNSLs were randomly divided to receive four courses of either methotrexate 3.5 g/m^2 on day 1 (n=40) or methotrexate 3.5 g/m^2 on day 1 plus cytarabine 2 g/m^2 twice a day on days 2-3 (n=39). Both regimens were administered every 3 weeks and were followed by whole-brain radiotherapy (WBRT). After chemotherapy, seven patients given methotrexate and 18 given methotrexate plus cytarabine achieved a complete remission, with a complete remission rate of 18% and 46% (p=0.006), and a 3-year OS of 32% and 46% (p=0.07) respectively. In patients aged 75 years and younger with PCNSL, the addition of high-dose cytarabine to high-dose methotrexate provides improved outcome with acceptable toxicity compared with high-dose methotrexate alone. Thiel et al. [8] aimed to investigate whether first-line chemotherapy based on high-dose methotrexate was non-inferior to the same chemotherapy regimen followed by WBRT for overall survival. Patients received high-dose methotrexate (4 g/m^2) on day 1 of six 14-day cycles; thereafter, patients received high-dose methotrexate plus ifosfamide (1.5 g/m^2) on days 3-5 of six 14-day cycles. In those assigned to receive first-line chemotherapy followed by radiotherapy, WBRT was given to a total dose of 45 Gy. 551 patients (median age 63 years) were enrolled and randomised, of whom 318 were treated per protocol. In the per-protocol population, median OS was 32.4 months in patients receiving WBRT (n=154), and 37.1 months in those not receiving WBRT (n=164), hazard ratio 1.06 (p=0.71). Median progression-free survival (PFS) was 18.3 months in patients receiving WBRT, and 11.9 months (p=0.14) in those not receiving WBRT. Treatment-related neurotoxicity in patients with sustained complete response was more common in patients receiving WBRT than in those who did not. No significant difference in OS was recorded when WBRT was omitted from first-line chemotherapy in patients with newly diagnosed PCNSL. The PFS benefit afforded by WBRT has to be weighed against the increased risk of neurotoxicity in long-term survivors. The results of this trial may indicate that WBRT can be omitted from first-line treatment of PCNSL.

4. Neurological toxicity

As survival of patients with PCNSL becoming long, the quality o life and mental function is now very important. Neurotoxicity typically is associated with significant cognitive, motor and autonomic dysfunction, and has a negative impact on quality of life. Delayed neurologic toxicity is a serious complication, especially occurring in patients older than 60 years [24]. MTX is a known neurotoxin and has the potential of producing leukoenceohalopathy as well as other types of neurotoxicities such as microangiopathy [25]. MTX is a folate antagonist inhibiting nucleic acid and methioine synthesis. Methionine is necessary for CNS myelination. The presence of a risk haplotype defined by polymorphisms influencing methionine metabolism referred a relative risk for CNS white matter changes [26]. MTX in combination with WBRT relates to its potential for causing delayed leukoencephalopathy. Radiation therapy prior to MTX administration increase the risk of leukoencephalopathy. While intrathecal, intravenous MTX and WBRT have the potential for producing leukoencephalopathy independently, when two or three of them are combined the risk will increase [27]. Nguyen et al. [28] reported late treatment-associated neurotoxicity in 15% of patients and was significantly associated with total radiation doses greater than 36 Gy. O`Brien et al. [29] reported 30% of neurotoxicity risk who were treated with MTX (1g/m^2) followed by WBRT. For patients aged>60 years the risk of neurotoxicity at 7 years was 58%. Correa et al. [30] reported the neuropsychological evaluation of 28 patients. These were of sufficient severity to reduce quality of life in half of the patient sample. Patients treated with WBRT+/- chemotherapy revealed more pronounced cognitive impairement, particularly in the memory and attention/executive domain. Extent of white matter disease correlated with attention/executive, memory, and language impairment. PCNSL survivors treated with WBRT+/- chemotherapy displayed more pronounced cognitive dysfunction than patients treated with MTX-based chemotherapy alone. Omuro et al. [31] described delayed neurotoxicity, analyzing 185 PCNSL patients. The 5-year cumulative incidence of neurotoxicity was 24%. Neurotoxicity presented as a rapidly progressive subcortical dementia characterized by psychomotor slowing, executive and memory dysfunction, behavioral changes, gait ataxia, and incontinence. Imaging findings revealed diffuse white matter disease and cortical-subcortical atrophy. Available autopsy data showed white matter damage with gliosis, thicking of small vessels, and demyelination. Older age, mental status changes at diagnosis, female sex, and radiotherapy predicted neurotoxicity on univariate analysis, but only radiotherapy remained significant in the multivariate setting. They conclude that the core pathophysiological mechanism is the interruption of frontal-subcortical circuits mediated by radiation damage, possibly caused by microvascular alterations, loss of oligodendrocyte progenitors, or oxidative stress. Fliessbach et al. [32] reported the impact of HD-MTX based chemotherapy alone on long term cognition and quality of life in patients with PCNSL. The median follow-up period was 44 months after diagnosis. In long-term follow-up 22 (95%) of 23 patients showed either preserved or improved cognitive functions as compared with pretreatment and immediate posttreatment baseline assessment. Eleven (48%) of 23 patients displayed at least mild cognitive deficits at long-term follow-up not related to therapy. Nineteen (83%) of 23 patients reported a good quality of life (QOL). They conclude that in patients with PCNSL treated with MTX-based chemotherapy alone, no gross cognitive decline has to be expected as a long-term treatment effect. Finally, formal neuropsychological examination guideline in PCNSL clinical trial should be established in the future.

5. Molecular biomarker

There are still many individual variations within the diagnostic and prognostic categories, resulting in a need for additional molecular biomarkers, partly because of the inability to recognize these patients prospectively. Although the clinical scoring model using age, Karnofsky Performance Status (KPS), and lactate dehydrogenase (LDH) level has prognostic value for PCNSL [33-35], it has not been used successfully to stratify patients for therapeutic trials. Molecular markers could improve the outcome prediction, discover potential targets for therapeutic intervention, and elucidate mechanisms that result in resistance to chemotherapy. The reason little progress in molecular analyses of PCNSL has been achieved so far is the very tiny sample amounts obtained for genetic analyses. A better understanding of PCNSL biology is crucial to improve its prognosis. However, only a few studies have been reported on gene expression profiles of PCNSLs. Rubenstein et al. [36] compared the gene expression signature of 23 PCNSL patients with that of nine nodal large B-cell lymphoma patients. They showed that individual cases of PCNSL were classified as GCB cell, ABC (activated B-cell-like) cell, or type 3 large B-cell lymphoma based on the cell-of-origin classification described by Alizadeh et al [37]. In addition, PCNSLs were distinguished from nodal B-cell lymphoma by high expression of regulators of the unfolded protein response signaling pathway by c-Myc and Pim-1. The IL-4 signaling pathway is associated with tumorigenesis and adverse prognosis in PCNSL patients [36]. Montesinos-Rongen et al. [38] reported the gene expression profile of 21 PCNSLs. They showed that PCNSLs resembled late GCB cells in their gene expression pattern, and that PCNSLs were distributed among the spectrum of systemic DLBCLs. Tun et al. [39] reported a gene expression comparison between 13 PCNSLs and 30 non-CNS DLBCLs. PCNSL was characterized by significant expression of multiple extracellular matrix- and adhesion-related pathways. Sung et al. [40] evaluated 12 PCNSL patients by comparative genomic hybridization and 7 out of the 12 patients by expression profiling. They selected eight candidate genes in which expression changes were associated with copy number changes.

Systemic DLBCLs comprise several diseases that differ in responsiveness to chemotherapy [41,42]. The GCB cell-like subgroup expressed genes characteristic of normal GCB cells and were associated with a good outcome, whereas the ABC cell-like subgroup expressed genes characteristic of activated B cells and were associated with a poor outcome. Gene expression analyses of PCNSLs have largely focused on normal lymphocyte development, and the cell-of-origin classification method was investigated so far. Kawaguchi et al. [43] developed a novel scoring system based on molecular markers. Expression profiling was performed on 32 PCNSLs. A gene classifier with 23 genes was developed using the random survival forests model. Based on this, Prognosis Prediction Score using immunohistochemical analysis is also developed and validated in another data set. Among the genes, BRCA1 protein expression was most strongly associated with patient survival. They have identified gene expression signatures that can accurately predict survival in patients with PCNSL.

6. Conclusion

Much more aggressive therapies, such as high-dose chemotherapy with stem cell implantation [44] or molecular targeted therapies that specifically target disabled pathways, might be tailored in those patients with a poor prognosis. In this regard, molecular biomarkers might not only predict the likelihood of short-term survival, but also yield clues on individual genes involved in tumor development, progression, and response to therapy. Moreover, the ability to distinguish PCNSLs will enable appropriate therapies to be tailored to specific tumor subtypes. Class prediction models based on defined molecular profiles allow classification of PCNSLs in a manner that will be better correlated with clinical outcomes. Therefore, identification of these molecular subclasses of PCNSLs could greatly facilitate prognosis prediction and ability to develop effective treatment protocols.

Author details

Ryuya Yamanaka*

Address all correspondence to: ryaman@cmt.kpu-m.ac.jp

Kyoto Prefectural University of Medicine, Graduate School for Health Care Science, Kamigyoku, Kyoto, Japan

References

[1] Panageas KS, Elkin EB, DeAngelis LM, Ben-Porat L, Abrey LE. Trends in survival from primary central nervous system lymphoma, 1975-1999: a population-based analysis. Cancer 2005;104(11):2466-72.

[2] Olson JE, Janney CA, Rao RD, Cerhan JR, Kurtin PJ, Schiff D, Kaplan RS, O'Neill BP. The continuing increase in the incidence of primary central nervous system non-Hodgkin lymphoma: a surveillance, epidemiology, and end results analysis. Cancer 2002;95(7): 1504-10.

[3] Haldorsen IS, Krossnes BK, Aarseth JH, Scheie D, Johannesen TB, Mella O, Espeland A. Increasing incidence and continued dismal outcome of primary central nervous system lymphoma in Norway 1989-2003 : time trends in a 15-year national survey. Cancer 2007;110(8):1803-14.

[4] Makino K, Nakamura H, Kino T, Takeshima H, Kuratsu J. Rising incidence of primary central nervous system lymphoma in Kumamoto, Japan. Surg Neurol 2006;66(5):503-6.

[5] Gavrilovic IT, Hormigo A, YahalomJ, DeAngelis LM, Abrey LE. Long-term follow-up of high-dose methotrexate-based therapy with and without whole brain irradiation for newly diagnosed primary CNS lymphoma. J Clin Oncol 2006;24(28):4570-4.

[6] Ferreri AJ, Reni M, Foppoli M, Martelli M, Pangalis GA, FrezzatoM, Cabras MG, Fabbri A, Corazzelli G, Ilariucci F, Rossi G, Soffietti R, Stelitano C, Vallisa D, Zaja F, Zoppegno L, Aondio GM, Avvisati G, Balzarotti M, Brandes AA, Fajardo J, Gomez H, Guarini A, Pinotti G, Rigacci L, Uhlmann C, Picozzi P, Vezzulli P, Ponzoni M, Zucca E, Caligaris-Cappio F, Cavalli F; International Extranodal Lymphoma Study Group (IELSG). High-dose cytarabine plus high-dose methotrexate versus high-dose methotrexate alone in patients with primary CNS lymphoma: a randomised phase 2 trial. Lancet 2009;374(9700):1512-20.

[7] Chamberlain MC, Johnston SK. High-dose methotrexate and rituximab with deferred radiotherapy for newly diagnosed primary B-cell CNS lymphoma. Neuro Oncol 2010;12(7):736-44.

[8] Thiel E, Korfel A, Martus P, Kanz L, Griesinger F, Rauch M, Röth A, Hertenstein B, von Toll T, Hundsberger T, Mergenthaler HG, Leithäuser M, Birnbaum T, Fischer L, Jahnke K, Herrlinger U, Plasswilm L, Nägele T, Pietsch T, Bamberg M, Weller M. High-dose methotrexate with or without whole brain radiotherapy for primary CNS lymphoma (G-PCNSL-SG-1): a phase 3, randomised, non-inferiority trial. Lancet Oncol 2010;11(11):1036-47.

[9] Fine HA, Mayer RJ. Primary central nervous system lymphoma. Ann Intern Med 1993;119:1093-104.

[10] Küker W, Nägele T, Korfel A, Heckl S, Thiel E, Bamberg M, Weller M, Herrlnger U. Primary central nervous system lymphomas (PCNSL): MRI features at presentation in 100 patients. J Neurooncol 2005; 72(2):169-77.

[11] Jahnke K, Korfel A, Komm J, Bechrakis NE, Stein H, Thiel E, Coupland SE.Intraocular lymphoma 2000-2005: results of a retrospective multicentre trial. Graefes Arch Clin Exp Ophthalmol 2006;244(6):663-9.

[12] Fischer L, Martus P, Weller M, Klasen HA, Rohden B, Röth A, Storek B, Hummel M, Nägele T, Thiel E, Korfel A. Meningeal dissemination in primary CNS lymphoma: prospective evaluation of 282 patients. Neurology 2008;71(14):1102-8.

[13] Herrlinger U, Schabet M, Eichhorn M, Petersen D, Grote EH, Meyermann R, Dichgans J. Prolonged corticosteroid-induced remission in primary central nervous system lymphoma: report of a case and review of the literature. Eur Neurol 1996;36: 241-3.

[14] Endo S, Zhang SJ, Saito T, Kouno M, Kuroiwa T, Washiyama K, Kumanishi T. Primary malignant lymphoma of the brain: mutation pattern of rearranged immunoglobulin heavy chain gene. Jpn J Cancer Res 2002;93(12):1308-16.

[15] Nelson DF. Radiotherapy in the treatment of primary central nervous system lymphoma (PCNLS). J Neurooncol 1999;43: 241-7.

[16] Nelson DF, Martz KL, Bonner H, Nelson JS, Newall J, Kerman HD, Thomson JW, Murray KJ. Non-Hodgkin's lymphoma of the brain: can high dose, large volume radiation therapy improve survival? Report on a prospective trial by the Radiation Therapy Oncology Group (RTOG): RTOG 8315. Int J Radiat Oncol Biol Phys 1992; 23: 9-17.

[17] Shibamoto Y, Ogino H, Hasegawa M, Suzuki K, Nishio M, Fujii T, Kato E, Ishihara S, Sougawa M, Kenjo M, Kawamura T, Hayabuchi N. Results of radiation monotherapy for primary central nervous system lymphoma in the 1990s. Int J Radiat Oncol Biol Phys 2005;62(3):809-13.

[18] DeAngelis LM, Yahalom J, Thaler HT, Kher U. Combined modality therapy for primary CNS lymphoma. J Clin Oncol 1992;10 : 635-43.

[19] Glass J, Gruber ML, Cher L, Hochberg FH. Preirradiation methotrexate chemotherapy of primary central nervous system lymphoma: long-term outcome. J Neurosurg 1994;81: 188-95.

[20] Abrey LE, Yahalom J, DeAngelis LM. Treatment for primary CNS lymphoma: the next step. J Clin Oncol 2000;18: 3144-50.

[21] Freilich RJ, Delattre JY, Monjour A, DeAngelis LM. Chemotherapy without radiation therapy as initial treatment for primary CNS lymphoma in older patients. Neurology 1996;46 : 435-9.

[22] O'Brien P, Roos D, Pratt G, Liew K, Barton M, Poulsen M, Olver I, Trotter G. Phase II multicenter study of brief single-agent methotrexate followed by irradiation in primary CNS lymphoma. J Clin Oncol 2000;18 : 519-26.

[23] Sandor V, Stark-Vancs V, Pearson D, Nussenblat R, Whitcup SM, Brouwers P, Patronas N, Heiss J, Jaffe E, deSmet M, Kohler D, Simon R, Wittes R. Phase II trial of chemotherapy alone for primary CNS and intraocular lymphoma. J Clin Oncol 1998;16:3000-6.

[24] Abrey LE, DeAngelis LM, Yahalom J. Long-term survival in primary CNS lymphoma. J Clin Oncol 1998;16: 859-63.

[25] Schlegel U, Pels H, Glasmacher A, Kleinschmidt R, Schmidt-Wolf I, Helmstaedter C, Fliessbach K, Deckert M, Van Roost D, Fimmers R, Bode U, Klockgether T. Combined systemic and intraventricular chemotherapy in primary CNS lymphoma: a pilot study. J Neurol Neurosurg Psychiatry 2001;71: 118-22.

[26] Linnebank M, Pels H, Kleczar N, Farmand S, Fliessbach K, Urbach H, Orlopp K, Klockgether T, Schmidt-Wolf IG, Schlegel U. MTX-induced white matter changes are associated with polymorphisms of methionine metabolism. Neurology 2005;64(5): 912-3.

[27] Bleyer WA, Griffin TW. White matter necrosis, mineralizing microangiopathy, and intellectual abilities in survivors of childhood leukemia: associations with central nervous system irradiation and methotrexate therapy. In Glibert HA, Kagan AR editors. Radiation damage to the nervous system. A delayed therapeutic hazard. New York: Raven;1980. p.155-74.

[28] Nguyen PL, Chakravarti A, Finkelstein DM, Hochberg FH, Batchelor TT, Loeffler JS. Results of whole-brain radiation as salvage of methotrexate failure for immunocompetent patients with primary CNS lymphoma. J Clin Oncol 2005;23(7):1507-13.

[29] O'Brien PC, Roos DE, Pratt G, Liew KH, Barton MB, Poulsen MG, Olver IN, Trotter GE. Trans-Tasman Radiation Oncology Group. Combined-modality therapy for primary central nervous system lymphoma: long-term data from a Phase II multicenter study (Trans-Tasman Radiation Oncology Group). Int J Radiat Oncol Biol Phys 2006;64(2):408-13.

[30] Correa DD, DeAngelis LM, Shi W, Thaler H, Glass A, Abrey LE. Cognitive functions in survivors of primary central nervous system lymphoma. Neurology 2004;62(4): 548-55.

[31] Omuro AM, Ben-Porat LS, Panageas KS, Kim AK, Correa DD, Yahalom J, Deangelis LM, Abrey LE. Delayed neurotoxicity in primary central nervous system lymphoma. Arch Neurol 2005;62(10):1595-600.

[32] Fliessbach K, Helmstaedter C, Urbach H, Althaus A, Pels H, Linnebank M, Juergens A, Glasmacher A, Schmidt-Wolf IG, Klockgether T, Schlegel U. Neuropsychological

outcome after chemotherapy for primary CNS lymphoma: a prospective study. Neurology 2005;64(7):1184-8.

[33] Ferreri AJ, Blay JY, Reni M, Pasini F, Spina M, Ambrosetti A, Calderoni A, Rossi A, Vavassori V, Conconi A, Devizzi L, Berger F, Ponzoni M, Borisch B, Tinguely M, Cerati M, Milani M, Orvieto E, Sanchez J, Chevreau C, Dell'Oro S, Zucca E, Cavalli F. Prognostic scoring system for primary CNS lymphomas: the International Extranodal Lymphoma Study Group experience. J Clin Oncol 2003;21(2):266-72.

[34] Abrey LE, Ben-Porat L, Panageas KS, Yahalom J, Berkey B, Curran W, Schultz C, Leibel S, Nelson D, Mehta M, DeAngelis LM. Primary central nervous system lymphoma: the Memorial Sloan-Kettering Cancer Center prognostic model. J Clin Oncol 2006;24(36):5711-5.

[35] Shenkier TN, Voss N, Chhanabhai M,Fairey R, Gascoyne RD, Hoskins P, Klasa R, Morris J, O'Reilly SE, Pickles T, Sehn L, Connors JM. The treatment of primary central nervous system lymphoma in 122 immunocompetent patients: a population-based study of successively treated cohorts from the British Colombia Cancer Agency. Cancer 2005;103(5):1008-17.

[36] Rubenstein JL, Fridlyand J, Shen A, Aldape K, Ginzinger D, BatchelorT, Treseler P, Berger M, McDermott M, Prados M, Karch J, Okada C, Hyun W, Parikh S, Haqq C, Shuman M. Gene expression and angiotropism in primary CNS lymphoma. Blood 2006;107(9):3716-23.

[37] Alizadeh AA, Eisen MB, Davis RE, Ma C, Lossos IS, Rosenwald A, Boldrick JC, Sabet H, Tran T, Yu X, Powell JI, Yang L, Marti GE, Moore T, Hudson J Jr, Lu L, Lewis DB, Tibshirani R, Sherlock G, Chan WC, Greiner TC, Weisenburger DD, Armitage JO, Warnke R, Levy R, Wilson W, Grever MR, Byrd JC, Botstein D, Brown PO, Staudt LM. Distinct types of diffuse large B-cell lymphoma identified by gene expression profiling. Nature 2000;403(6769):503-11.

[38] Montesinos-Rongen M, Brunn A, Bentink S,Basso K, Lim WK, Klapper W, Schaller C, Reifenberger G, Rubenstein J, Wiestler OD, Spang R, Dalla-Favera R, Siebert R, Deckert M. Gene expression profiling suggests primary central nervous system lymphomas to be derived from a late germinal center B cell. Leukemia 2008;22(2):400-5.

[39] Tun HW, Personett D, Baskerville KA,Menke DM, Jaeckle KA, Kreinest P, Edenfield B, Zubair AC, O'Neill BP, Lai WR, Park PJ, McKinney M. Pathway analysis of primary central nervous system lymphoma. Blood 2008;111(6):3200-10.

[40] Sung CO, Kim SC, Karnan S, Karube K, Shin HJ, Nam DH, Suh YL, Kim SH, Kim JY, Kim SJ, Kim WS, Seto M, Ko YH. Genomic profiling combined with gene expression profiling in primary central nervous system lymphoma. Blood 2011:117(4), 1291-300.

[41] Shipp MA, Ross KN, Tamayo P, Weng AP, Kutok JL, Aguiar RC, Gaasenbeek M, Angelo M, Reich M, Pinkus GS, Ray TS, Koval MA, Last KW, Norton A, Lister TA, Mesirov J, Neuberg DS, Lander ES, Aster JC, Golub TR. Diffuse large B-cell lymphoma

outcome prediction by gene-expression profiling and supervised machine learning. Nat Med 2002;8(1):68-74.

[42] Rosenwald A, Wright G, Chan WC, Connors JM, Campo E, Fisher RI, Gascoyne RD, Muller-Hermelink HK, Smeland EB, Giltnane JM, Hurt EM, Zhao H, Averett L, Yang L, Wilson WH, Jaffe ES, Simon R, Klausner RD, Powell J, Duffey PL, Longo DL, Greiner TC, Weisenburger DD, Sanger WG, Dave BJ, Lynch JC, Vose J, Armitage JO, Montserrat E, López-Guillermo A, Grogan TM, Miller TP, LeBlanc M, Ott G, Kvaloy S, Delabie J, Holte H, Krajci P, Stokke T, Staudt LM; Lymphoma/Leukemia Molecular Profiling Project. Lymphoma/Leukemia Molecular Profiling Project. The use of molecular profiling to predict survival after chemotherapy for diffuse large-B-cell lymphoma. N EnglJ Med 2002;346(25):1937-47.

[43] Kawaguchi A, Iwadate Y, Komohara Y, Sano M, Kajiwara K, Yajima N, Tsuchiya N, Homma J, Aoki H, Kobayashi T, Sakai Y, Hondoh H, Fujii Y, Kakuma T, Yamanaka R. Gene Expression Signature–Based Prognostic Risk Score in Primary Central Nervous System Lymphoma Patients. Clin Cancer Res (In press)

[44] Soussain C, Hoang-Xuan K, TaillandierL, Fourme E, Choquet S, Witz F, Casasnovas O, Dupriez B, Souleau B, Taksin AL, Gisselbrecht C, Jaccard A, Omuro A, Sanson M, Janvier M, Kolb B, Zini JM, Leblond V; Société Française de Greffe de Moëlle Osseuse-Thérapie Cellulaire. Intensive chemotherapy followed by hematopoietic stem-cell rescue for refractory and recurrent primary CNS and intraocular lymphoma: Société Française de Greffe de Moëlle Osseuse-Thérapie Cellulaire. J Clin Oncol 2008;26(15):2512-8.

Section 10

Neural Basis of Consciousness

Chapter 22

Contributions to the Understanding of the Neural Bases of the Consciousness

Leon Dănăilă and Mihail Lucian Pascu

Additional information is available at the end of the chapter

http://dx.doi.org/10.5772/52688

1. Introduction

Perhaps no concept is as difficult to define and understand as human consciousness. Its nature has been intensively debated for centuries by philosophers [1], for decades by psychologists [2], and by neuroscientists [3] as knowledge and techniques have advanced to the point where an experimental approach to such a complex issue is finally possible [4].

The cognitive revolution in psychology was paralleled by the development of the field of cognitive science, whose practitioners included neuroscientists, behavioral biologists, neurosurgeons, psychologists, psychiatrists, philosophers, linguists, sociologists, anthropologists and even physicists.

Over many centuries, philosophers and physicians, poets and priests have debated and written at great length on how mind may relate to brain.

And it is not surprising that neurosurgeons, from their unrivaled vantage point of dealing with the human brain, sometimes in conscious patients (as during epilepsy surgery), should seek answers to this seductive enigma.

There is no accepted definition of consciousness. While some take consciousness to be a unique substance, others say it is a special property, and still others claim it to be nothing more than the operation of the brain [5]. Other authors have shown that consciousness includes "what it is like" to be something. So, the role of subjectivity should be one component, if not the essential one in any definition of consciousness [6].

Consciousness has been also called "the last surviving mystery" [7]. Crick considered consciousness the central problem of biology [8]. According to [5], understanding consciousness implies to produce the quintessence of philosophy, psychology, neuroscience and several other fields of study.

Consciousness may be also defined as our awareness of our environment, our bodies and ourselves [9]. Awareness of ourselves implies an awareness of awareness, that is the conscious of being. Awareness of ourselves implies meta-cognition [9, 10]. Some authors emphasize consciousness as a momentary creation of a neural pattern which describes a relation between the organism and an object or event [11]. According to [12], consciousness is, quite literally, mind-boggling.

We consider that consciousness is an universal set of neurologic and mental or spiritual processes produced by the brain in awake state, which allows people to understand the mind of others (mind reading); it also allows an optimal social living to perform any kind of high normal behavior activity (social, political, professional, moral, ethic, religious, etc.) related to the self and the environment (family, society).

So, the two separate forms of consciousness are neurologic on one hand and mental or spiritual on the other. Although many theorists treat consciousness as single, all-or-nothing phenomenon, others distinguish between first-order consciousness and a meta-level of consciousness. For example, they may distinguish between consciousness and metaconsciousness [13], primary consciousness and higher-order consciousness [14], or core consciousness and extended consciousness [15]. Animals possess primary (core) consciousness which comprises sensory awareness, attention, perception, memory (or learning), emotion and action [12, 16]. In [16] it is also shown that every organism, even bacteria, would possess some degree of consciousness.

However, animals have got an inferior consciousness function. It is, of course, unclear at what phylogenetic level this assumption - about self-awareness and the environment - falls below the definition of consciousness as we noted it. According to [9], what differentiates humans from their fellow mammals, and gives humans what Edelman defines as secondary consciousness, depends upon language and the associated enrichment of cognition that allow humans to develop and to use verbal and numeric abstraction. Spoken and written language are human specializations. These mental capacities contribute to our sense of self as agents and as creative beings. This fact also determines the awareness of awareness that we assume our animal "collaborators" do not possess [9].

Many factors are involved in establishing the levels of consciousness commonly referred to as wakefulness and sleep. Such factors include the enormous driving of the cerebral cortex over the ascending activating and inhibiting systems and the influence of cyclic limbic activation of cerebral cortical areas. There are complex interconnections between these areas of the nervous system. But, the brain is such a complex structure that even now we know only a tiny portion of what is to be known about it. By dividing consciousness into various attributes - self-reflection, attention, memory, perception emotion, arousal, thoughts - and ordering these into a functional hierarchy, we can link anatomy and function. So, consciousness must be a function of numerous interacting systems. No single neural structure is necessary and sufficient for consciousness. Not all areas of the brain contribute equally to consciousness.

Our state of consciousness also includes accompanying autonomic responses such as changes in respiration, heart rate, or body temperature. Injuries that involve a considerable part of

http://dx.doi.org/10.5772/52688

tegmentum of the midbrain result in a profound coma because of the interruption of ascending multisynaptic activating system as well as descending hypothalamotegmental and dorsal longitudinal fasciculus path.

In humans, the complex system of mental and spiritual processes depends on, and is produced by the highest psychical activities, i.e. depends on, and is produced by the brain, making people to: use symbolic representation and language; reflect on the past and anticipate and plan for the future; transform thought into speech and action; logically record the personal experience and transmit it orally by writing and/or by drawing; participate in the progress and civilization; read other people's thoughts, judge correctly their intentions and act consequently; use abstractization and generalization to make new discoveries; know, spread and protect the ethical, moral and religious standards in order to live an optimal social life; organize behavior and extrapolate it in time; deal with cognitive novelty.

The prediction and comprehension of others' behavior are, evidently, very important aspects of social functioning.

The consciousness processes belong, in essence, to people who act by control mechanisms of psychological activities, generalization and abstractization mechanisms, exploring and handling of mental images to solve all the problems man is facing with.

In humans, the level of consciousness depends on the complexity of the brain ontogenetic evolution; the human brain makes culture and technology possible. We believe that the cerebral cortex is absolutely necessary for this function; machines that are responsive to sensory events and are capable of complex movements are not conscious. Some philosophers stress that the two defining characteristics of consciousness are: intentionality and subjectivity.

In [17] is pointed out that computers are not conscious because they lack intentionality. Computers have no clue about what exactly it is they are computing. In this respect, Searle [18] rebuts those who imagine that present-day computers (because their operations, in some ways, resemble mental processes) can already be considered to have the rudiments of consciousness. Searle emphasized that meaningful output from a computer, however sophisticated, cannot provide evidence for consciousness or self-awareness within it. Despite this argument, deflating simplistic assertions that extant machines exhibit rudimentary form of consciousness, Searle does not dispute the idea that in the future it is possible to construct conscious entities. Anyhow, machines that are responsive to sensory events and are capable of complex movements do not possess consciousness.

They do not refer to anything in the real world. Human mental computations are about something; they are grounded in reality. According to this point of view, the brainstem occupies the bottom of the totem pole, providing the basic arousal mechanism without which the higher brain regions cannot operate.

On the other hand, consciousness must be a function of numerous interacting systems. The major structures supposed to play a key role in the neural correlates of consciousness are: the brainstem, the midbrain, the cerebellum, the diencephalon (especially the hypothalamus and thalamus), the limbic system, and the cerebral cortex. There is the idea of being conscious versus unconscious.

Thus, the brain "language" can be conceptualized as the transmission of neural signals [19]. The "grammar" of the brain's language system concerns the proper timing of neuronal impulses. Neuronal impulse timing is based upon proper integration and balance of excitatory and inhibitory processes [20].

Consciousness is a product of all cortical areas, but it exists only in association with the passage of the impulses through ever-changing circuits of the higher brainstem, mesencephal, diencephal, cortex and their cognitive operations.

So, consciousness is a function of numerous interacting systems. Certainly, without higher brain stem and diencephalic integration it cannot exist.

In fact, consciousness is not a single process but a collection of many processes, such as those associated with language, thinking, memory, emotion, feelings, seeing, executive function and so on.

In sum, there are: consciousness of the self; consciousness of the environment; and social cognition. Social cognition is a learned consciousness that allows us to make sense of another person's actions and intentions.

Certainly, some anatomical formations and functional processes are much more important for consciousness than others.

Consciousness is not always the same. A person at different ages of his/her life is not thought to be equally conscious: young children are usually not considered to experience the same type of consciousness as healthy adults do. Indeed, part of the process of maturation is becoming fully conscious. Conscious state varies across the spam of a day as we pass through various states of sleep and waking [21].

The sleep is intrinsically reversible; sufficient stimulation will return the individual to a normal waking state.

2. Patients and methods

In our attempt to demonstrate the presence of the ascending inhibitory system, the consciousness disorders and its modular aspect, a group of fifteen patients has been subjected to evaluation or surgery within National Institute of Neurology and Neurovascular Diseases in Bucharest. Thirteen of them have been diagnosed, respectively, with brain tumor, one patient with limbic encephalitis, and another one with brain cysticercosis. Patients' average age was 41.5 years, the youngest being 21 and the oldest 73.

Ten (66.6%) of the patients were male. In 14 patients, the main examination was computed tomography (CT) and magnetic resonance imaging (MRI).

In the following, we will present the clinical symptomatology of every patient.

Case 1. A 21-year-old man presented himself with a sudden onset coma. MRI-scan revealed a bilateral ponto-mesencephalic hemorrhage triggered by a cavernoma. After total resection of

http://dx.doi.org/10.5772/52688

the cavernoma and hematoma, patient's status has improved significantly, presenting only a remaining minimal right side weakness and hemisensory deficit. Now the patient is a student, and his state is excellent.

Case 2. A 38-year-old woman was admitted with a history of logorrhea syndrome, with hyperkinesia, hyperwakefulness and hyperprosexia. The patient could sleep for only a short time, and then awake and was unable to fall back asleep. MRI-scan revealed a left petroclival meningioma which significantly compresses the superior part of the brainstem.

The postoperative evolution was very good. She remained for five weeks with mild hypoesthesia on the left face but logorrhea syndrome with hyperkinesia disappeared.

Case 3. A 36-year-old man presented with intermittent increased intracranial pressure, paralysis of the conjugate upward gaze (Parinaud's sign), pseudo-Argyll-Robertson pupil and arousal disorders. A contrast-enhanced CT-scan revealed a tumor of the pineal area. Only 15% of the patients with tumors of the pineal area, which are compressing the dorsal part of the mesencephalon, also experienced arousal disorders. Postoperative, the patient remained clinically intact and arousal disorders disappeared.

Case 4. A 27-year-old man was admitted in the department of neurosurgery with headache, memory impairment, endocrinopathy (gonadal insufficiency, loss of libido and reduced masculine hair growth) and bitemporal hemianopsia. Neurobehavioral abnormalities manifested with intermittent hypersomnia, apathy, depression, and flatting of affect. Preoperative MRI demonstrates a large supraselar, paraselar and intraselar mass with a few calcifications (craniopharingiomas). Symptoms reflect the tumor's close proximity to hypothalamic region, pituitary gland, optic apparatus, third ventricle and intracranial vessels.

The hypothalamus and its surrounding structures are especially important for the ascending activatory and inhibitory system and for the anatomy, physiology and pathology of the consciousness. Upward grown into the region of the hypothalamus, this tumor affected overall endocrine control.

After radical subfrontal resection, the patient remained in an excellent state and returned to full activity.

Case 5. A 29-year-old woman presented with left hemiparesis by compression of the adjacent internal capsule, palsies of vertical and lateral gaze, absence of convergence, retraction nystagmus, and mild sensory deficit in the opposite side of the body, including the trunk. Pain and thermal sensation were more affected than touch, vibration and position.

Involvement of ventral posterolateral and posteromedial nuclei of the thalamus causes loss or diminution of all forms of sensation on the opposite side of the body. Contrast medium-enhanced coronal and axial MRI shows a big right thalamic tumor.

The tumor was fully resected and thirty-five days after surgery was started radiation therapy using a 10 MeV linear accelerator. The clinical examination performed thirteen month after surgery, demonstrated a good health condition of the patient. However she remained with a mild sensory deficit and a hemiparesis, but she returned to an independent life.

Case 6. A 27-year-old woman complained of headaches which progressed to double vision, nausea and vomiting. At the neurologic examination, the presence of a slight Parinaud's syndrome was discovered.

Contrast-enhanced Tl-weighted magnetic resonance images show a well-demarcated and homogeneously enhanced pineal body tumor. After its surgical resection, the final histological diagnose was of pineocytoma. Immunohistochemistry for neurofilament (68 kDa) showed numerous positive cell processes.

Immunohistochemistry of GFAP showed strong positivity in interstitial cells. Post-surgical evolution was excellent.

Case 7. A 56-year-old man presented with a sudden onset of coma and fever. Coronal and axial Tl-weighted MRI scans revealed edematous, demyelination symmetrical infra- and supratentorial changes which involved the entire midbrain, both thalamic formations, bilateral basal ganglia, two-side temporo-occipital convolution and hippocampus; these were determined by encephalitis (limbic encephalitis). After 9 days of coma the patient died.

Case 8. A 56-year-old man, with a history of severe headaches, presented with taste and smell disorder, excessive euphoria accompanied by peculiar kind of compulsive, shallow and childish humor (moria), irritability, hypomania and puerilism.

The patient also shown disorders of attention and motility, distractibility, hyperreactivity, hyperkinesia, perseveration, emotional lability, cognitive dysfunction that impede the initiation and temporal organization of actions, and lack of initiative, wrong decision and instinctual disinhibition (sociopathy).

Contrast-enhanced computed tomography (CT) scan shows a giant size olfactory groove meningioma and displacement of anterior brain. Post-surgery, after complete resection of the tumor, the orbitofrontal syndrome disappeared almost completely.

Case 9. A 35-year-old woman was admitted to the department of neurosurgery with a bilateral meningioma of the anterior falx which compressed dorsolateral premotor and prefrontal cortex (Brodmann's areas 6, 8, 9, 10, and 46).

As symptoms, she had attention disorder directed to a particular item of sensorium or inner experience, and the capacity to suppress from inner experience items that can interfere with what is currently on focus. She was apathetic, disinterested in herself and in the world around her. Visuospatial neglect along with gaze abnormalities were also present because the lesion encroaches on area 8.

According to our experience, the apathy is present in all lateral-damage conditions, and is mostly apparent after large bilateral lesions of the frontal convexity.

Perseveration, dysexecutive syndrome with attention, working-memory and planning disorders were among the symptoms. Language disorders were directly linked to failure of temporal integration.

In this patient, depression was secondary to cognitive disorder. Postoperative, the frontal syndrome disappeared.

Case 10. A 42-year-old man presented with a 2-year history of subtle but progressive sensory aphasia, the inability to designate or name the different fingers of the two hands, and the inability to calculate and write (an incomplete Gerstmann's syndrome). The patient also showed constructional apraxia, alexia and misdirected and dissymmetric movement of the opposite limbs. MRI prior to surgery showed a left side parietal cystic astrocytoma. After extirpation of the tumor, all symptoms disappeared.

Case 11. A 39-year-old man was admitted with progressive left hemiparesis, tactile inattention, constructional apraxia, dressing apraxia, dysprosody, and anosodiaphoria. Preoperative CT-scan showed a tumor in the right parietal region.

Post-surgery, the patient improved his motor strength and was discharged after 3 weeks in a very good state, while the CT-scan demonstrates the complete removal of the tumor (fibrillary astrocytoma).

Case 12. A 46-year-old man was admitted with olfactory hallucination ("uncinate fits") often accompanied by a dreamy state of mind, auditory elementary hallucination when the patient heard the sound of running water, impaired recognition of melodies in the absence of words, and the usual tendency for the patient to report the current date as an earlier one. Coronal Tl-weighted, gadolinium-enhanced MRI prior to surgery showed a large right-sided temporo-basal tumor (astrocytoma).

After complete removal of the tumor, the patient remained in a very good state. The patient improved very much and was discharged after 2 weeks.

Case 13. A 42-year-old woman was admitted to the department of neurosurgery with a failure to precisely grasp or touch an object under visual guidance (optic ataxia). This optic ataxia was detected when she tried to reach for an object. Patients with such unilateral lesions typically demonstrate greater impairment when reaching for items located in the hemispace, that is contralateral to the lesion, using the contralateral hand. Another symptom was visual inattention (simultanagnosia) which affected mainly the periphery of the visual field. Simultanagnosia was considered to be a disruption in spatial attention, which was associated with the inability to direct one's attention to more than one or to a few objects at the time.

The presence of simultanagnosia was tested by asking the patient to carry out tasks such as looking at a series of objects, and connecting a series of dots by a line or to examine and describe the events depicted in a complex visual image. Once he focused on one object in his visual field, the patient ignored or neglected all the other objects.

Therefore, optic apraxia and visual inattention have been described within a single visual field contralateral to the right parieto-occipital lesion (areas 7 and 19) (incomplete Balint's syndrome). Generally, patients with Balint's syndrome display three classic symptoms including simultanagnosia (visual inattention), optic ataxia, and ocular apraxia, but this patient had only two symptoms, so an incomplete Balint's syndrome. After total extirpation of the tumor, the patient Balint's syndrome disappeared.

Case 14. A 73-year-old man was admitted with a coma and deceased within 18 hours. On autopsy, more than 110 bilateral cortical and intracerebral metastases have been discovered, originating from a melanocarcinoma situated in the right abdominal area, subject to surgery 7 months earlier.

Case 15. A 56-year-old man complained of headache, nausea, vomiting, cognitive dysfunction and drowsiness. The disease onset was sudden and progressive, with attention deficit (3 months before), memory disorder, disorientation, difficult walking and loss of continence. A magnetic resonance image showed multiple cysts in the parenchyma depicted as round hypointense lesions, sized at 5 mm at most. The respective lesions are disseminated bilaterally in the cortex and cerebral mass, surrounded by hyperintense areas with slight brain edema.

The histopathology examination based on a brain biopsy sample reported neurocysticercosis. The overall and neurological state of the patient deteriorated, and he deceased in the fifth day following in-hospital admission.

3. Results

From the analysis of the 15 presented cases, and also of those previously published in [22 - 24], we had ascertained several important results with reference to the state of consciousness and the alteration of the most important cerebral structures which are necessary for its achievement.

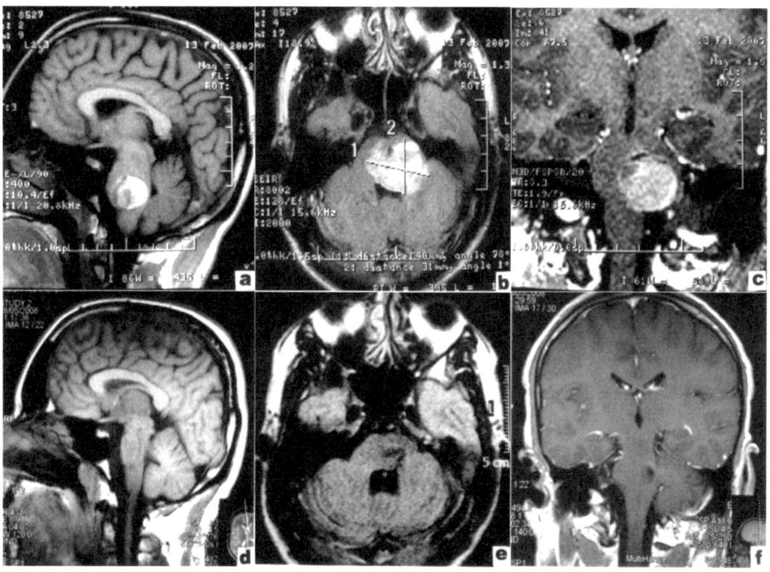

Figure 1. A 21-year-old man who presented with a history of sudden onset of coma. Sagittal (a), axial (b) and coronal (c) T1-weighted magnetic resonance imaging (MRI) scans revealed a gross pontine hemorrhage (1.9 cm) from a cavernous malformation that reached the surface of the floor of the fourth ventricle and in the cerebelopontine angle. The lesion was resected through a suboccipital approach. Sagittal (d), axial (e), and coronal (f) MRI scans, one year later, reveal no rest of the malformation. Two months after surgery, the patient presented with minimal right sided weakness and hemisensory deficits. (surgeon Leon Dănăilă) (case 1).

Hence, we had reasoned clinically that the existence of the ascending reticular activating system (ARAS, further called AAS) and of the ascending reticular inhibitory system (ARIS, further called AIS), which are functioning interdependently, are essential for the functioning of the Central Nervous System (CNS).

In Fig. 1 (case 1), the pontomesencephalic hemorrhage caused the development of coma, and in case 2 the extra-axial pontomesencephalic compression led to the development of the logorrhea syndrome with hyperkinesia.

The respective compression has induced the reduction or the abolition of the function of the ascending reticular activating system and the diminution, to a greater or lesser extent, of its influence on the cerebral and especially on the cortical functions.

Hereinafter we shall reproduce comments concerning the existence and the functioning of the 2 ascending activating and inhibiting systems.

3.1. The brainstem

The brainstem is the portion of the central nervous system rostral to the spinal cord and caudal to the cerebral hemispheres.

The net-like appearance of the brainstem neurons led to the designation as "reticular formation", a term that was originally used in a purely descriptive anatomical sense.

3.1.1. The reticular formation

The reticular formation (RF), beginning in the medulla and extending to the midbrain, plays a major role in the sleep-wakefulness cycles of animals and humans. It occupies a significant portion of the dorsal brainstem and forms a network of reticular fibers that synapse with, and modulate many ascending and descending fiber tracts.

Nuclei of RF receive afferent information from all sensory (visual, auditory, etc.) and motor systems as well as from other major structures of the brain, and project their axons upwards and downwards to virtually all parts of the nervous system. Through their connections with the thalamus, hypothalamus and directly to the cerebral cortex they can send information to, and receive it from all areas of the cortex. There are ascending (or forward) and descending (or backward) connections between them.

The RF is also known as the reticular activating system and the reticular inhibitory system [22, 23, 25]. The role of reticular formation is to awake or to get to sleep the cerebral cortex.

After waking, the cortex allows all modes of sensory processing (sight, hearing, touch, etc.) to combine with conscious thought and experience, in order to focus on some inputs and suppress others. Neuroscientists now recognize that the various nuclei within the brainstem serve many functions and that only a few participate in waking and sleeping.

Instead of being used in a descriptive analogical way, the reticular formation was promoted to a functional concept, a brainstem system, which, by virtue of its nonspecific connectivity, could act as a kind of volume control for the degree of conscious arousal and sleeping and as a homeostatic system.

3.1.2. Ascending (reticular) Activating System (AAS)

In [26] is reported the innovation of the electroencephalogram (EEG), which is closely correlated with the level of consciousness of the patients. Since Berger's first observation, the various ongoing brain oscillations have been used successfully to characterize mental status such as sleep, waking state or vigilance and mental pathologies such as epilepsy. Sensory evoked potentials (EEG signals triggered by an external stimulation) have demonstrated that such mental factors as sensation, attention, intellectual activity, and planning of movement, have distinctive electrical correlates at the surface of the skull [27]. Afterwards, in [28, 29] were examined the EEG waveforms in cats into which the lesions of the brainstem were placed. It was found that after a transection between the medulla and the spinal cord, a preparation that he called the encephale isolé, or isolated brain, animals showed a desynchronized (low-voltage, fast-wave) EEG pattern and appeared to be fully awake [27 – 29]. When the neuraxis between the superior and inferior colliculus was transected, a preparation called the cerveau isolé, or isolated cerebrum, the EEG showed a synchronized, or high-voltage, slow-wave pattern indicative of deep sleep and the animals were behaviorally unresponsive. Bremer concluded that the forebrain fell asleep due to the lack of somatosensory and auditory sensory inputs.

The reticular activating system obtained this designation in [30] were one reported that it was stimulated electrically in anesthetized cats and that it was found that the stimulation produced a waking pattern of electrical activity in cat's cortex. When the lesions were placed in the paramedian reticular formation of the midbrain, the animals showed cortical-evoked responses to somatosensory or auditory stimuli, but the background EEG was synchronized and the animals were behaviorally unresponsive. These observations emphasized the midbrain reticular core as relaying important arousing influences to the cerebral cortex and this pathway was labeled the ascending reticular activating system (today named AAS).

The most important reticular nuclei for arousal and consciousness are the raphe nuclei and the central nuclei. These groups receive significant converging sensory input from all sensory modalities and project to the thalamus (i.e., intralaminar nuclei), cholinergic basal forebrain nuclei, and the entire cerebral cortex. An important component of the central reticular activating system is thought to be the noradrenergic nuclei, particularly the locus coeruleus, at the pontomesencephalic junction.

The centromedian and parafascicular nuclei, two of the intralaminar nuclei of the thalamus representing the rostral extent of the AAS, receive inputs from the spinothalamic, trigeminothalamic and multisynaptic ascending pathways (of the reticular formation) relaying pain sensation. As a result of their diffuse cortical connections, they are involved in the maintenance of arousal.

The neurons of the locus coeruleus project to the thalamus, hypothalamus, basal cholinergic nuclei, and the neocortex [31, 32]. Immediate coma results from the destruction of the central reticular nuclei at or above the upper pontine level.

http://dx.doi.org/10.5772/52688

Anyhow, AAS acts on the cerebral cortex through the thalamus, directly, and through the arousal caudal hypothalamic neurons (tuberomammillary nucleus) which are connected with suprachiasmatic nuclei (Fig. 2).

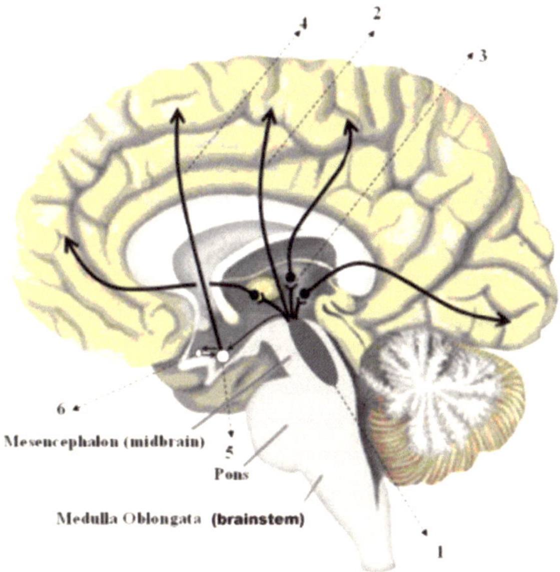

Figure 2. The Ascending Reticular Activating System (AAS) is found in the brainstem (1), and sends projections throughout the cortex: directly (2), through the thalamus (3), or through the hypothalamus (4), tuberomammillary neurons (5), which receive influence from suprachiasmatic nucleus (6).

As a result, the reticular formation comes to be known as the reticular activating system to maintain general arousal, and as the reticular inhibitory system for sleeping.

However, an exact physiologic role of the reticular activating system in consciousness is unclear. The awake condition, as well as the sleep, has many phases: a quick short phase, which is determined by the direct action of AAS on the cerebral cortex, a longer phase, during 24 hours, determined by indirect action of AAS on the cortex through the thalamus, and a rhythmical phase, determined by the AAS action on the cerebral cortex through the hypothalamus awaking system under the influence of the suprachiasmatic nucleus. These nuclei are serially interconnected with AAS not only in the forward, but also in the reverse direction (backward).

It is generally agreed that a key component of the reticular activating system is a group of cholinergic nuclei near the pons-midbrain junction that project to the thalamocortical neurons. The relevant neurons in the nuclei are characterized by high discharge rates during the waking. When stimulated, these nuclei cause "desynchronization" of the electroencephalogram (that is, a shift of EEG activity, from high-amplitude, synchronized waves to lower amplitude, higher-frequency, desynchronized ones).

In [33] it has been concluded that the intralaminar nuclei act not only as a thalamic pacemaker and as a relay for cortical arousal, but they are characterized also by the presence of cells responding to visual auditory and somesthetic stimuli. In [34] it is written "cortical and subcortical innervations of the intralaminar nuclei place them in a central position to influence distributed networks underlying arousal, attention, intention, working memory and sensori-motor integration, including gaze control". Thus, there are three main types of thalamic projections: the specific (for vision, audition), the diffuse, and the projection to striatum (essentially, all from intralaminar nuclei). Diffuse intralaminar nuclei efferents are widely, though sparsely, distributed to most of neocortex: this is the diffuse projection that has to do with consciousness. One can understand how intralaminar nuclei could directly influence ideation, as ideation is a function of cortex [35].

Activity of these neurons is not, however, the only neuronal basis of wakefulness: the noradrenergic neurons of the locus coeruleus; the serotoninergic neurons of the raphe nuclei; and histamine-containing neurons in the tuberomammillary nucleus (TMN) of the hypothalamus are also involved. The locus coeruleus and raphe nuclei are modulated by the TMN neurons located near the tuberal region that synthesize the peptide orexin (also called hypocretin). Orexin promotes waking, and thus may have useful applications in jobs where operators need to stay alert. On the other hand, antihistamines inhibit the histamine-containing TMN network, and thus tend to make people drowsy [36].

Arousal systems are regulated not only by external stimuli, but also by control systems of the brain. For example, the frontal cortex, particularly the orbitofrontal area, regulates the thalamic reticular nucleus and the cholinergic basal forebrain structures. Patients with lesions in this area show deficits in arousal [37]. Cortical control is not limited to cholinergic modulation. In a work on the norepinephrine system [32], it is demonstrated the role of locus coeruleus - norepinephrine system in the prefrontal cortex function and cognitive control.

The frontal cortex also exerts an influence on the limbic system, which regulates emotional arousal. The anterior cingulate region is important in the self-regulation of arousal through its connections with the cholinergic basal forebrain [37].

In sum, AAS can exert both direct and indirect action on the cerebral cortex. However, the reticular formation which appears to be responsible for maintaining cortical arousal is not the same with consciousness.

3.1.3. Ascending (reticular) Inhibitory System (AIS)

According to case 2, it is impossible that the two important functions of the central nervous system, arousal and sleep, or activation and inhibition, depend only on AAS. The two compulsory conditions (arousal and sleep) cannot be determined or explained by the AAS activity or inactivity only.

In [22, 23, 25] is clinically demonstrated that, besides the AAS, there is an ascending reticular inhibitory system (AIS) as well, whose lesion leads to the appearance of the logorrhea syndrome with hyperkinesia, hyperwakefulness, and hyperprosexia.

Normally, during the 24 daily hours, after arousal follows sleep, which is based on AIS. The two reticular systems (AAS and AIS) are under the influence of the suprachiasmatic nucleus and of the awake and sleep centers in the hypothalamus.

As much as awake is determined by AAS, sleep, considered the most profound natural alteration of consciousness, is determined by AIS. It acts on the cerebral cortex directly, through the thalamus, through the ventrolateral preoptic (VLPO) nucleus of the hypothalamus, which, in its turn, is under the influence of the suprachiasmatic nucleus, and through the basal ganglia.

The lateral group of the reticular formation, localized in the pons and rostral part of the brainstem, gives origin to AIS. When AIS is activated, the cerebral cortex becomes inactive and the person is asleep. This system receives inhibitory signals from the cerebellum and sends output signals to the thalamus, to the hypothalamic sleeping center, and directly to the cerebral cortex (Fig. 3).

The raphe nuclei, in the midline of the brainstem, use serotonin as their primary neurotransmitter and have diffuse connections to the cerebral cortex and subcortical gray matter [38].

Thus, the correlated activity between reticular neurons leads to a strengthened connection, both excitatory and inhibitory. In the absence of inhibition, any external input, weak or strong, would generate more or less the same one-way pattern, an avalanche of excitatory stimuli involving the whole population [39]. Cortical networks gain their nonlinearity and functional complexity primarily from the inhibitory interneuronal system [40]. The specific firing patterns of principal cells in a network depend on the temporal and spatial distribution of inhibition. Without inhibition, and dedicated neural formation, excitatory circuits cannot accomplish anything useful [41]. Fast coupling of the excitatory and inhibitory influences can bring about a submillisecond precision of spike timing [40].

Anyhow, reticular nucleus efferents terminate in the immediately underlying thalamic nuclei and the reticular nuclei efferents are GABA-ergic (the neurons in reticular nuclei are exclusively inhibitory, using GABA as their transmitter) [35, 42]. Thus, thalamocortical communication can be simultaneously inhibited by this reticular nucleus efferents that terminate in the underlying thalamic nuclei. In the brain, and particularly in the cerebral cortex, there are multiple influences, both inhibitory and facilitatory. When a performance has been lost because the competence has lost some facilitation, the re-emergence of the performance can result simply from the subsidence of inhibition [43, 44]. The main point is that a loss of performance is not necessarily the result of damage to the competence for that performance; it may result from unbalanced or excessive inhibition of the competence [42].

Generally, the reticular formation of the brainstem is, in turn, influenced by circadian clocks located in the suprachiasmatic nuclei and the arousal (tuberomammillary nucleus) and sleeping (ventrolateral preoptic nucleus) centers of the hypothalamus. The clock adjusts periods of sleep and wakefulness to appropriate duration along the 24-hours cycle of light and darkness. So, in all structures of the nervous system, inhibition plays a pivotal role.

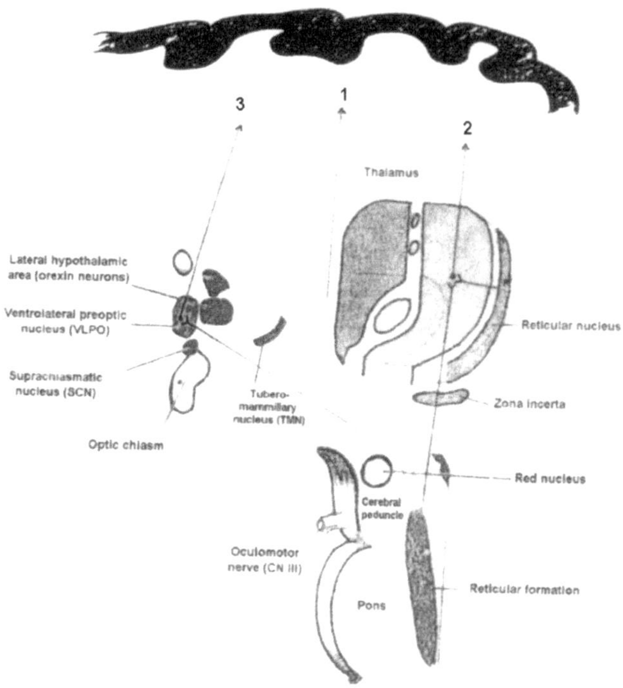

Figure 3. The Ascending Reticular Inhibitory System (AIS) is found in the brainstem, and sends projections throughout the cortex: directly (1), through the thalamus (2), or through the hypothalamus; ventrolateral preoptic nucleus - VLPO, (3), which receives influence from suprachiasmatic nucleus.

Thus, brain uses not only excitation, but also inhibition during its normal operations and behaviors. With no inhibitory cells in a network, depending on the temporal and spatial distribution and dedicated interneurons, excitatory circuits cannot accomplish anything useful [41]. Excitatory potentials dominate on the dendrites of principal cells, whereas only inhibitory postsynaptic potentials impinge upon the cell body (soma). Interneurons provide autonomy and independence to neighboring principal cells but they offer, at the same time, useful temporal coordination. The functional diversity of principal cells is enhanced by the domain-specific actions of GABA-ergic interneurons which can dynamically alter the qualities of the principal cells [41]. The separation of inputs in a network with only excitatory connections and circuits is not possible. Like all somatic functions, at all levels of the system, executive functions, beginning with attention, make use of inhibition for focus, contrast suppression of interference, order, and timeliness [45]. Inhibition enhances saliency and contrast. Inhibition appears essential for the control of impulsivity and a wide array of instinctual drives.

So, there are two opposing active processes that could summate, algebraically, a control excitatory reticular system and a control inhibitory one. Thus, the brain uses not only excitation, but also inhibition during its normal function.

Ascending output of the brainstem reticular formation not only subserves arousal and sleep but also contains information about other bodily states and other neural formation outside the reticular formation. This is why ARAS and ARIS might be named ascending activatory system (AAS) and, respectively, ascending inhibitory system (AIS).

3.1.4. Clinical aspects

It is important to distinguish between alertness and impairment of the wakeful state. It is possible to be awake and not conscious, but it is impossible to be conscious and not awake. A combination of clinical lesion studies and animal data has identified the following major mechanisms through which alterations in consciousness are produced: disturbance of the ascending reticular system; bilateral lesions of the midbrain and diencephalon; and bilateral involvement of the cerebral cortex (hemispheres). To which degree the same damage will render unconsciousness to a person or another, remains to be clarified.

3.1.4.1. Coma

Destructive lesions of the brainstem may occur as a result of vascular disease, tumor, infection, or trauma. Unlike compressive lesions, which can often be reversed by removing a mass, destructive lesions cannot be reversed. Between the conscious state of mind and coma there are multiple intermediary stages that manifest through: confusion or lethargy, drowsiness, stupor, semicoma (light coma), locked-in syndrome persistent vegetative state, loss of consciousness in concussion (diffuse axonal injury).

We will shortly discuss below the most important of them.

3.1.4.2. Persistent vegetative state

The term persistent vegetative state was introduced in [46] to describe the state of preservation of autonomic function and primitive reflexes, without the ability to interact meaningfully with external environment.

The vegetative state has been differentiated from the newly introduced category of minimally conscious state (MCS) [47, 48]. In MCS, patients may show islands of relatively preserved brain response [49, 50], as well as fragments of behavior interpretable as signs of perception and voluntary movement that preclude the diagnosis of vegetative state [27]. Both, the vegetative and minimally conscious states need to be distinguished from the locked-in syndrome in which the patient is fully conscious but, due to a circumscribed brainstem lesion, is unable to communicate in any way other than by the lid closure and the vertical eye movements.

Overall, brain metabolism is less reduced in locked-in patients [51].

3.1.4.3. Diffuse axonal injury (loss of consciousness in concussion)

The mechanism of the loss of consciousness with a blow to the head is not completely understood.

Brief loss of consciousness, which in humans is not usually associated with any changes in CT and MRI scan, may be due to the shearing forces transiently applied to the ascending arousal system at the mesodiencephalic junction. Physiologically, the concussion causes abrupt neural depolarization and promotes release of excitatory neurotransmitters. There is an efflux of potassium from cells with calcium influx into cells and sequestration in mitochondria leading to impaired oxidative metabolism. There are also alterations in the cerebral blood flow and in the glucose metabolism, all of which impair neuronal and axonal functions [52].

Concussion or hemorrhage into the dorsolateral mesopontine tegmentum may be visible on MRI, but diffuse axonal injury is generally not. Magnetic resonance spectroscopy may be useful in evaluating patients with diffuse axonal injury, who typically have a reduction in N-acetylaspartate as well as elevation of glutamate/glutamine and choline/creatinine ratio [53 - 55].

3.1.4.4. Logorrhea syndrome with hyperkinesia

The activity in the reticular formation is the mechanism that induces the sleep, awakens one from sleep and brings one back to full consciousness.

Thus, damage in the reticular formation typically sends a person into coma because this is an on/off switch for all higher brain centers or determines the logorrhea syndrome with hyperkinesia [22, 23, 25]. In a study on the behavior of patients with brainstem tumors and another neurosurgical conditions, reported in [22, 23], it was observed that, apart from the locked-in syndrome, persistent vegetative state or coma, the patients may also manifest various other states, especially logorrhea syndrome with hyperkinesia, hyperwakefulness and hyperprosexia (Fig. 4, Case 2). In our opinion, the logorrhea syndrome with hyperkinesia, hyperwakefulness and hyperprosexia reflect a hyperconsciousness or, in other words, a super-arousal determined by the release of the AAS from the influence of AIS which is damaged.

Thus, the logorrhea syndrome with hyperkinesia is produced by the lesion of the AIS and is an argument in favor of the existence of AIS. The lesions found in our cases (pons, rostral part of the brainstem) mark the location of the AIS. In [56] is described a syndrome of hemiballism and logorrhea determined by a hematome of the left subthalamic nucleus. The right hemiballism is explained by the influence on the subthalamic nucleus, but not the logorrhea. In our opinion, the image given in figure 1 of their article shows multiple subthalamic lesions which affect zona incerta; one knows that zona incerta has an inhibitory role [57].

So, we consider that in this case the logorrhea syndrome is given by the lesion produced to the zona incerta which is located in the immediate neighborhood of the subthalamic nucleus. AIS passes through zona incerta.

In sum, besides the other homeostatic systems, the reticular system (AAS and AIS) represents an actual regulator system of the entire neuraxis, as proven by its participation in the regulation of all the psychical processes (attention, memory, reasoning, behavior, etc.), speech, muscular tonus, and the physiognomy of movement.

In case 3, in spite of the presence of an important compression on the mesencephal, the respective patient has shown only a dorsal mesencephalic syndrome, without the alteration of the state of consciousness.

http://dx.doi.org/10.5772/52688

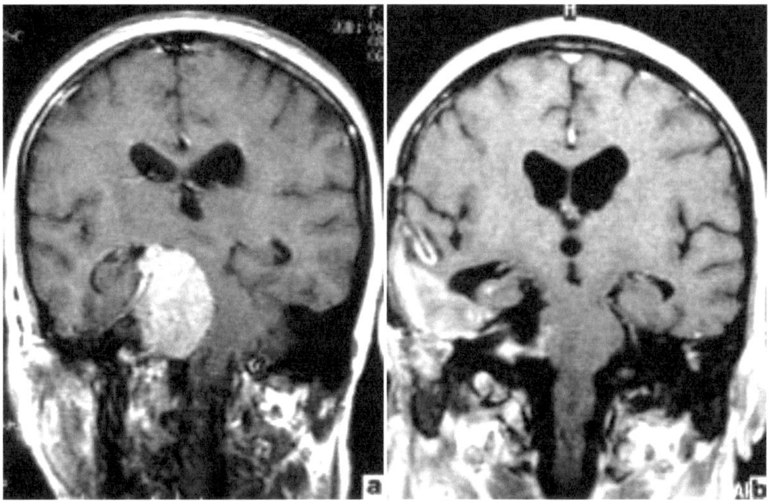

Figure 4. MRI studies of a petroclival meningioma (a) which compresses from outside the Brainstem and provokes logorrhea syndrome with hyperkinezia and hyperwakefulness. Postsurgery (b) this syndrome disappears (surgeon Leon Dănăilă) (case 2).

When the tumor is bigger and it exerts a higher compression on this upper part of the brainstem, we are also faced with the development of coma, besides the above mentioned syndrome.

3.2. The midbrain (Mesencephalon)

The midbrain is the short portion of the brain between the pons and the cerebral hemispheres. It consists of tectum, contains the four corpora quadrigemina and two cerebral peduncles with tegmentum and crus cerebri.

The cerebral aqueduct, surrounded by the central gray matter, separates the tectum from the tegmentum. The cerebral peduncle consists of two parts: (1) a dorsal part, the tegmentum, and (2) a ventral part, the crus cerebri. These two parts are separated from each other by substantia nigra.

The midbrain tegmentum contains the trochlear and oculomotor nuclei, neural structures concerned with ocular and visual reflexes, the mesencephalic reticular formation, the red nuclei and many scattered collections of cells.

3.2.1. Dorsal midbrain syndrome

The midbrain may be forced downward through the tentorial opening by a mass lesion impinging upon it from the dorsal surface (Fig. 5, case 3).

The most common causes are masses in the pineal gland, in the posterior thalamus, or in upward transtentorial herniation which kinks the midbrain.

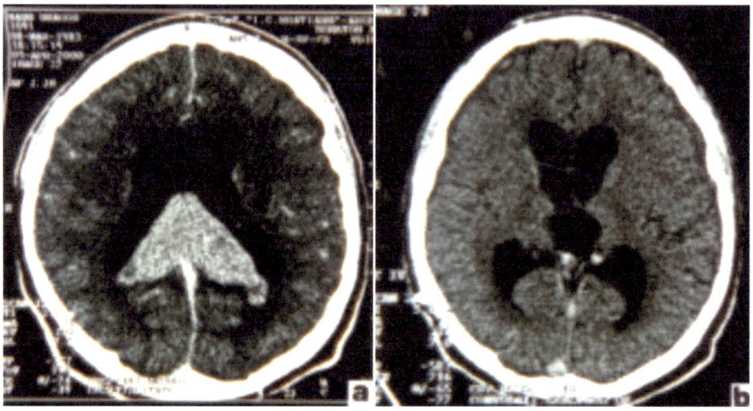

Figure 5. a) A contrast-enhanced axial CT-scan of a 36-year-old man with hydrocephalus and a large pineal region tumor, that was totally resected. Post-surgery, the patient remains clinically intact. (b) Axial CT-scan, 3 months postsurgery, confirming total removal of the tumor (germinoma) (surgeon Leon Dănăilă) (case 3).

Primary midbrain hemorrhages, which may be of either type, are rare. Most of such patients present themselves with acute headache, alteration of consciousness and abnormal eye signs. Most of them recover completely from bleeds from cavernous angiomas, but some remain with mild neurologic deficit.

Pressure from this direction produces the characteristic dorsal midbrain syndrome manifested first by limited upgaze. In severe cases, the eyes may be fixed in forced, downward position. There may be also a deficit of convergent eye movements and associated pupilloconstriction. The presence of retractory nystagmus, in which all of the eye muscle contracts simultaneously to pull the globe back into the orbit, is characteristic.

Motor responses are difficult to obtain or result in extensor posturing. Motor tone and tendon reflexes may be heightened, and plantar responses are in extension.

If the cerebral aqueduct is compressed sufficiently to cause acute hydrocephalus, however, an acute increase in supratentorial pressure may ensue. This may cause an acute increase in downward pressure on the midbrain, resulting in sudden lapse into deep coma [58]. Most patients in whom the herniation can be reversed suffer chronic neurologic disability [59 - 60].

After the midbrain stage becomes complete, it is rare for patients to fully recover.

3.3. Diencephalon

The diencephalon contains: hypothalamus, thalamus, subthalamus (substantia nigra, zona incerta, the nucleus of the tegmental fields of Forel, ansa lenticularis, Forel's field H1 -thalamic fasciculus - Forel's field H2 – lenticular fasciculus –, and subthalamic fasciculus), metathalamus (medial geniculate body, and lateral geniculate body), and epithalamus (pineal body, habenular trigones, stria medullaris, and roof of the third ventricle).

http://dx.doi.org/10.5772/52688

In the following, we shall deal only with the role of the hypothalamus and thalamus in sleep, arousal, and circadian rhythm.

3.3.1. Hypothalamus

Fig. 6 (Case 4) is considered important because in it the hypothalamus was affected. The compression of this important part of the brain led to the appearance of several specific hormonal disorders and also to the alteration of the state of consciousness manifested by apathy, depression, flattened affectations, hyposomnia, as well as the development of confusional states.

In this case it has been affected the tuberomammillary nucleus in the caudal hypothalamus, as well as the connections of the hypothalamus with the suprachiasmatic nucleus, causing the development of hypersomnia and circadian rhythm disorders.

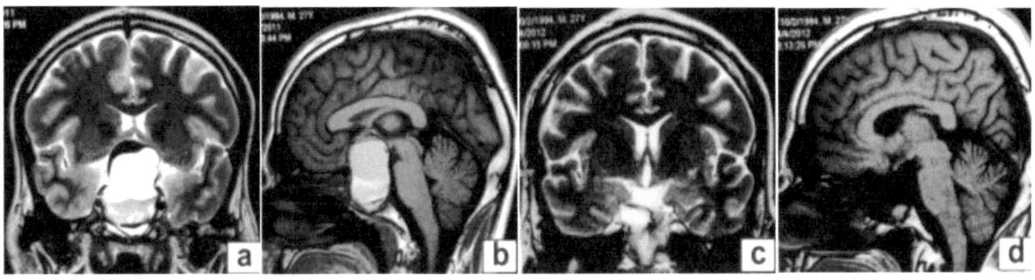

Figure 6. Preoperative T1-weighted coronal (a), and sagittal (b) magnetic resonance imaging (MRI)-scan demonstrates a large supraselar, paraselar, and intraselar mass. T2-weighted MRI-scan illustrates a few calcifications. MRI-scan (c and d) six months after radical subfrontal resection of the craniopharingiomas (surgeon Leon Dănăilă) (case 4).

We shall further present hereinafter several details concerning sleep and the hypothalamus function.

The hypothalamus is composed of about 22 small nuclei, the fiber system that passes through it and the pituitary gland. Although the hypothalamus comprises only about 0.3% of the brain weight, it takes part in nearly all aspects of motivated behavior, including sleeping, arousal, temperature regulation, emotional behavior, endocrine function, metabolism, sexual behavior, and movement [61, 62].

From our point of view, the ventrolateral preoptic nucleus (sleeping system), the tuberomammillary nucleus (arousal system), and the suprachiasmatic nucleus (day-night cycle system) are important.

The sleep is a circadian function, and although the suprachiasmatic nuclei are not essential for its generation, they are responsible for consolidation of sleep in cycles that occur within a circadian framework.

According to the results reported in [9], when humans go to sleep, they rapidly become less conscious. The initial loss of awareness of the external world that may occur when we are reading in bed is associated with the slowing of the EEG that is called Stage I. At sleep onset, although awareness of the outside world is lost, subject may continue to have visual imagery and associated reflective consciousness. Even in the depths of non-REM stage IV sleep, when consciousness appears to be largely obliterated, the brain remains highly active and it is still capable of processing its own information. From PET and single neuron studies, it can safely be concluded that the brain remains about 80% active in the depths of sleep. Most of the brain activity is not associated with consciousness. Non-REM, stage IV is characterized by low-frequency, high-amplitude EEG, in which subjects may report not only some thought-like mentation but also movie-like dreams [63].

The circuitry through which AIS influences the sleep is localized in the upper pons and rostral parts of the brainstem and includes the hypothalamic ventrolateral preoptic nuclei, suprachiasmatic nuclei, the thalamus, and the cerebral cortex. In [64] very good arguments are provided regarding the sleep and arousal. Nevertheless, in our opinion, the explanation of the sleep/wakefulness given by them as due to a flip-flop switch, to the influence of suprachiasmatic nucleus, to the homeostatic mechanism and to the allostatic mechanism is not enough. We believe that the explanation should also include the existence of the AAS and AIS, which are working also under the influence of the suprachiasmatic nucleus, homeostatic mechanisms, and allostatic mechanism, and which control the sleep.

The arousal, like sleep, exhibits more steps: a rapid one, which has a short lifetime and which is determined by the direct action of the AAS on the cerebral cortex; another, with a longer lifetime within the 24 hours, which is caused by indirect action of AAS on the cerebral cortex *via* thalamus; and the third, which is rhythmic and it is determined by the AAS action on the cerebral cortex *via* the hypothalamic arousal system that, in its turn, is found under the influence of the suprachiasmatic nucleus.

Some studies have demonstrated that the influence of the hypothalamus on arousal is not restricted to the tuberomammillary neurons in caudal hypothalamus. In particular, a prominent group of neurons confined to the lateral hypothalamus has been implicated in the sleep disorder known as narcolepsy [65].

These neurons express novel neuropeptides known as hypocretins or orexins and are differentially concentrated within the perifornical nucleus that surrounds the fornix in the tuberal hypothalamus. Mapping studies have shown that hypocretin (orexin) neurons are similar to tuberomammillary neurons in that they are confined to the hypothalamus and give rise to extensive projections throughout the neuraxis [66].

Human sleep occurs with circadian periodicity. Thus, humans have an internal "free-running clock" that operates even in the absence of information about the period of 24 hours [67 - 69]. This clock is controlled by the suprachiasmatic nucleus.

So, circadian rhythms provide temporal organization and coordination for physiological, biochemical, and behavioral variables in all eukaryotic organisms and in some prokaryotes. Circadian rhythms that are genetically determined, not learned [70- 72], are generated by an endogenous self-sustained pacemaker.

The pineal body synthesizes the sleep-promoting neurohormone melatonin and secretes it into the bloodstream where it modulates the sleep.

3.3.2. Thalamus

Although the thalamus is the first neurological structure at whose level begins the process of awareness, the result of the ablation of a single thalamus demonstrated that the female patient in Fig. 7 (case 5) has shown postoperatively only moderate sensitivity disorders on the opposite part of the body and a slight hemiparesis.

Nevertheless, the concomitant involvement of the right and left thalamus leads to the loss of consciousness and coma.

Although the thalamic physiology has been scarcely studied, and therefore limitedly understood, we present below several data concerning the extremely important and complex function of this component of the CNS.

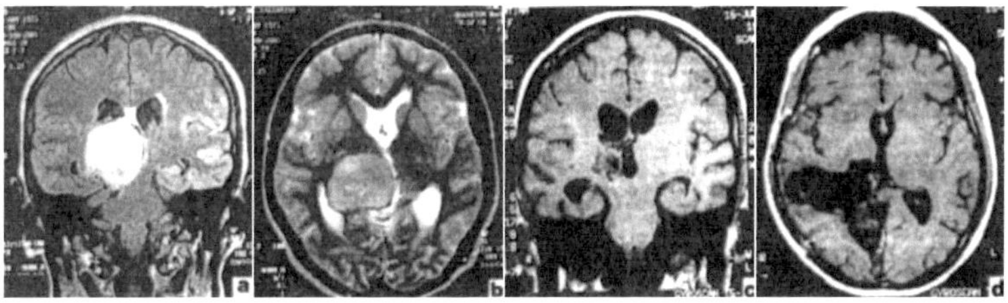

Figure 7. Contrast medium-enhanced coronal (a) and axial (b) magnetic resonance imaging showing a big right thalamic tumor that proved to be an astrocytoma. Thirteen months following resection and radiotherapy, coronal (c) and axial (d) magnetic resonance imaging demonstrates the absence of tumor. The patient was conscious and in good state (surgeon Leon Dănăilă) (case 5).

The fundamental function of the thalamus is that of relay and it modulates peripheral information to the cerebral cortex and to the basal ganglia, keeping the somatosensory, mental, and emotional activity of a living individual in harmony.

With the exception of the thalamic reticular nucleus, all thalamic subnuclei possess thalamic projection neurons that relay processed information to the cerebral cortex. In addition, the thalamic subnuclei also have inhibitory GABA-ergic interneurons whose cell bodies and processes are confined to a single subnucleus. The reticular nucleus of the thalamus is a continuation into the diencephalon of the reticular formation of the brainstem. It receives inputs from the cerebral cortex and thalamic nuclei. The former are collaterals of corticothalamic projections, and the latter are collateral of thalamocortical projections. The reticular nucleus projects to other thalamic nuclei. The inhibitory neurotransmitter of this projection is GABA. The reticular nucleus is unique amongst the thalamic nuclei because its axons do not leave the thalamus. Based on its connections, the reticular nucleus plays a role in integrating and gating activities of the thalamic nuclei.

As the termination site for the reticular ascending system is considered, it is not surprising that the thalamus has an important arousal and sleep-producing function [52, 73 – 75] and that it alerts, activates or inhibits a specific processing and response system. Its involvement in attention shows up in diminished awareness of stimuli impinging on the opposite side the lesion (unilateral inattention) [22, 23, 76 - 78].

The ascending input to intralaminar nuclei can help explain consciousness of primitive percepts (non-cognitive component). So, ascending output of the brainstem reticular formation not only subserves arousal but also contains information about other states. Thus, other input to reticular formation comes from the spinothalamic system, trigeminal complex, and dentate nuclei in the cerebellum conveying proprioceptive signals. There are also ascending inputs to intralaminar nuclei from deep layers of the periaqueductal gray, substantia nigra and amygdala with affective information, and from the vestibular nuclei with information about body position [33, 52, 79, 80].

Intralaminar nuclei. These nuclei, embedded in the internal medullary lamina, consist of centralis, lateralis, paracentralis, central medial nuclei (anterior group), and centromedial and parafasciculus nuclei (posterior group) (Ohye, 2002). The latter are often called the centromedian-parafascicular complex.

The anterior group receives different projections from the spinothalamic tract, deep cerebellar nucleus, brainstem reticular formation, etc. The posterior group has a reciprocal connection with the basal ganglia. The efferent connection with the cerebral cortex is very wide and it was thought to be a diffuse projection. The intralaminar nuclei were classified as representatives of the "nonspecific system" rather than of the "specific system", such as the thalamic station for the visual, auditory, or somatosensory system with definite modality - specific peripheral input.

3.3.3. Reticular nucleus

This nucleus is considered to be related to arousal, attention, cognitive function, etc. It plays a role in maintaining cortical activity in a disease state of epilepsy [52, 81, 82]. In [83] it was studied the human thalamus using microrecordings during stereotactic thalamotomy for dyskinesia and it was found verbal command neurons in this nucleus and in the adjacent area.

Surround-type inhibition mediated by thalamic reticular nuclei may selectively gate out extraneous stimuli while allowing focused relay important sensory data to the thalamocortical circuits, which endow a given neural activity pattern with the property of conscious perception [84]. But how is this neurophysiologic activity coordinated in time to produce a somewhat unified conscious stream? Data suggest the answer may lie in the acquisition of gamma synchrony, most commonly at approximately 40 Hz [85].

Gamma synchrony has also been hypothesized to "bind" disparate features of a given object, such as color, size, texture, and motion, into a temporally unified sensory stimulus [86].

On the other hand, thalamocortical neurons receive ascending projections from the locus coeruleus (noradrenergic), raphe nuclei (serotoninergic), reticular junction (cholinergic), TMN (histaminergic) and project to cortical pyramidal cells. In the tonic firing state, thalamocortical neurons transmit information to the cortex that is correlated with the spike trains encoding peripheral stimuli [87, 88]).

In brief, the control of sleep and wakefulness depends on the brainstem and hypothalamic modulation of the thalamus and cortex.

3.3.4. Epithalamus

Fig. 8 (Case 6) did not confirm the presence of the sleep/vigil rhythm disorder as we should have expected. As a conclusion, the pineal gland has not a relevant role in the evolution of the state of consciousness.

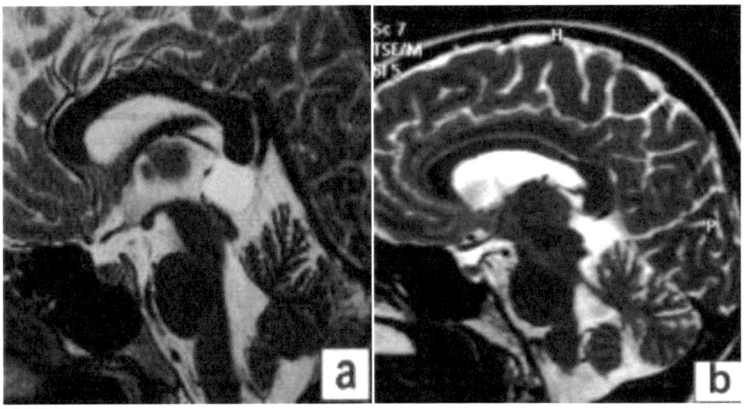

Figure 8. Sagittal (a) gadolinium-enhanced magnetic resonance images show a pineal body tumor (pineocytoma) before, and complete removal of it (b),(surgeon Leon Dănăilă) (case 6).

The function of the epithalamus is not well understood. The production of the pineal hormone melatonin is cyclic with high levels of synthesis occurring at night and low levels during the day.

3.3.5. A destructive disease of the diencephalon

Unilateral thalamic or diencephalic lesions (tumors, hemorrhage, etc.) do not determine coma.

Bilateral destructive lesions of the diencephalic region result in deep coma and death, despite an intact cortex.

Occasional inflammatory and infectious disorders may have a predilection for the diencephalon. Fatal familial insomnia, a prion disorder, is reported to affect the thalamus selectively, and this has been proposed as a cause of the sleep disorder although this produces hyperwakefulness, not coma [89]. Humans with bilateral damage to the region of the dorsal pons, midbrain, and thalamus (by trauma, brain tumor, viral or bacterial infection, ischemic or hemorrhagic stroke) may exhibit an impaired state of alertness, possibly becoming stuporose or comatose.

3.4. The limbic system and hippocampus

The bilateral limbic encephalitis lesions in Fig. 9 (case 7) where the cerebral cortex has remained unaffected by the above mentioned pathological process has led in a very short time to the development of coma and the death of the patient.

Broca first described and named the limbic lobe [90]. In a subsequent phase in speculation on the limbic lobe it was suggested that, in humans, this lobe is partially olfactory and is mainly concerned with emotional behavior. In addition, the amygdala was seen as part of limbic lobe [91, 92]. Finally, it was shown that the hippocampus projects *via* the fornix back to the hypothalamus [91]. This concept was developed further, insisting on the functional importance of certain regions of the neural axis, such as the septum, cingulate gyrus, orbitofrontal cortex, preoptic area, "limbic striatum" (including the nucleus accumbens, mesolimbic dopaminergic tract), nonspecific thalamic nuclei, hypothalamus and midbrain tegmental area, regions closely related to the amygdala and hippocampus [93]. These regions form a ring, or "limbus", around the base of the brain. Anterior cingulate cortex (ACC) is part of a neural circuit that mediates outcome-contingent changes in behavior [94 - 96] and processes fictive information in humans [97]. The ACC is interconnected with the orbitofrontal cortex which mediates fictive thinking in humans [98, 99].

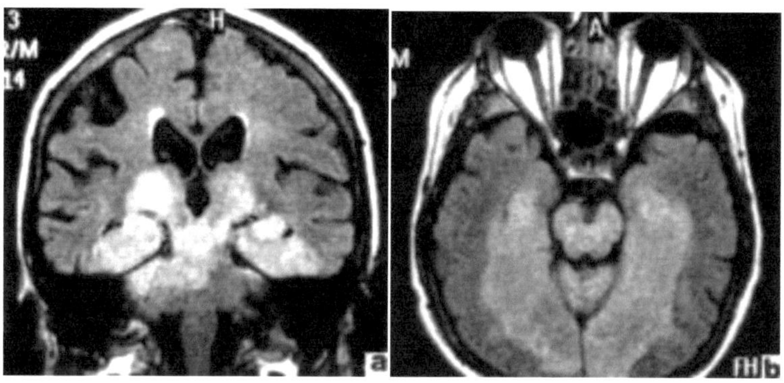

Figure 9. Coronal (a) and axial (b) T1-weighted magnetic resonance imaging scans revealed edematous, demyelination symmetrical changes infra- and supratentorial, which involve the entire midbrain, both thalamic formations, bilateral basal ganglia, two-side temporo-occipital convolution and hippocampus, determined by encephalitis (limbic encephalitis). After 9 days of coma, the patient died (case 7).

It was also hypothesized that neurons in the ACC, which monitors the consequences of actions and mediates subsequent changes in behavior, would respond to fictive reward information [100].

Generally, the hypothalamus allows to consider that the link between the limbic and endocrine system reasonable. The limbic system is now considered to be a functional unit. Areas around the limbic system are called paralimbic and have a more complex histologic structure. Anyhow, the limbic system makes a link between the external and the internal world.

3.4.1. Hippocampus

The hippocampus occupies the medial part of the floor of the temporal horn and is divided into three parts: head, body and tail. The hippocampus is bilaminar, consisting of the cornu Ammonis (or hippocampus proper) and the gyrus dentatus (or fascia dentata), with one lamina rolled up inside the other. The possible functions of the hippocampus are divided into four categories: (1) learning and memory, (2) regulation of emotional behavior, (3) certain aspects of motor control, and (4) regulation of hypothalamic functions [101]. The hippocampus and related diencephalic structures form and consolidate declarative memories that are ultimately stored elsewhere.

The hippocampus is also involved in the regulation of the hypothalamo-hypophyseal axis. Through its projections to the paraventricular hypothalamic nucleus, it may inhibit the hypophyseal secretion of adrenocorticotrophic hormone (ACTH)[102 – 105].

3.4.2. Amygdala

The amygdala is a complex mass of gray matter buried in the anterior-medial portion of the temporal lobe, just rostral to the hippocampus. The amygdala and its interconnections with an array of neocortical areas in the prefrontal cortex and anterior temporal lobe, as well as several subcortical structures, appear to be especially important in the higher order processing of emotion.

The amygdala links cortical regions that process sensory information with hypothalamic and brainstem effector systems. In a review of the role of the amygdala in emotional processing, there were identified five areas in which there is evidence coming out from studies regarding the cognition-emotion interactions involving the amygdala: implicit emotional learning and memory; emotional modulation of memory; emotional influences on perception and attention; emotion and social behavior; emotion, inhibition and regulation [106].

3.5. The cerebral cortex

We consider that the most important logical scheme to shape and analyze the consciousness has a modular structure. The inner structure of all our behavior acts is multimodular and it is subordinated to a main module, in agreement with [107]: " In the brain everything is connected to everything". In our opinion the module is one morphofunctional cortical specific unit (column, area, circumvolution, etc) related to selfconsciousness (physical, psychic), or to the structure and content of the external, objective environment (social, political, religious, physical, etc).

From the analysis of cases 8 - 15 it results that the injury of a part of the cerebral cortex or of a cerebral lobe leads to the partial alteration of certain components, or better said modules, of the state of consciousness. Thus, in Fig. 10 (case 8), where the orbital prefrontal region is compressed by the meningioma, there has been administered or has disappeared certain emotional functions such as response inhibition, stimulus significance, perception, memory and thought.

The reactivating process and the immediate memory has been the most affected. The moriatic orbitofrontal syndrome has asserted itself through emotional lability, impulsive behavior, sexual disinhibition, reduction of criticism, puerile euphoria, logorrhea, excessive joviality, urinary and stercoral gatism [108]. It has been shown that this region has a significant role in the social and emotional behavior, as well as in the build-up of the new memory data [45, 109, 110]. The orbitofrontal module of the state of consciousness has an extremely important role in the social life.

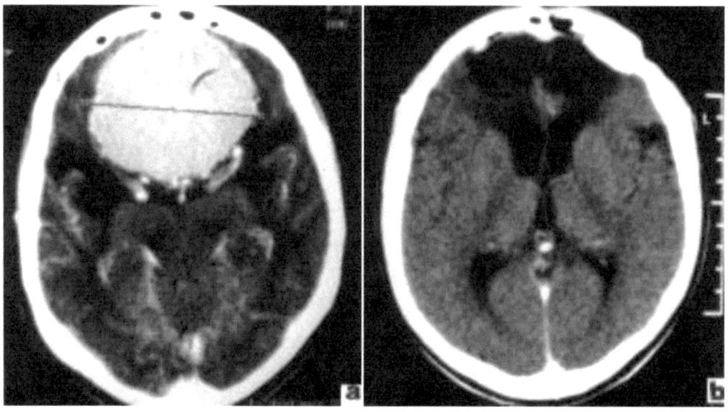

Figure 10. A preoperative contrast-enhanced computed tomographic (CT)-scan of a 56-year-old man shows a giant size olfactory groove meningioma, and displacement of anterior brain (a). The patient presented an orbitofrontal syndrome. Postoperative contrast-enhanced CT-scan showing no residual tumor (b) and the fact that the orbitofrontal syndrome disappeared (surgeon Leon Dănăilă) (case 8).

The patient with lesions of the orbitofrontal cortex does not have adequate social abilities, in spite of the fact that he shows an intact cognitive processing of multiple tasks which are performed with great difficulty. Occasionally, the behavioral syndrome is so severely affected that it has been introduced the term of "acquired sociopathy" [111, 112].

Fig. 11 (Case 9) demonstrates the loss of another consciousness module relative to the functionality of the lateral prefrontal cortex, namely the areas 8, 9, 10 and 46.

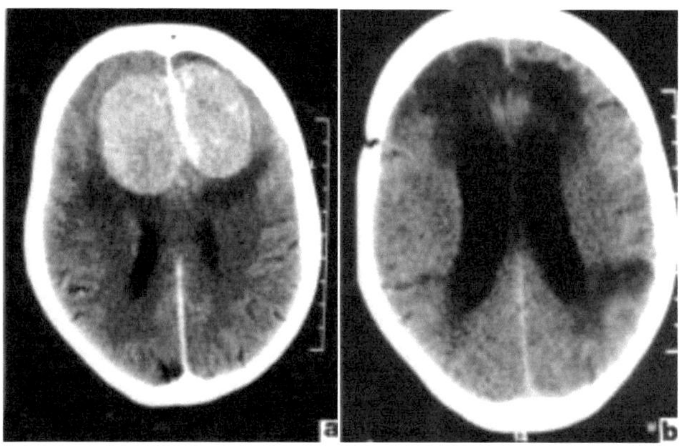

Figure 11. A preoperative contrast-enhanced computed tomographic (CT) scan of a 35-year-old woman shows a bilobed meningioma of the anterior falx (a). She has a dorsolateral frontal syndrome. Postoperative contrast-enhanced CT scan showing no residual tumor (b) and the fact that the frontal syndrome disappeared (surgeon Leon Dănăilă) (case 9).

The injury of these areas leads to the alteration of a wide range of cognitive processes, such as the sustained and concentrated attention, the fluency and flexibility of thought in generating solutions for new circumstances, and the purpose-oriented adjustment of the adaptive behavior [45, 112, 113].

In Fig. 12 (case 10), the left parietal cistic astrocytoma has led to the development of Gerstmann's syndrome, another consciousness module which is specific for this lobe.

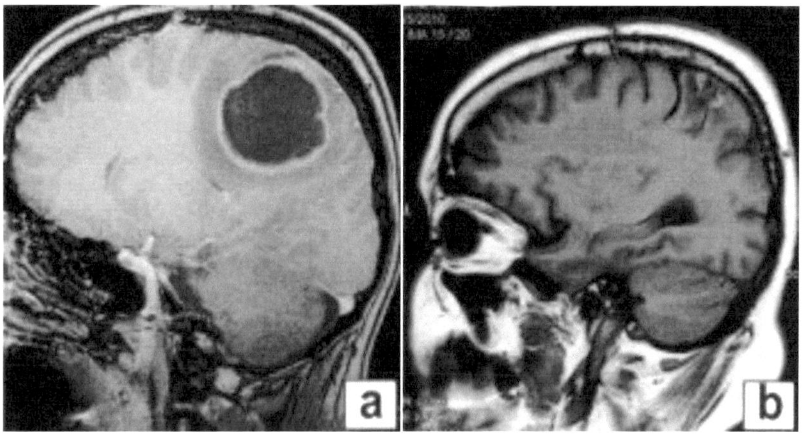

Figure 12. T1- enhanced sagital MRI (a) demonstrates a large parietal cystic tumor in a 42-year-old man, presented with a 3 months history of a subtle sensory aphasia and Gerstmann's syndrome (incompletely). Postoperative sagittal MRI (b) demonstrates total tumor removal of a cystic astrocytoma and Gerstmann's syndrome disappeared (surgeon Leon Dănăilă) (case 10).

If we consider the anterior (somatosensory) and posterior parietal zones as functionally distinct regions, we can identify two independent contributions of the parietal lobes. The anterior zone processes somatic sensations and perceptions; the posterior zone is specialized primarily for integrating sensory input from the somatic and visual regions and, to a lesser extent, from other sensory regions, mostly for the control of movement [21]. In 1924, Gerstmann described a patient with an unusual disorder subsequent to a left parietal stroke. Gerstmann's syndrome (left - right confusion, acalculia, and agraphia) provides the striking example of bilateral asomatognosia and is due to a left, or dominant parietal lesion [114].

The results of the examination of Fig. 13 (case 11) highlighted the right parietal module whose alteration leads to the occurrence of a series of symptoms which has been very well summarized by [115 - 117]. Tactile perseveration and hallucination of touch, cortical sensory loss, impaired recognition of objects, texture, two-point discrimination, stimulus localization, barognosis, vibratory sensation, position, sense, graphesthesia, hemianesthesia, tactile inattention, altered sensory adaptation time, anaesthoagnosia, asymboly for pain, pseudothalamic pain syndrome, unilateral asomatognosia (Anton Babinski syndrome), anosognosia, amorphosynthesis, ideomotor and ideational apraxia, dressing apraxia, stereoanesthesia, astereognosias tactile agnosia etc.

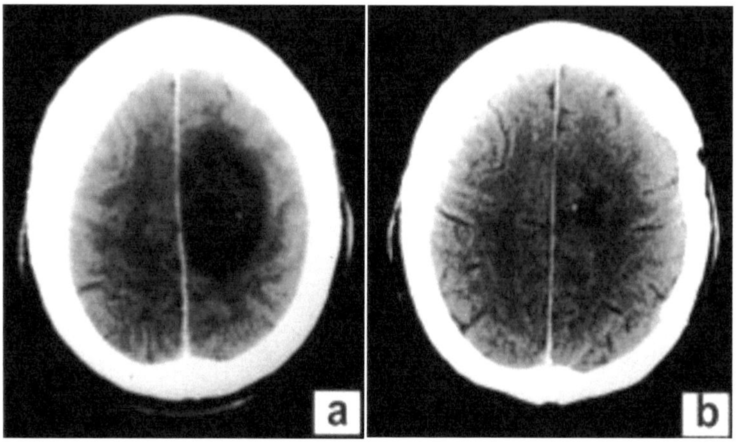

Figure 13. Preoperative CT-scan (a) of a 39-year-old man shows a tumor in the right parietal region. The patient was noted to have a left hemiparesis, tactile inattention and constructional apraxia, dysprosody, apraxia for dressing, and anosodiaphoria. Postoperative CT-scan (b) demonstrates the complete removal of the tumor (astrocytoma). Parietal syndrome disappeared (surgeon Leon Dănăilă) (case 11).

So, patient's appreciation of self in relation to the environment is distributed. Some disorder occurs in the state of continuous consciousness of parts of the body, which depends on the influx of sensations and their association with past memories, the stream-of-life experiences, and the feelings that keep us continuously aware of ourselves [116]. The patients have an altered way of feeling and experiencing. It is tempting to view all these elusive clinical phenomena as manifestations of more general disturbances of the body-environmental schemata, but the evidence to support this view is insufficient [116].

In Fig. 14 (Case 12), the right temporal tumor demonstrates the presence of another modular appearance of the state of consciousness. The temporal lobes do not have a unitary function, in that they house the primary auditory cortex (Heschl's gyrus with aria 41), the auditory association cortex, the visual cortex, the limbic cortex, and the amygdala and hippocampus.

Left temporal lesions are associated with deficits in processing speech sounds, whereas right temporal lesions are associated with deficits in processing certain aspects of music.

Right, but not left, temporal-lobe lesions lead to impairments in the recognition of face and facial expression. The temporal lobe is the great integrator of sensations, emotions, and behaviors and it is continuously active throughout life. So, the two sides play different roles in social recognition and have different effects on personality and consciousness.

The temporal lobe seems to be the site where all sensory modalities are integrated into ultimate self-awareness. The stream of thinking requires both language and memory function and both these functions involve the temporal lobes.

Long-term memory depends on the entire visual stream as well as on the paralimbic cortex of the medial temporal region.

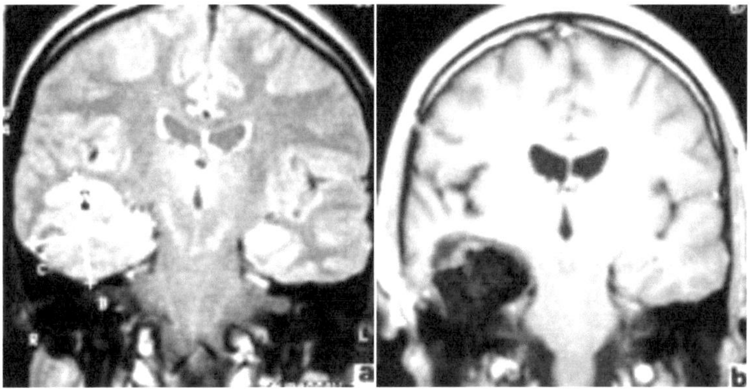

Figure 14. Preoperative coronal T1-weighted, gadolinium-enhanced magnetic resonance images (a) were obtained from a 46-year-old man and demonstrated a large right-sided temporo-basal astrocytoma; (b). image obtained after complete removal of the tumor. (surgeon Leon Dănăilă) (case 12).

Patients with left posterior temporal lesions may show dysphasic symptoms in which they can recognize the broader categorization but have difficulty with the more specific ones.

The amygdala contributes to normal and abnormal emotional responses and experiences [112, 118, 119]. Epilepsy is not an unitary phenomenon and there is no reason to expect patients with epilepsy to have a specific personality type.

So, psychomotor symptoms may be defined as a "state of clouding of consciousness" [120].

The results of the examination of Fig. 15 (case 13) have revealed the absence of another module of the state of consciousness known as Balint's syndrome. However, at the level of each lobe we can find several modules of the state of consciousness.

Their numbering and statistical assessment might lead to the calculation or estimation of the state of consciousness of each individual, in both normal and pathological states.

Hereinafter we shall underline the modular functions of the occipital lobe.

Extrastriate cortical areas are organized into two largely separate systems that eventually feed information into cortical association areas in the temporal and parietal lobe. Thus, the dorsal stream leads from the striate cortex into the parietal lobe. This system is responsible for spatial aspects of vision and for the speed of movement [121]. The ventral stream includes area V4 and leads from the striate cortex into the inferior part of the temporal lobe. This system is responsible for high-resolution form vision and object recognition, such as selectivity for shape, color, texture, and faces [121]. Some neuroimaging studies have implicated ventral occipito-temporal cortex in the nearly area, but distinct from fusiform face area, in the analysis of visual world form.

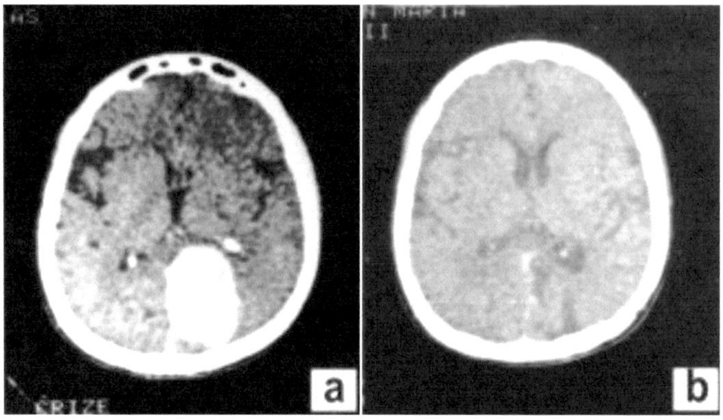

Figure 15. Preoperative contrast-enhanced CT-scan (a), showing a right side parasagittal parietooccipital meningioma in a 42-year-old woman who presented Balint's syndrome. Postoperative CT-scan demonstrates total removal of the tumor (b). After two months, Balint's syndrome disappeared (surgeon Leon Dănăilă) (case 13).

Primary visual cortex, also known as striate cortex (V1) is within, and adjacent to, the calcarine sulcus. V1 sends feedforward signals to many higher visual areas such as V2, V3, V4 and motion-sensitive area MT, to name a few [122].

So, in clinical description, a patient who suffered a stroke that damage the extrastriate region, thought to be comparable to area MT (middle temporal area) in the monkey, is unable to estimate the motion of objects.

Another example of a specific visual deficit as a result to extrastriate cortex is cerebral achromatopsia.

However, different cortical areas and neurons involved in processing specific kind of visual stimuli (color, orientation, motion, faces, objects, etc.), together with other cortical areas and subcortical structures (thalamus, hypothalamus, reticular formation, etc.) seem to play different roles in our conscious visual experience [123].

Combination of feedforward-feedback signals is important for awareness, because higher areas need to check the signals in nearly areas and confirm if they are getting the right message, or perhaps to link neural representation of an object to the specific features that make up the object [124].

Visual field deficits, visual agnosis, associative agnosia, apperceptive agnosia, simultanagnosia, prosopagnosia, visual object agnosia, disorder of reading, disorder of color processing, achromatopsia, color anomia, color agnosia, visual neglect, polyopsia, oscillopsia, cortical blindness (Anton's syndrome), topografical disorientation, defects in constructional skills, visual illusions (metamorphosias), visual hallucination, etc. are symptoms known by the neurologists for more than ninety years.

Brain lesions studies are important for understanding what brain areas may be necessary for certain kind of visual awareness - awareness of color, motion, faces, objects, or the capacity to be aware of seeing anything at all [124].

The results arising from the analysis of Fig. 16 (case 14) and of Fig. 17 (case 15) demonstrate that the bilateral cortical and subcortical lesions lead to the development of coma and death.

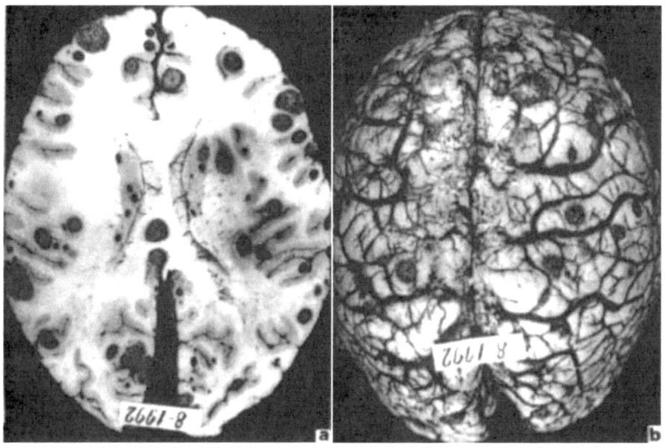

Figure 16. Bilateral, cortical and subcortical, showing more than 110 cerebral metastases (a) and (b). The primitive tumor was a melanocarcinoma (case 14).

The patients with catastrophic diseases and panhemispheric syndromes who are associated with intractable seizures, determined by Rasmussen's encephalitis, hemimegaencephalopaty, tuberous sclerosis, hamartomas, Sturge-Weber syndrome, and congenital hemiplegia or porencephaly, are subjected to hemispherectomy [125].

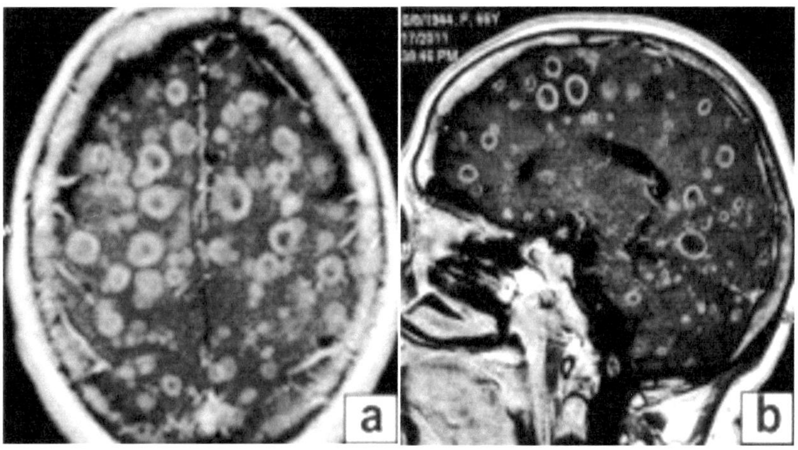

Figure 17. Fast spin-echo TI-weighted axial (a) and sagittal (b) images with enhanced contrast, reveal round, multiple parenchymal cysts in the acute encephalitic stage that are T2 hyperintense and TI hypointense. These lesions were associated with central nervous system cysticercosis. Scolex are rarely visible as a small point in the interior of certain cysts.

After hemispherectomy, the respective patients remain conscious, but with more or less important deficits, depending on the excised hemisphere.

As a conclusion, the involvement of a single hemisphere leads to the disappearance of some of the consciousness modules, but not to its total loss.

The cerebral cortex of the cerebral hemispheres, the convoluted outer layer of gray matter composed of tens of billions of neurons and their synaptic connections, is the most highly organized correlation center of the brain, but the specific of cortical structures in mediating behavior is neither clear-cut nor circumscribed [126, 127]. This multitude of neurons sends a large number of axons in all directions, covered by supportive myelin. This forms the white matter of the cortex fills the large subcortical space.

The cerebral cortex receives sensory information from internal/external environment of the organism, processes this information and then decides on and carries out the response to it.

In general, the cerebral cortex supply much of the content and registration function of consciousness, including language, abstract reasoning, somatosensory visual and spatial abilities, map of the physical dimensions of the self, executive function, complex emotion, feelings, memory and ability to read other's mind. While the cortex is vital for cognitive functions, it interacts constantly with major satellite organs, notably the thalamus, basal ganglia, hypothalamus, cerebellum, brainstem, and limbic regions, among others.

In order to be conscious, to operate at normal parameters, to record and potentiate the internal and external sensory data and to correctly process them based on the previous individual experience, and to answer adequately, it is necessary that the cerebral cortex should be integer and aroused by the ascending activating system.

These considerations suggest that there might be multiple conscious awareness systems each of them supporting conscious awareness in different mental domains.

3.5.1. Unilateral and diffuse, bilateral cortical destruction

Different regions of the cerebral cortex have modular specific functions (somatic sensory and motor, visceral sensory and motor, integrative cognitive functions, speech functions, etc.) responsible for the high-order cognitive processing or conscious mind. These correspond to the Brodmann areas, as well as to each of the four cerebral lobes.

Being aware of the somatic and visceral ego refers to the ability of being conscious of the components of one's body, concrete activities and their status. Thus, a lesion of the parietal lobe leads to a destruction of the ego, which manifests through agnosia, such as asomatognosia (denial of one's own body part), finger agnosia, tactile agnosia, hemiosomatognosia.

The ideational consciousness refers to the ability of one person to be aware of their concrete activities, ideas and thoughts that are expressed through spoken or written words. A lesion of the frontal, parietal, occipital, temporal lobe and of the callous body leads to apraxia, Gerstman's syndrome, Balint's syndrome, akinetic mutism, aphasia and agraphia. Emotional consciousness refers to the ability of being aware of emotions. The frontal lobe and the left parietal lobe coordinate positive emotions, whereas the ones on the right side coordinate negative emotions.

http://dx.doi.org/10.5772/52688

We stress on the existence of the same discrete modules in the brain for each possible neuropsychological capacity. Adjacent modules communicate with each other more than do non-adjacent modules. So, the term of modular or functional localization of consciousness is used to indicate that certain functions can be localized to particular areas of the cerebral cortex. The mapping of cortical functions began with the inference made from the deficits produced by cortical lesions in humans.

As we have noticed, partial lesion of some Brodmann specialized areas or of one of the lobes, leads to the modular loss of consciousness. When the entire cerebral cortex is destroyed as well as the white matter of the two hemispheres, that globally depress neuronal activity, the consciousness level decreases and coma is produced. These causes of diseases include cortical and subcortical tumors, hypoxia, sedatives, hypnotics, neurotransmitter receptor antagonists, neural toxins, infectious diseases and metabolic diseases. Careful studies of split-brain patients make it clear that the right hemisphere has a consciousness of its own, even if it lacks the ability to communicate its experiences verbally.

4. Discussion

The consciousness processes belong to people who act by control mechanisms of psychological activities, generalization and abstractization mechanisms, as well as by exploring and handling of mental images to solve all the problems man is facing with. The consciousness level depends on the complexity of the brain ontogenetic evolution. It must be a function of numerous interacting systems.

Data based on our experience support this statement. In Table 1 we present a synthesis of the lesions produced to the brain modules for the patients/cases analyzed in this paper. All the damaged modules or circuits have as direct consequences modifications of the respective consciousness state of the patients as described in detail in the chapter Results.

According to Tononi and Laureys, consciousness can be dissociated from other brain functions, such as responsiveness to sensorial inputs, motor control, attention, language, memory, reflection, spatial frames of reference, the body and perhaps even the self [128]. We consider this point of view to be incorrect because consciousness cannot appear without these functions. It cannot be dissociated from them. The respective functions represent modules of the consciousness. The consciousness results from the respective cerebral activities. Lesions of some functions lead to modular disorder of the consciousness.

The major structures supposed to play a key role in the neural correlates of consciousness are: the brainstem, the diencephalon (the hypothalamus and thalamus), the limbic system (especially the hippocampus and amygdala), basal ganglia, cerebellum, and the cerebral cortex. The brainstem is the source of massive reticular formation pathways that activate or inhibit higher and lower brain centers. They are the core of the basic arousal and sleeping cycle.

The hypothalamus, the thalamus and the cerebral cortex are likely closely intertwined with RF which plays a key role in consciousness. In general, there are an ascending activating system (AAS) and an ascending inhibitory system (AIS).

However, AAS which appears to be responsible for maintaining cortical arousal is not the same with consciousness.

Sleep is based on ascending reticular inhibitory system. The two reticular systems (AAS and AIS) are under the influence of the suprachiasmatic nucleus and of the awake and sleep centers in the hypothalamus. So, as much as awake is determined by AAS, sleep, considered the most profound natural alteration of consciousness, is determined by AIS. AAS and AIS are not the neurological basis of consciousness but they rather constitute the necessary substrate for consciousness to emerge.

Lesions of AIS produced the logorrhea syndrome with hyperkinesia, hyperwakefulness and hyperprosexia. Bilateral lesions/destructions of the neurological formations (brainstem, midbrain, diencephalon, limbic system and cerebral cortex) lead to the loss of consciousness. The ascending inhibitory system is important in explaining the sleep and many other behavior aspects.

On the other side, the cerebral cortex and consciousness have a modular structure. AAS and AIS reach the cerebral cortex directly, through the thalamus and the hypothalamus. In order to be conscious, it is necessary that the cerebral cortex should be integer and aroused. Thus, to be conscious is equivalent of having access to information about the self and the environment and to have the capacity to read another individual's intention. The consciousness is the most developed form of expressing the personality. The self, similar to the ego, the spirit, the soul is the main expert in primary knowledge. So, consciousness is not equal to the awakened state of mind, as it involves functions of almost the entire brain. But different brain structures and functions have a certain role in generating consciousness. The consciousness, as a result of functions from almost entire brain, is composed by modules which have different important values and features.

Injuring one module only leads to partial modification of the conscious state. Thus, attention, memory, sensorial input, motor output, language, introspection/reflection, space, body and self, perception, imagination, gnosia, etc. are necessary prerequisite of consciousness. The measurement scale of the (actual) level of consciousness of a person in the awakened state of mind and under ordinary life condition is composed of several modules such as: being aware of the somatic, visceral, cognitive, emotional and spiritual ego, and being aware of the physical, spatial, social, socio-relational extra ego.

In the following we will analyse a few data about the implication of the cerebellum in the consciousness.

Throughout the lifespan, the cerebellum plays an essential and fundamental role in organization and expression of higher-level cognitive functions and consciousness. Cerebello-cortical and cortico-cerebellar circuits represent the neuroanatomic substrate. So, the feed forward connections from cortex to cerebellum and the feedback connections from cerebellum to cortex are developed very early in life [129]. However, there is a topographical organization of the cerebellum, along antero-posterior and medial-lateral gradients. Thus, sensori-motor functions are primarily mapped in anterior regions of the cerebellum. Cognitive functions are primarily mapped in posterior and inferior cerebellar regions [130]. Lesions in the anterior lobes should generate motor deficits, and lesions in posterior lobes should result in cognitive impairment [131].

CASE / FIGURE IN THE TEXT	DAMAGED CIRCUITS OR MODULES
LESIONS OF AREA OR BRAIN CIRCUITS BETWEEN BRAINSTEM AND CEREBRAL CORTEX	
Case 1; Fig.1	*Via* the Ascending (reticular) activating system (AAS)
Case 2; Fig.4	*Via* the Ascending (reticular) inhibitory system (AIS)
LESIONS OF SOME SUBCORTICAL CENTERS	
Case 3; Fig.5	Pineal gland
Case 4; Fig.6	Hypothalamus
Case 5; Fig.7	Thalamus
Case 6; Fig.8	Pineal gland
Case 7; Fig.9	Limbic encephalitis
LESIONS OF BROADMANN CORTICAL CEREBRAL AREAS	
Case 8; Fig.10	Olfactory meningioma; lesions produced on cortical areas: 10; 11; 13; 14; 34; 35; 47.
Case 9; Fig.11	Bi-lobed meningioma of the anterior falx; lesions produced on cortical areas: 8; 9; 10; 46.
Case 10; Fig.12	Left parietal cystic astrocytoma; lesions produced on cortical areas: 7a, 7b and 5 which project the frontal areas 6, 8, 9.
Case 11; Fig.13	Right parietal fibrillary astrocytoma; lesions produced on cortical areas: 1; 2; 3a; 3b; 5; 7; 40.
Case 12; Fig.14	Right-sided temporobasal astrocytoma; lesions produced on cortical areas: 20; 28; 34; 36; 38.
Case 13; Fig.15	Right parieto-occipital meningioma producing lesions of the cortical areas: 7; 19.
Case 14; Fig.16	Cortical and intracerebral metastases producing lesions of all the cortical areas.
Case 15; Fig.17	Neurocysticercosis metastases producing lesions of all the cortical areas.

Table 1. Lesions produced in the brain modules shown by the reported cases

In addition, the medial-lateral gradient predicts that lesions within the vermal area should generate changes in affective/emotional functioning, while lesions in lateral region should result in cognitive deficits. Cognitive deficits include impairment in attention, planning, abstract thinking, and memory.

Children with involvement of the vermis, or "limbic cerebellum", develop changes in personality functioning, such as irritability, emotional lability, and even autistic-like cognitive and behavioral features [132].

So, the cerebellum contributes to consciousness.

The cerebellar cognitive affective syndrome with his group of cognitive, emotional, and behavioral symptoms is a module of consciousness [133]. The picture of cognitive and affective characteristics of this syndrome is impaired in patients with posterior involvement of the cerebellum and in patients demonstrating pathology within the vermis.

The type and level of impairment that these patients demonstrated was undistinguishable from that observed in individuals demonstrating pathology within the cerebral cortex, because the cerebellum regulates neural signals in these regions of the brain [129].

Disturbances have been identified in executive functioning, like impaired planning, set-shifting, verbal fluency, abstract reasoning, visuospatial organization, working memory, episodic memory, and attention. Blunting of affect or desinhibited and inappropriate behavior, are characteristic of patients with midline cerebellar involvement.

General intellectual functioning was also affected.

Visuospatial deficits are characteristic of patients with left cerebellar lesions and verbal memory difficulty, with particular problems in working memory and are also characteristic of patients with right cerebellar infarcts [134]. Deficiencies in the performance of non-verbal tasks and deficits in prosody follow left cerebellar lesions. Impairment in verbal intelligence and higher-level language skills typically follow right cerebellar lesions. In addition, the language deficit observed with right cerebellar involvement does not occur in isolation. It is accompanied by cognitive deficits such as impairment in the shifting of attention and thinking or persevering behavior, as well as impairment in problem-solving. Residual functional deficits are common [135, 136].

So, there were visuospatial deficits and dysprosodia with left cerebellar hemispheric infarct and language difficulties and executive function deficit with right cerebellar hemisphere infarct. These localizations of the previous phenomena have been reported in [133 – 135, 137, 138].

The left lateral cerebellum is more active in procedural learning through the ipsilateral hand, but the right lateral cerebellum is activated in procedural learning regardless of hand [139, 140]. The role of the right cerebellum has been related to the refinement or timing of signals within the left dorsolateral prefrontal cortex. Patients with either focal or atrophic cerebellar damage have also been described as demonstrating impairment in cognitive sequence learning [141, 142].

On the other hand, the discovery of the existence and functions of the mirror-neurons, reported in [143, 144] led to the explanation of the learning by imitation, of the empathy, of the reading of other people's thoughts and to the understanding of the connection between the individual and universal consciousness. The development of the multitude of the specific human abilities took place only when the mirror-neurons multiplied and became concentrated in well localized zones within the cerebral cortex and in particular in the pre-frontal lobes.

5. Conclusions

According to our results, two reticular systems: ascending activating system – AAS and ascending inhibitory system – AIS, may be introduced as functional units that seem to play an important role in consciousness. Observing and correlating the status of the "hardware" of the brain whose subunits are affected by neurological diseases/accidents and by related neuro-surgical interventions in humans with the induced modifications of the consciousness in the respective patients, we have been led to the conclusion: besides the already reported and accepted ascending activating system (AAS, formerly called ARAS) that has an important role in the consciousness state, an ascending inhibitory system (AIS) should be defined which acts so that in interaction with AAS the consciousness state may be controlled and kept under functional equilibrium. By points, our main conclusions are:

- The bilateral destruction of the reticular activating nuclei at the rostral pons and midbrain lead to loss of consciousness and the induction of coma.
- The damage of the ascending reticular inhibitory system leads to the appearance of the logorrhea syndrome with hyperkinesia, hyperwakefulness, and hyperprosexia.
- The ascending inhibitory system is very important in explaining the sleep and many other behaviors.
- AAS and AIS reach the cerebral cortex by three distinct ways: directly, through the thalamus, and through the hypothalamus.
- The sleep is controlled by the action of the AAS-AIS dipole.
- With respect to its functioning, the cerebral cortex may be compared to a continuous chess game between of the two systems, AAS and AIS, which act in perfect equilibrium, in order to perform all functions and behaviors of the individual.
- The cerebral cortex and consciousness have a modular structure.

Related to our conclusions, in Table 2 we present a more detailed synthesis of the relations between the lesions produced in the brain by the tumors operated neurosurgically and the modifications of the consciousness observed before and after operations. In this table are shown the specific connections between the brain (AAS and AIS included) lesions/tumors and the consciousness alterations, for each of the operated cases. The connections are made between the brain modules numbers (as generally known) [24, 25], the modules of the consciousness and their denominations on one hand (first two columns). On the other hand, are presented in the columns 3, 4 and 5, respectively, the case number and the corresponding figure, the modules of the consciousness that suffered modifications due to the lesions produced in the brain modules (in each operated case), and the coma/disease cases. As for the brain modules 9 and 10, in Table 2 no operated cases were shown by us in this chapter.

MODULE NUMBER**	CONSCIOUSNESS MODULE DENOMINATION	CASE ORDER / FIG. NUMBER	CONSCIOUSNESS MODULE(S) WHICH SUFFERED LESIONS	COMA / DECEASE***
ONE	COGNITIVE MODULE Discrimination, Identification, Classification, Elaboration, Plan & Decision taking	Case 1; Fig.1	All modules	Coma
		Case 2; Fig.4	2; 5; 9	-
TWO	MODULE FOR COMUNICATION AND LANGUAGE Mediates and Processes Information about the Self and the Environment	Case 3; Fig.5	6; 9	-
		Case 4; Fig.6	6; 7; 9; 10	-
THREE	AXIOLOGIC MODULE Socio-Cultural Standards, System of Individual Values and Individual Character	Case 5; Fig.7	9; 10	-
		Case 6; Fig.8	9; 10	-
FOUR	ADAPTATION MODULE Collection, Processing and Stocking Information about the Self and the Environment	Case 7; Fig.9	All modules	Coma and Decease
		Case 8; Fig.10	1; 3; 4; 5; 7; 10	-
FIVE	VOLITIVE MODULE Regulates the Superior Function of the Consciousness and the Function of Adjustment of the Subject to the External Challenges	Case 9; Fig.11	3; 7; 8; 9; 10	-
		Case 10; Fig. 12	1; 2; 10	-
SIX	MOTIVATION MODULE Internal and Homeostatic Reasons and the Signaling of the Internal States related to the Start-up of the Behavior devoted to satisfy the Physiological, Moral, Esthetic, Religious, Knowledge Needs.	Case 11; Fig. 13	1; 7; 9; 10	- -
		Case 12; Fig. 14	1; 10; 12	-
SEVEN	AFECTIVE MODULE Regulates Positive and Negative Emotions	Case 13; Fig. 15	9; 10	-
		Case 14; Fig. 16	All modules	Coma and Decease
EIGHT	MEMORY MODULE Up-dates Knowledge Need to cope with the Current Tasks	Case 15; Fig. 17	All modules	Coma and Decease
NINE	MOTOR MODULE Mental Schemes and Programs that Control the Movements	No cases reported in this paper.		
TEN	SENTITIVO – SENZORIAL MODULE Contains Records of the Mental Schemes related to the Self and the Environment	No case reported in this paper		

* AAS and AIS act on Cerebral Cortex and Hypothalamus, in opposition to each other. Ex.: AAS acts on wakefulness center/ AIS acts on sleep activating center.

**The Module number refers to the generally defined consciousness modules.

***Lesions of all modules lead to coma with or without decease. Unless specified, coma/decease are not produced.

Table 2. Relations between lesions of the brain and modifications of the consciousness in thecases described in this paper*

http://dx.doi.org/10.5772/52688

From the data and the analysis dedicated to the description and understanding of the neurological bases of the consciousness it became obvious for us that this subject is not completely elucidated and there is still the need to further develop systematic and systemic research on this topic.

Author details

Leon Dănăilă[1] and Mihail Lucian Pascu[2*]

*Address all correspondence to: mihai.pascu@inflpr.ro

1 National Institute of Neurology and Neurovascular Diseases, Bucharest

2 National Institute for Laser, Plasma and Radiation Physics, Bucharest

References

[1] Haldane, E. S. Ross GRT. The philosophical works of Descartes. (translated by ES Haldane and GRT Ross, University Press, (1911).

[2] Gray, J. A. The contents of consciousness: A neuropsychological conjecture. Behavioral and Brain Science (1995). , 18, 659-722.

[3] Crick, F, & Kock, C. Toward a neurobiological theory of consciousness. Seminars in Neuroscience (1990). , 2, 263-275.

[4] Grossman, R. G. Are current concepts and methods in neuroscience adequate for studying the neural basis of consciousness and mental activity? In: HM Pinsker, WD Willis Jr. (eds), Information processing in the nervous system. New York, Raven Press, (1980).

[5] Dietrich, A. Introduction to Consciousness. Palgrave-Macmillan, (2007).

[6] Nagel, T. What is it like to be a bat? Philosophical Review (1974). , 83, 435-451.

[7] Dennett, D. C. Consciousness Explained, Little Brown, (1991).

[8] Crick, F. The Astonishing Hypothesis. New York, Scribner, (1994).

[9] Hobson, J. A. State of consciousness: normal and abnormal variation. In: PD Zelazov, M Marcovitch and E Thompson (ed), The Cambridge Handbook of Consciousness, Chapter 16. Cambridge, University Press, Cambridge, New York, (2007). , 435-444.

[10] Lewis, M. The development of self-consciousness. In: J Roessler and N Eilan (eds) Agency and self-awareness. Oxford, Oxford University Press, (2003). , 275-295.

[11] Damasio, A, & Mayer, K. Consciousness: An Overview of the Phenomenon and of Its Possible Neural Bassis. In: Layers S, Tononi G (eds). The neurology of consciousness. Cognitive Neuroscience and Neuropathology. Academic Press, Amsterdam, Boston, Heidelberg, London, (2009). , 3-14.

[12] Dehaeme, S. The eternal silence of neuronal spaces. Science (2012). , 336, 1507-1508.

[13] Schooler, J. W. Representing consciousness: dissociations between experience and meta-consciousness. Trends in Cognitive Sciences (2002). , 6, 339-344.

[14] Tononi, G, & Edelman, G. Consciousness and complexity. Science (1998). , 282, 1846-1851.

[15] Damasio, A. R. The feeling of what happens. New York, Harcourt Press, (1999).

[16] Edelman, G. M. Bright air, brilliant fire: On the matter of the mind. New York: Basic Books, (1992).

[17] Searle, J. R. The Rediscovery of the Mind. Cambridge, MA: MIT Press, (1992).

[18] Searle, J. R. In Discussion, Toward a Science of Consciousness Conference. Tucson, AZ, (2000).

[19] Yamazaki, T, & Tanaka, S. The cerebellum as a liquid state machine. Neural Networks (2007). , 20, 290-297.

[20] Hatta, T, Masui, T, Ito, E, Hasegawa, Y, & Matsuyama, Y. Relation between the prefrontal cortex and cerebro-cerebellar functions: evidence from the results of stabilometrical indexes. Apply Neuropsychology (2004). , 11, 153-160.

[21] Kolb, B, & Whishaw, Q. I. Fundamentals of Human Neuropsychology. Fifth Edition, World Publishers, New York, (2003). , 345-369.

[22] Danaila, L. Clinical and experimental study on the reticular substance psychopathology (Romanian language). Graduating thesis, Faculty of Philosophy, University of Bucharest, 110, (1972).

[23] Arseni, C, & Danaila, L. Logorrhea syndrome with hyperkinesia. Eur Neurol (1977). , 15, 183-187.

[24] Danaila, L, & Pascu, M. L. Lasers in Neurosurgery. Ed Acad Romane, Bucharest, (2001).

[25] Danaila, L, & Pascu, M. L. Second International Symposium on Coma and Consciousness: Clinical, Social and Ethical Implications, Berlin, June, EU COST ACTION BM0605. Abst. 21, (2009). , 4-5.

[26] Berger, H. Ueber das electroenkephalogramm des menschen. Arch Psychiatr Nervenkr (1929). , 87, 527-570.

[27] Zeman, A. Consciousness. Brain (2001). Pt. 7), 1263-1269.

[28] Bremer, F. Cerveau isolé et physiologie du someil. Comp. Rend. Soc. Biol (1935). , 118, 1235-1242.

[29] Bremer, F. Nouvelles recherches sur le mécanisme du sommeil. Comp Rend Soc Biol (1936). , 122, 460-464.

[30] Moruzzi, G, & Magoun, W. H. Brainstem reticular formation and activation of the EEG. Electroencephalography and Clinical Neurophysiology (1949). , 1, 455-473.

[31] Moore, R. Y, & Bloom, F. E. Central catecholamine system: Anatomy and physiology of the norepinephrine and epinephrine systems. Ann Rev Neurosci (1979). , 2, 113-168.

[32] Minzenberg, M. J, Watrous, A. J, Yoon, J. H, Ursu, S, & Carter, C. Modafinil shifts human locus coeruleus to low-tonic, high-phasic activity during functional MRI. Science (2008). , 322, 1700-1702.

[33] Mcguiness, C. M, & Krauthamer, G. M. The afferent projections to the centrum medianum of the cat as demonstrated by retrograde transport of horseradish peroxidase. Brain Research (1980). , 184, 255-269.

[34] Schiff, N. D, & Plum, F. Web forum: The neurology of impaired consciousness: Global disorder and implied models.(1999). http://athena.english.vt.edu/egi-bin/netforum/nic/a/

[35] Bogen, J. E. The thalamic intralaminar nuclei and the property of consciousness. In: PD Zelazov, M Moscovitch, E Thompson (eds), The Cambridge Handbook of Consciousness, Cambridge Univ, Press, (2007). , 775-807.

[36] Willie, J. T, Chemelli, R. M, & Sinton, C. M. Distinct narcolepsy syndromes in orexin receptor-2 and orexin null mice: Molecular genetic dissection of non- REM and REM sleep regulatory processes. Neuron (2003). , 38, 715-730.

[37] Marrocco, R. T, & Field, B. A. Arousal. In: V.S. Ramachandran (ed) Encyclopedia of the Human Brain. Amsterdam, Boston, London etc., Academic Press, (2002). , 223-236.

[38] More, R. Y, Halaris, A. E, & Jones, B. E. Serotonin neurons of the midbrain raphe: Ascending projections. J Comp Neurol (1978). , 180, 417-438.

[39] Hopfield, J. J, & Tank, D. W. Computing with neural circuits: A model. Science (1986). , 233, 625-633.

[40] Pouille, F, & Scanziani, M. Enforcement of temporal fidelity in pyramidal cells by somatic feed-forward inhibition. Science (2001). , 293, 115-116.

[41] Buzsaki, G. Diversity of cortical functions is provided by inhibition. In: G. Buzsaki (ed), Rhythms of the Brain, Oxford University Press, Cycle 3; (2006). , 61-79.

[42] Bogen, J. E. Some neurophysiologic aspects of cons. Semin Neurol (1997). , 17, 95-103.

[43] Sherrington, C. S. Inhibition as a coordinative factor. Elsevier, Amsterdam, (1932).

[44] Von Monakow, C. ed). Localization of brain functions. Springfield, IL: CC Thomas. (1911).

[45] Fuster, J. M. The Prefrontal Cortex. Fourth Edition. Amsterdam, Boston, Heidelberg, Academic Press Elsevier, (2009).

[46] Jennet, B, & Plum, F. Persistent vegetative state after brain damage: A syndrome in research of a name. Lancet (1972). , 1, 734-737.

[47] Giacino, J. T, Ashwal, S, & Childs, N. The minimally conscious state. Definition and diagnostic criteria. Neurology (2002). , 58, 349-353.

[48] [48].Giacino, J. T. The minimally conscious state: defining the border of consciousness. Progress in Brain Research (2005). , 150, 381-395.

[49] Schiff, N. D, Ribary, U, & Moreno, D. R. Residual cerebral activity and behavioural fragments can remain in the persistently vegetative brain. Brain (2002). , 215, 1210-1234.

[50] Bly, M, Faymonville, M. E, & Peigneux, P. Auditory processing in severely brain injured patient: differences between the minimally conscious state and the persistent vegetative state. Archives of Neurology (2004). , 61, 233-238.

[51] Levy, D. E, Sidtis, J. J, Rottenberg, D. A, & Jarden, J. O. Differences in cerebral blood flow and glucose utilization in vegetative versus locked-in patients. Annals of Neurology (1987). , 22, 673-682.

[52] Giza, C. C, & Hovda, D. A. The neurometabolic cascade of concussion. J Athl Train (2001). , 36, 228-235.

[53] Adams, J. H, Graham, D, & Jennett, B. The neuropathology of the vegetative state after an acute brain insult. Brain (2000). , 123-1327.

[54] Brooks, W. M, Friedman, S. D, & Gasparovic, C. Magnetic resonance spectroscopy in traumatic brain injury. J. Head Trauma Rehabil (2001). , 16-149.

[55] Schutter, L, Tong, K. A, & Holshouser, B. A. Proton MRS in acute traumatic brain injury: role for glutamate/glutamine and choline for outcome prediction. J Neurotrauma (2004). , 21, 1693-1705.

[56] Trillet, M, Vighetto, A, & Croisile, N. Hémiballisme avec libération thymo-affective et logorrhée par hématome du noyau sous-thalamique gauche. Rev. Neurol (Paris) (1995). , 151, 416-419.

[57] Jones GJEThe Thalamus. Second edition Vol I and II. Cambridge, New York, Melborne. Cambridge, University Press, (2007).

[58] Posner, J. B, Saper, C. B, Schiff, N. D, & Plum, F. eds). Plum and Posner's Diagnosis of Stupor and Coma. Fourth Edition. Chapter 3. Structural causes of stupor and coma. Oxford University Press, (2007). , 88-118.

[59] Brendler, S. J, & Selverstone, B. Recovery from decerebration. Brain (1970). , 93, 381-392.

[60] Zervas, N. T, & Hedley-whyte, J. Successful treatment of cerebral herniation in five patients. N Engl J Med (1972). , 286, 1075-1077.

[61] Gaus, S. E, Strecker, R. E, Tate, B. A, Parker, R. A, & Saper, C. B. Ventrolateral preoptic nucleus contains sleep-active, galaninergic neurons in multiple mammallian species. Neuroscience (2002). , 115, 285-294.

[62] Szymusiak, R, Alam, N, Steininger, T. L, & Mcginty, D. Sleep-waking discharge patterns of ventrolateral preoptic anterior hypothalamic neurons in rats, Brain Res (1998). , 803, 178-188.

[63] Bosinelli, M. Mind and consciuosness during sleep. Behavioural Brain Research (1995). , 69, 195-201.

[64] Saper, C. B, Scammell, T. E, & Lu, J. Hypothalamic regulation of sleep and circadian rhythns. Nature (2005). , 437, 1257-1263.

[65] Card, J. P, Swanson, L. W, & Moore, R. Y. The hypothalamus: An overview of regulatory system. In: Fundamental Neuroscience (M Zigmond, FE Bloom SC Landis, L Roberts, LR Squire Eds), Academic Press, San Diego, (1999). , 1013-1026.

[66] Parent, A. Hypothalamus. In: Carpenter's Human Neuroanatomy, 9th ed, Williams and Wilkins, Baltimore, (1997). , 706-743.

[67] Aschoff, J. Circadian rhythms in man. Science (1965). , 148, 1427-1432.

[68] Hobson, J. A. Sleep. New York, Scientific American Library, (1989).

[69] Colwell, C. S, & Michel, S. Sleep and circadian rhythms: Do sleep centers talk to the clock? Nature Neurosci (2003). , 10, 1005-1006.

[70] Hall, J. C. Genetics of circadian rhythms. Ann. Rev Genet (1990). , 24, 659-694.

[71] Rosato, E, Piccin, A, & Kyriacou, C. P. Molecular analysis of circadian behavior. Bioassays (1997). , 19, 1075-1082.

[72] Von Schantz, M, & Archer, S. N. Clocks, genes and sleep. J Roy Soc Med (2003). , 96, 486-489.

[73] Green, S. Physiological psychology. New York, Routlege and Kegan Paul, (1987).

[74] Steriade, M, Jones, E. G, & Linas, R. R. Thalamic oscillations and signaling. New York, Wiley, (1990).

[75] La Berge DNetworks of attention. In: MS Gazzaniga (ed). The new cognitive neuroscience (2nd ed). Cambridge MA, MIT Press, (2000).

[76] Ojemann, G. A. Common cortical and thalamic mechanisms for language and motor functions. American Journal of Physiology (1984). , 246, 901-903.

[77] Posner, M. I. Structures and functions of selective attention. In: Boll and BK Bryant (eds), Clinical neuropsychology and brain function: Research, measurement, and practice. Washington DC, American Psychological Association, (1988).

[78] Heilman, K. M, Watson, R. T, & Valenstein, E. Neglect and related disorders. In: KM Heilman and E Valenstein (eds), Clinical neuropsychology (4th ed). New York, University Press, (2003).

[79] Kaufman, E. F, & Rosenquist, A. C. Afferent connections of the thalamic intralaminar nuclei in the cat. Brain Research (1985). , 335, 281-296.

[80] Royce, G. J, Bromley, S, & Gracco, C. Subcortical projections to the centromedian and parafascicular thalamic nuclei in the cat. Journal of Comparative Neurology (1991). , 306, 129-155.

[81] Ohye, C. Thalamus. In: The Human Nervous System (G. Paxinos ed.) Academic Press, San Diego, (1990). , 439-468.

[82] Ohye, C. Thalamotomy for Parkinson's disease and other types of tumor. Part 1: Historical background and technique. In: Textbook of Stereotactic and Functional Neurosurgery (PL Gildenberg, RR Tasker Eds),McGraw-Hill, New York, (1998). , 1167-1178.

[83] Ohye, C. Thalamus and thalamic damage. In: VS Ramachandran (ed), Encyclopedia of the human brain Academic Press, Amsterdam, Boston, London, (2002).,4, 575-597., 4

[84] Ames, C, & Marshall, L. Differential diagnosis of altered states of consciousness. In: HR Winn (ed), Youmans Neurological Surgery. Fifth Edition, Saunders, Philadelphia. Pennsylvania, (2003), 1, 277-299., 1

[85] Gray, C. M. Viana di Prisco G. Stimulus dependent neuronal oscillations and local synchronization in striate cortex of the alert cat. J Neurosci (1997). , 17, 3239-3253.

[86] Singer, W, & Gray, C. M. Visual feature integration and the temporal correlation hypothesis. Ann Rev Neurosci (1995). , 18, 555-586.

[87] Steriade, M. Basic mechanisms of sleep generation. Neurol (1992). , 42, 9-18.

[88] Steriade, M. Coherent oscillations and short-term plasticity in corticothalamic networks. TINS (1999). , 22, 337-345.

[89] Della Porta PMaiolo AT, Negri VU. Cerebral blood flow and metabolism in therapeutic insulin coma. Metabolism (1964). , 13, 131-140.

[90] Broca, P. Anatomie comparée des circonvolutions cérébrales. Le grand lobe limbique et la scissure limbique dans la série des mammifères. Rev Anthropol (1878). , 1, 385-398.

[91] Papez, J. W. A proposed mechanism of emotion. Arch Neurol Psychiatry (1937). , 38, 725-743.

[92] Brodal, A. The hippocampus and the sense of smell. A review. Brain (1947). , 70-179.

[93] Nauta WJHHippocampal projections and related neural pathways to the midbrain in the cat. Brain (1958). , 81, 319-340.

[94] Ito, S, Stuphorn, V, Brown, J. W, & Schall, J. D. Performance monitoring the anterior cingulate cortex during saccade countermanding. Science (2003).

[95] Kerns, J. G, & Cohen, J. D. MacDonald AW, Cho YR, Stenger AV, Carter SC. Anterior cingulate conflict monitoring and adjustments in control. Science (2004). , 303, 1023-1026.

[96] Kennerley, S. W, Walton, M. E, Behrens, E. J, & Buckley, M. Rushworth MSF. Optimal decision making and the anterior cingulate cortex. Nature Neurosscience (2006). , 940-947.

[97] Chiu, P. H, Lohrent, T. M, & Montague, P. R. Smokers' brains compute, but ignore, a fictive error signal in a sequential investment task. Nature Neuroscience (2008). , 11, 514-520.

[98] Camille, N, Coricelli, G, Sallet, J, Pradat-diehl, P, Duhamel, J. R, & Sirigu, A. The involvement of the orbitofrontal cortex in the experience of regret. Science (2004). , 1167-1170.

[99] Ursu, S, & Carter, C. S. Outcome representations, counterfactual comparisons and the human orbitofrontal cortex: implications for neuroimaging studies of decision-making. Cognitive brain research (2005).

[100] Hayden, B. Y, Pearson, J. M, & Platt, M. L. Fictive reward signals in the anterior cingulate cortex. Science (2009). , 324, 948-950.

[101] Duvernoy, H. M. The Human Hippocampus. Third Ed, Springer Verlag, Berlin, Heidelberg, (2005).

[102] Jacobs, M. S, Mc Farland, W. L, & Morgane, P. J. The anatomy of the brain of the bottlenose dolphin (Tursiops truncatus). Rhinic lobe (rhinencephalon): the archicortex. Brain Res Bull (1979). Suppl 1,, 1-108.

[103] Teyler, T. J, Vardaris, R. M, Lewis, D, & Rawitech, A. B. Gonadal steroid: effects of excitability of hippocampal pyramidal cells. Science (1980). , 209, 1017-1019.

[104] Herman, J. P. Schäfer MKH, Young EA, Thompson R, Douglas J, Akil H, Watson SJ. Evidence for hippocampal regulation of neuroendocrine neurons of the hypothalamo-pituitary-adrenocortical axis. J Neurosci (1989). , 9, 3072-3082.

[105] Diamond, D. M, Fleshner, M, Ingersoll, N, & Rose, G. M. Psychological stress impairs spatial working memory: relevance to electronophysiological studies of hippocampal function. Behav. Neurosci (1996). , 110, 661-672.

[106] Phelps, E. A. Le Doux JE. Contributions of the amygdala to emotion processing from animal models to human behavior. Neuron (2005). , 48, 175-187.

[107] Laurente De No RThe structure of the cerebral cortex. In J.F. Fulton (ed.). Physiology of the nervous system. Ed.3. Oxford Univ. Press, New York, (1949). , 288-330.

[108] Roberts, A. C, Robbins, T. W, & Weiskrantz, L. The Prefrontal Cortex Executive and Cognitive Functions. Oxford University Press, New York, (1998).

[109] Morecraft, R. J, & Yeterian, E. Prefrontal cortex. Enciclopedia of Human Brain (2002). , 4, 11-26.

[110] Miller, B. L, & Cummings, J. L. The Human Frontal Lobe. Functions and Disorders. Second Edition. The Guilford Press. New York, London, (2007).

[111] Damasio, A. R. Descartes' error: Emotion, reason, and the human brain. New York, Putnam, (1994).

[112] Danaila, L, & Golu, M. Handbook of Neuropsychlogy, (in Romanian) Editura Medicală Bucureşti, (2006)., 2, 15-74., 2

[113] Duncan, J, & Emslie, H. Williams. Intelligence and the frontal lobe: the organization of goal-directed behavior. Cogn Psychol (1996). , 30, 257-303.

[114] Gerstmann, J. Fingeragnosie: eine umschriebene Störung der Orientierung am eigenen Körper. Wien Klin Wschr (1924). , 37, 1010-1012.

[115] Critchley, M. The Parietal Lobes. London, (1953).

[116] Adams, R. D, Victor, M, & Ropper, A. H. Principles of Neurology. Sixth Edition. McGraw-Hill, New York, St Louis, San Francisco, (1997). , 454-459.

[117] Bradley, W. G, Daroff, R. B, & Fenichel, G. M. Marsden CD (eds), Neurology in Clinical Practice. Principles of Diagnosis and Management. 1, 703-706.

[118] Buchtel, H. A. Temporal Lobes. In: VS Ramachandran (ed.), Encyclopedia of the Human Brain. Academic Press, Amsterdam, Boston, London, (2002).,4, 569-574., 4

[119] Danaila, L, & Craciun, E. Neuropsychology (in Romanian), Ed. Renaissance, Bucureşti, (2008).

[120] Fenton, G. W. Psychiatric Disorders of Epilepsy: Classification and Phenomenology. In: EH Reynolds and MR Trimble, Epilepsy and Psychiatry, Churchill Livingstone, Edinburgh, (1981).

[121] Purves, D, Augustine, G. J, & Fitzpatrick, D. Central visual pathways. In: D Purves, Augustine GJ, Fitzpatrick D et al., (eds), Neuroscience. Third Edition. Chapter 11, Sinauer Associates Inc Publishers. Sunderland, Massachusets USA, (2004). , 259-282.

[122] Felleman, D. J, & Van Essen, D. C. Distributed hierarchical processing in the primate cerebral cortex. Cerebral Cortex (1991). , 1, 1-47.

[123] Rees, G, Kreiman, G, & Koch, C. Natural correlates of consciousness in human. Nat Rev Neurosci (2002). , 3, 261-270.

[124] Tong, F, & Pearson, P. Vision. In: BJ Bass and MN Gage (eds.), Cognition, Brain and Consciousness. Amsterdam, Boston, Heidelberg. Academic Press, (2007). , 149-182.

[125] Cramer, J. A, Perrine, K, & Devinsky, O. Development and cross-cultural translation of a 31-item quality of life in epilepsy inventory. Epilepsia (1998). , 39, 81-88.

[126] Collins, R. C. Cerebral Cortex. In: AL Pearlman and RC Collins (eds.), Neurobiology of disease, New York, Oxford University Press, (1990).

[127] Franckowiak RSJFriston KJ, Frith CD, Dolan RJ, Mazziota JC. Human brain function. San Diego, Academic Press, (1997).

[128] Tononi, G, & Laureys, S. The neurology of consciousness: an overview. In: S Laureys and G Tononi (eds), The Neurology of Consciousness: Cognitive Neuroscience and Neuropathology. Academic Press, Amsterdam, Boston, Heidelberg, (2009). , 375-412.

[129] Koziol, L. F, & Budding, D. E. Subcortical structures and cognition. Springer, New York, (2009). , 125-165.

[130] Kalashnikova, L. A, Zueva, Y. V, Pugacheva, O. V, & Korsakova, N. K. Cognitive impairments in cerebellar infarcts. Neuroscience and Behavior Physiology (2005). 35, 773-779.

[131] Hu, D, Shen, H, & Zhou, Z. Functional asymmetry in the cerebellum: a brief review, Cerebellum (2008).

[132] Guzzetta, F, Mercuri, E, & Spano, M. Congenital lesions of cerebellum. In: A Benton, E De Renzi,D Riva (eds). Localization of brain lesions and development functions. London, John Libbey, (2000). , 147-152.

[133] Schmahmann, J. D. Disorders of the cerebellum. Ataxia, dysmetria of thought, and the cerebellar cognitive affective syndrome. Journal of Neuropsychiatry and Clinical Neurosciences (2004). , 16, 367-378.

[134] Hokkanen, L. S, Kauranen, V, Roine, R. O, Salonen, O, & Kotila, M. Subtle cognitive deficits after cerebellar infarcts. Eur J Neurol (2006). , 13, 161-170.

[135] Riva, D, & Giorgi, C. The contribution of the cerebellum to mental and social functions in developmental age. Fiziol Cheloveka (2000). , 26, 27-31.

[136] Steinlin, M, Imfeld, S, & Zulauf, P. Neuropsychological long-term sequelae after posterior fossa tumour resection during childhood. Brain (2003). , 126, 1998-2008.

[137] Riva, D, & Giorgi, C. The cerebellum contributes to higher functions during development: Evidence from series of children surgically treated for posterior fossa tumours. Brain (2000). , 123, 1051-1061.

[138] Gordon, N. The cerebellum and cognition. European Journal of Pediatric Neurology (2007). , 11, 232-234.

[139] Torriero, S, Oliveri, M, & Koch, G. Interference of left and right cerebellar γTMS with procedural leading. Journal of Cognitive Neuroscience (2004). , 16, 1605-1611.

[140] Torriero, S, Oliveri, M, & Koch, G. Cortical networks of procedural learning: Evidence from cerebellar damage. Neuropsychologia (2007). , 45, 1208-1214.

[141] Leggio, M. G, Todesco, A. M, & Chiricozzi, F. R. Cognitive sequencing impairment in patients with focal or atrophic cerebellar damage. Brain (2008). , 131, 1332-1343.

[142] Edelman, G. M, & Tononi, G. An universe of consciousness. New York: Basic Books, (2000).

[143] Rizzolatti, G, Foggassi, L, & Gallese, V. Neurophysiological mechanisms underlying the understanding and imitation of action. Nature Review: Neuroscience (2001). , 2, 661-670.

[144] Rizzolatti, G, & Craighero, L. The mirror-neurons system. Annual review of Neuroscience (2004). , 27, 169-192.

Section 11

Antioxidants in Brain Tumors

Chapter 23

The Stance of Antioxidants in Brain Tumors

Pinar Atukeren and M. Ramazan Yigitoglu

Additional information is available at the end of the chapter

http://dx.doi.org/10.5772/54791

1. Introduction

The incidence of brain tumors and other types of cancer have been evidently increasing during the last few decades. Due to the well documented fact that the cancer cells are under high levels of oxidative stress, the relevance between oxidative stress and cancer has been the main topic of intense discourse (Powis & Baker, 1997; Pervaiz & Clement, 2004). Elevated levels of intrinsic oxidative stress has been emphasized in different types of tumors, possibly due to the clustering of factors such as enhanced metabolism, mitochondrial mutation, inflammation and cytokines (Mumper, 2009). Cellular damage on account of oxidative stress has been indicated in a range of disorders such as cancer (Floyd, 1990) diabetes mellitus (Dandona, et al.,1996), atherosclerosis (Valko, et al., 2007), neurodegenerative disorders such as Alzheimer's disease and Parkinson's disease (Jenner, 1997) autoimmune disorders such as arthritis and has also been indicated to be involved in aging (Ames & Shigenaga, 1992)

Oxidation is a natural process of cellular metabolism, but oxidation is what creates these destructive reactive oxygen species (ROS). ROS are constantly produced during oxidative metabolism and can have deleterious effects on cell function and viability due to their ability to induce damage to the cells. The formation of ROS is a consequence of aerobic metabolism (Castro, 2001). ROS are generated in many compartments and by numerous enzymes in cells (Fig. 1).

In normal conditions, the countenance in the intracellular ROS levels is maintained with the contribution of antioxidant scavenging systems and defense components. Yet, in some disorders such as cancer, the balance between the ROS and the antioxidant status falls off. Brain tissue also displays higher susceptibility to oxygen and glucose necessity, which are required to support normal function through glycolysis and oxidative phosphorylation thus the brain is particularly susceptible to oxidative damage since does not have much antioxidant storage. Additionally, the brain has a high amount of fatty acids. All these attributes lead to brain cell damage. Thereby human brain encounters intense percentage of oxygen consumption, eventually generates an excessive amount of reactive oxygen species (ROS) when compared with other tissues.

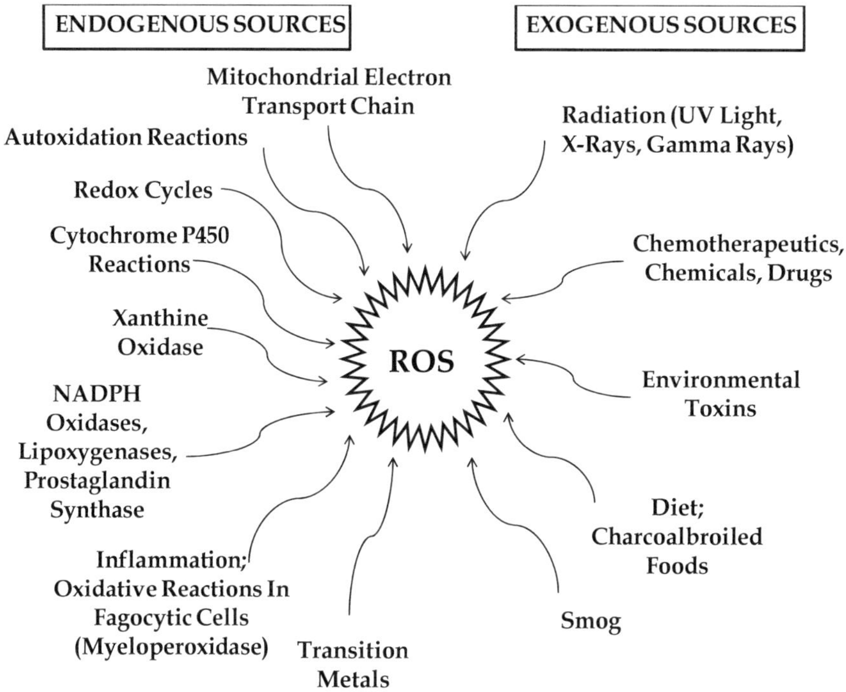

Figure 1. Sources of reactive oxygen species in the human body

Oxidative stress can be defined as the disturbance in the oxidant-antioxidant balance (Chandra, et al., 2000). The cancer cells exposed to oxidative stress tend to heavily interpret adaptation mechanisms and may deplete cellular antioxidant capacity. The generated excessive ROS cannot be neutralized by cellular antioxidants and oxidative stress endures (Pervaiz, 2006). The redox status related to the production of intracellular ROS in cancer cells has also been denoted to control the aggression of cancer cells. The reason of the induced oxidative stress in cancer cells is a result of the lower levels of antioxidant enzymes such as SOD, glutathione peroxidase, glutathione reductase, and catalase (Anshul, 2009). The reduced ROS combout is known in conjunction with tumor growth and metastasis.

The enhanced oxidative stress can lead to modification of cellular targets and induce cell damage and death. Nuclear and mitochondrial DNA single strand breaks, mitochondrial inner membrane damage resulting with the loss of cellular ATP storage and initiation of lipid peroxidation in membrane phospholipids can be seen (Farber, et al., 1990). The cell damage and the following deficiency in cellular repair processes due to the constant oxidative damage are correlated with carcinogenesis(Behrend, et al., 2003; Federico, et al.,

2007; Nair & Nair, 2007). Such as, guanine nucleotide base oxidation in DNA results in the formation of 8- hydroxy-2-deoxyguanosine (8-OHdG), which alters DNA and eventuates as mutagenesis and cause carcinogenesis (Gate, et al., 1999). ROS interaction with DNA results in fragmentation with the loss of bases and causes DNA strand breaks (Imlay, 1988; Farber, et al., 1990; Farber, 1994). When DNA strand breaks accumulates in cells, this can lead oncogenic transformation depending on the intensity of cellular repair processes (Federico, et al., 2007). At this level, cells exposed to excessive ROS stress either undergo apoptosis or in some cases the cells start to proliferate and thus are irreversibly turn into malignant cells (Fruehauf & Meyskens, 1997) and maintain excessive oxidative stress compared to normal cells. Thus the strategy of producing further ROS stress in malignant cells could be a successful anti-cancer strategy (Anshul, 2009).

On the other hand, ROS also subserve for the regulation of cellular functions and normal metabolism (Poli, et al., 2004). Adversely, low concentrations of ROS serve a variety of important cellular functions such as the activation and modulation of the signal transduction pathways (Monteino & Stern, 1996), modulation of the activities of the redox sensitive transcription factors (Li, et al., 1998; Oberley, 2002) regulation of apoptosis (Nulton-Persson, 2001; Fang & Iyer, 2007) and the regulation of mitochondrial enzyme activities (Nulton-Persson, 2001; Oberley, 2002). Increased ROS production is well displayed in transformed cells (Toyokuni, et al., 1995; Burdon, 1995; Storz, 2005; Kryston, et al., 2011) and growing evidence suggests that ROS act as second messengers in intracellular signaling pathways (Liou & Storz, 2010).

Recently, oxidative stress has been related with the etiology and the prospective treatment of cancer (Powis & Baker, 1997; Pervaiz & Clement, 2004). Cells have developed a number of antioxidant defense systems to confront the hazardous effects of endogenous ROS production and accumulation to protect against cellular oxidative damage. Antioxidants in the cells form a heterogeneous group including low molecular weight substances which are water or lipid soluble, being inclusive in the body through nutrition, also a number of endogenous metabolites own antioxidant activities.

Malignant gliomas account for the most diagnosed primary brain cancers (Behrend, et al., 2003). Despite of exquisite treatment approaches the prognosis remains poor. There is a well-documented association between increased consumption of antioxidants and decreased incidence of cancer. Antioxidant supplements are recommended as part of a cancer prevention diet. Even though cells have endogenous antioxidant enzymes, most human cancer cells have decreased antioxidant enzyme levels compared to their normal tissue counterparts. It is found that; cruciferous vegetables such as broccoli, horseradish, brussels, decreased the risk of anaplastic astrocytomas which is a type of aggressively growing brain tumor. One of the important functions of apoptosis is disposing of preneoplastic and neoplastic cells which appears when a damage or malfunction is recognized and signaling cascades are initiated so caspases and endonucleases that kill the cell are activated. In cell suicide, the signaling cascade avails ROS as messenger molecules. Thats why antioxidants are ascendant in the inhibition of apoptosis. So, the removal of antioxidants from the diet can be suggested as this may enhance apoptosis and inhibit tumor growth. The tumor cell survives in an ROS rich environment depending on the overexpression of antioxidant enzymes and the excessive levels of nonenzymatic antioxidant scavengers. A range of complementary and alternative therapies can be inclusive for the treatment of brain cancer. Nutrients and herbs are believed to protect against side effects of conventional therapies, they may also enhance chemotherapy and support anticancer activities. At that, normal cells protect themselves when exposed to high doses of antioxidants while cancer cells can not adapt and they suffer damage caused by the antioxidants. Thus, high doses of antioxidants may be toxic to cancer cells but not to normal cells. Antioxidants which are active in the brain tissue, can cross the blood brain barrier and prevent oxidative damage, so this can also be taken into consideration as a good treatment and prevention strategy of brain cancer.

2. The redox status of the brain

Brain is considered enormously vulnerable to oxidative damage so is the target for oxidative stress damaging effects than the other tissues. One of the reasons is its having high oxygen consumption (Sah, et al., 2002) and this is around 20% of the total metabolic activity (Dal-Pizzol, et al., 2000). Also, the brain tissue contains much amounts of polyunsaturated fatty acids, which are particularly sensitive to free radical attacks and prooxidative transition metals such as high levels of iron which is a triggering factor in lipid peroxidation of the cell membranes and also the brain has a comparatively low antioxidant capacity (Sies, 1993; Bellissimo, et al. 2001; Freitas, et al., 2004) and glucose deprivation, which are needed to support normal metabolic functions through glycolysis and oxidative phosphorylation.

Massive neuronal death is the outcome of the secondary injury response, creating an excessive pool of ROS, which triggers a cascade of reactive oxygen chain reactions. The free metal concentrations are also controlled in the nervous system by transport proteins such as ferritin (Sies, 1993) and this limits the non-enzymatic catalysis of hydroxyl radical formation. The nervous system contains antioxidant enzymes; including Cu/Zn- and Mn dependent SOD and GPx which are expressed in higher quantities than CAT (Shivakumar et al., 1991; Hussain et al., 1995). It was shown that the zinc, iron and selenium concentrations were found significantly lower in cancer patients and the copper concentrations were found to be either elevated or significantly elevated, as 2-3 fold, when compared to age matched samples of normal tissues (Kuo, et al., 2002; Zuo, et al., 2006). It has been also shown that the Cu/Zn, Cu/Se and Cu/Fe ratios were found higher in cancer patients when compared to normal subjects.

Cancer cells display increased glycolysis rate combined with a reduced respiration rate (Spitz, 2000). The enhanced requirements for ATP; generates oxygen free radicals and this causes oxidative stress conditions to come out which eventually promotes cell death. Neurons and cancer cells consume glucose as energy source to respond this issue and glycolytic metabolism rules over in tumor cells. The release of cytochrome c couples with the pentose phosphate pathway and this initiates cytochrome c mediated apoptosis (Vaughn &Deshmukh, 2008). Caspase activation is initiated by cytochrome c when released from mitochondria during apoptosis. So, the cancer cells and neurons control apoptosis through regulation of cytochrome c release, while utilizing glucose as a source of energy (Dajas, 2012). This marked changes in metabolism have been shown to be related with increased oxidative stress which is emphasized to be due to increased mitochondrial superoxide radical production (Oberley, et al., 1981). A more oxidizing redox status of the transforming cell occurs and this streamlines immortalization, increases cell proliferation and supports development of the malignant cell (Spitz, et al., 2000). In the initial steps of carcinogenesis, a relatively prooxidant intracellular environment is developed and entails the mutation of tumor suppression genes and the activation of the oncogenes. Thus, the loss of normal redox control in cell growth and development occurs (Blackburn, et al., 1999).

Oxidative stress in the brain is known to increase the glutamate release in the hippocampus, and this affects ionic homeostasis and neurotransmission (Costa, 2004). The glutamate receptors are activated subsequently so acidification occurs in neurons because of Ca^{2+} entry and this can be associated with the death of central neurons (Reynolds & Hastings, 1995; Bellisimo, et al., 2001). This countenance can be altered by increased ROS production or decreased intracellular antioxidant defense systems (Tejada, et al., 2006).

Studies have been done to evaluate antioxidant enzyme activities in different types of brain tumors. However, most studies have emphasized decreased levels of antioxidant enzymes and vitamins in diverse malignancies (Rao, et al., 2000; Manju, et al., 2002; Gromadzinska, et al., 2003) but still the results are inconsistent (Hennekens, et al., 1996).

2.1. Mitochondrial changes in tumor cells

Mitochondrial DNA is more vulnerable to mutation when compared with nuclear DNA. Conversely to nuclear DNA, mitochondrial DNA is in close proximity to the electron transport system where ROS are produced, and it doesn't have any protective histones and chromatin structure, also its repair capabilities are limited, and it doesn't have any introns (Copeland, et al., 2002). Many studies have established mitochondrial DNA changes in different cancer types related to these features (Lu, et al., 1992; Savre-Train, et al., 1992; Polyak, et al., 1998; Modica, et al., 2002; Modica, et al., 2007). Cancer specific mitochondrial DNA mutations have been identified. Recent studies, associating the alterations in mitochondrial DNA and cancer risk, suggest mitochondrial DNA changes during cancer development are more complicated than estimated (Ebner, et al., 2011; Lam, et al. 2012).

Mitochondria are highly prospered with antioxidants such as GSH and antioxidant enzymes such as superoxide dismutase and GPx, which exist on both sides of their membranes to minimise oxidative stress in the organelle because mitochondria are the major zone of free radical generation (Cadenas & Davies, 2000). Superoxide radicals are ascendantly detoxified into hydrogen peroxide and into water by Cu/ZnSOD and MnSOD. The redox components of the cell comprises mitochondrial redox indicators which are glutathione (GSH/GSSG), thioredoxin (Trx/TrxR), glutaredoxin (Grx) and peroxiredoxin (Prx) systems dependent merely on NADPH generation via reduction of $NADP^+$ by mitochondria.

In some apparent cases, when mitochondrial oxidative stress increases, over generation of the antioxidant defences above a certain threshold may lead to cell death. In normal cells, the same process would take longer to happen as mitochondrial oxidative stress would be in basal levels and lower. Indeed, most of the anti tumor agents are known to act as prooxidant agents and they disturb the mitochondrial respiratory chain and this leads to an increase in mitochondrial oxidative stress levels (Chou, et al., 2004).

Relying on glycolysis other than oxidative phosphorylation for glucose oxidation and enhanced usage of glutamine as an energy source are the the two common metabolic reprogramming processes in cancer. Excessive upregulation in glutamine consumption is seen in tumor cells which is a second shift in energy metabolism (Barbosa, et al., 2012). Mitochondria are the the main energy producers via oxidative phosphorylation in normal cells and they produce various metabolic intermediates, and they mediate various apoptotic pathways (Weinberg & Chandel, 2009). Mitochondria exhibits same essential roles in cancer cells, too. Though, mitochondria undergo massive changes during oncogenesis, and this mostly result with a change in the energy metabolism, a resistance to apoptosis and enhanced ROS production.

Because the cancer cells have different metabolic and mitochondrial needs other than their normal counterparts, metabolic and mitochondrial changes in cancer cells may suggest an efficient and selective anti cancer therapy opportunity. This fact can be taken into consideration when targeting tumor mitochondria in terms of therapy.

3. Antioxidant defence systems

ROS are detoxified by exhaustive antioxidant defence systems. When the balance between ROS and antioxidant status is disturbed, cellular defences can be reeled causing an abnormal cell growth and this leads in turn to tumor cell forming (Wang, et al., 2011). Mammalian cells have developed a number of antioxidant defense systems to withstand the detrimental effects of ROS and they protect against cellular oxidative damage (Aoyama, et al., 2008). Antioxidants comprise of a highly heterogeneous group. They involve water or lipid soluble low molecular weight substances and enzymes such as CAT, SOD, GPx and GR. Also, a number of endogenous metabolites have antioxidant activities (Table 1).

Superoxide dismutase enzyme decomposes superoxide radicals into H_2O_2 and O_2. The most important H_2O_2 scavenging enzymes and concerned proteins having antioxidant capacity comprise CAT, GPx, GR enzymes associated with the synthesis of reduced GSH (Halliwell & Gutteridge, 1996) and a group of cysteine containing proteins known as thioredoxins, thioredoxin peroxidases (peroxiredoxins), and glutaredoxins (Kumar & Holmgren, 1999; Rhee, et al., 1999; Powis, et al., 2000; Holmgren, 2000). When ROS production is enhanced, the antioxidant scavenging capacity is disturbed and this results in the development of oxidative stress which leads to tissue injury and apoptosis activation (Todorova, et al., 2004).

GSH is a low molecular weight thiol and it has a key role in maintaining the intracellular redox balance. Cellular glutathione appears mainly in the reduced form as GSH, while some of the total GSH exists in its oxidized disulfide form as GSSG. Depletion of

GSH and an eventual decrease in the GSH/GSSG ratio may be seen in oxidizing conditions, yet peroxidise coupled reactions can mediate its antioxidant activity. GSH also amends signaling pathways and some cellular events. In oxidative stress, GSH is depleted hereby the GSH pool is affected (Dickinson & Forman, 2002; Circu & Aw, 2008; Biswas & Rahman, 2009; Forman et al., 2009; Yuan & Kaplowitz, 2009).

ANTIOXIDANTS

Enzymatic antioxidants

Superoxide dismutase (SOD)
Catalase (CAT)
Glutathione peroxidase (GPx)
Glutathione reductase (GR)
Glutathione-S-transferase (GST)

Non-enzymatic antioxidants

Vitamin E	Flavonoids	Albumin	Haptoglobin
Vitamin C	Melatonin	Glutathione	Ceruloplasmin
Vitamin A	Uric acid	Ubiquinone	Transferrin
α-Lipoic acid	Bilirubin	Selenium	Lactoferrin

Table 1. Antioxidants

Vitamin E, vitamin C and carotenoids can be defined as traditional antioxidant nutrients when consumed with diet, also they have antioxidant and anti inflammatory properties along with multiple other bioactive phytochemicals. The phytochemicals that includes phenolic acids and their derivatives, flavonoids and different types of coumarins and tannins consist of a large and heterogeneous group (Liu, 2004).

The phenolic compounds have recently been attracting attention conversely to antioxidant vitamins and carotenoids (Gescher, et al., 2001) and still most have not been tested in placebo controlled cancer prevention strudies. Curcumin, a phenolic acid derivative obtained from the spice turmeric; resveratrol, a polyhydroxylated stilbene found in grapes ; and genistein, an isoflavone readily isolated from soy have been pointed out for future studies (Gullet, et al., 2010). These compounds are known to have antioxidant and anti inflammatory features (Djuric, et al., 2001; Leu, et al., 2006; Brisdelli, et al., 2009), and they are implied as promising in cancer prevention depending on in vitro and in vivo animal experiments (Sarkar, et al., 2006; Sarkar, et al., 2010; Kelkel, et al., 2010; Patel, et al., 2010; Slusarz, et al., 2010). Resveratrol; having a hydroxylated structure, is a well identified antioxidant. It can act both as free radical scavenger and as metal chelator. Moreover, it also amends many enzymes in the regulation of redox status which are CAT, SOD, GR, NADPH oxidase, xanthine oxidase and (Delmas et al., 2005; Pervaiz & Holme, 2009). Flavonoids are polyphenols and isoflavones and anthocyanidines as the subclasses of flavonoids. They have a strong antioxidant activity because of their free radical scavenging and metal chelating features, also they can interact with enzymatic and non enzymatic mechanisms of the regulation of redox status (Heim et al., 2002; Laguerre et al., 2007; Aron & Kennedy, 2008) (Fig.2).

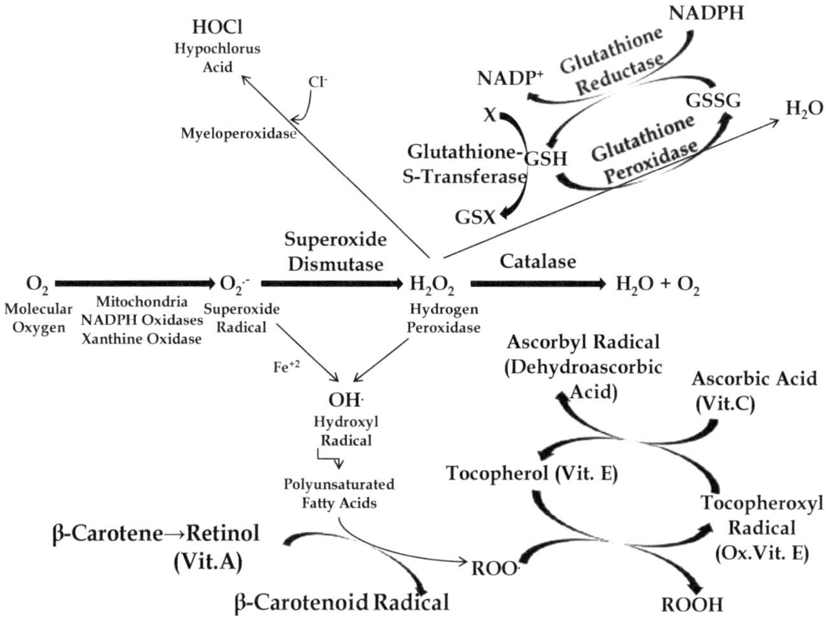

Figure 2. Antioxidant defence systems

Antioxidant molecules has been known as also beneficial in the induction of endogenous protective antioxidant enzymes and in the modulation of various of cellular signaling pathways (Valko et al., 2007). They can quickly oxidize spontaneously or induced by the biological microenvironment.

Antioxidant enzymes can antagonize initiation and promotion steps of carcinogenesis and they are reduced in cancer. Mitochondrial Mn-SOD is the most frequently decreasing enzyme and this suggests that MnSOD may be a new type of tumour suppressor gene. On the other hand, studies also suggest that the deficiency of the MnSOD enzyme activity depends on a defect in the expression of the related gene. Transition metal ions such as Mn and Fe have been found to be significantly lower in some tumours. It can be thought that, an impairment in the signal transduction may cause the defect in the MnSOD gene expression in the early stage of carcinogenesis (Mates, et al., 2000).

Studies are present implying low antioxidant status and enhanced oxidative stress in cancer patients, even before chemotherapy starts. Low activities of Cu, Zn-SOD, MnSOD, CAT, and GPx are shown in different types of tumor cells when compared with their normal counterparts (Sykes, et al., 1978). Some studies show that administration of antineoplastic agents during cancer therapy results in a higher level of oxidative stress rather than the stress induced by cancer itself (Conklin, 2000). Chemotherapeutic agents are thought to cause increase in ROS generation by affecting mitochondrial respiration chain (Carew, et al., 2003; Pelicano, et al., 2003).

In chemotherapy, an increase in lipid peroxidation products and a significant decrease in some plasma antioxidants such as Vitamin E, Vitamin C and carotenes are shown (Jeanne, et al., 2003). The increase in oxidative stress during chemotherapy may exceed the oxidative defense in cancer cells and this may initiate lipid peroxidation. Enhanced lipid peroxidation inhibits cancer cell proliferation and intervenes chemotherapy. Thus, the antioxidant status in cancer may play an important role in response to chemotherapy (Papageorgiou, et al., 2005).

3.1. Antioxidant status of the brain

Tumor cells frequently demonstrate a change in redox status. The alterations in the redox environment enhancing oxidation can induce some of the factors that cause cell proliferation and malignant transformation.

Elevated MnSOD levels were shown in the serum samples of neuroblastoma patients in a study (Kawamura, et al., 1992). In recent studies, MnSOD was found to be associated with loss of differentiation and increased clinical malignancy in neuroepithelial origined brain tumors (Landriscina, et al., 1996; Ria, et al., 2001). MnSOD was found significantly positive in Grade IV astrocytomas and medulloblastomas and negative in normal brain samples (Cobbs, et al., 1996). It can be said that MnSOD is overexpressed in most brain tumor types and enhanced MnSOD expression is related with a poor prognosis. MnSOD seems to be a tumor suppressor in the proliferative stage. When tumor progresses more aggressive, MnSOD is upregulated. MnSOD level positively correlates with increased metastasis so MnSOD has an oncogene role (Hempel, et al., 2011; Dhar, et al., 2011). Increase in MnSOD level was seen during the progression of different types of tumors, including brain, to the metastatic stage. Tumorigenesis and metastasis are dependent on the levels of ROS. A cell having low levels of MnSOD is vulnerable to oxidative stress then it may turn its progression to a tumor cell (Miriyala, et al., 2012). Oxidative gene polymorphism and brain tumor risk seems associated, the increased risk of glioma and meningioma type brain tumors were found to be related with variants in some antioxidant enzyme genes (Rajaraman et al., 2008) and in a study, MnSOD tissue expression is said to be a prognostic marker for glioblastoma (Park et al., 2009). SOD and GPx activities showed a clear decrease proportionally with tumor malignancy, decrease of SOD activity with the increasing grades of malignancy in brain tumors were implied.

The GSH redox cycle is one of the most important antioxidative systems (Arrick & Nathan, 1984; Mitchell, et al., 1989; Tedeschi, et al., 1990). GSH is a primary endogenous neuroprotectant for the brain. GSH protects neuron cells from lipid peroxidation and brain cells from peroxynitrite mediated oxidative damage (Mark et al., 1997; Koppal et al., 1999). GSH, also has roles in the activation of transcription factors, DNA repair, regulation of enzyme activity and many other metabolic processes (Meister, 1995). GSH synthesis, usage and export are the processes on which GSH homeostasis is dependent in glial and neuronal cells (Anderson, 1998). The main path for chemotherapy metabolism is through the conjugation of the xenobiotic with GSH. The removal of the GSH conjugates from the cell causes cellular GSH depletion and cellular redox balance disruption.

GSH content depends on the substrate availability in the brain and cysteine is the rate limiting substrate for neuronal GSH biosynthesis (Dringen, et al., 1999). Astrocytes provide neighbour cells the needed precursor amino acids for GSH synthesis (Hirrlinger, et al., 2010). GSSG levels and the GSH/GSSG ratios can be restored through the GR mediated pathway and flow of GSSG leaded by ATP dependent multi drug resistance-associated protein-1 (Mrp1) transporter in astrocytes and neurons (Hirrlinger, et al., 2001; Casagrande, et al., 2002; Minich, et al., 2006). Cultured astrocytes have high levels of reduced GSH (Dringen & Hamprecht, 1998) while oligodendrocyte precursors have high levels of iron but lower levels of cellular GSH when compared with astrocytes or neurons (Hussain & Juurlink, 1995; Thornburne & Juurlink, 1996), also oligodendrocyte precursors are more sensitive to oxidative stress induced death in relation to GSH depletion (Back, et al., 1998). The GSH neutralization system has been shown also in the chemoresistance of medulloblastoma (Colvin, et al., 1993). GSH and GST are prevalantly seen in brain tissue, thus highly expressed in various primary brain tumors (Bredel, 2001). GSH content and GST expression was shown to be related to tumor response to nitrogen mustard therapy in human brain neoplasms (Evans, 1993). Also in another study it was indicated that the cytotoxic effect of BCNU in human brain tumor cells seems associated with the GSH content (Ali-Osman, et al., 1989). When GST isoenzymes in neoplastic and non-neoplastic astroglia were compared, GST3 isoenzyme was seen to be significantly higher in tumors (Strange, et al., 1992). It is said that GST expression levels in brain tumors seems in association with the tumor histology as some tumor types express enhanced levels but some show only slight rise or decrease when compared to normal cells (Bredel, 2001). GST was found to be active in high levels in benign tumors such as meningioma but only two, three folds higher compared to normal tissue but it was slightly increased in astrocytoma (Matsumoto, et al., 1992). In glioblastomas, GSH levels were found significantly lowered compared to normal tissue and merely elevated in meningioma (Kudo, et al., 1990).

It has been reported that elevation of intracellular GSH in tumour cells is associated with mitogenic stimulation (Shaw & Chou, 1986), that GSH controls the onset of tumour-cell proliferation by regulating protein kinase C activity and intracellular pH (Terradez et al., 1993). GPx and GR decrease and protein oxidation increases in patients with glioblastoma multiforme and transitional meningioma and clear different oxidative status was found in the two kinds of tumors which represent specially one of the most malignant and most benign tumors respectively (Tanriverdi et al., 2007) and it was shown that there is a complex relationship between pro- and anti-apoptotic molecules in glioblastoma multiforme pathogenesis, thus targeting multiple pathways with advanced chemotherapeutic agents or radiotheraupetic regimens following total resections might be helpful in patients with glioblastoma multiforme (Atukeren et al., 2010).

Antioxidant enzymes activity and concentration of nonenzymatic antioxidants in human brain tumours were evaluated and significant increases in all enzyme activities and decreases in GSH and ascorbate levels were observed in brain tumors (Dudek et al., 2004) and consistent differences in the levels of antioxidants in different types of brain tumors were emphasized in different studies (Hanimoglu et al., 2007; Tanriverdi et al., 2007; Tuzgen et al., 2007; Zengin et al., 2009).

Serum β-carotene and α-tocopherol levels were found to be decreased in brain tumor patients when compared to healthy subjects and also more less in malign tumors than the benign types (Potishman, et al., 1991; Zheng, et al, 1993; Palan, et al., 1996). Few studies have been done to compare the levels of these antioxidants in various histological types of brain tumors. It was seen that β-carotene and α-tocopherol levels decreases when malignancy grade increases and the decrease was found significant for oligodendroglioma grade I-II, glioblastoma multiforme and medulloblastoma. The protective antioxidant effects of these two vitamins are suggested (Brigelius–Flohe, et al., 2002). The decreased antioxidant levels in brain tumor patients reflect the enhanced oxidative damage and increased cancer developing possibility, stating the role of antioxidants in cancer prevention and role of oxidative injury as the of cancer (Aggarwal, et al., 2006).

4. The potential therapy in brain tumors regarding antioxidants

Antioxidant consumption is appraised if it can be a pledging therapeutic approach in preventing or minimizing neuronal oxidative damage (Halliwell, 2001; Uttara et al., 2009). A relationship between excessive antioxidant consumption or high blood levels and a low cancer incidence was found in many studies (Comstock, et al., 1992; Van den Brant, et al., 1992). Also the importance of exogenous utilization of antioxidants with malignant glioma was shown in various studies (Il'yasova et al., 2009; DeLorenze et al., 2010) yet antioxidant supplementation by cancer patients during treatment is quite contentious. Indeed, a distinct declination or recommendation for the simultaneous use of antioxidants with chemotherapy has not been verified currently. The prospective antioxidant therapeutic approaches should involve either inhibiting the ROS generation or scavenging. Recently, new strategies for antioxidant consumption have been studied carefully in order to maximize the influence and safety by improving drug release and site specific targeting and to limit the adverse effects (Ratnam, et al., 2006). Cancer cells' having a a weak antioxidant defense system against oxidative stress brings about a theoretical basis for the use of ROS generating systems in treatment (Laurent, et al., 2005). Knowing that ROS have stimulating effects on tumor metastasis, the scavenging of ROS is also a reasonable strategy to inhibit metastasis (Nishikawa, et al., 2006). Main strategies as a potential treatment are the inhibition of the antioxidant enzymes and molecules in cancer cells and the production of ROS leading to apoptosis (Lopez-Lazaro, 2007; McCarty, et al., 2007). Recent studies involving ROS producing agents implied that their anti cancer and cytotoxic effects are limited to cancer cells and no toxicity was seen in the surrounding normal tissue (Yoshikawa, et al., 1995). The main mechanism of most chemotherapy drugs is via ROS formation, but also free radicals production during chemotherapy is a serious side effects (Block, et al., 2008). Interactions between chemotherapeutic compounds and antioxidants are quite complicated and also the dose, the localization and the metabolism of the drug have different effects. Furthermore, some antioxidants may act as oxidative molecules related with their relative concentration (Badajatia, et al., 2010).

The coexpression of catalase was shown to revert malignancy (Hempel, et al., 2011). The overexpression of catalase protected cancer cell from excessive peroxide production as a result of combined menadione/ascorbate anticancer treatment (Glorieux, et al., 2011). Also, the ability of ascorbate to radiosensitize primary human glioblastoma cells and mouse astrocytes and astrocytoma, was investigated and it was concluded that pharmacological concentrations of ascorbate radiosensitize glioblastoma primary cells more than astrocytes and this can be of clinical significance in therapeutic approach (Herst, et al., 2012). Besides, the activation of ferroptosis was shown to be resulted in the nonapoptotic destruction of some cancer cells and inhibiting this process by ferrostatin-1 seems to protect from neurodegeneration (Dixon, et al., 2012).

4.1. Targeting GSH pathway

GSH and the GSH related enzyme system might be a distinctive factor for the susceptibility of several brain tumors to different chemotherapeutic agents (Backos, et al., 2012). Studies have shown that drug resistance mediated by the GSH/GST system mediated drug resistance in brain tumors might be the outcome of a change in a GSH related enzyme system and increased GSH level (Ali-Osman, et al., 1989; Freidman, et al., 1992). Chemotherapeutics, thereby chemoresistance, were shown to be related with increased cellular GSH content in brain tumor cell lines (Ali-Osman, et al., 1989; Ali-Osman, et al., 1990). The increased GSH content is related with tumor drug resistantance so exhaustion of cellular GSH can restore the sensitivity to the cytotoxic effect of an anticancer agent (Barbosa, et al., 2012). So, it can be suggested that the depletion of GSH content may increase the sensitivity to different chemotherapeutics. The multidrug resistance-associated proteins (Mrp) can function as GSH, GSSG and GSH conjugate carrier (Jedlitschky, et al., 1994; Muller, et al., 1994). Expelling these drug metabolites conjugated with GSH ; changes the intracellular GSH levels distinctly. Mrps are considered to have a role in resistance development to chemotherapeutics in most human brain tumors (Bredel & Zentner, 2002). Mrp overexpression is associated with drug resistance in gliomas (Abe, et al., 1998) and conversely with clinical outcome in neuroblastoma (Norris, et al., 1996). Astrocytes have a potent GSH biosynthesis and antioxidant coupling is substantial in sustaining neuronal GSH status and conserving neurons from ROS (Dringen R & Hirrlinger, 2003). Even the concerned GST polymorphisms have been found to be associated with the survival (Kilburn, et al., 2010), decreased GSH levels seems to play an important role in the increased sensitivity of oligodendrogliomas to chemotherapy due to decreased GSH needed for detoxification. The elevated iron levels in these cells also makes them daintily exquisite to ROS generation based on chemotherapeutics (Yonezawa, et al., 1996). In a study, alantolactone which inhibits tumor growth and triggers apoptosis and GSH depletion in glioblastoma, is suggested as a potential lead compound for antiglioma therapy (Khan, et al., 2012).

4.2. Targeting mitochondria

Cancer cells have distinct metabolic and mitochondrial needs from their normal counterparts so mitochondrial alterations in the context of metabolic reprogramming are an appealing target for different therapeutic approaches. Most anti tumor agents act as prooxidants and they disturb mitochondrial respiratory chain and enhance mitochondrial oxidative stress (Chou, et al., 2004). Considering that ROS have a role in activating signaling pathways thereby guiding to metabolic remodeling; mitochondrial oriented antioxidants involving MitoQ may donate to normalizing the metabolic phenotype in cancer cells. This antioxidant molecule has already been indicated to diminish the hypoxic stimulation of ROS and to impair HIF-1alpha protein by decreasing its transcriptional activity (Sanjuan-Pla, et al., 2005).

Occasionally, overloading the antioxidant system by increasing mitochondrial oxidative stress over a certain threshold can be encountered leading to cell death. The same process would take longer to come up in normal cells because the basal mitochondrial oxidative stress would be lower. In a recent study, sulforaphane, having antioxidant and anti tumor features is suggested to provide antitumor activity in malignant glioma cells via mitochondria and caspase dependent pathways (Huang, et al., 2012).

4.3. Therapy via natural antioxidants

A great number of plants are good sources of phytochemical antioxidants and which have been estimated having cancer fighting ability (Wang, et al., 2011). There is a reasonable scientific and commercial interest in espialling new anti cancer molecules from natural sources, involving secondary plant metabolites (Kinghorn, et al., 2003). Phytochemical antioxidants existing in foods exhibit their anticancer properties via reducing ROS induced oxidative damage by either scavenging or by increasing endogenous antioxidants (Du, et al., 2007). Natural antioxidants have the ability to modulate signal transduction pathways by the activating or inhibiting multiple redox sensitive transcription factors which is asserted as their potential use as chemopreventive agents for therapy. They can act a part in initiation, promotion and progression stages of carcinogenesis to prevent cancer progress (Sporn, 1991).

Recently potential chemopreventive activities of dietary polyphenols was shown in most studies (Thomasset, et al., 2007). The effects of flavonoids being natural polyphenolic antioxidant compounds in brain development, neuroprotection and glial tumor formation are mentioned and developing new therapeutic approaches was discussed (Nones et al.; 2010). Epigallocatechin-3-gallate (EGCG) from green tea, curcumin from turmeric, and resveratrol from grapes are some examples of polyphenols.

Resveratrol has the ability to block the activation of carcinogens and induce their detoxification, thus to prevent ROS damage and alleviate inflammatory responses and to reduce the proliferation of cancer cells which reflect its chemopreventive property (Aggarwal, et al., 2004; Shankar, et al., 2007). The chemotherapeutic potential of resveratrol is refered to its blocking angiogenic and metastatic processes of tumor progression and relieving chemotherapy resistance (Aggarwal, et al., 2004; Fulda & Debatin, 2006). The potential therapeutic effect of resveratrol being a dietary phytochemical antioxidant, is investigated in glioma type brain tumors (Gangliano et al., 2010) and glioblastoma multiforme cells exhibited variable responses to resveratrol depending on the brain associated sulfonation activity of the cells and resveratrol seemed to have value in glioblastoma treatment (Sun, et al., 2012). Also the combination of resveratrol with alkylating agent temozolomide was shown to improve the efficacy of chemotherapy for brain tumors (Herst, et al., 2012). EGCG also exhibited the same effect with temozolomide like as resveratrol in another study, in brain tumor therapy (Chen, et al., 2011). Curcumin as a polyphenol gets attention in blocking brain tumor formation in a study. The chemopreventive and anticarcinogenic action of curcumin is shown and suggested as this might be due to its ability to inhibit proteins that initiate protective signals (Purkayastha, et al., 2009).

Different studies implied the importance of using nutritional antioxidants. Lycopene, present in tomato, was shown for its potential therapeutic benefit in the adjuvant management of high grade gliomas (Puri et al., 2010). Gynostemma pentaphyllum extract selectively shifted H_2O_2 concentration in glioma tumor cells to toxic levels due to increased SOD activity so can be suggested for cancer therapy (Schild et al., 2010) and the apoptotic effect of γ-Mangostin in Garcinia mangostana fruit was shown and it was suggested as a prospective anti brain tumor agent (Chang et al., 2010).

5. Conclusion

The incidence of brain tumors is obviously increasing recently. The occurance of ROS are the inevitable outcome of the metabolism and they have important roles in many biochemical processes but they must be precisely kept under control. Antioxidant molecules are that delay, prevent, or remove the existing oxidative damage to a target molecule. The brain is quite vulnerable to ROS damage because of its low antioxidant levels. To get over ROS damage, the brain needs a sufficient supply of antioxidants and it seems convinent that working up with ROS signaling pathways would provide a great neuroprotective effect. The development of the suitable antioxidant compounds seems a challenging and pledging strategy for brain tumor treatment but plenty of work has to be done to emphasize the exact role of antioxidants for therapy in clinical use.

Adjusting the antioxidant dose and scheduling of the administration or combining different antioxidants and exploring a more potent and specific antioxidant should be the main theme. Also the preventive and therapeutic molecule should target multiple biochemical pathways comprising the processes entailing malignancy and restrain the unwanted side effects and toxicity in the normal tissue counterparts. In the same time should attend a beneficial task in stimulating the therapeutic effect of chemotherapy and diminishing certain side effects. It is clear that there is a deficient evidence concerning the prospective antioxidant therapies in brain tumors. Regarding to the fact that there is little knowledge concerning complementary therapy with antioxidant molecules and their effects or side effects, there is a crucial need for further research of these treatment strategies.

Acknowledgements

We would like to dedicate this chapter to brain cancer patients.

Author details

Pinar Atukeren[1] and M. Ramazan Yigitoglu[2]

1 Istanbul University, Cerrahpasa Medical Faculty, Department of Biochemistry, Istanbul, Turkey

2 Turgut Ozal University, Medical Faculty, Department of Biochemistry, Ankara, Turkey

References

[1] Abe, T.; Mori, T.; Wakabayashi, Y.; Nakagawa, M.; Cole, SP; Koike, K; Kuwano, M. & Hori, S. (1998). Expression of multidrug resistance protein gene in patients with glioma after chemotherapy, *J. Neurooncol.*, Vol. 40, pp.11-8 1998;40:11–8

[2] Aggarwal, BB.; Bhardwaj, A.; Aggarwal, RS.; Seeram, NP.; Shishodia, S. & Takada, Y. (2004). Role of resveratrol in prevention and therapy of cancer: preclinical and clinical studies, *Anticancer Res.*, Vol. 24, pp. 2783–2840

[3] Aggarwal, S.; Subberwal, M.; Kumar, S. & Sharma. M. (2006). Brain tumor and role of ß-carotene, α- tocopherol, superoxide dismutase and glutathione peroxidase, *J. Cancer Res.*, Vol. 2(1), pp. 24-7

[4] Ali-Osman, F.; Caughlan, J. & Gray, GS. (1989). Decreased DNA interstrand cross-linking and cytotoxicity induced in human brain tumor cells by 1,3-bis(2-chloroethyl)-1-nitrosourea after in vitro reaction with glutathione, *Cancer Res.*, Vol. 49, pp.5954–8

[5] Ali-Osman, F.; Stein, DE. & Renwick A. (1990). Glutathione content and glutathione-S – transferase expression in 1,3-bis(2-chloroethyl)-1-nitrosourea-resistant human malignant astrocytoma cell lines, *Cancer Res.*, Vol. 50, pp. 6976–80

[6] Ames, BN. & Shigenaga, MK. (1992). Oxidants are a major contributor to aging, *Ann. NY Acad. Sci.*, Vol. 663, pp. 85–96

[7] Anderson ME. (1998). Glutathione: an overview of biosynthesis and modulation, *Chem. Biol. Interact.*, Vol.11, pp.1-112

[8] Aoyama, K.; Watabe, M. & Nakaki, T. (2008). Regulation of neuronal glutathione synthesis, *J. Pharmacol. Sci.*, Vol. 108, pp. 227–38

[9] Aron, P. M., & Kennedy, J. A. (2008). Flavan-3-ols: nature, occurrence and biological activity, *Mol. Nutr. Food Res.*, Vol. 52(1), pp.79–104

[10] Arrick, B. A. & Nathan, C. F. (1984). Glutathione metabolism as a determinant of therapeutic efficacy: a review, *Cancer Res.*, Vol. 44, pp. 4224-4232

[11] Atukeren, P.; Kemerdere, R.; Kacira, T.; Hanimoglu, H.; Ozlen, F.; Yavuz, B.; Tanriverdi, T.; Gumustas, K. & Canbaz, B. (2010). Expressions of some vital molecules: glioblastoma multiforme versus normal tissues, *Neurol Res.*, Vol.32, No.5, pp. 492-501

[12] Badajatia, N.; Satyam, A.; Singh P.; Seth, A. & Sharma, A. (2010). Altered antioxidant status and lipid peroxidation in Indian patients with urothelial bladder carcinoma, *Urol. Oncol.*, Vol. 28, pp. 360–7

[13] Back, SA.; Gan, X.; Li, Y.; Rosenberg, PA. & Volpe, JJ. (1998). Maturation-dependent vulnerability of oligodendrocytes to oxidative stress-induced death caused by glutathione depletion, *J. Neurosci.*, Vol.18, pp. 6241–53

[14] Backos, DS.; Franklin, CC. & Reigan, P. (2012). The role of glutathione in brain tumor drug resistance, *Biochemical Pharmacology*, Vol. 83, pp. 1005–1012

[15] Barbosa, IA.; Machado, NG.; Skildum, AJ.; Scott, PM. & Oliveira, OJ. (2012). Mitochondrial remodeling in cancer metabolism and survival: Potential for new therapies, *Biochimica et Biophysica Acta*, Vol. 1826, pp. 238–254

[16] Block, K.; Koch, A. & Mead, M. (2008). Impact of antioxidant supplementation on chemotherapeutic toxicity: A systematic review of the evidence from randomized controlled trials, *Int. J. Cancer*, Vol. 123, pp. 1227–39

[17] Bredel, M. & Zentner J. (2002). Brain-tumour drug resistance: the bare essentials, *Lancet Oncol.*, Vol. 3, pp. 397–406

[18] Behrend, L.; Henderson, G. & Zwacka, RM. (2003). Reactive oxygen species in oncogenic transformation, *Biochem. Soc. Trans.*, Vol. 31, pp. 1441–4

[19] Bellissimo, MI.; Amado, D.; Abdalla, DS.; Ferreira, EC., Cavalheiro, EA. & Naffah-Mazzacoratti, MG. (2001). Superoxide dismutase, glutathione peroxidase activities and the hydroperoxide concentration are modified in the hippocampus of epileptic rats, *Epilepsy Res.*, Vol. 46, pp. 121–128

[20] Biswas, S. K., & Rahman, I. (2009). Environmental toxicity, redox signalling and lung inflammation: the role of glutathione., *Mol. Aspects Med.*, Vol. 30(1–2), pp. 60–76

[21] Blackburn, R. V.; Spitz, D. R.; Liu, X.; Galoforo, S. S.; Sim, J. E.; Ridnour, L. A.; Chen, J. C.; Davis, B. H.; Corry, P. M.; Lee, Y. J. (1999). Metabolic oxidative stress activates signal transduction and gene expression during glucose deprivation in human tumor cells, *Free Radic. Biol. Med.*, Vol. 26, pp. 419– 430

[22] Bredel, M. (2001). Anticancer drug resistance in primary human brain tumors, *Brain Research Reviews*, Vol. 35, pp. 161–204

[23] Brigelius–Flohe, R.; Kelly, FJ. & Salonen, JT. (2002). The Europeon perspective on vitamin E: current knowledge and future research, *Am. J. Clin. Nutr.*, Vol. 76. pp. 703–16

[24] Brisdelli, F.; D'Andrea, G. & Bozzi, A.(2009). Resveratrol: a natural polyphenol with multiple chemopreventive properties, *Curr. Drug Metab.*, Vol. 10, pp. 530–546

[25] Burdon, RH. (1995). Superoxide and hydrogen peroxide in relation to mammalian cell proliferation, *Free Radic. Biol. Med.*, Vol. 18, pp. 775–794

[26] Cadenas, E. & Davies KJA. (2000). Mitochondrial free radical generation, oxidative stress, and aging, *Free Rad. Biol. Med.*, Vol. 29, pp. 222–230

[27] Carew, JS.; Zhou, Y.; Albitar, M.; Carew, JD.; Keating, MJ. & Huang P. (2003). Mitochondrial DNA mutations in primary leukemia cells afterchemotherapy: clinical significance and therapeutic implications, *Leukemia,* Vol. 17, pp 1437–47

[28] Casagrande, S.; Bonetto, V.; Fratelli, M.; Gianazza, E.; Eberini, I.; Massignan, T.; Salmona, M.; Chang, G.; Holmgren, A. & Grezzi, P. (2002). Glutathionylation of human thioredoxin: a possible crosstalk between the glutathione and thioredoxin systems, *Proc. Natl. Acad. Sci.*, Vol., 99, pp. 9745–9

[29] Castro, L. (2001). Reactive oxygen species in human health and disease, *Nutrition,* Vol. 17, pp. 161–5

[30] Chandra, J.; Samali, A. & Orrenius, S. (2000). Triggering and modulation of apoptosis by oxidative stress, *Free. Rad. Med. Biol.*, Vol.29, pp. 323–33

[31] Chang, HF.; Huang, WT.; Chen HJ. & Yang LL. (2010). Apoptotic Effects of γ-Mangostin from the Fruit Hull of Garcinia mangostana on Human Malignant Glioma Cells, *Molecules,* Vol. 7, No. 15(12), pp. 8953-66

[32] Chen, TC.; Wang, W.; Golden, EB.; Thomas, S.; Sivakumar, W.; Hofman, FM.; Louie, SG. & Schönthal, AH. (2011). Green tea epigallocatechin gallate enhances therapeutic efficacy of temozolomide in orthotopic mouse glioblastoma models, *Cancer Lett.,*Vol. 302(2), pp. 100-8

[33] Chou, WC.; Jie, C.; Kenedy, AA.; Jones, RJ.; Trush, MA. & Dang, CV. (2004). Role of NADPH oxidase in arsenic-induced reactive oxygen species formation and cytotoxicity in myeloid leukemia cells, *Proc. Natl. Acad. Sci.*, Vol. 101(13), pp. 4578-83

[34] Circu, M. L., & Aw, T. Y. (2008). Glutathione and apoptosis, Vol. 42(8), pp. 689–706

[35] Cobbs, CS.; Levi, DS.; Aldape, K. &Israel, MA. (1996). Manganese superoxide dismutase expression in human central nervous system tumors, *Cancer Res.,*Vol. 56, pp. 3192–3195

[36] Colvin, OM.; Friedman, HS.; Gamcsik, MP.; Fenselau, C. & Hilton J.(1993). Role of glutathione in cellular resistance to alkylating agents, *Adv. Enzyme Regul.,* Vol. 33, pp. 19–26

[37] Comstock, GW.; Bush, TL. & Helzlsouer, K. (1992). Serum retinol. beta-carotene, vitamin E and selenium as related to subsequent cancer of specific sites, *Am. J. Epidemiol.,* Vol. 135, pp. 115-121

[38] Conklin, KA. (2000). Dietary antioxidants during cancer chemotherapy: impact on chemotherapeutic effectiveness and development of side effects, *Nutr Cancer.,* Vol. 37, pp. 1–18

[39] Copeland, WC.; Wachsman, JT.; Johnson, FM. & J.S. Penta. (2002). Mitochondrial DNA alterations in cancer, *Cancer Invest.*, Vol. 20, pp.557–569

[40] Costa, MS.; Rocha, JB.; Perosa, SR.; Cavalheiro, EA. & Naffah-Mazzacoratt, G. (2004). Pilocarpine-induced status epilepticus increases glutamate release in rat hippocampal synaptosomes, *Neurosci. Lett.*, Vol. 356, pp. 41–44

[41] Dajas, F. (2012). Life or death:Neuroprotective and anti cancer effects of quercetin, *Journal of Ethnopharmacology*, Doi: 10.1016/j.jep.2012.07.005

[42] Dal-Pizzol, F.; Klamt, F.; Vianna, MM.; Schroder, N.; Quevedo, J.; Benfato, MS.; Moreira, JC. & Walz, R. (2000). Lipid peroxidation in hippocampus early and late after status epilepticus induced by pilocarpine or kainic acid in Wistar rats, *Neurosci. Lett.*, Vol. 291, pp. 179–182

[43] Dandona, P.; Cook, S.; Synder, B. & Makowski, J.(1996). Oxidative damage to DNA in diabeted mellitus, *Lancet*, Vol. 347, pp. 444–5

[44] Delmas, D., Jannin, B., & Latruffe, N. (2005). Resveratrol: preventing properties against vascular alterations and ageing. *Mol. Nutr. Food Res.*, Vol. 49(5), pp. 377–395

[45] DeLorenze, GN.; McCoy, L.; Tsai, AL.; Quesenberry, CP Jr.; Rice, T.; Il'yasova, D. & Wrensch M. (2010). Daily intake of antioxidants in relation to survival among adult patients diagnosed with malignant glioma, *BMC Cancer*, Vol.19, pp. 10-215

[46] Dhar, SK.; Tangpong, J.; Chaiswing, L.; Oberley, TD. & St Clair, DK. (2011). Manganese superoxide dismutase is a p53-regulated gene that switches cancers between early and advanced stages, *Cancer Res.*, Vol. 71, pp. 6684–6695

[47] Dickinson, D. A., & Forman, H. J. (2002). Cellular glutathione and thiols metabolism, *Biochem. Pharmacol.*, Vol. 64(5–6), pp. 1019–1026

[48] Dixon, SJ.; Lemberg, KM.; Lamprecht, MR.; Skouta, R.; Zaitsev, EM.; Gleason, CE.; Patel, DN; Bauer, AJ.; Cantley, AM.; Yang, WS.; Morrison, B 3rd. & Stockwell, BR. (2012). Ferroptosis: an iron-dependent form of nonapoptotic cell death, *Cell*, Vol. 25;149(5), pp. 1060-72

[49] Djuric, Z.; Chen, G.; Doerge, D. R.; Heilbrun, L. K. & Kucuk, O. (2001). Effect of soy isoflavone supplementation on markers of oxidative stress in men and women, *Cancer Lett.*, Vol. 172, pp. 1–6

[50] Dringen, R. & Hamprecht, B. (1998). Glutathione restoration as indicator for cellular metabolism of astroglial cells, *Dev. Neurosci.*, Vol. 20, pp. 401–7

[51] Dringen, R. & Hirrlinger J. (2003). Glutathione pathways in the brain, *Biol. Chem.*, Vol. 384, pp. 505–16

[52] Dringen, R.; Pfeiffer, B. & Hamprecht, B. (1999). Synthesis of the antioxidant glutathione in neurons: supply by astrocytes of CysGly as precursor for neuronal glutathione, *J. Neurosci.*, Vol. 19, pp. 562–9

[53] Du, Y., Guo, H., & Lou, H. (2007). Grape seed polyphenols protect cardiac cells from apoptosis via induction of endogenous antioxidant enzymes, *Journal of Agricultural and Food Chemistry*, Vol. 55, pp. 1695–1701

[54] Dudek, H.; Farbiszewski, R.; Rydzewska, M.; Michno, T. & Kozłowski A. (2004). Evaluation of antioxidant enzymes activity and concentration of non-enzymatic antioxidants in human brain tumours, *Wiad Lek.*, Vol. 57, No. 1-2, pp. 16-9

[55] Ebner, S.; Lang, R.; Mueller, EE.; Eder, W.; Oeller, M.; Moser, A.; Koller, J.; Paulweber, B.; Mayr, JA.; Sperl, W. & Kofler, B. (2011). Mitochondrial haplogroups, control region polymorphisms and malignant melanoma: a study in Middle European Caucasians, *PLoS One,* Vol 6(12), pp. e27192.

[56] Evans, VG. (1993). Multiple pathways to apoptosis, *Cell Biol. Int.,* Vol. 17, pp. 461–476

[57] Fang, J. & Iyer, AK. (2007). Tumor-targeted induction of oxystress for cancer therapy, *J. Drug Targ.,* Vol. 15, pp. 475–86

[58] Farber, JL.; Kyle, ME. & Coleman, JB. (1990). Mechanisms of cell injury by activated oxygen species, *Lab. Invest.* Vol. 62, pp. 670–9

[59] Farber, JL. (1994). Mechanism of cell injury by activated oxygen species, *Env. Health Perspect.,* Vol. 102, pp. 17–24

[60] Federico, A.; Tuccillo, C.; Ciardiello, F. & Loguercio, C. (2007). Chronic inflammation and oxidative stress in human carcinogenesis, *Int .J. Cancer,* Vol. 121, pp. 2381–6

[61] Floyd, RA. (1990). Role of oxygen free radicals in carcinogenesis and brain ischemia, *FASEB J.,* Vol. 4, pp. 2587–97

[62] Forman, H. J., Zhang, H., & Rinna, A. (2009). Glutathione: overview of its protective roles, measurement, and biosynthesis, *Mol. Aspects. Med.,* Vol. 30(1–2), pp. 1−12

[63] Friedman, HS.; Colvin, OM.; Kaufmann, SH.; Ludeman, SM.; Bullock, N.; Bigner, DD. & Griffith, OW. (1992). Cyclophosphamide resistance in medulloblastoma, *Cancer Res.,* Vol.52, pp. 5373–8

[64] Freitas, RM.; Nascimento, VS.; Vasconcelos, SM.; Sousa,FC.; Viana, GS. & Fonteles, MM. (2004). Catalase activity in cerebellum, hippocampus, frontal cortex and striatum after status epilepticus induced by pilocarpine in Wistar rats, *Neurosci. Lett.,* Vol. 365, pp. 102–105

[65] Fruehauf, JP. & Meyskens, FL. (2007). Reactive oxygen species: A breath of life or death?, *Clin. Cancer. Res.,* Vol. 13, pp. 789–94

[66] Fulda, S. & Debatin, KM. (2006). Resveratrol modulation of signal transduction in apoptosis and cell survival: a mini-review, *Cancer Detect. Prev.,* Vol. 30, pp. 217–223

[67] Gangliano, N; Aldini, G.; Colombo, G.; Rossi, R.; Colombo, R; Gioia, M.; Milzani, A.; & Dalle-Donne, I. (2010). The potential of resveratrol against human gliomas, *Anticancer Drugs.,* Vol.21, No.2, pp. 140-50

[68] Gate, L.; Paul, J.; Ba, GN.; Tew, KD. & Tapiero H. (1999). Oxidative stress induced in pathologies: the role of antioxidants. *Biomed. Pharmcother.,* Vol. 53, pp. 169–80

[69] Gescher, AJ.; Sharma, RA. & Steward, WP. (2001). Cancer chemoprevention by dietary constituents: a tale of failure and promise, *Lancet Oncol.,* Vol. 2, pp. 371–379

[70] Glorieux, C.; Dejeans, N.; Sid, B.; Beck, R.; Calderon, PB. & Verrax, J. (2011). Catalase overexpression in mammary cancer cells leads to a less aggressive phenotype and an altered response to chemotherapy, *Biochem. Pharmacol.,* Vol. 82, pp. 1384–1390

[71] Gromadzinska, J.; Wasowicz, W.; Rydzynski, K. & Szeszenia–Dabrowska, N. (2003). Oxidative stress markers in blood of lung cancer patients occupationally exposed to carcinogens, *Biol. Trace. Elem. Res.,* Vol. 91, pp. 203–15

[72] Gullett, N. P.; Ruhul Amin, A. R.; Bayraktar, S.; Pezzuto, J. M.; Shin, D. M.; Khuri, F. R.; Aggarwal, B. B.; Surh, Y. J. & Kucuk, O.(2010). Cancer prevention with natural compounds, *Semin. Oncol.,* Vol. 37, pp. 258–281

[73] Halliwell, B. (2001). Role of free radicals in the neurodegenerative diseases: therapeutic implications for antioxidant treatment, *Drugs Aging,* Vol. 18, No. 9, pp. 685-716

[74] Halliwell, B. & Gutteridge, JMC. (1996). Free radicals in biology and medicine. Oxford: Clarendon

[75] Hanimoglu, H.; Tanriverdi, T.; Kacira, T.; Sanus, GZ.; Atukeren, P.; Aydin, S.; Tunali, Y.; Gumustas, K. & Kaynar, MY. (2007). Relationship between DNA damage and total antioxidant capacity in patients with transitional meningioma, *Clin Neurol Neurosurg.,* Vol. 109, No. 7, pp. 561-6

[76] Heim, KE., Tagliaferro, AR., & Bobilya, D J. (2002). Flavonoid antioxidants: chemistry, metabolism and structure–activity relationships, *J. Nutr. Biochem.,* Vol. 13(10), pp. 572–584

[77] Hempel, N.; Carrico, PM. & Melendez, JA. (2011). Manganese superoxide dismutase (Sod2) and redox-control of signaling events that drive metastasis, *Anti-cancer Agents. Med. Chem.,* Vol. 11, pp. 191–201

[78] Hennekens, CH.; Buring, JE.; Manson, JE.; Stsmpfer, M. & Rosner, B. (1996). Lack of effect of long term supplementation with β–carotene on the incidence of malignant neoplasms and cardiovascular disease, *N. Eng. J. Med.,* Vol., 334, pp. 1145–9

[79] Herst, PM.; Broadley, KW.; Harper, JL.; McConnell, MJ. (2012). Pharmacological concentrations of ascorbate radiosensitize glioblastoma multiforme primary cells by increasing oxidative DNA damage and inhibiting G2/M arrest, *Free Radic. Biol. Med.,*Vol.52(8), pp. 1486-93

[80] Hirrlinger, J. & Dringen R. (2010). The cytosolic redox state of astrocytes: maintenance, regulation and functional implications for metabolite trafficking, *Brain Res. Rev.,* Vol. 63, pp. 177–88

[81] Hirrlinger, J.; Konig, J.; Keppler, D.; Lindenau, J.; Schulz, JB. & Dringen, R. (2001). The multidrug resistance protein MRP1 mediates the release of glutathione disulfide from rat astrocytes during oxidative stress, *J. Neurochem.*, Vol., 76, pp. 627–36

[82] Holmgren, A. (2000). Antioxidant function of thioredoxin and glutaredoxin systems, *Antioxid. Redox Signaling,* Vol. 2, pp. 811– 820

[83] Huang, TY., Chang, WC.; Wang, MY.; Yang, YR. & Hsu, YC. (2012). Effect of sulforaphane on growth inhibition in human brain malignant glioma GBM 8401 cells by means of mitochondrial- and MEK/ERK-mediated apoptosis pathway, *Cell Biochem. Biophys.,* Vol. 63(3), pp. 247-59

[84] Husain, J. & Juurlink, BH. (1995). Oligodendroglial precursor cell susceptibility to hypoxia is related to poor ability to cope with reactive oxygen species, *Brain Res.,* Vol. 698, pp. 86–94

[85] Hussain, S.; Slikker, Jr W. & Ali, SF. (1995). Age-related changes in antioxidant enzymes, superoxide dismutase, catalase, glutathione peroxidase and glutathione in different regions of mouse brain, *Int. J. Dev. Neurosci.,* Vol. 13, pp. 811- 817

[86] Il'yasova, D.; Marcello, JE.; McCoy, L.; Rice, T. & Wrensch, M. (2009). Total dietary antioxidant index and survival in patients with glioblastoma multiforme, *Cancer Causes Control,* Vol.20, No. 8, pp. 1255-60

[87] Imlay, JA. (1988). DNA damage and oxygen radical toxicity. *Science*, (New York, NY), Vol. 240, pp. 1302–9

[88] Jeanne, A.; Drisko, JA.; Chapman, J. & Hunter, VJ. (2003). The use of antioxidant therapies during chemotherapy, *Gynecol. Oncol.,* Vol. 88, pp. 434–9

[89] Jedlitschky, G.; Leier, I.; Buchholz, U.; Center, M. & Keppler D. (1994). ATP-dependent transport of glutathione S-conjugates by the multidrug resistance-associated protein, *Cancer Res.,* Vol. 54, pp. 4833–6

[90] Jenner P. (1994).Oxidative damage in neurodegenerative diseases, *Lancet,* Vol.344, pp. 796–8

[91] Kawamura, N.; Suzuki, K.; Ishikawa, M.; Iizuka, S.; Miyake, M.; Mino, M. & Taniguchi, N. (1992). High levels of Mn-superoxide dismutase in serum of patients with neuroblastoma and in human neuroblastoma cell lines, *Free Radic. Biol. Med,* Vol. 12, pp. 281–286

[92] Kelkel, M.; Jacob, C.; Dicato, M. & Diederich, M. (2010). Potential of the dietary antioxidants resveratrol and curcumin in prevention and treatment of hematologic malignancies, *Molecules,* Vol. 15, pp. 7035–7074

[93] Khan, M.; Yi, F.; Rasul, A.; Li, T.; Wang, N.; Gao, H.; Gao, R. & Ma, T. (2012). Alantolactone induces apoptosis in glioblastoma cells via GSH depletion, ROS generation, and mitochondrial dysfunction, *IUBMB Life.,*Vol. 64(9), pp. 783-94

[94] Kilburn, L.; Okcu, MF.; Wang, T.; Cao, Y.; Renfro-Spelman, A.; Aldape, KD.; Gilbert, MR. & Bondy, M. (2010). Glutathione S-transferase polymorphisms are associated with survival in anaplastic glioma patients, *Cancer,* Vol. 116, pp. 2242–9

[95] Kinghorn, AD.; Farnsworth, NR.; Soejarto, DD.; Cordell, GA.; Swanson, SM.; Pezzuto, JM.;Wani, MC.; Wall, ME.; Oberlies, NH.; Kroll, DJ.; Kramer, RA.; Rose, WC.; Vite, GD.; Fiarchild, CR.; Peterson, RW. & Wild, R. (2003). Novel strategies for the discovery of plant-derived anticancer agents, *Pharmaceut. Biol.,* Vol. 41, pp. 53–67

[96] Koppal, T.; Drake, J. & Butterfield, DA. (1999). In vivo modulation of rodent glutathione and its role in peroxynitrite-induced neocortical synaptosomal membrane protein damage, *Biochim. Biophys. Acta,* Vol. 1453, pp. 407–411

[97] Kryston, TB.; Georgiev, AB.; Pissis, P. & Georgakilas, AG. (2011). Role of oxidative stress and DNA damage in human carcinogenesis, *Mutat. Res.,* Vol. 711, pp. 193–201

[98] Kudo, H.; Mio, T.; Kokunai, T.; Tamaki, N.; Sumino, K. & Matsumoto, S. (1990). Qunatitative analysis of glutathione in human brain tumors, *J. Neurosurg.,* Vol. 72, pp. 610–615

[99] Kumar, S. & Holmgren, A. (1999). Induction of thioredoxin, thioredoxin reductase and glutaredoxin activity in mouse skin by TPA, a calcium ionophore and other tumor promoters, *Carcinogenesis,* Vol. 20, pp. 1761– 1767

[100] Kuo, KW.; Chen, SF.; Wu, CC.; Chen, DR. & Lee, JH. (2002). Serum and tissue trace elements in patients with breast cancer in Taiwan, *Biol. Trace Elem. Res.,* Vol. 89, pp. 1–11

[101] Laguerre, M., Lecomte, J., & Villeneuve, P. (2007). Evaluation of the ability of antioxidants to counteract lipid oxidation: existing methods, new trends and challenges, *Prog. Lipid Res.,* Vol. 46(5), pp. 244–282

[102] Lam, ET.; Bracci, PM.; Holly, EA.; Chu, C.; Poon, A.; Wan, E.; White, K.; Kwok, PY.; Pawlikowska, L. & Tranah, GJ. (2012). Mitochondrial DNA sequence variation and risk of pancreatic cancer, *Cancer Res.,* Vol. 72, pp. 686–695

[103] Landriscina, M.; Remiddi, F.; Ria, F.; Palazzotti, B.; De Leo, M. E.; Iacoangeli, M.; Rosselli, R.; Scerrati, M. & Galeotti, T. (1996). The level of MnSOD is directly correlated with grade of brain tumours of neuroepithelial origin, *Br. J. Cancer,* Vol. 74, pp. 1877–1885

[104] Laurent, A.; Nicco, C.; Chereau, C.; Goulvestre, C.; Alexandre, J.; Alves, A.; Levy, E.; Goldwasser, F.; Panis,Y.; Soubrane, O.; Weill, B. & Batteux, F. (2005). Controlling tumor growth by modulating endogenous production of reactive oxygen species, *Cancer Res.,* Vol. 65, pp 948–956

[105] Leu, T. H. & Maa, MC. (2002). The molecular mechanisms for the antitumorigenic effect of curcumin, *Curr. Med. Chem. Anticancer Agents,* Vol. 2, pp. 357–370

[106] Li, JJ.; Fan, M. & Colburn, NH. (1998). Inhibition of AP-1 and NF-kappa B by manganese-containing superoxide dismutase in human breast cancer cells, *FASEB J.*, Vol. 12, pp. 1713–23

[107] Lin, CJ.; Lee, CC.; Shih, YL.; Lin, TY.; Wang, SH.; Lin, YF. & Shih, CM. (2012). Resveratrol enhances the therapeutic effect of temozolomide against malignant glioma in vitro and in vivo by inhibiting autophagy, *Free Radic. Biol. Med.,*Vol. 52(2), pp. 377-91

[108] Liu, RH. (2004). Potential synergy of phytochemicals in cancer prevention: mechanism of action, *J. Nutr.,* Vol. 134, 3479S–3485S.

[109] Liou, GY. & Storz, P. (2010). Reactive oxygen species in cancer, *Free. Radic. Res.,* Vol. 44, 479–496

[110] Lopez-Lazaro, M. (2007). Dual role of hydrogen peroxide in cancer: Possible relevance to cancer chemoprevention and therapy, *Cancer Lett.,* Vol. 252, pp. 1–8

[111] Lu, X.; Walker, T.; MacManus, JP. & Seligy, VL. (1992). Differentiation of HT-29 human colonic adenocarcinoma cells correlates with increased expression of mitochondrial RNA:effects on trehalose on cell growth and maturation. *Cancer Res.,* Vol. 52(13), pp. 3718-25

[112] Manju, V.; Kalaivani Sailaja J. & Nalini N. (2002). Circulating lipid peroxidation and antioxidant status in cervical cancer patients:a case–control study, *Clin. Biochem.,* Vol. 35, pp. 621–5

[113] Mark, RJ.; Lovell, M.; Markesbery, WR.; Uchida, K. & Mattson, MP. (1997). A role for 4- hydroxynonenal, an aldehydic product of lipid peroxidation, in disruption of ion homeostasis and neuronal death induced by amyloid beta-peptide, *J. Neurochem.,* Vol. 68, pp. 255–264

[114] Mates, JM. & Sanchez-Jimenez, FM. (2000). Role of reactive oxygen species in apoptosis: implications for cancer therapy, *The International Journal of Biochemistry & Cell Biology,* Vol. 32, pp. 157-170

[115] Matsumoto, Y.; Sasaoka, N.; Tsuchida, T.; Fujiwara, T. & Nagao, S. (1992). Quantitative analysis of glutathione and glutathione *S*-transferase in human brain tumors, C6 rat glioma cells and drug resistant C6 cells, *No Shinkei Geka,* Vol. 20, pp. 1069–1074

[116] McCarty, MF.; Barraso-Aranda, J. & Contreras, F. (2007). A two phase strategy for treatment of oxidant dependent cancers, *Med. Hypothesis,* Vol. 69, pp. 489–96

[117] Meister, A. (1995). Mitochondrial changes associated with glutathione deficiency, *Biochim Biophys Acta,* Vol. 1271, pp. 35–42

[118] Minich, T.; Riemer, J.; Schulz, JB.; Wielinga, P.; Wijnholds, J. & Dringen, R. (2006). The multidrug resistance protein 1 (Mrp1), but not Mrp5, mediates export of glutathione and glutathione disulfide from brain astrocytes, *J Neurochem,* Vol. 97, pp. 373–84

[119] Mitchell, JB.; Cook, JA.; DeGraff, W.; Glatstein, E. & Russo, A. (1989). Keynote address: Glutathione modulation in cancer treatment: will it work? *Int. J. Radiat. Oncol. Biol. Phys.*, Vol. 16, pp. 1289-1295

[120] Miriyala, S.; Spasojevic, I.; Tovmasyan, A.; Salvemini, D.; Vujaskovic, Z.; St. Clair, D. & Batinic-Haberle, I. (2012). Manganese superoxide dismutase, MnSOD and its mimics, *Biochimica et Biophysica Acta*, Vol. 1822, pp. 794–814

[121] Modica-Napolitano, JS. & Singh, KK. (2004). Mitochondrial dysfunction in cancer, *Mitochondrion*, Vol. 4, pp. 755–762

[122] Modica-Napolitano, JS.; Kulawiec, M. & Singh, KK. (2007). Mitochondria and human cancer, *Curr. Mol. Med.*, Vol. 7, pp. 121–131

[123] Monteiro, HP. & Stern, A. (1996). Redox modulation of tyrosine phosphorylation-dependent signal transduction pathways, *Free Rad. Biol. Med.*, Vol. 21, pp. 323–33

[124] Muller, M.; Meijer, C.; Zaman, GJ.; Borst, P.; Scheper, RJ.; Mulder, NH.; de Vries, EG. & Jansen, PL. (1994). Overexpression of the gene encoding the multidrug resistance-associated protein results in increased ATP-dependent glutathione S-conjugate transport, *Proc. Natl. Acad. Sci. USA*, Vol. 91, pp. 13033–7

[125] Mumper, AGRJ. (2009). Elevated copper and oxidative stress in cancer cells as a target for cancer treatment, *Cancer Treatment Reviews*, Vol. 35, pp. 32– 46

[126] Muthu, MS.; Kulkarni, SA.; Xiong, J. & Feng, SS. (2011). Vitamin E TPGS coated liposomes enhanced cellular uptake and cytotoxicity of docetaxel in brain cancer cells, *Int. J. Pharm.*, Vol. 421(2), pp. 332-40

[127] Nair, U. & Nair J. (2007). Lipid peroxidation-induced DNA damage in cancer-prone inflammatory diseases: a review of published adduct types and levels in humans, *Free Rad. Biol. Med.*, Vol. 43, pp. 1109–20

[128] Nishikawa, M. & Hashida, M. (2006). Inhibition of tumour metastasis by targeted delivery of antioxidant enzymes, *Expert Opin. Drug Deliv.*, Vol. 3, pp. 355–369

[129] Nones, J.; Stipursky, J.; Costa, SL.; Gomes, FC. (2010). Flavonoids and astrocytes crosstalking: implications for brain development and pathology, *Neurochem. Res.*, Vol. 35, No. 7, pp. 955-66

[130] Norris, MD.; Bordow, SB.; Marshall, GM.; Haber, PS.; Cohn, SL. & Haber, M. (1996). Expression of the gene for multidrug-resistance-associated protein and outcome in patients with neuroblastoma, *N. Engl. J. Med.*, Vol. 334, pp. 231–8

[131] Nulton-Persson, AC. (2001). Modulation of mitochondrial function by hydrogen peroxide, *J. Biol. Chem.*, Vol. 276, pp. 23357–61

[132] Oberley, TD. (2002). Oxidative damage and cancer, *Am. J. Path.*, Vol. 160, pp. 403–8

[133] Oberley, LW.; Oberley, TD. & Buettner, GR. (1981). Cell division in normal and transformed cells: the possible role of superoxide and hydrogen peroxide. *Med. Hypoth.*, Vol. 7, pp. 21– 42

[134] Orrenius, S. (2007). Reactive oxygen species in mitochondria-mediated cell death, *Drug Metab. Rev.*, Vol. 39, pp. 443–55

[135] Palan, P.; Mikhail, M.; Goldberg, G.; Runowicz, C. & Romney, S. (1996). Plasma levels of â– carotene, lycopene, canthaxanthin, retinol, and á and ã tocopherol in cervical intraepithelial neoplasia and cancer, *Clin. Cancer Res.*, Vol. 2, pp. 181–5

[136] Papageorgiou, M.; Stiakaki, E.; Dimitriou, H.; Malliaraki, N.; Notas, G.; Castanas, E. & Kalmanti, M. (2005). Cancer chemotherapy reduces plasma total antioxidant capacity in children with malignancies, *Leukemia Research*, Vol. 29, pp. 11–16

[137] Park, CK.; Jung, JH.; Moon, MJ.; Kim, YY.; Kim, JH.; Park, SH.; Kim, CY.; Paek, SH.; Kim, DG.; Jung, HW. & Cho, BK. (2009). Tissue expression of manganese superoxide dismutase is a candidate prognostic marker for glioblastoma, *Oncology*, Vol.77, No. 3-4, pp. 178-81

[138] Patel, VB.; Misra, S.; Patel, BB. & Majumdar, AP. (2010). Colorectal cancer: chemopreventive role of curcumin and resveratrol. *Nutr. Cancer*, Vol. 62, pp. 958–967

[139] Pelicano, H.; Feng, L.; Zhou, Y.; Carew, JS., Hileman, EO.; Plunkett. W.; Keating, MJ. & Huang, P. (2003). Inhibition of mitochondrial respiration: a novel strategy to enhance drug-induced apoptosis in human leukemia cells by a reactive oxygen species-mediated mechanism, *J. Biol. Chem.*, Vol., 26, pp. 37832–9

[140] Pervaiz, S. & Clement, MV. (2004). Tumor intracellular redox status and drug resistance-serendipity or a causal relationship?, *Curr. Pharm. Des.*, Vol. 10, pp. 1969–77

[141] Pervaiz, S. (2006). Pro-oxidant milieu blunts scissors: insight into tumor progression, drug resistance, and novel druggable targets, *Curr. Pharm. Chem.*, Vol. 12, pp. 4469–77

[142] Pervaiz, S. & Holme, AL. (2009). Resveratrol: its biologic targets and functional activity, *Antioxid Redox Signal*, Vol. 11(11), pp. 2851–2897

[143] Poli, G.; Biasi, F. & Chiarpotto, E. (2004). Oxidative stress and cell signaling, *Curr. Med. Chem.*, Vol. 11, pp. 1163–82

[144] Polyak, K.; Li, Y.; Zhu, H.; Lengauer, C.; Willson, JK., Markowitz, SD., Trush, MA.; Kinzler, KW. & Vogelstein, B. (1998). Somatic mutations of the mitochondrial genome in human colorectal tumors, *Nat. Genet.*, Vol. 20(3), pp. 291-3

[145] Potishman, N.; Herrero, R.; Brinton, LA.; Reeves, WC. & Stacewicz–Sapuntzakis, M. (1991). A case control study of nutrient status and invasive cervical cancer. II. Serological indicators, *Am. J. Epidemiol.*, Vol. 134, pp. 1347–55

[146] Powis, G. & Baker, A. (1997). Redox signaling and the control of cell growth and death, *Adv. Pharmacol.*, Vol. 38, pp. 329–59

[147] Powis, G.; Mustacich, D. & Coon, A. (2000). The role of the redox protein thioredoxin in cell growth and cancer, *Free Radic. Biol. Med.,* Vol. 29, pp. 312– 322

[148] Puri, T.; Goyal, S.; Julka, PK.; Nair, O.; Sharma, DN & Rath, GK. (2010). Lycopene in treatment of high-grade gliomas: a pilot study, *Neurol India,* Vol. 58, No. 1, pp. 20-23

[149] Purkayastha, S.; Berliner, A.; Fernando, SS.; Ranasinghe, B.; Ray, I.; Tariq, H. & Banerjee, P. (2009). Curcumin blocks brain tumor formation, *Brain Res.,* Feb 10 (in press).

[150] Rajaraman, P.; Hutchinson, A.; Rothman, N.; Black, PM.; Fine, HA.; Loeffler, JS.; Selker, RG.; Shapiro, WR.; Linet, MS. & Inskip, PD. (2008). Oxidative response gene polymorphisms and risk of adult brain tumors, *Neuro Oncol.,* Vol. 10, No. 5, pp. 709-715

[151] Ratnam, DV.; Ankola, DD.; Bhardwaj, V.; Sahana, DK. & Kumar, MN. (2006). Role of antioxidants in prophylaxis and therapy: a pharmaceutical perspective. *J Control Release.,* Vol. 20;113 pp. 189-207

[152] Rao, GM.; Rao, AV.; Raja, SN. & Rao, A. (2000). Role of antioxidant enzymes in brain tumors, *Clin. Chim. Acta,* 2000;Vol. 296, pp. 203–12

[153] Reynolds, IJ. & Hastings, TG. (1995). Glutamate induces the production of reactive oxygen species in cultured forebrain neurons following NMDA receptor activation, *J. Neurosci.,* Vol. 15, pp. 3318–3327

[154] Rhee, SG.; Kang, SW.; Netto, LE.; Seo, MS. & Stadtman, ER. (1999). A family of novel peroxidases, peroxiredoxins, *Biofactors,* Vol. 10, 207– 209

[155] Ria, F.; Landriscina, M.; Remiddi, F.; Rosselli, R.; Iacoangeli, M.; Scerrati, M.; Pani, G.; Borrello, S. & Galeotti, T. (2001). The level of manganese superoxide dismutase content is an independent prognostic factor for glioblastoma. Biological mechanisms and clinical implications, *Br. J. Cancer,* Vol. 84, pp. 529– 534

[156] Sagara, J.; Makino, N. & Bannai, S. (1996). Glutathione efflux from cultured astrocytes, *J Neurochem,* Vol. 66, pp. 1876–81

[157] Sah, R.; Galeffi, F.; Ahrens, R.; Jordan, G. & Schwartz-Bloom, RD. (2002). Modulation of the GABA(A)-gated chloride channel by reactive oxygen species, *J. Neurochem.,* Vol. 80, pp. 383–391

[158] Sanjuan-Pla, A.; Cervera, AM.; Apostolova, N.; Garcia-Bou, R.; Victor, VM.; Murphy, MP. & McCreath, KJ. (2005). A targeted antioxidant reveals the importance of mitochondrial reactive oxygen species in the hypoxic signaling of HIF-1alpha, *FEBS Lett,* Vol. 579, pp. 2669–2674

[159] Sarkar, FH.; Adsule, S.; Padhye, S.; Kulkarni, S. & Li, Y. (2006). The role of genistein and synthetic derivatives of isoflavone in cancer prevention and therapy, *Mini Rev. Med. Chem.,* Vol. 6, pp. 401–407

[160] Sarkar, FH.; Li, Y.; Wang, Z. & Kong, D. (2010). The role of nutraceuticals in the regulation of Wnt and Hedgehog signaling in cancer, *Cancer Metastasis Rev.,* Vol. 29, pp. 383–394

[161] Savre-Train, I.; Piatyszek, MA. & Shay, JW. (1992). Transcription of deleted mitochondrial DNA in human colon adenocarcinoma cells, *Hum. Mol. Genet.*, Vol. 1, pp. 203–204

[162] Schild, L.; Chen, BH.; Makarov, P.; Kattengell, K.; Heinitz, K. & Keilhoff, G. (2010). Selective induction of apoptosis in glioma tumour cells by a Gynostemma pentaphyllum extract, *Phytomedicine,* Vol. 17, No. 8-9, pp. 589-597

[163] Shankar, S.; Singh, G. & Srivastava, RK. (2007). Chemoprevention by resveratrol: molecular mechanisms and therapeutic potential, *Front. Biosci.*, Vol. 12, pp. 4839–4854

[164] Shaw, JP. & Chou, IN. (1986). Elevation of intracellular glutathione content associated with mitogenic stimulation of quiescent fibroblasts, *J. Cell. Physiol.*, Vol. 129, pp. 193–198

[165] Shivakumar, BR.; Anandatheerthavarada, HK. & Ravindranath, V. (1991). Free radical scavenging systems in developing rat brain. *Int. J. Dev. Neurosci.,* Vol. 9, pp. 181-185

[166] Sies, H. (1993). Strategies of antioxidant defense, *Eur. J. Biochem.,* Vol. 215, pp. 213-219

[167] Slusarz, A.; Shenouda, NS.; Sakla, MS.; Drenkhahn, SK.; Narula, AS.; MacDonald, RS.; Besch-Williford, CL. & Lubahn, DB. (2010). Common botanical compounds inhibit the hedgehog signaling pathway in prostate cancer, *Cancer Res.,*Vol. 70(8), pp.3382-90

[168] Spitz, DS.; Sim, JE.; Ridnour, LA.; Galoforo, SS. & Lee, YJ. (2000). Glucose deprivation-induced oxidative stress in human tumor cells: a fundamental defect in metabolism?, *Ann. N. Y. Acad. Sci.,* Vol. 899, pp. 349–362

[169] Sporn, MB. (1991). Carcinogenesis and cancer: different perspectives on the same disease, *Cancer Res.,* Vol. 51, pp. 6215–6218

[170] Storz, P. (2005). Reactive oxygen species in tumor progression, *Front. Biosci.,* Vol. 10, pp. 1881–1896

[171] Strange, RC.; Fryer, AA.; Matharoo, B.; Zhao, L.; Broome, J.; Campbell, DA.; Jones, P.; Pastor, IC. & Ringh, RV. (1992). The human glutathione *S*-transferases: comparison of isoenzyme expression in normal and astrocytoma brain, *Biochim. Biophys. Acta,* Vol. 1139, pp. 222–228

[172] Sun, Z.; Li, H.; Shu, XH.; Shi, H.; Chen, XY.; Kong, QY.; Wu, ML. & Liu, J. (2012). Distinct sulfonation activities in resveratrol-sensitive and resveratrol-insensitive human glioblastoma cells, *FEBS J.,* Vol. 279(13), pp. 2381-92

[173] Sykes, JA.; McCormack Jr., FX. & O'Brien, TJ. (1978). A preliminary study of the superoxide dismutase content of some human tumors, *Cancer Res.,* Vol. 38, pp. 2759–2762

[174] Tanriverdi, T.; Hanimoglu, H.; Kacira, T.; Sanus, GZ.; Kemerdere, R.; Atukeren, P.; Gumustas, K, Canbaz, B. & Kaynar, MY. (2007). Glutathione peroxidase, glutathione reductase and protein oxidation in patients with glioblastoma multiforme and transitional meningioma, *J. Cancer Res. Clin. Oncol.,* Vol. 133, pp. 627–633

[175] Tedeschi, M.; Bohm, S.; Di Re, F.; Oriana, S.; Spatti, GB.; Tognella, S. & Zunino, F. (1990). Glutathione and detoxification, *Cancer Treat. Rev.,* Vol. 17, pp. 203-208

[176] Tejada, S.; Roca, C.; Sureda, A.; Rial, RV.; Gamund´ı, A. & Esteban, S. (2006). Antioxidant response analysis in the brain after pilocarpine treatments, *Brain Research Bulletin,* Vol. 69, pp. 587–592

[177] Terradez, P.; Asensi, M.; Lasso de la Vega, MC.; Puertes, I.; Vin˜a, J.; Estrela, JM. (1993). Depletion of tumour glutathione in vivo by buthionine sulfoximine: modulation by the rate of cellular proliferation and inhibition of cancer growth, *Biochem. J.,* Vol., 292, pp. 477–483

[178] Thomasset, SC.; Berry, DP.; Garcea, G.; Marczylo, T.; Steward, WP. & Gescher,AJ. (2007). Dietary polyphenolic phytochemicals—promising cancer chemopreventive agents in humans? A review of their clinical properties, *Int. J. Cancer,* Vol. 120, pp. 451–458

[179] Thorburne, SK. & Juurlink, BH. (1996). Low glutathione and high iron govern the susceptibility of oligodendroglial precursors to oxidative stress, *J. Neurochem.,* Vol.67, pp. 1014–22

[180] Todorova, VK.; Harms, SA.; Kaufmann,Y.; Luo, S.; Luo, KQ.; Babb, K. & Klimberg, VS. (2004). Effect of dietary glutamine on tumor glutathione levels and apoptosis-related proteins in DMBA-induced breast cancer of rats, *Breast Cancer Res. Treat.,* Vol. 88, pp. 247–256

[181] Toyokuni, S.; Okamoto, K.; Yodoi, J. & Hiai, H. (1995). Persistent oxidative stress in cancer, *FEBS Lett.,* Vol. 358, pp. 1–3

[182] Tuzgen, S.; Hanimoglu, H.; Tanriverdi, T.; Kacira, T.; Sanus, GZ.; Atukeren, P.; Dashti, R.; Gumustas, K.; Canbaz, B. & Kaynar, MY. (2007). *Relationship between DNA damage and total antioxidant capacity in patients with glioblastoma multiforme, Clin Oncol (R Coll Radiol).,* Vol. 19, No. 3, pp. 177-81

[183] Uttara, B.; Singh, A. V.; Zamboni, P.; Mahajan, RT. (2009). Oxidative stress and neurodegenerative diseases: a review of upstream and downstream antioxidant therapeutic options, *Curr.Neuropharmacol.,* Vol. 7, No. 1, pp. 65-74

[184] Valko, M.; Leibfritz, D.; Moncol, J.; Cronin, MTD.; Mazur, M. & Telser, J. (2007). Free radicals and antioxidants in normal physiological functions and human disease, *Int. J. Biochem. Cell Biol.,* Vol. 39, pp. 44–84

[185] Valko, M.; Leibfritz, D.; Moncol, J.; Cronin, MT.; Mazur, M. & Telser, J. (2007). Free radicals and antioxidants in normal physiological functions and human disease, *Int J Biochem Cell Biol.,* Vol. 39(1), pp. 44–84

[186] Van den Brandt, PA.; Goldbohm, RA.; Van't Veer, P.; Bode, P.; Dorant, E.; Hermus, RJ.; Sturmans, F. (1993). A prospective cohort study on selenium status and the risk of lung cancer, *Cancer Res.,* Vol. 53, pp. 4860-4865

[187] Vaughn, AE. & Deshmukh, M. (2008). Glucose metabolism inhibits apoptosis in neurons and cancer cells by redoxin activation of cytochrome c, *Nature Cell Biology*, Vol. 10, pp. 1477–1483

[188] Wang, S.; Meckling, KA.; Marcone, MF.; Kakuda, Y. & Tsao, R.(2011). Can phytochemical antioxidant rich foods act as anti-cancer agents?, *Food Research International,* Vol. 44, pp. 2545–2554

[189] Weinberg, F. & Chandel, NS. (2009). Mitochondrial metabolism and cancer, *Ann. NY. Acad. Sci.,* Vol. 1177, pp. 66–73

[190] Yonezawa, M.; Back, SA.; Gan, X.; Rosenberg, PA. & Volpe, JJ. (1996). Cystine deprivation induces oligodendroglial death: rescue by free radical scavengers and by a diffusible glial factor. *J. Neurochem.,* Vol. 67, pp. 566–73

[191] Yoshikawa, T.; Tainaka, K.; Naito, Y. & Kondo, M. (1995). A novel cancer therapy based on oxygen radicals. *Cancer Res.,* Vol. 55, pp. 1617–20

[192] Yuan, L. & Kaplowitz, N. (2009). Glutathione in liver diseases and hepatotoxicity. *Mol. Aspects Med.,* Vol. 30(1–2), pp. 29–41

[193] Zengin, E.; Atukeren, P.; Kokoglu, E.; Gumustas, MK. & Zengin, U. (2009). Alterations in lipid peroxidation and antioxidant status in different types of intracranial tumors within their relative peritumoral tissues, *Clin Neurol Neurosurg.,* Vol. 111, No. 4, pp. 345-51

[194] Zheng, W.; Blot, WJ.; Diamond, EL.; Norkus, EP. & Spate, V. (1993). Serum micronutrients and the subsequent risk of oral and pharyngeal cancer. *Cancer Res.,* Vol. 53, pp. 795–8

[195] Chen, JM.; Zhou, X.; Li, XZ. & Mei, GY. (2006). Levels of selenium, zinc, copper and antioxidant enzyme activity in patients with leukemia, *Biol. Trace. Elem. Res.*, Vol. 114, pp. 41–54

Section 12

Anesthesia for Patients with a Brain Tumor and Pregnancy

Chapter 24

Management of Brain Tumor in Pregnancy — An Anesthesia Window

Hala M. Goma

Additional information is available at the end of the chapter

http://dx.doi.org/10.5772/54250

1. Introduction

Brain tumor surgery during pregnancy has a great concern in Egypt now days. High prevalence of brain tumors during pregnancy y was noticed. There is no accurate statics for the prevalence. The most common tumors are pituitary tumors, menegioma, gliomas, metastis of breast carcinomas. Many problems affects anesthesia, as the interaction between many different factors, as the physiological changes during pregnancy, including, cardiovascular, respiratory changes [1]. Problems occur, during diagnosis, and treatment of tumors. Also problems during surgery are, drug interactions with the anesthesia drugs, blood loss and transfusion, prevention preterm labour, and anesthesia for urgent cesarean section during surgery for removal of brain tumor, in the chapter I tried to summary all these factors from anesthesia point of views did many cases for brain resection during pregnancy,I hope to give this experience for any young anesthesit how may facing such cases

1.1. Common tumors during pregnancy

1.1.1. Meningiomas

The incidence of meningiomas is approximately twice as high in women as in men. Specifically, intracranial meningiomas are twice as common and intraspinal meningiomas nine times as common in females [2]. Meningiomas also seem to have a relationship to sex hormones with accelerated growth of these tumors during the luteal phase of the menstrual cycle and during pregnancy [3]. There may also be an increased incidence of meningiomas in women with breast cancer, although one study contests this relationship. A large number of studies have examined the role of androgen, estrogen and progesterone receptors in meningiomas with most finding progesterone and androgen receptors in a high proportion and low levels of estrogen receptors in a small proportion of meningioma specimens obtained at the time of initial surgery and at recurrence [4].

1.1.2. Pituitary tumors

Pituitary tumors account for approximately 15% of all primary intracranial neoplasms and occur in higher frequency in women, mainly in the child-bearing years [4].

The female preponderance of these tumors is due to the increased frequency of prolactinomas in women in the second and third decades. Women are affected four times as commonly as men and account for 78% of all prolactinomas [5].

1.2. Cranial metastases

1.2.1. Breast cancer

Breast cancer is the most common malignancy among women in North America accounting for 27% of all cancers. Approximately 181,000 new cases of breast cancer were diagnosed in 1992 and 46,000 women died from the disease the same year. Neurologic complications occur in approximately 25% of patients with metastatic breast cancer although autopsy studies have demonstrated central nervous system involvement in 31-57% of examinations [6,7].

2. Problems in management of brain tumors with pregnancy

2.1. Problems in diagnosis

Symptoms of increased intracranial pressure including headache, nausea and vomiting are similar to the symptoms of early pregnancy, or pregnancy related hypertensive diseases(eclampsia or preeclampsia).

The use of Neuro imaging of the pregnant patient with these symptoms become necessary. In the first trimester it is preferred to be avoided.the MRI is the procedure of choice as there is no exposure to ionizing radiation. Although there is no evidence that MRI affects the fetus there is exposure to powerful electromagnetic fields and this imaging modality should be avoided if possible in the first trimester.Similarly, there is very little evidence regarding the safety of the ferromagnetic contrast agent gadolinium and this is not sanctioned for use in pregnancy and should be avoided if possible. In the patient with rapid neurologic deterioration computerized tomography (CT) may be necessary. This does involve radiation exposure of approximately 2.5 to 3 rads to the head of the patient and a fetal exposure estimated to be approximately 1 mrad or less per slice which can be reduced by appropriate shielding of the uterus with a lead apron. [9] At fetal exposures less than 10 rads no adverse effects in excess of the background rate of spontaneous abnormalities in 3% of livebirths and the spontaneous abortion rate of 30% in all pregnancies. Medically indicated exposures of up to 5 rads are considered acceptable in pregnancy when unavoidable. There has been limited experience with the use of iodinated contrast agents during pregnancy and the risks are not precisely defined. Such agents should be avoided in the first trimester.

2.2. Problems during treatment

Treatment of brain tumors or their complications may be necessary during pregnancy. Cerebral edema and increased intracranial pressure may require the use of glucocorticoids and mannitol. Glucocorticoids have been used during pregnancy for other reasons including the prevention of neonatal respiratory distress syndrome and there is no evidence of growth, physical, motor or developmental deficiencies within the first three years of life. However, fetal adrenal suppression may occur with long-term, high dose therapy during any part of pregnancy and necessitates the use of supplemental steroids in the peri-partum period. Although mannitol does cross the placenta and is excreted by the fetal kidney into the amniotic fluid no adverse effects have been reported [10].

Cranial irradiation exposes the fetus to higher doses of radiation than diagnostic imaging. In general, radiation exposure in utero carries a risk of adverse fetal outcomes including spontaneous abortion, anatomic malformation, growth and mental retardation and possibly childhood cancer with the latter risk highest in the first trimester The exposure to the fetus from scatter is low when conventional radiation therapy is delivered to parts distant from the uterus and such exposure carries low risk. Strategies to reduce fetal exposure include the use of focal rather than whole brain irradiation, radiation dose reduction, substitution of heavy charged particles for photons and deferring radiation until after delivery [11].

Chemotherapy typically involves agents which are teratogenic in the first trimester and associated with adverse fetal outcomes. Properties of chemotherapeutic agents which improve permeability across the blood brain barrier also facilitate transport across the placenta making these drugs especially hazardous. Although there is data to suggest that certain chemotherapeutic agents are associated with minimal risk in the second and third trimesters, chemotherapy for malignant brain tumors should be avoided during pregnancy. Meningiomas are tumors that are thought to arise from meningothelial cells which make up the arachnoid villi of the meninges. These lesions account for approximately 20% of all intracranial and 25% of all intraspinal tumors and the incidence increases with age [11].

2.3. Problems during anesthesia for brain tumor surgery

Altered maternal physiology.

Respiratory system and acid-base balance changes

a. Alveolar ventilation increases 25% by the fourth month of gestation and 45% to 70% by term. This results in a chronic respiratory alkalosis, with a $Paco_2$ of 28 to 32 mm Hg, a slightly alkaline pH (e.g., approximately 7.44), and decreased levels of bicarbonate and buffer base.

b. oxygen consumption increases during gestation, Pao_2 usually increases slightly or remains within the normal range.

c. Functional residual capacity (FRC) decreases by approximately 20% as the uterus expands, which results in decreased oxygen reserve and the potential for airway closure.

d. obesity; perioperative intraabdominal distention; placement of the patient in the supine, Trendelenburg, or lithotomy positions), airway closure may be sufficient to cause hypoxemia

e. Failed intubation (which is the leading cause of maternal death from anesthesia) is as much a risk during nonobstetric surgery as it is during cesarean section.

f. rapid development of hypoxemia and acidosis during periods of hypoventilation or apnea due to decreased FRC, increased oxygen consumption, and diminished buffering capacity.

g. induction of general anesthesia occurs more rapidly during pregnancy, because alveolar hyperventilation and a decreased FRC allow faster equilibration of inhaled agents.

h. Acceleration in the induction of anesthesia is the approximately 30% decrease in the minimum alveolar concentration (MAC) for volatile anesthetic agents that occurs even during early gestation.

Cardiovascular system changes

a. Cardiac output increases by 30% to 50% during pregnancy because of increases in heart rate and stroke volume; both systemic and pulmonary vascular resistance decrease.

b. By eight weeks' gestation, 57% of the increase in cardiac output, 78% of the increase in stroke volume, and 90% of the decrease in systemic vascular resistance that typically are achieved by 24 weeks' gestation.

c. During the second half of gestation, the weight of the uterus compresses the inferior vena cava when the mother lies supine; this decreases venous return and cardiac output by approximately 25% to 30%.

d. Although upper extremity blood pressure may be maintained by compensatory vasoconstriction and tachycardia, uteroplacental perfusion is jeopardized whenever the mother lies supine.

e. Frank hypotension also can occur in the supine parturient, especially when regional or general anesthesia attenuates or abolishes normal compensatory mechanisms. is essential to displace the uterus laterally during any operation performed after the twentieth week of pregnancy.

Factors that can alter uteroplacental blood flow

1. Uterine Contraction
2. Decreased Uterine Blood Flow
3. Pathological Conditions
4. Pharmacological Agents

Intravenous induction agents

5. Inhalation agents (Desflurane and sevoflurane)
6. Antihypertensive agents
7. b-adrenergic blocking drugs
8. Tocolytic drugs
9. Epidural and subarachnoid opiates
10. Local anesthetics
11. Pharmacological agent added to the local anesthetic
12. Vasopressors

Maintenance of uteroplacental blood flow is the hallmark for fetal well-being; hence an in-depth knowledge of this subjectis essential for individuals taking care of pregnant women.

Uterine blood flow is determined by the equation.Hence any condition that will significantly decrease mean [14,15]

$$\frac{\text{Uterine arterial pressure} - \text{Uterine venous pressure}}{\text{Uterine vascular resistance}} \tag{1}$$

So when maternal arterial pressure decreases or significantly increase uterine vascular resistance will decrease utero placental blood flow and, ultimately, umbilical blood flow.At term, 10% of the cardiac output (700 mL/min) supplies the uterus. The placental vasculature remains maximally [16,17,18].

Changes in blood volume and blood constituents

- Blood volume expands in the first trimester and increases 30% to 45% by term. A smaller increase in red blood cell volume than in plasma volume results in a dilutional anemia.
- moderate blood loss is well tolerated during pregnancy, preexisting anemia decreases the patient's reserve when significant hemorrhage occurs. Fresh blood transfusion is needed to compensate blood loss during brain tumor surgery [18].
- Pregnancy induces a hypercoagulable state, with increases in fibrinogen; factors VII, VIII, X, and XII; and fibrin degradation products. Pregnancy is associated with enhanced platelet turnover, clotting, and fibrinolysis, and there is a wide range in the normal platelet count; thus pregnancy represents a state of accelerated but compensated intravascular coagulation. During the postoperative period, pregnant surgical patients are at high risk for thromboembolic complications.
- It is great challenge to Induce hypotensive technique and to maintain the placental perfusion pressure [19].

Gastrointestinal system changes

- Incompetence of the lower esophageal sphincter and distortion of gastric and pyloric anatomy result in an increased risk of esophageal reflux and aspiration pneumonitis.
- It seems prudent to consider any pregnant patient at risk for aspiration after 18 to 20 weeks' gestation.
- Rapid sequence induction to avoid aspiration and deep anesthesia to prevent increase in the intracranial pressure during brain tumor surgery is another problem.
- preoperative antiacid,sodium citreate, meteclopramid,muscle relaxant as rocuronium.
- complete recovery is needed before extubation.

Altered Responses to Anesthesia

- The decrease in MAC for inhaled anesthetic agents,
- thiopental requirements begin to decrease early in pregnancy.
- Plasma cholinesterase levels decrease by approximately 25% from early in pregnancy until the seventh postpartum day. Cautions in use of remifentanil and succinylcholine.
- *The anesthesiologist should monitor neuromuscular blockade with a nerve sti*mulator to ensure adequate reversal before extubation.
- Decreased protein binding associated with low albumin concentrations during pregnancy may result in a greater fraction of unbound drug, with the potential for greater drug toxicity during pregnancy.
- Antiepileptic drugs as **Carbamazepine** and, Phenytoin may potentiate effects of anesthetic drug used [20,21,22].

Risk of teratogenicity

- *Teratogenicity* has been defined as any significant postnatal change in function or form in an offspring after prenatal treatment. Concern about the potential harmful effects of anesthetic agents stems from their known effects on mammalian cells. These occur at clinical concentrations and include reversible decreases in cell motility, prolongation of DNA synthesis, and inhibition of cell division.Despite these theoretical concerns, no data specifically link any of these cellular events with teratogenic changes.

Anticonvulsants

- All anticonvulsants cross the placenta. Pregnant women with epilepsy who ingest anticonvulsant drugs have a fetal congenital anomaly rate of 4% to 8%, which is higher than the 2% to 3% background incidence quoted for the general population.
- **Carbamazepine**
- **Phenobarbital** is used in the treatment of partial and generalized tonic-clonic seizures and status epilepticus

- **Valproic acid** (Depakene, Depakote) is used to treat absence and generalized tonic-clonic seizures [23,24,25].

Tranquilizers

Some studies have suggested that first-trimester exposure to diazepam increases the risk of cleft lip.

Lithium

In the International Registry of Lithium Babies, (11.5%) of 217 infants exposed to lithium during the first trimester of pregnancy were malformed.Eighteen infants had cardiovascular anomalies.

Antidepressants

The selective serotonin reuptake inhibitors include sertraline (Zoloft), paroxetine (Paxil), fluoxetine (Prozac), and citalopram (Celexa). No increased risk of major malformations or developmental (language and behavior) abnormalities has been identified.

Nitrous oxide

In vivo and embryo culture studies in rats have confirmed that nitrous oxide produces several adverse reproductive effects, each of which results from exposure at a specific period of susceptibility [21].

Use of electronic fetal monitoring for assessing fetal well-being has become universal, used by both physicians and nurses. Monitoring the fetal heart rate is used to determine adequate cerebral oxygenation of the fetus. As the brain modulates the heart, a decrease in fetal heart rate is believed to reflect inadequate fetal cerebral oxygenation.External fetal heart ratemonitors use a Doppler detective device with computerized logic to interpret,and count the Doppler signals,whereas internal fetal heart rate monitors involve placement of an electrodeon the fetal scalp. The presenceof fetal heart tones as well as their rate and rhythm are well-recognized indicators of fetal well-being. A normal fetal heart rate tracing reveals a rate of 110–160 beats/min with minimal to moderate beat-to-beat variability with or without accelerations. Apretermfetus is expected to have a more rapid rate with little or no beat-to-beat variabilityand no accelerations (an increasein fetal heart rate over baseline, usually occurring with fetal movement.

The goal of antepartum fetal surveillance is to document fetal wellbeing,allowing the pregnancy to continue without concern for fetal death.Several antepartum techniques in use include fetal movement, nonstress test, contraction stress test, biophysical profile, and umbilical artery Dopplerflow velocimetry [26,27,,28,29,30]

Prevention of preterm labor

Fetal movement is the easiest means for documenting fetal well-being. The mother can perceive fetal movements,which serve as a basis for assessment.A diminution in the perception of fetal movement often precedes fetal death. Perception of 10 distinct movements in a period of up to 2 hours is considered reassuring. Heart rate reactivity is thought to be a good indicator of normal fetal autonomic function. Loss of reactivity is associated most commonly with fetal sleep but also may result from any central nervous system depression. A nonstress test involves connecting themother to the fetal heart rate monitor and observing. Non stress test results can be categorized as reactive or nonreactive.

The non stress test is considered *reactive* (normal) if two or more fetal heart rate accelerations are observed within a 20-minute period. The non stress test is considered *nonreactive* when no accelerations are observed [32,33]

Guidelines for the management of preterm delivery.

- Confirm diagnosis of preterm labor
- Exclude contraindications to expectant management and/or tocolysis
- Administer corticosteroids, if indicated
- Group B *Streptococcus* chemoprophylaxis, if indicated
- Pharmacologic tocolysis
- Consider transfer to tertiary care center

There is increased incidence of abortion and preterm delivery. volatile halogenated agents depress myometrial irritability The prophylactic use of tocolytic agents is controversial; they are not without risk, and it is unclear whether they affect outcome. Selective administration to those patients at greatest risk (e.g., those undergoing cervical cerclage) has been suggested [34,35].

Anesthetic management

1. Unlike other operations wherein thepatient is primarily concerned with him or herself, the pregnant woman usually is concerned for her baby'swelfare.
2. The anesthesia provider must beaware of the various physiologic changes of pregnancy and incorporatethem into the anesthetic plan.
3. These physiologic changes have implications for various diseases and must be considered.
4. The central nervous system effect of pregnancy include a reduced local anesthetic requirement when these agents are given intrathecally or epidurally.
5. Pregnant patients are at increased risk for aspiration during general anesthesia.
6. There is some suggestion that surgery during the first trimester is linked to central nervous defectsduring surgery.
7. Fetal heart rate monitoring is possible during some surgical procedures but is not universally used in theUnited States.
8. Preterm delivery remains the leading cause of perinatal morbidity and mortality in the United States. Preterm labor is difficult to control with medication; the most promising medications are the calcium channel-blocking drugs. Magnesium sulfate is frequently

used and is associated with prolonged depolarizing and nondepolarizing neuromuscularblockade.

9. The etiology of preeclampsia remains to be elucidated but is believedto be triggered by a paternal antigen in a susceptible mother.
10. Magnesium sulfate is the most effective medication for the prevention of seizures in women with preeclampsia.
11. Labetalol is the preferred medicationfor the control of blood pressure in mothers with preeclampsia.
12. The two causes of antepartum hemorrhage are placenta previa and placental abruption. Associated with the increase in cesarean sections isa high risk of placenta accreta in patients with placenta previa.
13. Perinatal transmission of HIV is low if the viral load is <1,000 copies/mL, and patients with these levels do not require cesarean section. If theviral load is greater, cesarean section may decrease the risk of perinatal transmission [36,37].

3. Preoperative management

Premedication may be necessary to allay maternal anxiety. Precautions against acid aspiration should include administration of an H_2-receptor antagonist and 30 mL of a clear antacid before the induction of anesthesia.

4. Choice of anesthesia

The choice of anesthesia should be guided by maternal indications and should take into consideration the site and the nature of the surgery. No study has correlated improved fetal outcome with any anesthetic technique. When possible, local or regional anesthesia (with the exception of paracervical block) is preferred; this permits the administration of drugs with no laboratory or clinical evidence of teratogenesis. In addition, maternal respiratory complications occur less frequently with local and regional anesthetic techniques. These techniques are suitable for cases involving cervical cerclage, urologic or lower extremity procedures, and operations on the arm or hand. Most abdominal operations require general anesthesia, because the incision typically extends to the upper abdomen, which creates an unacceptable risk of aspiration in a pregnant patient with an unprotected airway [38,39].

5. Prevention of aortocaval compression

Beginning at 18 to 20 weeks' gestation, the pregnant patient should be transported on her side, and the uterus should be displaced leftward when she is positioned on the operating table.

6. Monitoring

Maternal monitoring should include noninvasive or direct blood pressure measurement, electrocardiography, pulse oximetry, capnography, temperature monitoring, and the use of a nerve stimulator. The FHR and uterine activity should be monitored both during and after surgery when technically feasible.

7. Anesthetic technique

General anesthesia mandates endotracheal intubation beginning at approximately 18 to 20 weeks' gestation or earlier if gastrointestinal function is abnormal. Denitrogenation (i.e., preoxygenation) should precede the application of cricoid pressure, rapid-sequence induction, and endotracheal intubation. Drugs with a history of safe use during pregnancy include thiopental, morphine, meperidine, fentanyl, succinylcholine, and most of the nondepolarizing muscle relaxants. Many obstetric anesthesiologists would now add propofol to the list of "safe" drugs for use during pregnancy.

A commonly used technique employs a high concentration of oxygen, a muscle relaxant, and an opioid and/or a moderate concentration of a volatile halogenated agent. Scientific evidence does not support avoiding nitrous oxide during pregnancy, particularly after the sixth week of gestation. Omission of nitrous oxide may increase fetal risk if inadequate anesthesia results or if a high dose of a volatile agent results in maternal hypotension. A cautious approach would restrict nitrous oxide administration to a concentration of 50% or less and would limit its use in extremely long operations. Hyperventilation should be avoided; rather, end-tidal CO_2 should be maintained in the normal range for pregnancy.

Before the administration of spinal or epidural anesthesia, rapid intravenous infusion of 1 L of crystalloid seems prudent, although the anesthesiologist should not assume that this will prevent maternal hypotension. Appropriate vasopressors should be available to treat hypotension if it occurs. The usual precautions must be taken to guard against a high block and systemic local anesthetic toxicity.

Regardless of the technique used, avoidance of hypoxemia, hypotension, acidosis, and hyperventilation are the most critical elements of anesthetic management.

8. Postoperative management

8.1. Postoperative management

The FHR and uterine activity should be monitored during recovery from anesthesia. Adequate analgesia should be obtained with systemic or spinal opioids. Prophylaxis against venous thrombosis should be considered [38,39,40,41].

Case study:

- Pregnant woman 30 weeks of pregnancy, she was complained from multiple menegiomas, conservative treatment was used throughout pregnancy period. this patient developed sever continuous vomiting,and rapid deterioration of nutritional status,neuro surgery team decided urgent operation for decompression of the brain, the patient was referred for obstetric,and anesthesia consultant.

- Anesthesia examination revealed that :

Patient 35 years old 65 Kg, this the first baby,she complained from infertility for 15 years,she was hypertensive 150/90 on aldomit.anticovasant drugs was admintsred,liver enzymes was 2 folds,albumen was 2,5, prothrombin was 65% kidney function within normal range. Hb was 6,5gm/dl, Obesteric examination revealed that baby nearly mature,his weigt is under weight.

- Preoperative preparation:

Anesthesia consultant recommended blood transfusion for 4 units of packed RBCs,4 units of human albumen, 4 units of fresh plasma 2 days before surgery. Preparations of another for units of fresh blood were for intraoperative losses Preoperative antacid was administered. Obstetric Preparations was for urgent cesarean section. Pediatric preparing to receive the premature neonate if urgent cesarean section was needed

- Anesthesia management:

- Monitoring:

Invasive blood pressure, ECG,endtidal CO2,pulse oximetry, uterine contraction monitor, fetal Doppler. Postioning: Supine with left lateral tilt,

8.2. Induction of anesthesia

3-5 mg/kg sodium thiopental, rocuronium 04 meg/kg, fentanyl 1mg/kg. Intubation by rapid sequence, the precautions mentioned above were considered

The operation was long 5 hours, blood loss was replaced, fetal heart was declined at third hour,urgent cesarean section was done,the pediatric consultant intubated the neonate,and he was incubated,for 2 weeks,he extubated and he is still living.mother was in intensive care unit for 3 days.

Author details

Hala M. Goma*

Address all correspondence to: Ahmeda1995@yahoo.com

Faculty of Medicine,Cairo University, Cairo, Egypt

References

[1] Simon, R. H. Brain tumors in pregnancy. Semin Neurol (1988). , 8(3), 214-221.

[2] Roelvink NCAKamphorst W, van Alphen HAM et al. Pregnancy-related primary brain and spinal tumors. Arch Neurol (1987). , 44, 209-215.

[3] (Schlehofer B, Blettner M, Wahrendorf J. Association between brain tumors and menopausal status. J Natl Cancer Inst 1992; 84 [17]: 1346-1349. 1983; 56: 974-977). 56, 974-977.

[4] Harris, J. R, Morrow, M, & Bonadonna, G. Cancer of the breast. In DeVita VT, Hellman S, Rosenberg SA (eds). Cancer Principles and Practice of Oncology (ed 4]. Philadelphia: J B Lippincott, (1993). , 1993, 1264-1332.

[5] Haas, J. F, Janisch, W, & Staneczek, W. Newly diagnosed primary intracranial neoplasms in pregnant women: a population-based assessment. J Neurol Neurosurg Psychiatry (1986). , 49, 874-880.

[6] Cifuentes, N, & Pickren, J. W. Metastases from carcinoma of mammary gland: an autopsy study. J Surg Oncol (1979). , 11, 193-205.

[7] Anderson, N. E. Neurological complications of breast cancer. In Wiley RG (ed). Neurological Complications of Cancer. New York: Marcel Dekker, (1995). , 1995, 311-332.

[8] Hall, S. M, Buzdar, A. U, & Blumenschein, G. R. Cranial nerve palsies in metastatic breast cancer due to osseous metastasis without intracranial involvement. Cancer (1983). , 52, 180-184.

[9] Greenberg, H, Deck, M, & Vikram, B. Metastasis to the base of the skull: clinical findings in 43 patients. Neurology (1981). , 31, 530-537.

[10] Doll, D. C, Ringenberg, S, & Yarbro, J. W. Management of cancer during pregnancy. Arch Intern Med (1988). , 148, 2058-2064.

[11] Glick, R. P, Penny, D, & Hart, A. The pre-operative and post-operative management of the brain tumor patient. In Morantz RA, Walsh JW (eds). Brain Tumors. New York: Marcel Dekker, (1994). , 1994, 345-366.

[12] Carpenter, T. M. Murlin JR: The energy metabolism of mother and child just before and just after birth. *AMA Arch Intern Med* (1911). , 7, 184-222.

[13] Root, H. Root HK: The basal metabolism during pregnancy and the puerperium. *Arch Intern Med* (1923). , 32, 411-424.

[14] Sandiford, I, & Wheeler, T. The basal metabolism before, during, and after pregnancy J Bio Chem. lxii: , 329-52.

[15] Caton, D, Henderson, D. J, & Wilcox, C. J. Barron DH: *Oxygen consumption of the uterus and its contents and weight at birth of lambs*. In: Longo LD, Reneau DD, ed. Fetal and Newborn Cardiovascular Physiology, 2. New York: Garland STPM Press; (1978). vv28., 1978, 123-134.

[16] Yankowitz, J. *Use of medications in pregnancy: General principles, teratology, and current developments*. In: Yankowitz J, Niebyl JR, ed. *Drug Therapy in Pregnancy*, Baltimore: Lippincott Williams & Wilkins; (2001).

[17] Bain, M. D, Copas, D. K, & Landon, M. J l. In vivo permeability of the human placenta to inulin and mannitol. J Physiol (1988). , 399, 313-319.

[18] Basso, A, Fernandez, A, Althabe, O, et al. Passage of mannitol from mother to amniotic fluid and fetus. Obstet Gynecol (1977). , 49(5), 628-631.

[19] Evaluation of the Pregnant Patient *Robert Gaiser MD* ANESTHESIOLOGY Edited By:David E. Longnecker, MD, FRCARobert D. Dripps David L. Brown, MD Mark F. Newman, MD,Warren M. Zapol, MD Copyright © (2008). by The McGraw-Hill Companies, Inc.. CHAPTER 21 358

[20] Buehler, B. A, Delimont, D, & Van Waes, M. Finnell RH: Prenatal prediction of risk of the fetal hydantoin syndrome. N Engl J Med (1990). , 322, 1567-1572.

[21] Teratology Society Public Affairs CommitteeFDA classification of drugs for teratogenic risk. Teratology (1994). , 49, 446-447.

[22] Friedman JM: Report of the Teratology Society Public Affairs Committee Symposium on FDA Classification of DrugsTeratology (1993). , 48, 5-6.

[23] Doering, P. L, Boothby, L. A, & Cheok, M. Review of pregnancy labeling of prescription drugs: Is the current system adequate to inform of risks?. Am J Obstet Gynecol (2002). , 187, 333-339.

[24] Malone, F. D, & Alton, D. ME: Drugs in pregnancy: Anticonvulsants. *Semin Perinatol* (1997). , 21, 114-123.

[25] Morrell MJ: Guidelines for the care of women with epilepsy *Neurology* (1998). suppl 4):SS27., 21.

[26] Shapiro, S, Hartz, S. C, Siskind, V, et al. Anticonvulsants and parental epilepsy in the development of birth defects. Lancet (1976). i:, 272-275.

[27] Holmes, L. B, Rosenberger, P. B, Harvey, E. A, et al. Intelligence and physical features of children of women with epilepsy. *Teratology* (2000). , 61, 196-202.

[28] Holmes, L. B, Harvey, E. A, Cull, B. A, et al. The teratogenicity of anticonvulsant drugs. *N Engl J Med* (2001). , 344, 1132-1138.

[29] American College of Obstetricians and GynecologistsTeratology. ACOG Educational Bulletin April (1997). (236)

[30] Sever, L. E. Mortensen ME: *Teratology and the epidemiology of birth defects: Occupational and environmental perspectives*. In: Gabbe SG, Niebyl JR, Simpson JL, ed. *Obstetrics: Normal and Problem Pregnancies*, 3rd edition. New York: Churchill Livingston; (1996).

[31] American College of Obstetricians and GynecologistsAssessment of risk factors for preterm birth. ACOG Practice Bulletin October (2001). Liver to perinatal mortality. Br Med J 1976;, 2(31), 965-968.

[32] Villar, J, Ezcurra, E. J, De La Fuente, V. G, & Canpodonico, L. Pre-term delivery syndrome: the unmet need. Res Clin Forums (1994). , 16, 9-33.

[33] Tucker, J. M, Goldenberg, R. L, Davis, R. O, et al. Etiologies of preterm birth in an indigent population: is prevention a logical expectation? ObstetGynecol (1991). , 77, 343-347.

[34] Curtin, S. C. Recent changes in birth attendant, place of birth, and the use of obstetric interventions: United States,J Nurse Midwifery (1999). , 1989-1997.

[35] Goodlin, R. C. History of fetal monitoring.Am J Obstet Gynecol (1979).

[36] Kelso, I. M, Parsons, R. J, Lawrence, G. F, et al. An assessment of continuous fetal heartrate monitoring in labor: a randomized trial. Am J Obstet Gynecol (1978).

[37] Reuwer, P. J, Bruinse, H. W, & Stoutenbeek, T. Doppler assessment of the fetoplacentalcirculation in normal and growth-retardedfetuses. Eur J Obstet Gynecol Reprod Biol(1984).

[38] Vintzileos, A. M, Nioka, S, Lake, M, et al. Transabdominal fetal pulse oximetry with near-infrared spectroscopy. Am J Obstet Gynecol (2005).

[39] Martin, J. A, Hamilton, B. E, Sutton, P. D, et al. Births: Final Data for 2002; National Vital Statistics Reports, Hyattsville, MD: National Center forHealth Statistics, (2003). , 52(10)

[40] Hack, M, & Fanaroff, A. A. Outcomes ofextremely immature infants: a perinatal dilemma. N Engl J Med (1993).

[41] Mccormick, M. C. The contribution of low birth weight to infant mortality and childhood morbidity. N Engl J Med (1985).

Section 13

Surgical Management Issues

Chapter 25

Interdisciplinary Surgical Management of Orbital and Maxillo-Ethmoidal Complex Disorders

Jarosław Paluch, Jarosław Markowski, Jan Pilch, Agnieszka Piotrowska – Seweryn, Robert Kwiatkowski, Joanna Lewin-Kowalik, Czesław Zralek and Agnieszka Gorzkowska

Additional information is available at the end of the chapter

http://dx.doi.org/10.5772/53486

1. Introduction

Surgical management of the orbital and of maxillo-ethmoidal complex disorders is usually performed in patients with trauma, inflammation and/or neoplasms. Depending on the destructed craniofacial region rhinotomy, sinusotomy, orbitotomy, maxillectomy and other types of operations are performed. In case of skull base extension the situation becomes more complicated leading to the necessity of co-operation of several specialists as well as modifications of surgical technique. Surgical procedures on eyeball are undertaken mainly by opthalmologists,but no particular specialty has been yet dedicated for surgical treatment of other orbital regions. However, an attempt is made by surgeons, such as maxillo-facial surgeons, ENT surgeons, neurosurgeons, trauma surgeons, oncologic surgeons and rarely opthalmologists. Patients, in whom operation is performed, are 'border-line' patients and the anatomical structures that are traumatised belong topographically to above specialties. It is very uncommon that there is an interdisciplinary team of surgeons available permanently in hospital to treat the described cases.

In the chapter the authors present as follows: interdisciplinary surgical management of orbital region and anterior cranial fossa, then maxillo-ethmoidal complex and anterior cranial fossa. Additionally, diagnostic problems and treatment of traumas and inflammatory diseases of the pterygopalatine fossa and infratemporal fossa with their histo-clinical characteristics are thoroughly described (Fig.1-2). According to nosologic classification epidemiology, etiology, diagnosis and surgical techniques including own modifications and clinical results, especially in reference to neoplastic tumors is elaborated in both subsections. An integral part of the chapter consists of histo-clinical characteristic of the tumors of described region. A separate subdivision is dedicated to orbital complications and of anterior cranial fossa in the course of pansinusitis. Blow - out fracture is also mentioned in the chapter.

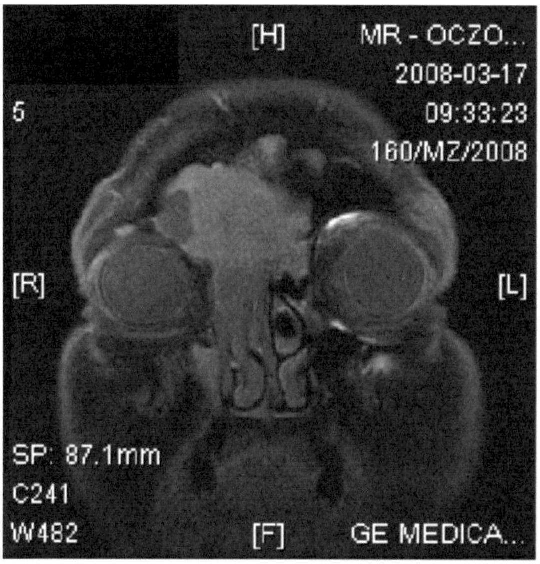

Figure 1. Massive inflammatory infiltration in maxillar sinus, ethmoidal sinus, frontal sinus with extension to anterior cranial fossa – MRI scan (own archives)

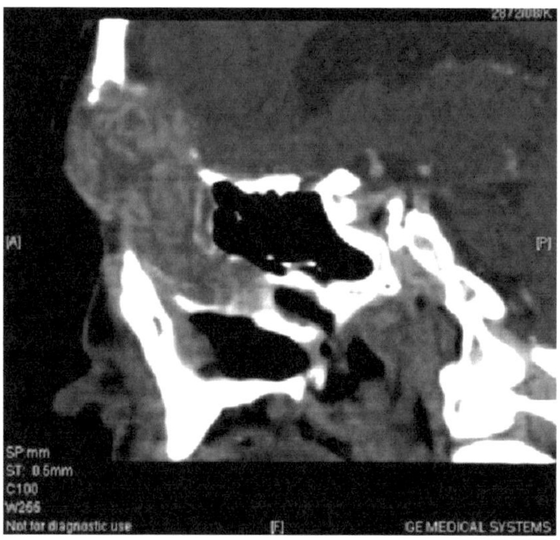

Figure 2. Malignant neoplasm of the orbit with extension to infratemporal fossa CT scan (own archives)

http://dx.doi.org/10.5772/53486

2. Epidemiology

Nowadays, **pansinusitis** is one of the most common diseases that occurs almost as often as arthritis and high blood preassure. Morbidity of chronic pansinusitis is 10,9% (according to Hastan D et al.).

Traumas and intoxications are the third causes of deaths in Poland. Higher mortality present cardiovascular diseases and neoplasms. Traumas of head and neck are responsible for 60-72% of multi-organ traumas. They usually affect elderly men. They occur mainly due to collapses and accidents.

According to Szyfter et al. 3% of head and neck **neoplasms** and 05% of all neoplasms is localized in maxillo-ethmoidal complex. They occur mainly in men, in their 60s-80s. They infiltrate maxillar sinus in 50-70% of cases, nasal cavity in 15-30 and ethmoidal sinus in 10-20%. According to anatomical topography and terminology neoplasms of maxillo-ethmoidal complex and orbit with skull base extension expand in the region above Ohngren's plane that divides the maxillary sinus into an anterior-inferior part and superior-posterior. Tumors that arise in the first part have better prognosis.

3. Diagnostic methods

Diagnosis of traumas, inflammatory diseases and carcinomas of the described region has to be very precise in order to use appropriate surgical approach. Apart from basic diagnostic methods such as thorough anamnesis and examination, the authors emphasise a great role of nasal and nasopharyngeal endoscopy perfectly suited for the assessment of inflammatory and tumor penetration of nasal cavity and paranasal sinuses. However, in terms of carcinomas of orbit and the maxillo-ethmoidal complex with skull base penetration it is recommended to use imaging techniques that improve both the preclinical research and clinical treatment, such as computed tomography (CT), magnetic resonance imaging (MRI), positron emission tomography (PET) and ultrasound imaging. Recently various modalities of these techniques have been introduced to investigate the progression and treatment results of brain tumors. Among them we can name CT three-dimensional reconstruction, electron beam CT, dynamic CT enhancement, CT angiography, CT perfusion enhancement, high-reslution computed tomography (HRCT), diffusion-weighted imaging (DWI-MR), diffusion tensor imaging (DTI-MR) and many others. However, due to financial reasons conventional CT and MRI remains the most common diagnostic imaging method in the management of diseases of the described region.

Also, the authors focus on a great role of fine-needle biopsy as a determinant in diagnosis of orbital neoplasms and of infratemporal fossa. It has been found that histological types of maxillo-ethmoidal complex including pterygopalatine fossa and infratemporal fossa are as follows: pseudotumor, angioma, lymphoma, malignant epithelial neoplasms, neuromas and neurofibromas. Histological classification of intraorbital tumors has been thoroughly described by Handerson.

Histopathological results of biopsied tumors are essential for the following treatment, especially surgical management.

3.1. Fine-needle aspiration biopsy of orbital tumors

Fine-needle aspiration biopsy of orbital tumors verifies whether the tumor is neoplastic or non-neoplastic as well as it gives information about its malignancy. The most common orbital tumors are pseudotumors. The possibility to perform a biopsy depends on the localization of a tumor. In case of meningiomas localized in orbital conus in patient with good vision biopsy should be avoided due to the risk of damaging the optic nerve. Also, biopsy of cavernous hemangioma might develop complications such as bleeding and even haemorrhage.

A 25G hollow needle (length- 25 or 40mm)is used in fine-needle biopsy. The place of its insertion into the examined mass is verified with palpatation. The insertion is carried out through the skin of eyelids without local anaesthesia. In case of impalpable tumors CT or MRI is used and the needle is continuously inserted until the resistance.

The consistence od most orbital tumors is solid. In case of cyst there is a liquid found and in teratomas – sebaceous masses.

The authors emphasise that diagnostic results obtained by fine-needle aspiration biopsy are not unequivocal and in lymphomas immunohistochemical examination is essential.

Also, it is worth mentioning that the described diagnostic methods are limited by 'diagnostic window' (short time in traumas, more time in inflammatory diseases and neoplasms).

4. Surgical management

Surgical treatment in cases of trauma of craniofacial region, pterygopalatine fossa and infratemporal fossa is undertaken using an approach that gives access to damaged structures

4.1. Common approaches

There are several approaches performed in the operation of described regions that are commonly used. Depending on the main disease (trauma, inflammation, primary tumor, metastases) and the operated area (nasal cavity, paranasal sinuses, pterygopalatine fossa, infratemporal fossa) we can name different types of rhinotomy, orbitotomy,sinusotomy, maxillectomy and craniotomy (Fig.3).

Rhinotomy enables an approach to nasal cavity, ethmoidal sinuses, maxillar sinuses as well as nasopharynx. The first lateral rhinotomy incision was introduced by Moure in 1902 (Fig.4).

Since than some other scientist has improved the method, for instance Weber-Ferguson, whose incision and extensions enable medial maxillectomy(Fig.5-6), sometimes with orbital exenteration.

http://dx.doi.org/10.5772/53486

1) Primarytumorsofmaxillo-ethmoidalcomplexwithskullbasepenetration

Lateralrhinotomyby PietroAntoniod'Lima(uni-orbilateral),eventuallysuborbitalcraniotomy

2) Primaryorbitaltumorswithskullbasepenetration

↓

Orbitotomy,eventuallysuborbitalcraniotomyand/orrhinotomy

3) Primarytumorsofpterygopalatinefossawithskullbasepenetration

↓

Fairbanks-Barbosa'sapproach,eventuallylateralcraniotomy

+and/ororbitotomybyKroenlein-Reese-Berkeand/orsuperior/inferiororbitotomy

+and/orlateralrhinotomy

Figure 3. Possible surgical approaches in primary tumors of different regions with skull base penetration

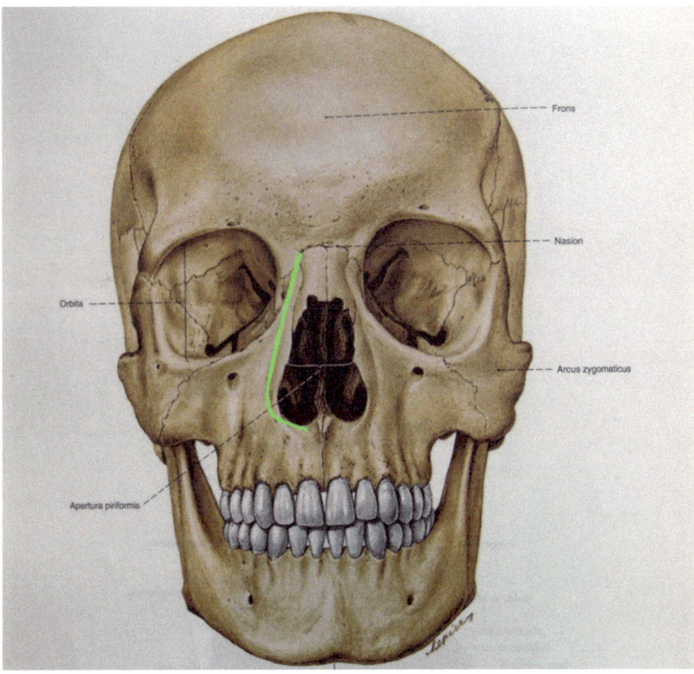

Figure 4. Lateral rhinotomy- Moure's approach (the line indicates skin incision)

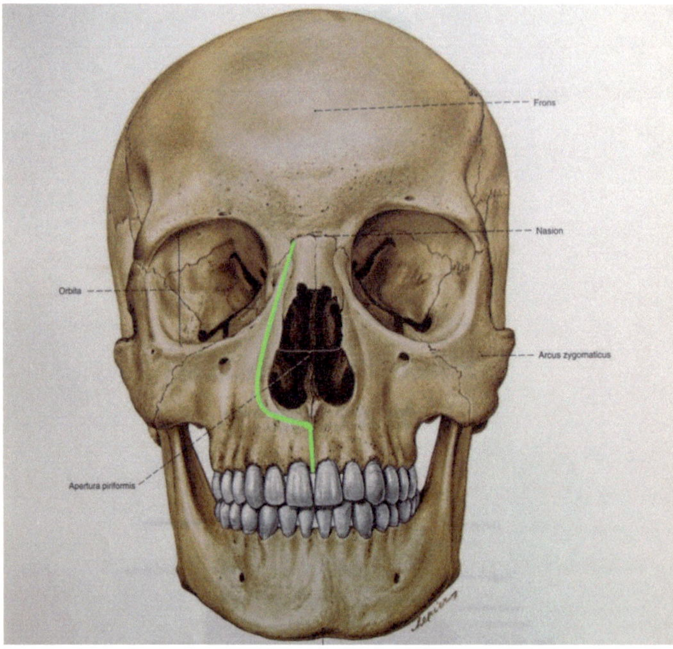

Figure 5. Weber-Ferguson incision. Lateral rhinotomy with inferior extension (the line indicates skin incision).

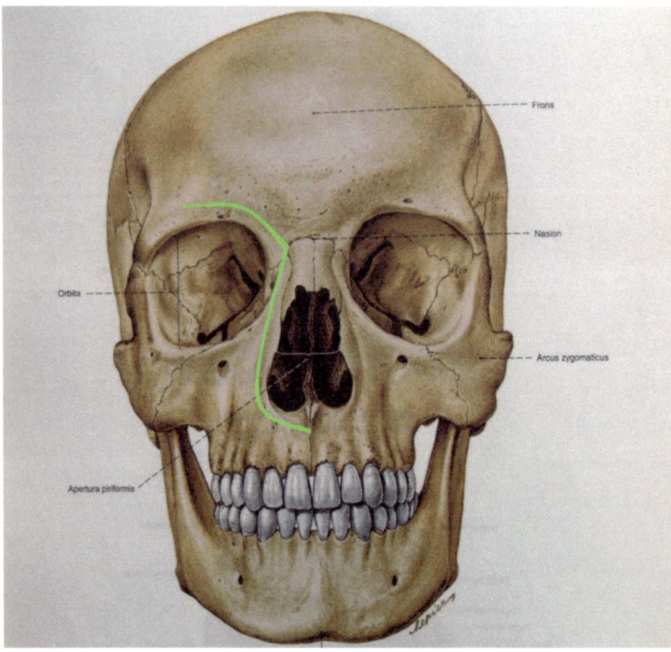

Figure 6. Weber-Ferguson incision. Lateral rhinotomy with superior extension (the line indicates skin incision).

http://dx.doi.org/10.5772/53486

Bechara Y. Ghorayeb has gone further, modifying Weber-Ferguson's incision. Namely, he created a V-shaped flap above the medial canthus in order to prevent scar retraction (Fig.7)

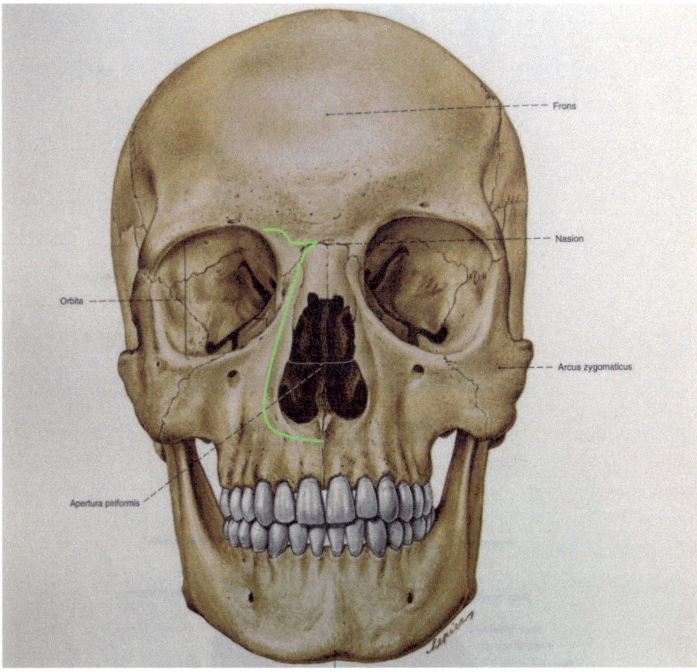

Figure 7. Modification of Weber-Ferguson insicion- by Bechara Y. Ghorayeb (the line indicates skin incision).

Common approaches to **maxillar sinus** include:

- Caldwell – Luc approach in fossa canina
- Denker's operation of maxillar sinus with resection of the anterior wall of maxillar sinus and lateral wall of the nasal cavity

In middle 80s of the twentieth century transcaruncular **orbitotomy** was performed at UCLA University and it is known as Baylis's approach. Later, Lynch described his medial orbitotomy (Fig. 8), which gives access to medio-superior part of the orbit and ethmoidal sinus and sphenoid sinus. Among other orbitotomies there is an anterior orbitotomy (Fig.9), lateral orbitotomy by Kroenlein-Reese-Berke (Fig.10-11) and posterior inferior orbitotomy, in which the technique is carried out through a standard Caldwell-Luc approach through the maxillary sinus. The posterior inferior orbital wall is removed and the inferior rectus is retracted either laterally or medially to gain access to the tumor, which is removed microsurgically.

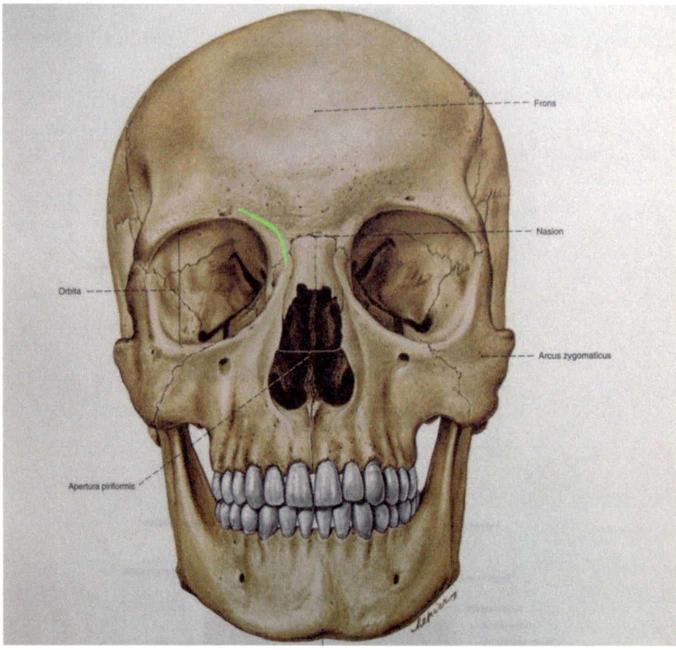

Figure 8. Lynch's medial orbitotomy (the line indicates skin incision)

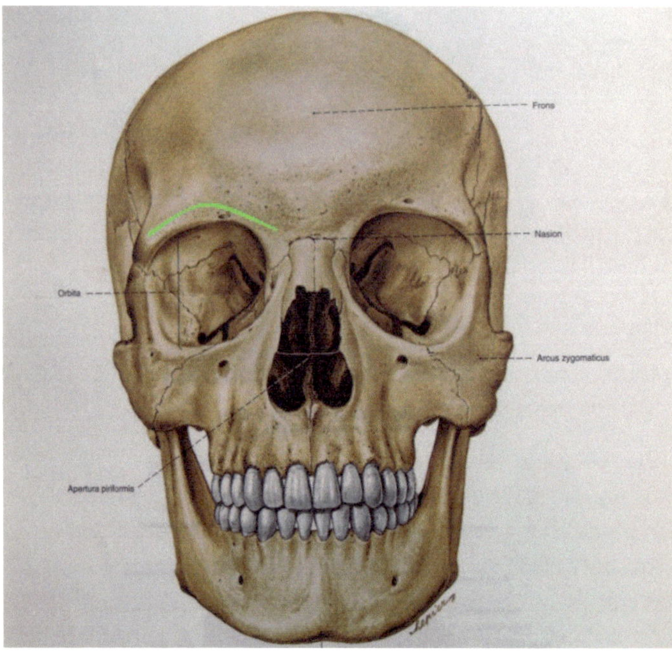

Figure 9. Anterior orbitotomy – incision in supracilial line (the line indicates skin incision)

http://dx.doi.org/10.5772/53486

In case of orbitotomy with bone removal, it is worth mentioning the names of particular operation, depending on the bone removed:

- Naffziger – removal of superior orbital wall
- Sewell – removal of medial orbital wall (ethmoidal sinus)
- Hirsch – removal of inferior orbital wall
- Kroenlein – removal of lateral orbital wall

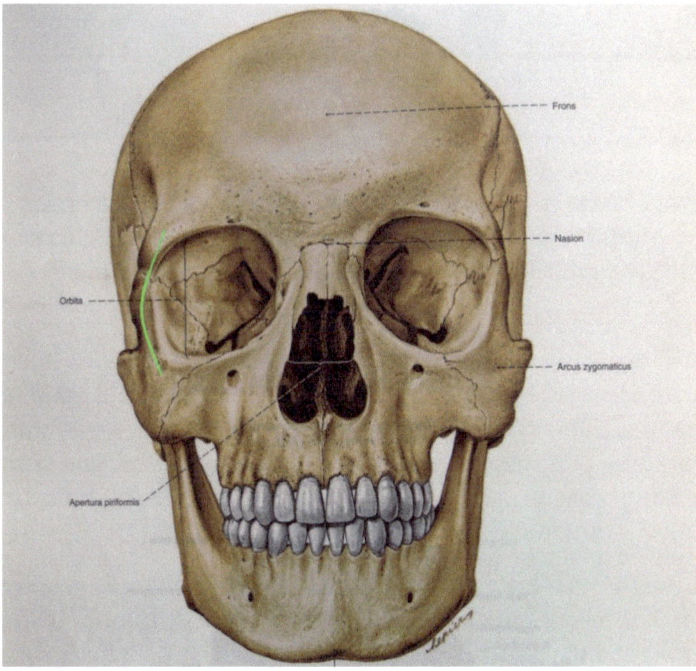

Figure 10. Kroenlein- Reese-Berke lateral orbitotomy (the line indicates skin incision).

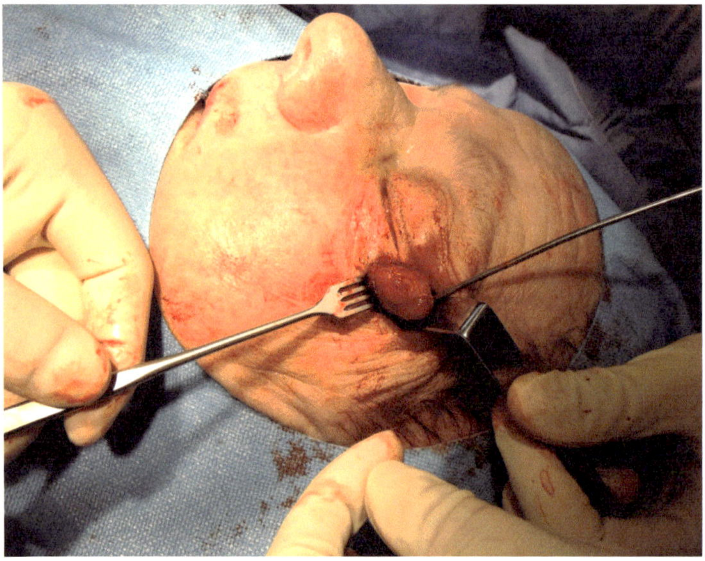

Figure 11. Lateral Kroenlein – Roose - Berke oribtotomy. Lipoma (own archives).

As far as operations on **frontal sinus** are concerned, it is essential to mention Kuemmel-Beck frontal trephine, which provides diagnostic information about the contents of the sinus and the function of the ostium.However, nowadays there are more and more endoscopic operations on the frontal sinus.

More complicated operations that provide wide access to nasal cavities, inferior and medial part of maxilla, infratemporal fossa and pterygopalatine fossa include **midfacial degloving** and **cranio-facial resection.** While midfacial degloving leaves no scars, cranio-facial resection gives wider access to upper parts of nasal cavity, frontal sinus and skull base and it is usually performed by a team of ENT surgeons and neurosurgeons. If the orbit is involved orbital exenteration is carried out.

Surgical procedures are the basic method of treatment of tumors of anterior cranial fossa. This kind of surgical management is usually performed by a team of both ENT surgeons and neurosurgeons and the common approaches can be divided into **extracranial, intracranial and endoscopic**. Among intracranial approaches, transcranial-transbasal one should be mentioned. It is a frontal craniotomy which gives access to tumors of ethmoidal sinuses infiltrating skull base and sphenoid sinus as well as clival tumors. Subcranial approach is a modification of this technique. Apart from common orbitotomies we also have orbito-temporal and orbito-zygomatic approaches. Extracranial approaches are usually transshenoidal. A separate group of operations on anterior cranial fossa is created by a combination of the two approaches- extra-and intracranial (known as cranio-facial resection= anterior fossa cranio-facial resection – AFCFR).

4.2. Own modifications of common approaches

Surgical treatment in cases of trauma of craniofacial region, pterygopalatine fossa and infratemporal fossa is performed with an approach that gives access to damaged structures. Presented surgical procedures are performed with internal approaches due to extensive character of inflammation/neoplasm. Therefore endoscopic techniques dedicated for limited diseases are not elaborated in the chapter.

In case of tumors, the resection is conditioned by clinical staging- from endoscopic endonasal tumorectomy, through endoscopic surgery of orbit and pterygopalatine fossa up to advanced resections like own modification of "scalp" approach to half of viscerocranium (lateral rhinotomy+ superior/inferior orbitotomy + Fairbanks- Barbosa's approach) (Case.1-Fig.12-16, Case.2 –Fig. 17-20, Case 3 – Fig. 21-23).

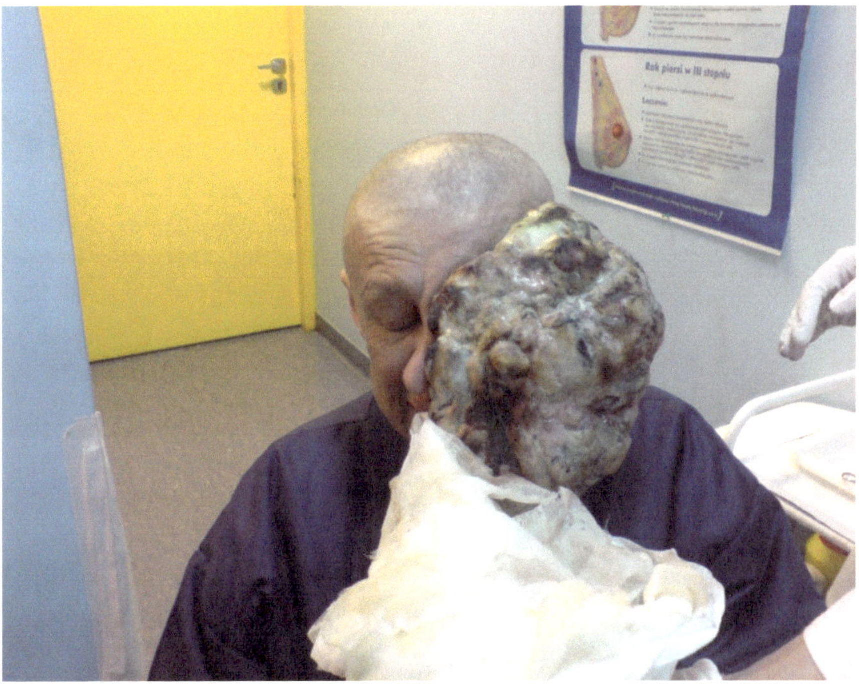

Figure 12. Case 1. Massive orbital carcinoma with co-existing active tuberculosis. (The photo was taken on patient's agreement)

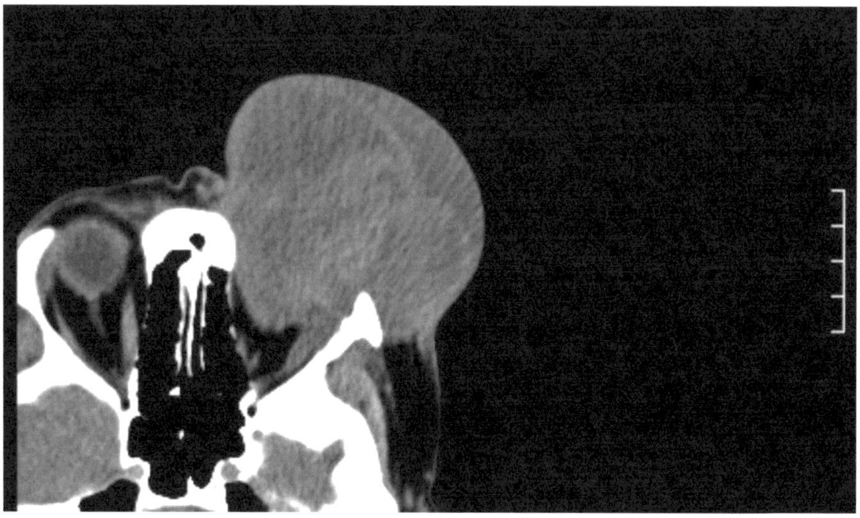

Figure 13. Case 1. Massive orbital carcinoma with co-existing active tuberculosis –preoperative CT scan.

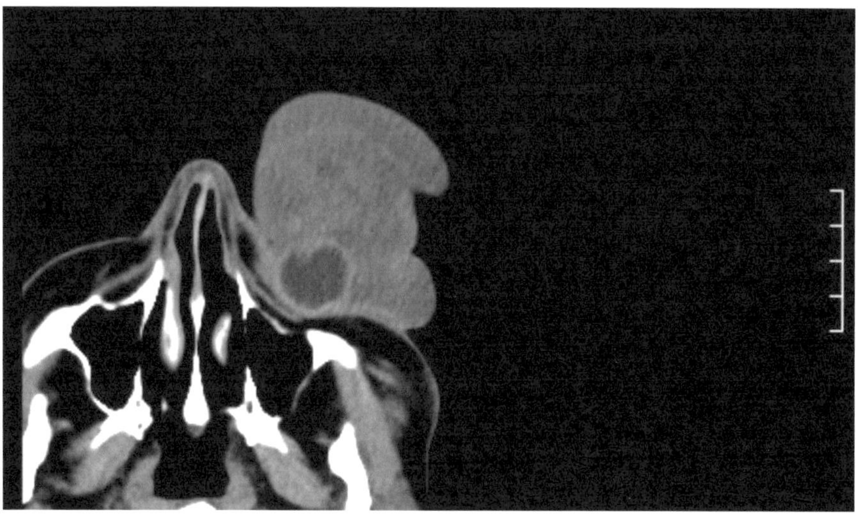

Figure 14. Case 1. Massive orbital carcinoma with co-existing active tuberculosis– preoperative CT scan.

http://dx.doi.org/10.5772/53486

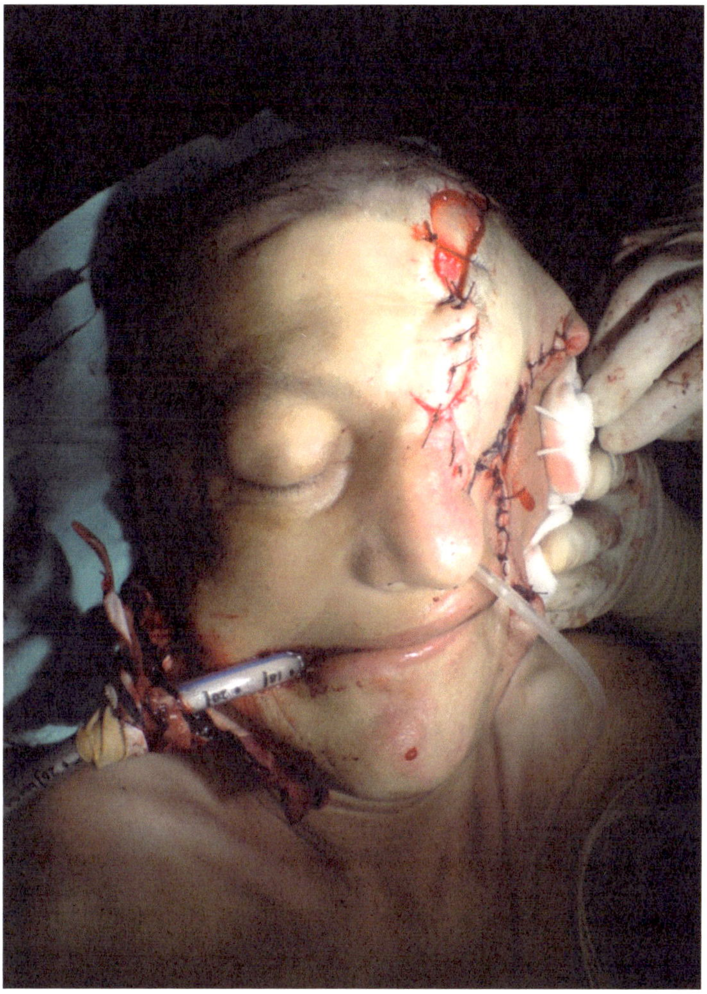

Figure 15. Case 1. Massive orbital carcinoma with co-existing active tuberculosis– intraoperative view. Lateral rhinotomy + superior orbitotomy + subfrontal approach (The photo was taken on patient's agreement).

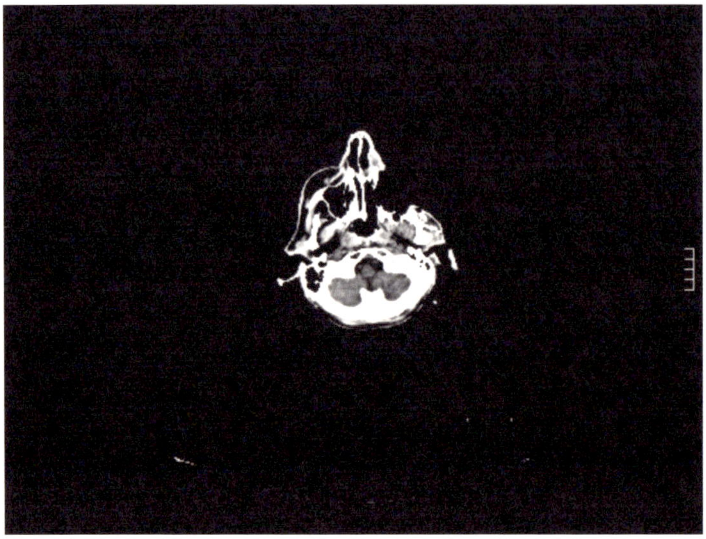

Figure 16. Case 1. Massive orbital carcinoma with co-existing active tuberculosis– postperative CT scan.

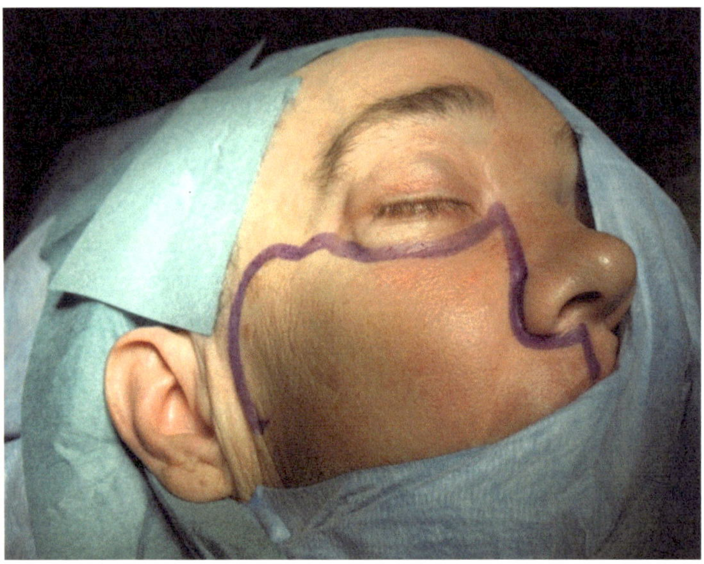

Figure 17. Case 2. Incission line (lateral rhinotomy+ infrerior orbitotomy + Fairbanks- Barbosa's approach)of modified approach to massive carcinoma of maxillo-ethmoidal complex – pre-operative image (The photo was taken on patient's agreement).

http://dx.doi.org/10.5772/53486

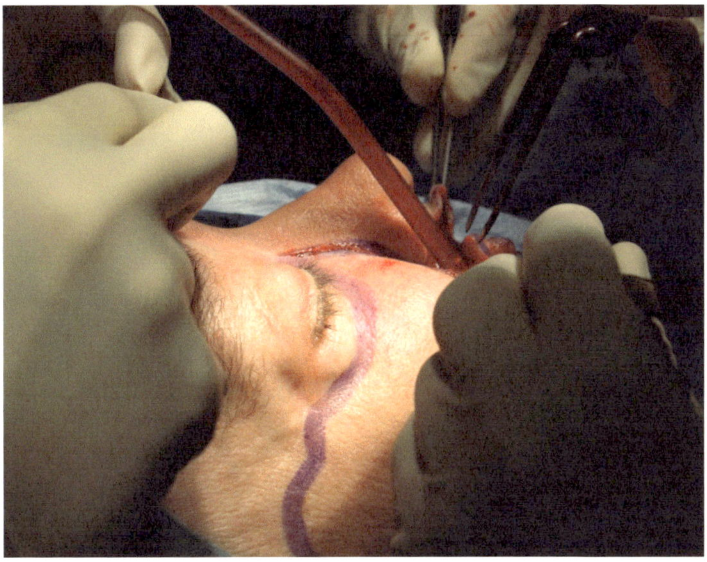

Figure 18. Case 2. Incission line of modified approach to massive carcinoma of maxillo-ethmoidal complex – interoperative image

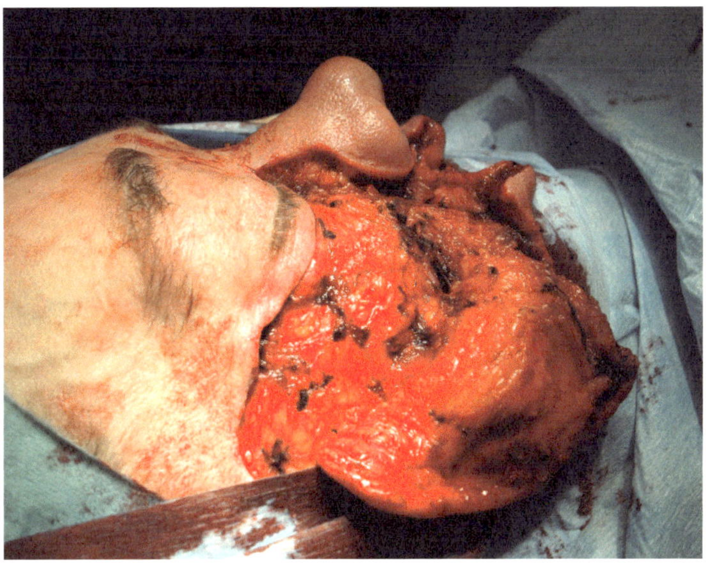

Figure 19. Case 2. Incission line (lateral rhinotomy+ infrerior orbitotomy + Fairbanks- Barbosa's approach)of modified approach to massive carcinoma of maxillo-ethmoidal complex – interoperative image

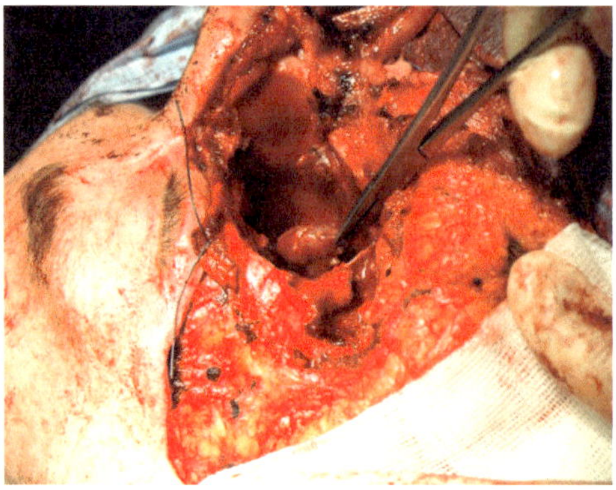

Figure 20. Case 2. Incission line (lateral rhinotomy+ infrerior orbitotomy + Fairbanks- Barbosa's approach)of modified approach to massive carcinoma of maxillo-ethmoidal complex – interoperative image. The surgical tool indicated neoplastic tissue.

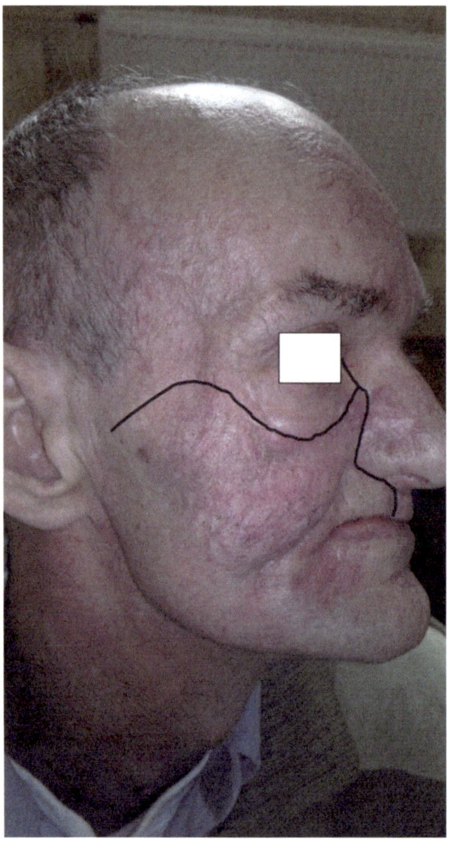

Figure 21. Case 3.Incission line of modified approach to massive carcinoma of maxillo-ethmoidal complex – post-operative image (The photo was taken on patient's agreement).

http://dx.doi.org/10.5772/53486

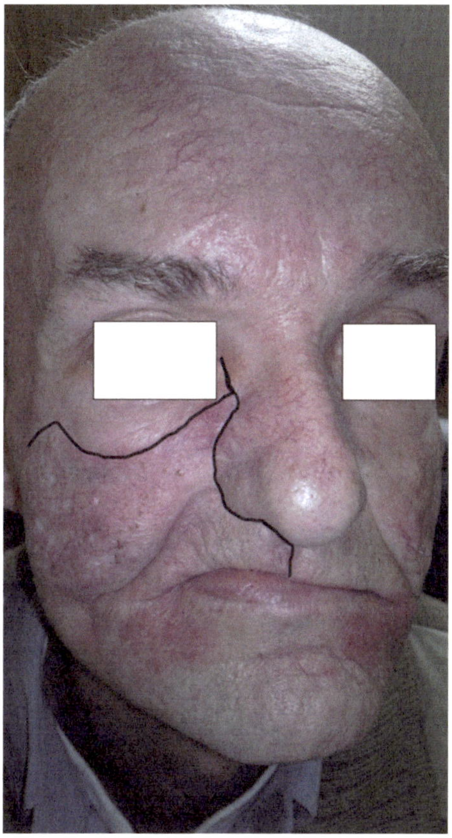

Figure 22. Case 3.Incission line of modified approach to massive carcinoma of maxillo-ethmoidal complex – post-operative image (The photo was taken on patient's agreement)

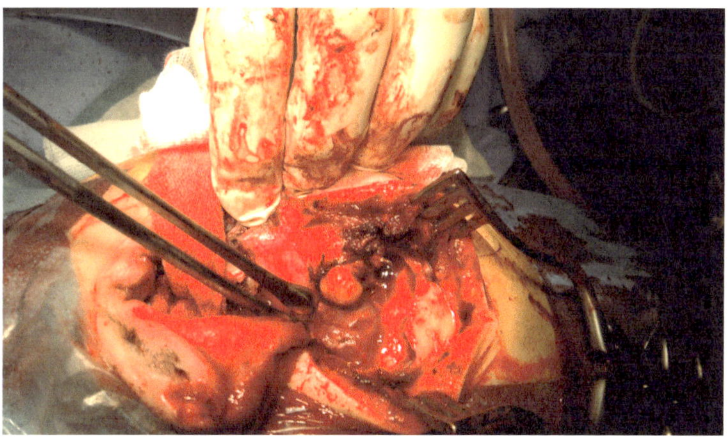

Figure 23. Case 3 - Intraoperative image (own archives)

In order to receive access to maxillo-ethmoidal complex and frontal sinus as well as anterior cranial fossa lateral rhinotomy combined with Uffenorde's approach can be performed (Fig. 24-25)

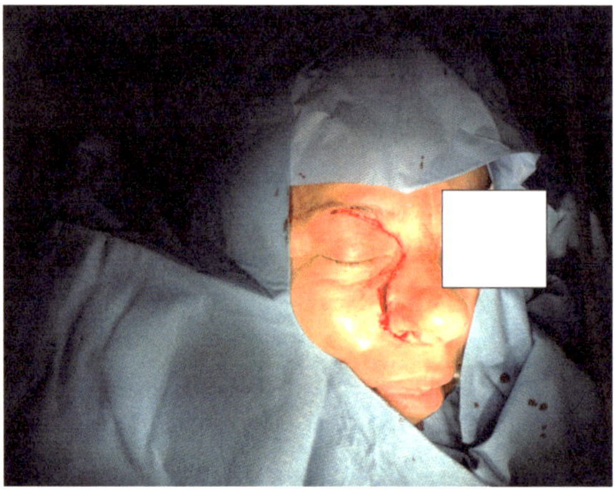

Figure 24. Case 4. Lateral rhinotomy + Uffenorde scission line- intraoperative image (own archives).

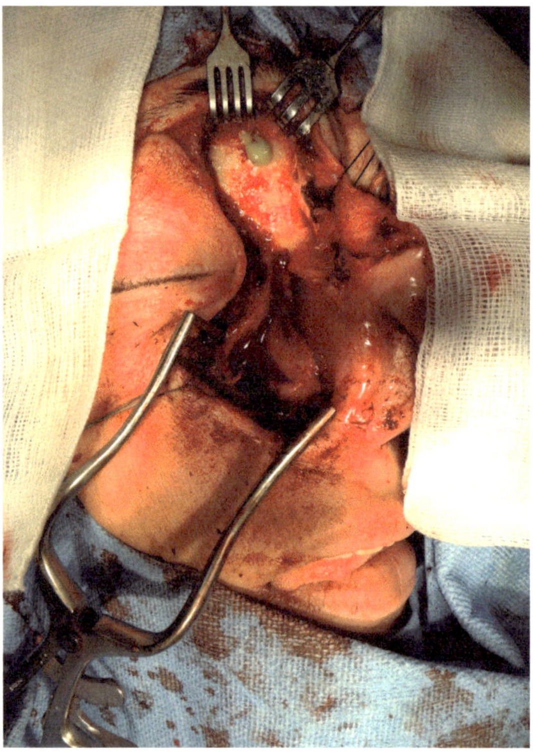

Figure 25. Case 4. Lateral rhinotomy + Uffenorde section line – intraoperative image. Pus in frontal sinus. (own archives).

http://dx.doi.org/10.5772/53486

Another modification, such as Fairbanks-Barbossa's approach and lateral pharyngotomy can be used in order to perform surgical management of pathologies localized in the inferior part of Ohrngren's plane (Fig.26-28)

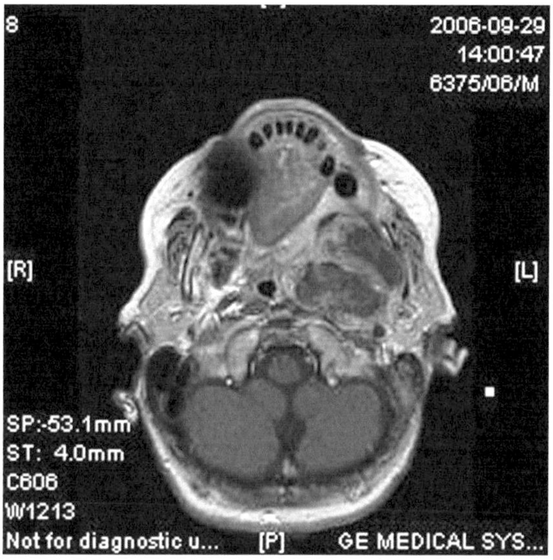

Figure 26. Case 5. A preoperative MRI scan showing tumour mass in left parapharyngeal region with pterygopalatine fossa and skull base penetration. Tumour reaches the level of lower wall of left maxillary sinus and infratemporal region.

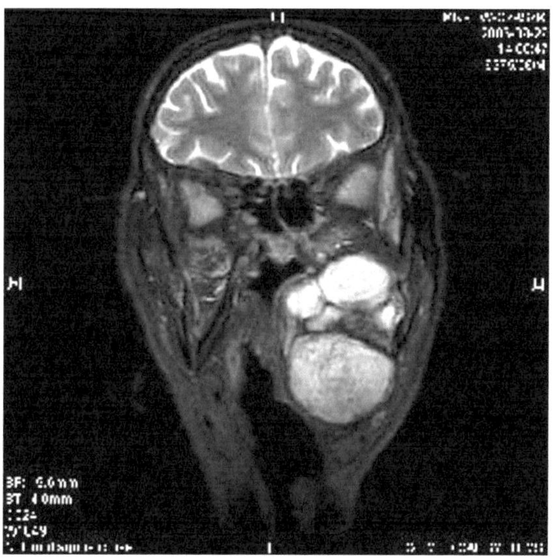

Figure 27. Case 5. A preoperative MRI scan showing a substantial mass effect – tumour mass bulges towards nasopharynx and mesopharynx causing compression and displacement of those structures.

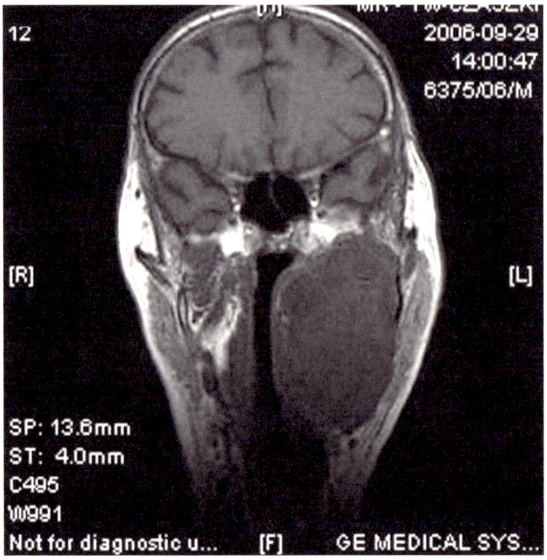

Figure 28. Case 5. A preoperative MRI scan showing tumour mass directly adjacent to the sphenoid bone and left parotid gland.

4.3. Other surgical aspects

In advanced neoplasms the operation is combined with simultaneous reconstruction of damaged areas, while in case of residual tissues an implantation of intraoperative applicators for brachytherapy might be used (Fig.29.). It is also possible to initiate adjuvant radiotherapy without reconstructive surgery.

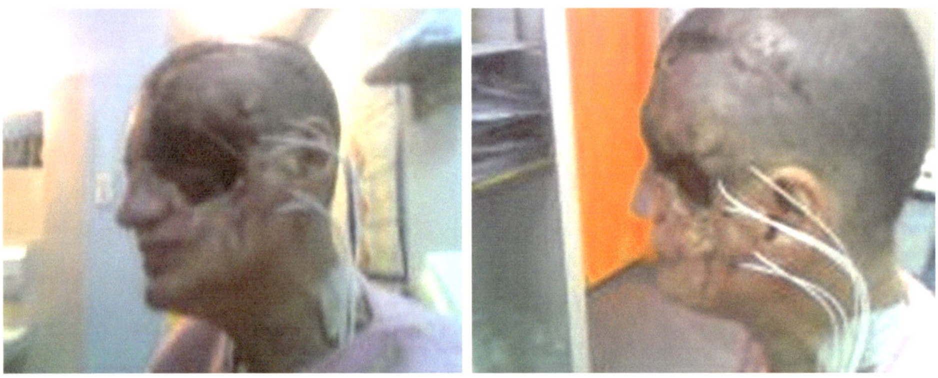

Figure 29. Case 1. Applicators of brachytherapy implanted intraoperatively. Teletherapy was impossible to be performed due to active tuberculosis. Follow-up- 2,5 years without recurrence.

http://dx.doi.org/10.5772/53486

However, reconstructive surgery with vascular microanastomosis seems to be the priceless method of treatment, resulting in good functional and aesthetic effect.

Occasionally, it is essential to obliterate mechanically the vessel providing blood to traumatised region and/or use temporary or permanent endovascular embolization (esp. internal jugular vein) as the first step of therapeutic procedure. A wide drainage to nasal cavities is crucial for proper healing of inflammations or inflammatory complications of orbit and pterygopalatine fossa.

Also, the authors indicate that in the described region there is a risk of expanding the neoplastic and/or inflammatory tissue into 'critical structures' such as meninges, optic nerve, internal carotid artery, facial nerve and sinus cavernosus limits safe course of surgical procedures. The situation reveals due to natural extension of neoplastic and/or inflammatory tissue, intraoperative failure or high-dose radiotherapy. The presence of critical structures limits safe course of surgical procedure.

It is also worth mentioning that in the course of chronic and, rarely, acute pansinusitis orbital complications are observed in 3,7-11 % of all patients hospitalized due to pansinusitis and they are associated with symptoms such as blurred vision, diplopia, deterioration of visual acuity, oedema of palpebra and oedema of the tissues of medial angle of the eye. In advanced situations exophthalmia may occur. The process can extend into extraorbital structures resulting in their oedema and phlegmons and/or abscess of the orbit. HRCT plays the greatest role in diagnosis. Surgical treatment consists of external opening of many sinuses and excision of the pathological tissues in the orbit. Opthalmological examination with assessment of visual acuity, morphology of the eyeball and possible damage of optical nerve is essential in preoperative diagnosis of above cases. Optic nerve and sinus cavernosus are 'critical structures in surgical management of this limited region.

A separate subdivision should be dedicated to blow-out fracture which is an orbital floor fracture due to blunt trauma of the head. Very fine bones of this region, in case of their fracture, cause an entrapment of the orbital content (i.e.extraocular muscles, esp.inferior rectus and inferior oblique) in maxillar sinus. A damage of infraorbital canal with infraorbital nerve is often observed and in such case numbness in the region of lower eyelid, cheek, lateral part of nose, upper labium, upper teeth and gingivia can be diagnosed.

Symptoms include:

- enopthalmos
- diplopia
- pain during eye movement
- limited movements of eyeball

Computed tomography scanning is preferred in diagnosis of blow-out fractures (Fig.30)

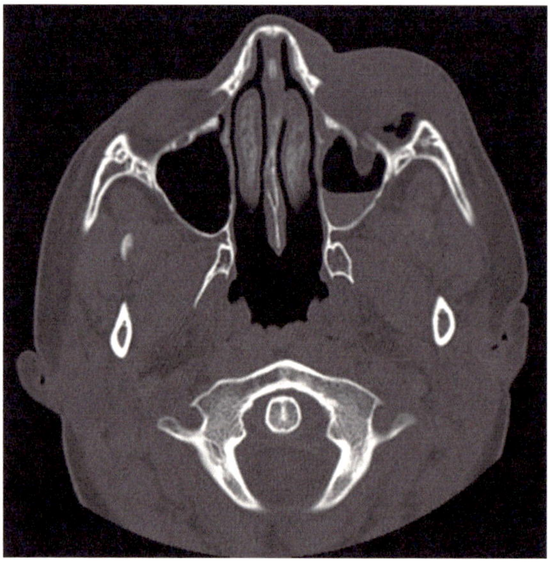

Figure 30. CT scan- blow-out fracture.

In surgical management of blow-out fractures resection of the injured bone is performed by orbitotomy or an approach through maxillar sinus. Reconstruction consists of autogenic grafts (fascia, bone graft) or allogenic ones (silicon, Teflon) (Fig.31.)

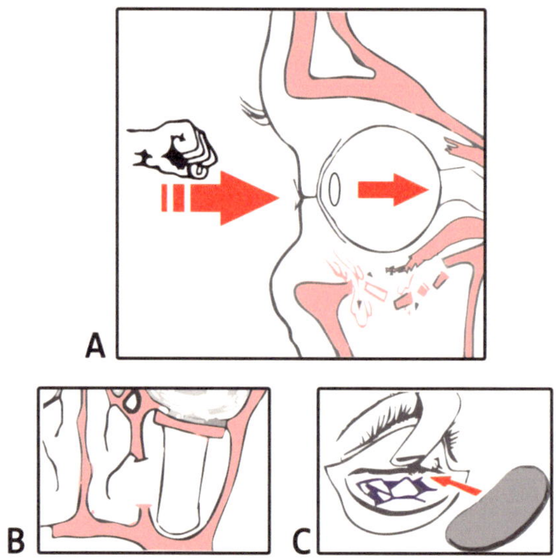

Figure 31. A- Blow-our fracture- patomechanism, B- bone graft inserted through nasal cavity, C- allogenic graft inserted subciliarily

http://dx.doi.org/10.5772/53486

In most cases oculoplastic surgeons will wait 10-14 days following the trauma in order to enable an associated oedema and/or heamorrage to be absorbed.

5. Results

The results of surgical management of tumors of described region depend on primary clinical staging assessed with TNM scale, the stage of malignancy, presence of associated disorders and patient's age. Survival rates depend on above factors and application of adjuvant oncologic treatment utilizing teletherapy, brachytherapy, chemical cytoreduction and combination of suggested methods.

In summary the authors emphasise the necessity of interdisciplinary treatment of orbit and maxillo-ethmoidal complex.

Author details

Jarosław Paluch[1], Jarosław Markowski[1], Jan Pilch[1], Agnieszka Piotrowska – Seweryn[1], Robert Kwiatkowski[2], Joanna Lewin-Kowalik[3], Czesław Zralek[4] and Agnieszka Gorzkowska[5]

1 Department of Laryngology, Medical University of Silesia, Katowice, Poland

2 Radiotherpay Division, Katowice, Poland

3 Department of Physiology, Medical University of Silesia, Katowice, Poland

4 Department of Neurosurgery, Medical University of Silesia, Katowice, Poland

5 Department of Neurology, Medical University of Silesia, Katowice, Poland

References

[1] Bulsara, Ketan R.; Al-Mefty: Skull Base Surgery for Benign Skull Base Tumors; Ossama.Journal of Neuro-Oncology vol. 69 issue 1-3 August 2004. p. 181 – 189.

[2] Byron J.Bailey : Head and neck surgery – Otolaryngology, Volume Two, J.B. Lippincott Company Philadalphia, 1993, 1110-1125

[3] Chen T. William: Oculoplastic surgery. The essentials; Thieme New York 2001; ISBN 1-58890 – 027-4; 419-451

[4] Handerson J.W.: Orbital Tumors, ed 3. New York: Raven Pres, 1994

[5] Hastan D, Fokkens WJ, Bachert C et al. Chronic rhinosinusitis in Europe - an underestimated disease. A GA2LEN study. Allergy 2011; Published online ahead of print, May 2011

[6] Hussain A, Hulmi OJ, Murray DP: Lateral rhinotomy through nasal aesthetic subunits. Improved cosmetic outcome; J Laryngol Otol. 2002 Sep;116(9):703-6.

[7] Kennerdell JS, Maroon JC, Celin SE. :The posterior inferior orbitotomy; Ophthal Plast Reconstr Surg. 1998 Jul;14(4):277-80.

[8] Kyuha C., Taeyun K., Kyungsun C., Myunghwan C., Jonghee Y., Chulhee C.: Diagnostic Techniques and Surgical Management of Brain Tumors, Current Optical Imaging Techniques for Brain Tumor Research: Application of in vivo Laser Scanning Microscopy Imaging with a Cranial Window System, ISBN: 978-953-307-589-1 , InTech 2011:155-172

[9] Lund VJ, Stammberger H, Nicolai P, Castelnuovo P, Beal T, Beham A, Bernal-Sprekelsen M, Braun H, Cappabianca P, Carrau R, Cavallo L, Clarici G, Draf W, Esposito F, Fernandez-Miranda J, Fokkens W, Gardner P, Gellner V, Hellquist H, Hermann P, Hosemann W, Howard D, Jones N, Jorissen M, Kassam A, Kelly D, Kurschel-Lackner S, Leong S, McLaughlin N, Maroldi R, Minovi A, Mokry M, Onerci M, Ong YK, Prevedello D, Saleh H, Sehti DS, Simmen D, Snyderman C, Solares A, Spittle M, Stamm A, Tomazic P, Trimarchi M, Unger F, Wormald PJ, Zanation A; European Rhinologic Society Advisory Board on Endoscopic Techniques in the Management of Nose, Paranasal Sinus and Skull Base Tumours: European position paper on endoscopic management of tumours of the nose, paranasal sinuses and skull base; Rhinol Suppl. 2010 Jun 1;(22):1-143.

[10] Margarino G., Scala M. , Mereu P., Comandin D.i, Schenone G., Galli A., Francaviglia N., Gipponi M.: Combined craniofacial approach to facial tumours involving the anterior skull base; European Journal of Surgical Oncology (EJSO)Volume 22, Issue 4, August 1996, Pages 361–365

[11] Mingkun Y., Wei Y., Xiangqian Q, Jun Q., Zhenyang L., Wenfeng F. : "Diagnostic Techniques and Surgical Management of Brain Tumors", Imaging Techniques in Brain Tumor, ISBN 978-953-307-589-1, InTech 2011:43-66

[12] Morioka M, Hamada J, Yano S, Kai Y, Ogata N, Yumoto E, Ushio Y, Kuratsu J: Frontal skull base surgery combined with endonasal endoscopic sinus surgery; Surg Neurol. 2005 Jul;64(1):44-9; discussion 49.

[13] Neumann H.H., Tardy M.E.,Jr, Kastenbauer E.R.: Head and Neck Surgery.Volume 1, Face, Nose and Facial Skull,Part II; Georg Thieme Verlag, Stuttgart, New York 1995, ISBN 3-13-547102-0, ISBN 0-86577-586-9: 476-498, 555-609

[14] Paluch J., Markowski J., Gierek T., Pencak P., Witkowska M., Kajor M., Gorzkowska A., Piotrowska A.: Resonance Tractography in Neuroradiological Diagnostic Aspects, Diagnostic Techniques and Surgical Management of Brain Tumors, ISBN 978-953-307-589-1, InTech 2011: 199-204

[15] Silver C.E. Atlas of Head and neck surgery; Churchill Livingstone, New York, Edinburgh, London, Melbourne 1986

[16] Słoniewski P., Dzierżanowski J, Lipowski P.,Szmuda T., Czapiewski P.: Orbital tumours operated by orbito-cranial ap roaches– results of treatment of 38 patients; Ann. Acad. Med. Gedan., 2010, 40, 81–89

[17] Snyderman CH, Carrau RL, Kassam AB, Zanation A, Prevedello D, Gardner P, Mintz A: Endoscopic skull base surgery: principles of endonasal oncological surgery; J Surg Oncol. 2008 Jun 15;97(8):658-64.

[18] Spaeth G.L:. Chirurgia okulistyczna. Wyd.I polskie pod redakcją Jerzego Szaflika, Urban & Partner, Wrocław 2006, ISBN -10-8389581-1, ISBN -13-978-83-89581-53-2; 457-471

[19] Szyfter W.:Nowotwory w otorynolaryngologii; Termedia Wydawnictwa Medyczne, Poznań 2012, ISBN: 978-83-62138-80-7; 139-144, 366-369

[20] Ulgen T, Turhan T, Yurtseven T, Oner K.: Simple anterior orbitotomy; Minim Invasive Neurosurg. 2004 Apr;47(2):115-8.

[21] Zhou W, Fang J, Ni X, Huang Z, Wang Q, Chen X, Chen XZ, Xu H: The modified rhinotomy for treatment of tumors involving skull base; Lin Chung Er Bi Yan Hou Tou Jing Wai Ke Za Zhi. 2010 Apr;24(7):301-3.

Section 14

Epidemiology of Brain Tumors

Chapter 26

The Epidemiology of Paediatric Brain Cancer — Descriptive Epidemiology and Risk Factors

Adrianna Ranger

Additional information is available at the end of the chapter

http://dx.doi.org/10.5772/52427

1. Introduction

Cancer is the most frequently diagnosed disease-related cause of death among children and adolescents [1]. Of all paediatric cancers, those involving the central nervous system (CNS), and especially the brain, are collectively among the most common, ranking as the most common solid tumor and either first or second overall (second only to leukaemia) in the United States (USA) [1]- [5], Canada [6], and Mexico [7]. For example, in the USA in 2004, 555 cases of CNS cancer-related death were confirmed among children, and 566 for leukemia, representing 25.0% and 25.5%, and therefore accounting, between them, for more than half of the total number of cancer deaths in individuals under age 20 [1]. Similar numbers through 2011 are published in an on-line report of the National Cancer Institute [5]. Since in excess of 90% of primary CNS cancers in children originate within the brain [4], from this point onward, this chapter will generally be limited to primary brain cancers. The *American Brain Tumor Association* has claimed that approximately 4,200 children younger than age 20 will be diagnosed with a primary brain tumor in the year 2012, of whom 3,020 will be under the age of 15 [8].

Survival rates from brain cancer have improved dramatically over the past forty years, presumably due to a combination of improved treatments and earlier detection [9]. However, there are concerns that the incidence of brain cancer has increased and/or is destined to increase due to the emergence of a host of new risk factors with almost universal exposure, especially in industrialized countries. Among these novel risk factors is the exponentially increasing use of hand-held electronic devices like cell phones, iPods, iPads and other electronic reading devices [10]- [12].

But is the incidence of brain cancer really increasing? Is this increase universal or just in certain countries and regions? Are these new devices playing a role? This chapter reviews the descriptive epidemiology of brain cancer in the paediatric age group, specifically looking at trends over time, followed by an examination of known and suspected risk factors. The first question is: Is the incidence of brain cancer really increasing?

2. Descriptive epidemiology

2.1. The incidence of paediatric brain cancer: Trends over time

Before discussing its incidence, it is necessary first to define what is meant by *paediatric brain cancer*. For the purposes of this chapter, only primary cancers of the brain will be considered, excluding metastases to brain from other sources, like lung and breast. Brain tumors are quite heterogeneous, in terms of both their histology and clinical course and prognosis. There also are exceedingly rare forms that stem from highly specialized cells, in addition to types that are more common. Most research on brain cancer has focused on the most common, which also tend to be the most lethal forms.

Cancers involving neurons themselves are quite rare, the majority of brain cancers involving cells that originate within the glial cell line [4]. Such glial cell cancers include astrocytomas in all their different forms and grades, from pilocytic astrocytomas to glioblastoma multiforme; oligodendrogliomas; other gliomas, and ependymomas. Primitive neuroectodermal tumors (PNET), which arise from primitive neuroectodermal tissues and include medulloblastomas, are another relatively common brain neoplasm that tends to arise in very young children; PNET account for approximately 20% of malignant CNS tumors in children [4]. Together, astrocytomas, oligodendrogliomas and other gliomas, ependymomas, and PNETs account for roughly 97% of all malignant paediatric brain tumors [4]. All remaining brain tumors are either very rare, usually benign, or both; and they all are especially uncommon in children. Primary CNS lymphomas that arise from the cells and tissues that comprise the CNS lymphatic system comprise one to two percent of all primary brain tumors, with patients whose immunity is compromised (e.g., AIDS patients and organ transplant recipients) at especially high risk. Other brain tumors that can be malignant but are usually benign include meningiomas, that are quite common, and pituitary and pineal tumors, which are much rarer, especially in children and adolescents. In this chapter, all brain cancers will be discussed; but the majority of research that has been conducted on risk factors for brain cancer in children has involved astrocytomas, oligodendrogliomas and other gliomas, ependymomas, and PNETs [4].

Despite its obvious importance as a medical issue, publications on general population studies (as opposed to case-control studies) assessing brain cancer incidence trends over time, and especially on its incidence in children, have been surprisingly rare. Almost all published general population data are at least a decade old, harkening back to a time when there was considerable concern that the incidence of brain cancer was increasing [4], [13]- [17]. Exceptions are longitudinal studies in the United Kingdom [18] and in India [19]. In the USA, between 1973 and 2001, the overall age-adjusted incidence of brain cancers was 6.1 cases per 100,000 person-years, of which roughly 46% (2.8 cases per 100,000 person-years) were the most malignant form, glioblastoma multiforme [13]. The incidence in children was 2.5 per 100,000 person-years. Overall, brain cancer rates increased steadily between 1973 and 1987, but then declined steadily afterwards; however, across all ages, the incidence of glioblastoma in 2001 was greater than the mean incidence over the 28 years of observation (3.0 versus 2.8 per 100,000). Though mortality across all brain cancers declined over the study period, survival did not improve for glioblastomas [13]. Data specifically on US children under age 15 between 1975 and 1995 reveal a clear increase in brain cancer incidence throughout the study period, rising from a low of under 2.5 per 100,000 person-years in 1975 and 1976 to highs of roughly 3.2 per 100,000 in 1987 and 1993 [4]. Further analysis of this trend identified, rather than a steady increase, a marked 'jump' in rate between the periods before and after 1985 [20], which corresponds to the marked increase in the availability of magnetic resonance imaging (MRI) for brain cancer detection in the mid 1980s and consistent with the lack of any significant increase in brain cancer mortality rate [4]. Interestingly, the noted increase was site specific, with incidence more than doubling in the brainstem and increasing by more than 50% in the cerebrum, but actually declining in the cerebellum and increasing by a mere 6% across all other sites [20]. Similarly, in the Northeastern U.S., certain brain cancers were noted to increase in incidence between 1954 and 1998 more than others, with annual increases of 1% in pilocytic astrocytomas, 1% in primitive neuroectodermal tumors, and 2.3% in miscellaneous gliomas [21].

The *Surveillance Epidemiology and End Results* database initially was created by the U.S. *National Cancer Institute* (NCI) in 1973 as the coalescence of 9 regional cancer registries to generate epidemiological data on cancer in the U.S. [22] It has since expanded to collect data on a broad array of cancers from registries representing 26% of the total U.S. population, and data on specific cancers are available for 1975 through 2009, including brain and other nervous system cancers [23]. SEER data demonstrate an overall incidence of brain and other nervous system cancers (invasive) of 5.85 across both sexes and all ages and races in 1975, with subsequent peak incidences of 6.51 in 1981, 7.05 in 1990, and 6.91 in 1999, with a gradual decline afterwards to 6.58 in 2009, for an overall incidence over the 35 years of data collection of 6.60 per 100,000 [24], and an average of 6.50 over the five years 2005 through 2009 [25]. Data by age are currently only listed for 2005 through 2009, and average 3.1 per 100,000 for those 19 and under, versus 19.6 for those 65 and older [25].

In other countries over roughly the same time period, roughly a 25% increase in cancer incidence was noted in Austria between 1970 and 2002, with mortality from brain cancer peaking in 2002 [14]; in Brazil between 1980 and 1998, age-adjusted brain cancer mortality rates across all age groups increased by approximately 50% (from 2.24 to 3.35 10^5) [16]; in Norway between 1970 and 1999, the overall rate of brain and CNS tumors increased from 6.49 to 12.02 cases per 100,000 person-years, an 85% increase, with a trend of continuing increase from 1995-1999, especially in children 0-4 years old and in those 60 years and older [17]; and in India between 1982 and 2003, statistically-significant 3.1 to 4.7% increases in incidence were noted at three of five major centres (Mumbai, Bangalore and Chennai) for both males and females across all ages, while incidence remained stable in Delhi and Bhopal [19]. Over a somewhat earlier period, incidence and mortality from brain cancer rose significantly in Canada between

1959 and 1987, though this was most marked in elderly males [26], and incidence doubled between 1948 and 1988 in New Zealand [27].

Contrary to these increases, in the United Kingdom between 1998 and 2007, no significant time trends were noted in overall incidence of brain cancers for either gender, or for any specific age group [18]. Site-specific increases were noted for the temporal lobe in men (0.04 new cases per year) and women (0.02 per year), accompanied by decreases in the rates of cancers involving the parietal lobe (-0.03 per year), cerebrum (-0.02 per year) and cerebellum (-0.01 per year), but in men only. The authors conjectured that the observed increase in the rate of temporal lobe cancers, if caused by mobile phone use, would constitute less than one additional case per 100,000 people over the observation period.

Consequently, though clear increases in the incidence of brain cancer were evident internationally into the 1990s, since that time there appears to have been relative stabilization, at least in the U.S and the U.K. Unfortunately, a lack of readily-accessible international data over the past decade precludes any assumptions beyond these two countries.

2.2. Trends in mortality from brain cancer

Brain cancer is the second leading disease-related (non-traumatic) cause of death among children and adolescents, behind leukemia, generally accounting for between 500 and 600 deaths per year in the USA since the year 2000 [1], [5]. However, in contrast with trends towards increasing incidence in many populations, overall there has been a decline in mortality from brain neoplasms over the past three to four decades, and this decline has been relatively continuous, even over periods of time when incidence has appeared to rise [4], [13], [20], [28]. In the U.S., this trend has been especially evident in children [4], [13], [20], [28], [29], with five-year relative survival rates from all brain cancers rising in those under age 15 from 59% between 1975 and 1984 to 67% between 1985 and 1994 [4] to over 70% by 2012 [30]. In terms of absolute numbers, mortality rates from brain malignancies declined from 1.0 per 10 [5] children in the 1970s, to 0.8 per 100,000 children in the 1990s, and then to roughly 0.6 per 100,000 from 2005 through 2009 in the SEER database [25].

Improvements in survival have been observed with certain neoplastic types much more than others, with survival rates from ependymomas increasing from 39 to 56% and from gliomas from 46 to 57% between these two time intervals. Overall improvements in survival generally have not extended to PNETs/medulloblastomas, with survival increasing only 3%, from 52 to 55% between 1975 and 1994 [4]. Nor have significant improvements been noted with glioblastomas [13], for which 1-year and 5-year survival rates have consistently fallen below thirty-five and five percent, respectively [4], [13], [31], [32]. Fortunately, as previously stated, children are much more likely than adults to have low-grade astrocytomas, in particular pilocytic astrocytomas and other low-grade gliomas that are almost never fatal and often cured, depending upon their location and surgical accessibility [33]- [35]. They also are far less likely to have virtually universally-fatal glioblastomas than adults, in whom they are the most common brain tumor type [8], [35]. Diffuse pontine gliomas, which account for roughly 15% of paediatric brain malignancies and arise anytime from infancy through adolescence, peaking in those between the ages of 7 and 9 years old, have a universally dismal prognosis, with median survival times of 12 months or less, irrespective of tumor grade; this is because their diffuse nature renders them unresectable [3] [6], and they tend to be unresponsive to either radiation or chemotherapy [37], [38].

At all ages, pediatric brain cancer survival rates have typically been much better than for adults [4], [13], a fact that largely can be explained by the much higher percentage of low-grade astrocytomas and gliomas, and much lower percentage of high-grade astrocytomas seen in children [8], [35]. Even among pediatric patients, however, survival rates vary with age, with older adolescents (ages 15 to 19) generally having fared better than children under age five, in whom low survival rates are especially noted for ependymomas and PNETs. This has been true not only in terms of current rates of survival (between 1986 and 1994, overall survival from all brain cancers was 77% in those 15 to 19 years old, versus just 45% in those under one year of age, and 59% in those between 1 and 4 years old), but also in terms of improvement in survival over time [4].

It must be considered, however, that long-term survival in children with brain cancer does not necessarily equal 'cure', and that low-grade neoplasms are not necessarily curable. How children do long-term is largely dependent upon the location and size of the tumor, its surgical accessibility, and its potential for re-growth [33], [34]. For example, even low-grade optic gliomas, localized brainstem gliomas, and medulloblastomas might never be cured, merely because of their location and associated high risks of surgical intervention. Moreover, even with lesions for which curative surgery is successful, considerable post-operative morbidity can result secondary to neurological damage caused by the tumor, especially if fast growing, and to the surgery itself [33], [34], [39]. Radiation therapy, classically used to de-bulk brain tumors prior to attempted resection, has been virtually contra-indicated in infants and preschool children, because of the adverse effects of radiation on the developing brain.

3. Known risk factors

3.1. Demographic variables (age, gender, and race)

Though relatively few data exist specifically addressing the association between various demographic factors and childhood brain cancers, the overall relationship between brain cancer incidence and mortality and patient age, gender and race have been well-established via a number of published studies [4], [13]- [19], [26]- [28], [40]- [42], as well as the SEER database [22]- [25]. In those under age twenty, age predicts not only overall incidence of and mortality from brain cancer, but also the incidence of and rate of survival from specific cancer types, and the risk of cancer at specific brain locations. From 2005 through 2009, the overall incidence of brain and other nervous system cancers was 3.7 per 100,000 in infants under one year of age, peaked to 3.9 in those 1 to 4 years old, and then steadily declined to 2.1 per 100,000 in adolescents between 15 and 19 [13], [25]. These numbers parallel earlier figures for 1986 through 1994, when incidence was 3.6 per 100,000 in infants, peaked to almost 4.0 by age 4, and then steadily declined to under 1.7 per 100,000 by age 19 [4]. In terms of lesion location, cerebellar lesions were much more common in children nine years old and under, at 0.93 and 0.97 per 100,000 for those under 5 and 5-9 years old, respectively, than in older children, being just 0.37 per 100,000 in children over 15 [4]. Similar patterns were evident for brain stem lesions and brain sites other than the brainstem, cerebellum and cerebrum [4]. Cerebral lesions, however, predominated among those over age 10 (see Figure 1).

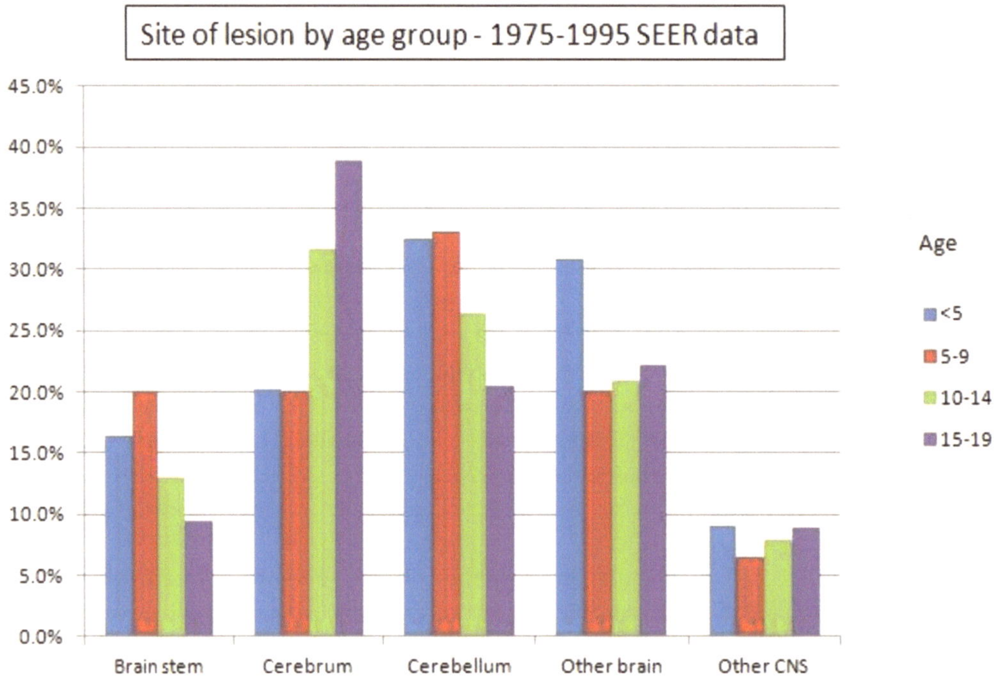

Figure 1.

Age also influences the types of brain cancer seen, especially in terms of ependymomas, most of which initially present in children under five years of age; and PNET, the incidence of which decreases steadily with age, from over 1.1 per 100,000 in the first year of life to roughly 0.2 per 100,000 in older teens [4]. The relatively poor prognosis of ependymomas and PNET, relative to the often low-grade gliomas and astrocytomas of childhood and adolescence, result in higher mortality rates among those under age five in both the U.S. and the U.K. [4], [41]; but other studies have also noted lower survival rates in younger versus older children with the same tumor; for example, low-grade astrocytomas [43] and ependymomas [41], [44].

Being male is considered a moderate risk factor for brain cancer. In the SEER database, over the entire period from 1975 through 2009, the incidence of CNS cancers was 7.90 per 100,000 in males versus 5.55 per 100,000 in females, and this disparity between the two sexes was evident every year, the rates being 7.72 and 5.60 per 100,000 in 2009 [24]. Over the entire time period, the incidence in males averaged 42% higher than in females, and this was relatively consistent. Similar population-based excess in brain cancers among males have been reported in Canada [26], the U.K. [18], Norway [17], Austria [14], India [19], New Zealand [27], and in 69 populations from a subset of cancer registries included in the *Cancer Incidence in Five Continents* database, in which male/female incidence rate ratios varied by age, but not by World Area, suggesting that the observed male versus female difference in brain cancer incidence is biologically based [45]. At least in the U.S. among children, this gender discrepancy largely is secondary to male predominance in certain neoplasms more than others, especially in medulloblastomas and ependymomas [4]. To date, however, no clear association between gender and cancer mortality rates has been established, especially among children.

Another very clear demographic predictor of brain cancer incidence, mortality, and type is race. Using the SEER database, between 1975 and 2009, whereas the overall incidence of brain and other nervous system cancers was 7.18 per 100,000 in whites, it was just 4.08 per 100,000 in blacks [24], 43% lower. This discrepancy between the races persists over the most recent 5-year data block from 2005-2009, in which the rates were 7.1 and 4.0 per 100,000 (44% lower), respectively [25]. A similar difference is observed for mortality, with mortality rates among whites and blacks being 4.6 and 2.5 per 100,000 over the same 2005-2009 time period, making mortality from brain cancer 46% lower in blacks. The incidence of astrocytic glioma and medulloblastoma are particularly more prevalent in whites than blacks [46]. A similar low rate of brain cancer and brain cancer mortality, relative to Caucasians, has been identified for Hispanics and Asians. In California, for example, in data gleaned from the State Cancer Registry for 1988-1997, the odds of CNS cancer was 0.70 among blacks (i.e., 70% of the rate among whites), 0.64 among Asians, and 0.57 among Hispanics relative to Whites. [42] Not all non-Caucasian populations are protected, however. In New Zealand, at least as of 1988, the native Maori population exhibited a fourfold increase in their incidence of ependymomas versus Caucasians, as well as a significant overall increase in all brain cancers [27].

3.2. Family history of cancer or other CNS disease

As will be discussed in the next section, there is a clear association between certain familial syndromes and brain malignancy. Even beyond this, however, studies support an association between family history and brain cancer, albeit less conclusive than for age, sex and race, and generally for brain cancers in general and not just pediatric brain cancers. For example, Farwell and Flannery compared the occurrence of cancer in parents, siblings, and offspring of 643 patients who had had a CNS tumor in childhood, as recorded in the Connecticut Tumor Registry, with its occurrence among the parents, siblings, and offspring of 360 controls matched for sex, birth date, and birthplace [47]. Overall cancer incidence was comparable in the two groups, but 11 CNS tumors were identified in the relatives of cases, versus none in the relatives of controls ($p = 0.0005$). The rate hematopoietic-lymphatic system tumors also was increased ($p = 0.003$). In addition, nine siblings of cases but only one sibling of a control had had cancer as a child. Medulloblastoma and glioblastoma multiforme were overrepresented in the group of children whose relatives had CNS tumors. Overall, a fivefold increase in CNS or hematopoietic-lymphatic malignancies was identified in cases versus controls.

In another study in which the nationwide Swedish Family-Cancer Database for the years 1958 through 1996 was used to analyze the risk of brain tumors in offspring ages 15-61 and siblings via parental cancer probands, among brain tumor patients, standardized incidence ratios (SIR) were statistically elevated to 1.7, 2.4, and 2.5 for all brain tumors, astrocytomas, and meningiomas, respectively. In addition, parental endometrial cancer and melanoma were associated with offspring astrocytoma, and parental breast and thyroid cancers with offspring ependymoma and neurinoma, respectively [48]. In a case-control study in Maryland, subjects with a family history of stomach cancer (odds ratio, OR, 2.2; 95% CI, 1.0-4.6), colon cancer (1.4; 0.9-2.2), prostate cancer (2.1; 1.1-3.8) or Hodgkin's disease (2.4; 0.9-6.3) all had an increased odds of glioma [49], while increased risk of meningioma was noted among those reporting a family history of benign brain tumor (4.5; 1.0-21.0) or melanoma (4.2; 1.2-15.0), and a family history of breast cancer was associated with an elevated meningioma risk among subjects 18 to 49 years old, but not older (3.9; 1.4-11.0) [50].

More recently, using the Utah Population Data Base (UPDB), among first degree relatives of a proband with brain cancer, the relative risk (RR) was found to be almost 4 (3.8) for astrocytomas, 2.3 for glioblastomas, and 3.3 for both, each of these RR values statistically greater than 1.0; among second degree relatives, only astrocytomas had a relative risk greater than 1.0 (RR = 1.9) [51]. Finally, in the Ohio Brain Tumor Study (OBTS), Ostrom et al. identified a significant association between a family brain cancer history and both malignant (e.g., malignant gliomas) and benign brain tumor subtypes, like meningiomas, acoustic neuromas, and pituitary adenomas [52]. Overall, the increased risk of brain cancer if a parent or sibling has had brain cancer has been estimated to be between 3 and 9-fold [4].

Some data also exist that support an association between brain cancer and a family history of epilepsy [53], [54], and between brain cancer and a family history of mental retardation [53], though these data are less conclusive. For example, in the 1991-1995 San Francisco Bay Area Adult Glioma Study, in which both personal and family histories were examined in 462 adults newly-diagnosed with glioma versus 443 controls, past epilepsy or seizures only were identified as a personal risk factor, the only family history risk factor identified being brain cancer, and only when both confirmed and probable family brain cancer cases were considered (OR 2.3; 95% confidence interval 1.0-5.8) [55]. Cancer in general, and a host of other health conditions were not significant predictors of glioma cases, either in personal or family history.

3.3. Genetics

Central nervous system cancers occur within a broad range of familial clinical syndromes including what some consider the prototype CNS tumor syndromes – neurofibromatosis, types I and II - but also other skin conditions that, along with neurofibromatosis, are collectively known as the *phakomatoses*. These additional syndromes include disorders like tuberous sclerosis, Von Hippel Lindau Disease, and basal cell nevus syndrome. Other familial disorders have been clearly linked to increased CNS cancer risk as well, like Li-Fraumeni syndrome, a congenital condition linked to germ-line mutations of the p53 tumor suppressor gene, and familial polyposis disorders, like Turcot syndrome. Finally, this author has already published several papers describing the association between CNS tumors and dyschondroplasia syndromes, in particular Ollier's disease and Maffucci's syndrome. A list of this broad array of genetic familial syndromes associated with increased CNS tumor risk is provided below.

http://dx.doi.org/10.5772/52427

• **Phakomatosis syndromes**	
	• Neurofibromatosis (types 1 and 2, and segmental forms)
	• Tuberous sclerosis
	• Von Hippel Lindau disease
	• Basal cell nevus syndrome
• **Other familial syndromes**	
	• Li Fraumeni syndrome
	• Familial polyposis syndromes (e.g., Turcot syndrome)
	• Rubenstein-Taybi syndrome
• **Dyschondroplasia syndromes**	
	Ollier's disease
	Maffucci's syndrome

Table 1. Familial Syndromes Associated with CNS Malignancies

4. Neurofibromatosis and other phakomatosis syndromes

The phakomatoses are characterized by the presence of pathological lesions involving the skin, eyes and central and peripheral nervous system (CNS) [56], all tissues of ectodermal origin. The phakamotoses otherwise share the features of being autosomal dominant, with variable expression but high penetrance; and all involving mutations of a tumor suppressor gene. Initially conceptualized by the ophthalmologist van der Hoeve in the early nineteenth century [57], they were assumed to primarily consist of three disorders: neurofibromatosis, tuberous sclerosis, and what we now know as von Hippel-Lindau syndrome. Over time, each of these three disease labels has been recognized as a collective term for multiple disorders; for example, neurofibromatosis is not one disease, but a collection of quite distinct diseases. On occasion, two distinct phakomatosis syndromes (for example, neurofibromatosis and tuberous sclerosis) have been described in the same patient [58]; but this is rare and may be the result of chance rather than some increased risk for both conditions. In terms of the current chapter, these three disorders, as well as more-recently described phakomatoses, share the property of being associated with an increased risk of malignancies involving the central and, sometimes, peripheral nervous system.

Neurofibromatosis (NF), which is now recognized not to be one, but at least two distinct disorders - neurofibromatosis type 1 (NF-1) and neurofibromatosis type 2 (NF-2) [59] - is the most common of all the phakomatosis syndromes, having been initially described by Frederick von Recklinghausen in the year 1882 [60]. Each of these two syndromes has its own diagnostic criteria that are very different; and whereas the characteristic lesion in NF-1 is the neurofibroma, the characteristic lesion in NF-2 is a peripheral nerve Schwannoma or neurolemoma [59], [61]- [63].

Neurofibromatosis type 1 (NF-1) is the most common form of disease, affecting one in roughly 2500 to 5000 live births [64]- [66]. This renders it more than ten times more common than NF-2 [64], [65]. Though autosomal dominant, up to 50% of cases arise spontaneously from a gene mutation that occurs on chromosome 17q11.2, which encodes for a large protein called *neurofibromin* [64], [66]. This NF-1 gene is a classical tumor suppressor gene, with tumor growth requiring the loss of BOTH alleles. Neurofibromatosis type 1 has a classical combination of clinical signs [67], for which the mnemonic CHANSOR has been used. These signs include Café au lait macules; Hamartomas of the iris (called Lisch nodules); Axillary and Inguinal Freckling; Neurofibromas; Skeletal lesions – like sphenoid wing dysplasia and thinning of long bone cortices; Optic gliomas; and in increased Risk of other CNS and systemic tumors. The disorder is diagnosed using National Institutes of Health (NIH) Consensus Criteria for the Diagnosis of NF-1 [65]. Besides the classic neurofibroma - which is generally an extra-cranial lesion that occurs both in paraspinal areas and in peripheral nerves [62], [67], [68] and, though benign, may transform into a neurofibrosarcoma - numerous other brain tumors are frequently observed in patients with NF-1. Most common are optic-hypothalamic gliomas, which manifest in roughly 15% of NF-1 patients. These lesions are categorized into those that involve just the optic nerve(s), lesions also involving the optic chiasm, and lesions that extend all the way into the hypothalamus. [69] Hemispheric and cerebellar gliomas are less common than lesions involving the optic tract [70]. Most are benign or only exhibit low-grade malignant potential; but all grades of malignancy have been reported [70]. Most are resectable. Brainstem gliomas also occur, as a heterogeneous group of lesions, with at least three main subtypes: (1) a diffuse area of brainstem enlargement; (2) focal enhancing nodules with or without cystic areas; and (3) peri-aqueductal gliomas. All subtypes generally have a very indolent course that usually does not require treatment, though MRI monitoring is indicated until their indolent course is confirmed. Some lesions regress on their own [70]. Though controversial, diffuse brainstem enlargement is presumed to represent gliomatous change, though these lesions have a more indolent course than brainstem gliomas seen outside of NF-1, such that adjuvant treatment only is required in that minority of patients whose lesions progress. This being said, these gliomas occasionally do progress to more malignant forms of astrocytoma, including glioblastoma [70], [71]. The focal enhancing nodules, with or without cystic areas, generally are thought to represent pilocytic astrocytomas, given their imaging characteristics. Like pilocytic astrocytomas elsewhere, they generally are indolent; but their course is unpredictable and the brainstem so susceptible to major deficits, relative to the cerebral hemispheres, that ongoing monitoring is required. Small, focal intrinsic lesions may enlarge and then regress spontaneously. Exophytic tumors often are more aggressive and require treatment.

Finally, peri-aqueductal gliomas occur adjacent to the aqueduct of Sylvius between the 3rd and 4th ventricles in the midbrain. They typically manifest with late-onset aqueductal stenosis, leading to hydrocephalus. Presumably, they represent low-grade gliomas or glial hamartomas, and typically are indolent. However, because of their location, shunting often is necessary. Resection is usually not necessary for any of the brainstem gliomas seen in NF-1 [70], [71].

Neurofibromatosis type 2 (NF-2) is much less common than NF-1, with a prevalence that has been estimated as roughly one in 25,000 to 50,000 [64], [65], [67]. NF-2 is caused by a mutation affecting chromosome 22q12 and the gene product *merlin* (a moesin-, erzin-, and radixin-like protein), which sometimes is called *schwannomin.* Merlin encodes for a polypeptide that may affect cell growth and motility; more interesting, in terms of its presence in NF-2, is that it is a tumor inhibitor that often is absent in brain tumors [72]- [74]. In addition, the same chromosomal abnormality is found in spontaneous spinal schwannomas, which suggests that a single location causes Schwann cell tumor growth [75]. Clinically, NF-2 is a combination of features that always entails at least one eighth cranial nerve (CN-VIII) neurilemoma, in addition to a variety of other tumors (e.g., neurofibromas, meningiomas, gliomas, neurilemomas), juvenile posterior sub-capsular cataracts, and occasional other lesions like café au lait spots. Like NF-1, it is diagnosed using NIH Consensus Criteria, initially proposed in 1988 [76], but modified in 1997 [77]. Cranial nerve neurolemomas, especially of the eighth cranial nerve (CN-VIII), are the hallmark lesion of NF-2, with CN-VIII lesions present in roughly 95% of patients with NF-2; when bilateral, they are diagnostic of NF-2 [63], [67]. As a rule, spinal lesions are more common in NF-2 than in NF1, while brain lesions are less common in NF-2 than NF-1. In NF-2, this includes extracranial neurilemomas and meningiomas. But also among the various tumors are brain neoplasms, particularly ependymomas that are the most common malignancy in NF-2, versus astrocytomas in NF-1 [62], [63], [70]. These ependymomas usually are well-circumscribed, and therefore often quite resectable. Their surgical and post-operative management (like the use of adjuvant therapy) is the same as for intramedullary spinal tumors in patients without neurofibromatosis.

Tuberous sclerosis, which also is called tuberous sclerosis complex (TSC) and Bourneville's disease, is the second most common phakomatosis syndrome, after neurofibromatosis type 1. It affects anywhere from one in 6000 to one in 30,000 people [78]- [80], with marked variations in penetrance rendering all estimates somewhat unreliable. The syndrome is autosomal dominant, but up to 60% of cases arise from spontaneous mutations [78], [80], [81]. Two tumor-suppressor genes, TSC-1 (tuberous sclerosis complex-1) and TSC-2, are responsible for TS. Roughly 80-90% of mutations involve TSC-2, while just 10-20% of mutations involve TSC-1 [81]. The genetic locus for TSC-1 is chromosome 9q34, and the TSC-1 gene product is called *hamartin.* The genetic locus for TSC-2 is chromosome 16p13.3, and the TSC-2 gene product is called *tuberin.* Both hamartin and tuberin appear to have roles in cell differentiation, proliferation and migration. The disorder effects cellular differentiation, proliferation and migration during early development, leading to various diffuse hamartomas and neoplastic lesions that can affect virtually any body organ [81], [82]. It can present at any age, but most commonly appears during childhood, especially late childhood. Though skin, heart, lung and renal involvement are common, neurological involvement is the most common cause of morbidity and mortality from TS, and the most common cause of death in patients under 30 years old. Problems stem from a broad variety of intra-cerebral tumors, which include cortical tubers, subependymal nodules, and subependymal giant cell astrocytomas (SEGA). Subependymal giant cell astrocytomas develop in between 5 and 15% of TS patients [83], typically developing in the region of the foramen of Monro, where they frequently cause obstructive hydrocephalus. Though they are slow-growing and rarely undergo malignant transformation, these tumors are problematic because of their location and relative inaccessibility for resection. Death primarily results from intractable seizures or SEGA-induced obstructive hydrocephalus; and, overall, the long-term prognosis is poor.

The average age at first presentation with Von Hippel-Lindau Disease is 26 years, and the average age at diagnosis 31 [84]. Nonetheless, pediatric cases are not uncommon. Von Hippel-Lindau disease is autosomal dominant, with 97-99% of cases familial and only 1-3% occurring as a result of spontaneous mutations. It is associated with inactivation of the tumor-suppressor gene VHL (Von Hippel Lindau), which is found on chromosome 3p25 [84], [85]. Decreased levels of the VHL protein, which is important in a critical pathway helping cells to adapt to hypoxic stress, lead to over-expression of a hypoxia-inducible transcription factor (HIF-1) which, in turn, results in increased cell proliferation, and the over-expression of several growth factors, ultimately manifesting as multiple, multi-systemic benign and malignant tumors, which sometimes are bilateral (e.g., both eyes) [86]. These tumors include haemangioblastomas of the cerebellum, spine, brainstem and retina (the most common tumor identified); renal clear cell carcinomas; pheochromocytomas; pancreatic and renal cysts; endolymphatic sac tumors (ELSTs, of the petrous bone at the cerebellopontine angle) [87]; papillary cystadenomas of the epididymus or broad ligament; and haemanigiomas of the adrenal glands, liver and lungs. As with all the other phakomatosis syndromes, the diagnosis is made on clinical grounds using established, published criteria. Central nervous system manifestations are highly prevalent [88], [89], with CNS haemangioblastomas occurring in 60 to 80% of patients. Moreover, they are more likely to be multiple and present at an earlier age than when they occur sporadically, being a presenting feature in roughly 60% of VHL patients [90]. These lesions may occur anywhere along the cranioaxial axis, but only 1% of these tumors are supratentorial [90]. The site of lesion determines the symptoms with which the patient presents. The cerebellum and brainstem are the most common sites of haemangioblastomas in VHL syndrome [90], where patients present with headaches, vomiting, lethargy, dysmetria, ataxia, papilloedema, polycythemia from tumor production of erythropoietin, and/or enlarging cysts that may cause brainstem compression (solid tumors generally do not cause such compression in VHL syndrome).

As with almost all the phakomatoses, basal cell nevus syndrome (BCNS) is autosomal dominant, the offending gene, called PTCH1, localized to chromosome 9q31 in about 85% of cases. The PTCH1 gene product is a trans-membrane receptor that binds to and regulates a protein called Sonic the hedgehog homolog (SHH), one of three proteins in the mammalian signalling pathway family called 'hedgehog', and one which plays a key role in the regulation of organ development in vertebrates, including the growth of fingers and toes and the organization of the central nervous system. It also controls cell division in adult stem cells and has been implicated in oncogenesis. Mutations in the PTCH1 gene result in uncontrolled SHH activation [91]. This rare condition, which affects roughly one in 50 to 60 thousand live births [84], is characterized by multiple basal cell cancers, often presenting in adolescence. Despite the relatively innocuous-sounding name, there is a wide range of non-neurological manifestations, including numerous other benign and malignant tumors, both non-CNS and CNS, including melanomas, leukaemia, lymphoma, lung and breast cancers, medulloblastomas, and meningiomas [92]. Like virtually all the familial cancer syndromes, basal cell nevus syndrome is diagnosed using diagnostic criteria.

5. Other familial syndromes associated with CNS malignancies

Other familial syndromes associated with paediatric CNS malignancies include Li-Fraumeni Syndrome (LFS), a very rare autosomal dominant disease that is caused by a germ line mutation of chromosome p53 in roughly 70% of families in which the syndrome is diagnosed [93]. Patients exhibit a variety of carcinomas and sarcomas, including premenopausal breast cancers, osteosarcomas, soft tissue sarcomas, acute leukaemia, cancer involving the adrenal cortex, and primitive neuroectodermal tumors (PNET) like medulloblastoma. This increased risk of several malignancies likely stems from deactivation of p53, which normally controls apoptosis and the repair of damaged DNA. Patients present not only with a variety of cancers, but with cancers at a very early age, with the mean age at presentation of brain tumors being 25 years. The diagnosis of so-called 'classic LFS' is made in any patient under 45 years who presents with a bone or soft-tissue sarcoma, plus one first-degree relative who presents with any cancer before age 45, plus one further first or second-degree relative of the same lineage who has had any cancer before age 45 or a sarcoma at any age [94]. More recently, a related syndrome, called Li-Fraumeni-like syndrome, has been described, defined as a proband with any childhood tumor or any sarcoma, brain or adrenocortical tumor before 45 years of age, who has a first- or second-degree relative with any cancer before the age of 60 [95], [96]. Interestingly, whereas p53 germ-line mutations are found in 70% to 80% of families with classic Li-Fraumeni syndrome, they only are identified in between 20% and 40% of families with Li-Fraumeni-like syndrome [8][4]. The CHK2 checkpoint homolog gene, CHEK2, which is located on the long (q) arm of chromosome 22, also has been implicated in some families with classic Li-Fraumeni syndrome. Recently, mutation of another gene, which encodes for the breast cancer 2 (BRCA2) susceptibility protein, has been found with increased frequency in the non-classic syndrome [96]. It should be noted that p53 mutations are rare in sporadically occurring medulloblastomas. Overall, about 10% of LFS patients will develop a glioma before the age of 45, and another 5% a supratentorial primitive neuroectodermal tumor (PNET), like a medulloblastoma, or choroid plexus carcinoma [97].

A Canadian surgeon named Jacques Turcot is accredited with having characterized Turcot syndrome, one of the several familial polyposis syndromes associated with familial, in this case autosomal recessive, inheritance and the presence of multiple colonic adenomas and adenocarcinomas [98]. An additional feature of Turcot syndrome is its association with several different neuroepithelial tumors of the central nervous system, including astrocytomas, medulloblastomas, pineoblastomas, gangliogliomas, and ependymomas [84]. Turcot syndrome has been categorized into types 1 and 2, with type 1 characterized by glioblastoma, no familial adenomatous polyposis, but often hereditary non-polyposis-related colorectal carcinoma. Germ-line mutations in a few DNA mismatch repair genes – PMS2, MLH1 and MSH2 – are associated with type-1 Turcot syndrome. Interestingly, type-1 Turcot syndrome also is associated with café au lait spots [84]. Conversely, type-2 Turcot syndrome families have medulloblastomas as their most common CNS malignancy, and multiple adenomatous polyps that often undergo malignant transformation [99]. Unfortunately, medulloblastomas, glioblastomas and anaplastic astrocytomas are the most common CNS tumors observed in Turcot's syndrome, the three combined accounting for 95% of all CNS tumors in these families [100]; and the latter two are inevitably fatal. In addition, they tend to occur early, with medulloblastomas typically diagnosed in children less than 10 years old, and gliomas in those under age 30 [84], [101]- [103]. As such, and because some die of metastatic colon cancer that sometimes presents quite early in childhood or the second decade of life, many die as adolescents or young adults. In one tragic case, for example, doctors in Pittsburgh reported the case of a girl who developed a medulloblastoma at the age of 5 years. Ten years later, she developed adenocarcinoma of the colon. Then, seven months after resection of a Dukes' C2 adenocarcinoma, she presented with a second primary CNS tumor, this time a glioblastoma multiforme [101].

Rubenstein-Taybi syndrome is an autosomal dominant disorder that is associated with numerous anatomical/functional abnormalities that include abnormal facies, microcephaly, broad thumbs, big toes and moderate to severe intellectual impairment. There also is an increased incidence of neuroepithelial tumors - in particular medulloblastomas, meningiomas, and oligodendrogliomas [104], though other CNS tumors have been described [105]. A germline mutation in one allele of CRE binding protein (CBP, a transcriptional co-activator for several c-AMP regulated genes) has been implicated in many cases. CBP binds to the activated form of GLI, a transcription factor that is important in the regulation of the Sonic the hedgehog homolog (SHH) that, as stated earlier, controls cell division in adult stem cells and has been implicated in oncogenesis. The GLI gene is downstream of the PTCH1 gene that is mutated in basal cell nevus syndrome.

6. Ollier's disease and Maffucci syndrome

Enchondromatosis, also called dyschondroplasia, is a hamartomatous proliferation of chondrocytes within the metaphysis of bone [106]. Though often asymptomatic and only diagnosed as an incidental X-ray finding, it can lead to significant deformities, reduced bone length [107], [108], and occasional pathologic fractures [108]. Moreover, just like the phakomatoses and familial syndromes like Li-Fraumeni and Turcot syndrome, enchondromatosis appears to confer a substantial increased risk of a variety of CNS and other malignancies, at least through the sixth decade of life and as early as the first decade. These tumors include chondrosarcomas that result from sarcomatous transformation of the enchondromas themselves, as well as other histologically-distinct malignancies like angiosarcomas, osteosacrcomas, ovarian tumors, various leukaemias, and a variety of glial-cell based central nervous system tumors (ranging from stage I to stage IV astrocytomas) [109]. This association with malignancy appears to be particularly true in instances of multiple enchondromatoses, as in Ollier's disease and Maffucci's syndrome [110], two very rare conditions [111], [112].

Since Boinet first reported CNS malignancy in a patient with multiple enchondromatosis, [113] 45 additional patients with either Ollier's disease (OD) or Maffucci's syndrome (MS) and some form of intracranial malignancy have been reported in the medical literature, ranging from 6 to 58 years old [114]. Ollier's disease patients appear to contract their neoplasms at a particularly early age, including very young childhood [109], [114], [115]. What causes this persistent increase in malignancy potential is not yet known. We do know that single enchondromas, outside some greater syndrome, are associated with an elevated risk of malignant change. Altay *et al* [116], for example, conducted an 18-year retrospective analysis of 627 cartilage-forming benign bone tumors, and found that 32 patients had experienced malignant transformation, with 14 of these 32 patients initially having had a solitary osteochondroma, ten multiple osteochondromas, six a solitary enchondroma, one Ollier's disease, and one Maffucci's syndrome. The one patient with Ollier's disease had two chondrosarcomas; and the single patient with multiple osteochondroma had three chondrosarcomas. The overall rate of malignant transformation for cartilage-originating tumors was 5.1%, being 4.2% for solitary osteochondromas, 9.2% for multiple osteochondromas, and 4.2% for solitary enchondromas. A variety of chromosomal abnormalities also have been reported in isolated cases of OD or MS and chondrosarcoma. These abnormalities include, for example, the interstitial deletion, del(1)(p11p31.2), as the only chromosomal abnormality identified in a low-grade chondrosarcoma in a patient with Ollier's disease [117]. Also, Bovée *et al* [118] identified (1) the loss of heterozygosity (LOH) in a tibial chondrosarcoma and its metastases, exclusively on chromosome bands 13q14 and 9p21, with the LOH not identified in a femoral enchondroma that was analyzed; and (2) p53 over-expression in a tibial chondrosarcoma and its metastases, not present in a femoral enchondroma. Meanwhile, Chang *et al* [119] identified identical male twins with OD who both developed astrocytomas within their cerebral cortex during their early twenties; and Robinson *et al* [120] found evidence of mitogenic neurotransmitters within both enchondromas and soft tissue hemangiomas in a patient with Maffucci's syndrome, implying that the bone and vascular lesions, and possibly malignant tumors, might be related to an underlying neural abnormality. Having said all this, to date, no consistent chromosomal abnormalities have been identified in these patients, and all theories regarding the cause of malignancies in these syndromes remain unproven.

6.1. Ionizing radiation

The first report of a radiation-induced CNS tumor was by Mann et al in 1953 [121]. He described the case of a 3 year-old girl, born in 1942, who presented with a left optic nerve astrocytoma that was excised and then irradiated with a total dose over time of 6,500 rads. Six years later, at age 9, she presented with her first episode of recurring frontal meningiomas, which subsequently underwent malignant change, leading to her death at age 10. At about the same time, two independent groups were reporting on the 1.5 to 2-fold increased risk of cancers, including brain cancers, in children exposed to X-rays *in utero* [53], [122]- [124]. Subsequently, more than 280 radiation-induced intracranial tumors have been reported in the literature, the most common being meningiomas, sarcomas, and gliomas, though ependymomas, Schwannomas, PNETs, and pituitary adenomas have been described as well [125]. Consequently, the association between therapeutic radiation to the head and the subsequent risk of brain cancer has been well-established, especially since a landmark study performed in Israel and published in 1988 [126]. In this study, the relationship between radiotherapy in childhood for tinea capitis and the later development of tumors of the brain and nervous system was evaluated in 10,834 patients treated between 1948 and 1960. Benign and malignant tumors were identified from the pathology records of all Israeli hospitals and from Israeli national cancer and death registries. Doses of radiation were estimated retrospectively for each patient (mean, 1.5 Gy). The incidence of tumors was 1.8 per 10,000 persons per year, and the estimated relative risk (RR) versus 10,834 matched general-population controls and 5392 non-irradiated siblings 6.9 (95% confidence interval 4.1-11.6) for all tumors and 8.4 (4.8-14.8) for neural tumors of the head and neck. Increased risks were observed for meningiomas (RR = 9.5), gliomas (2.6), nerve-sheath tumors (18.8), and other neural tumors (3.4). Moreover, a strong dose-response relationship was identified, with relative risk approaching 20 beyond estimated doses of 2.5 Gy. Radiotherapy also was associated with an increased risk of death from tumors of the head and neck, including brain cancers (RR = 3) and leukemia (RR = 2.3) [127].

In an earlier case-control study, 2,215 patients in New York who during childhood had been given x-ray therapy for tinea capitis between 1940 and 1959 were compared against 1,395 persons matched for age, sex, and race and also treated for tinea capitis over the same period without x-ray therapy [128]. Excess incidence was noted in irradiated cases of tumors of the head and neck, including the skin, brain, thyroid, and parotid. However, there was no increased mortality from malignant neoplasms or any other cause. In another study, diagnostic X-rays of the head and neck increased the odds of brain tumors by 64% (OR 1.64; 95%CI, 1.04-2.58). [129] Thierry-Chef et al has estimated that the life-time increase in brain cancer risk among pediatric patients receiving radiation to the brain ranges from 2 to 80%, depending upon the dose and conditions of exposure [130]. There is, however, a huge range in the latency time between irradiation and subsequent brain tumor development, from 4 to 47 years among 27 cases described by Chowdhary et al. [125] Clearly, some such tumors may arise in childhood, and others much later.

7. Suspected/possible risk factors

In addition to risk factors that have been established through consistent results across several studies, there are several suspected or possible risk factors for which data are either scarce or conflicting. Difficulties that arise from the study of these risk factors include their somewhat ubiquitous exposure (e.g., electromagnetic fields), difficulties measuring exposure (e.g., diet, parental occupation), and their relative novelty (e.g., cell phones and other hand-held electric devices).

7.1. Electromagnetic fields

Over the past few decades, considerable research has been compiled supporting the association between electromagnetic field (EMF) exposure and childhood leukemia, such that the International Agency for Research on Cancer has classified extremely-low-frequency magnetic field exposure as a possible human carcinogen [131]. However, data linking EMF exposure and brain cancer are much less conclusive [131]- [135]. Most older studies suffered from various methodological issues, like the problem of inadequate blinding of those evaluating EMF exposure, and crude measurements of actual exposure [53]. The first studies to overcome these short-falls were conducted in Denver, Colorado by Savitz et al. who, in their initial study, had blinded assessors evaluate the power-line configurations of the homes of all 356 residents in the five-county 1970 Denver, Colorado Standard Metropolitan Statistical Area between 0 and 14 years of age who had been diagnosed with any form of cancer between 1976 and 1983; among them were 59 confirmed cases of brain cancer [136]. The odds ratio comparing very high and high wire codes versus very low, low, and buried wire codes was 1.5 (95% CI = 1.0-2.3) for total cases, with OR = 2.0 for brain cancer. Subsequently, this same group studied the effect on childhood cancer of prolonged exposure to 60-H magnetic fields from electric appliances comparing Denver area children 0-14 years old whose incident cancers had been diagnosed between 1976 and 1983 versus controls selected by random digit dialing, matched for age, sex, and telephone exchange area. Parents of 252 cases and 222 controls were interviewed at home about the use of electric appliances by the mother during pregnancy (prenatal exposure) and by the child (postnatal exposure). After adjusting for income, prenatal electric blanket exposure was associated with a significant increase in the incidence of childhood brain cancer (OR = 2.5, 95% CI 1.1-5.5) [137]. Subsequently, Savitz et al assessed for risk in the same Denver population by comparing risks by high wire code (HWC) versus low wire code (LWC) classifications using the Wertheimer-Leeper coding method, modified by eliminating the distinction between thick and thin primaries, distinguishing only between open and spun secondaries, and reducing the number of categories from five to three [138]. The association between the modified code and measured magnetic fields was similar to the association with the original wire code. Residences assigned the high wire code had odds ratios of 1.9 for total cancers (95% CI: 1.1-3.2), 2.9 for leukemias (1.5-5.5), and 2.5 for brain cancer (1.1-5.5), after adjusting for all other measured potential risk factors for childhood cancer.

In 2001 [134] and again in 2010 [139], Kheifets et al reviewed all major studies published on the association between EMF and childhood brain cancers published to date and found that, where the earlier studies by investigators like Wertheimer and Leeper [140], Savitz et al [136]- [138] and Tomenius [141] identified an association between EMF exposure and increased brain cancer risk, later studies and reviews by investigators like Preston-Martin et al [142], Gurney et al [132], Feychting et al [143], Kheifits et al [133] generally failed to confirm this risk. In their 2010 meta-analysis of brain cancer risk with extremely low-frequency EMF, Kheifits et al subdivided studies in terms of both the methodology of EMF measurement (long-term, calculated fields, or spot measurement) and the type of home exposure (home at the time of cancer diagnosis, longest-lived-in home, and birth home) and found no significantly elevated odds ratios for any of the six categories, even with exposures $\geq 4\mu T$ [139]. This conclusion, that there are no conclusive data linking EMF exposure with brain cancer risk has been echoed by others [144], [145].

Relatively few papers have looked at the use of computers, *per se*. Both Mutnik et al and Wood specifically assessed the risk of computer use in terms of brain cancer development, and neither identified any significant risk [146], [147]. However, both papers were written in the 1990s, before the recent surge in home computer use, and long before prolonged exposures (e.g., 10 years or greater) to home computers could have occurred.

In one clever paper in which the pros and cons of the association between EMFs and childhood brain cancer were debated by two teams, each composed of eight international experts, using 12 pre-determined questions, arguments on both sides ultimately concluded that further research is necessary, an opinion vigorously championed by Carpenter in his paper *Electromagnetic fields and cancer: the cost of doing nothing* [10]. However, contributing to the confusion regarding EMF exposure are a number of methodological issues pertaining to the measurement of EMF, both in and around residences and in the workplace, issues that have sparked almost as much debate and research as the question of EMF exposure's role in disease [143], [148]- [154]. Such issues include questions about the accuracy of EMF measurements, how to avoid bias in subject selection, where best to measure EMF exposure (e.g., a child's bedroom versus elsewhere in or around the home), how to deal international variations in wiring techniques, how to interpret changes in electrical wiring over time and their effects, and how to adjust for the myriad of other potential confounders like other household exposures and exposures, EMF and otherwise, outside of the home. This last issue is, in fact, a problem with virtually all of the suspected or potential risk factors that are discussed here, including cell phones and other hand=held electronic devices, which are the topic of the next section.

7.2. Cell phones and other hand-held devices

Over the past 15 years, there has been a virtual explosion in the use of hand-held cellular devices like cell phones, iPods, iPads, Kindles, and other electronic reading devices. For example, whereas uncommon in use in 1995, as of 2011, there were more than 4.6 billion active mobile telephone subscriptions worldwide [155]. This has led to considerable concern regarding the impact such devices might have upon health and, in particular because of the issues raised with EMFs, upon brain cancer and leukemia rates.

Over the last decade, most data on cell-phone use and cancer risk have come from the 13-country INTERPHONE Study, and from Sweden, and the results from these two sources have been somewhat conflicting. In Sweden, most of the data has been collected by the research group of Hardell et al. [129], [156] In their most recent study, analysis was performed pooling data from two case-control studies on patients with malignant brain tumors diagnosed from 1997 through 2003 compared against matched controls alive at the time of study inclusion, and a third case-control study on deceased patients and controls diagnosed over the same time period [157]. In total, 1,251 (85%) cases and 2,438 (84%) controls were identified. Brain cancer risk was noted to increase with latency period and cumulative use in hours, both for mobile and cordless phones. The greatest level of risk was identified for astrocytoma, the odds ratio (OR) for the longest (>10 year) latency group for mobile phone use equal to 2.7 (95% CI, 1.9-3.7) and for cordless phone use 1.8 (1.2-2.9). The risk of astrocytoma was highest in the group with first use of a wireless phone before the age of 20 (mobile phone use OR = 4.9, 95% CI = 2.2-11; cordless phone use OR = 3.9, 95% CI = 1.7-8.7). Earlier, Hardell et al had reported on their comparison of mobile phone use in deceased brain cancer cases relative to controls who had died from another type of cancer other than brain tumor, and to controls who had died from other diseases. Exposure was assessed by a questionnaire sent to the next-of-kin. Replies were obtained for 346 (75% participation rate) cases, 343 (74%) cancer controls and 276 (60%) controls with other diseases. Use of mobile phones was associated with an increased risk of brain cancer that was highest in the >10-year latency group, with an odds ratio of 2.4, (1.4-4.1). The risk increased with cumulative number of lifetime hours for use, and was highest in those with more than 2,000 hours of mobile phone use (OR = 3.4; 1.6-7.1). No clear association was found for the use of cordless phones, though OR was 1.7 (0.8-3.4) among those with >2,000 h of cumulative use [158]. These findings were interpreted as supporting earlier findings by this group in other studies.

The INTERPHONE Study has been a multinational case-control study designed to investigate whether mobile phone use increases the risk of cancer and, more specifically, whether the RF fields emitted by mobile phones are carcinogenic [159]. As such, the study has focused on tumors that arise within those tissues most exposed to the RF fields emitted by mobile phones on the same (ipsilateral) side as phone use. In addition to collecting detailed histories on mobile phone use, information has been collected on a number of known and potential risk factors for these tumors. The study has been conducted in 13 countries: Australia, Canada, Denmark, Finland, France, Germany, Israel, Italy, Japan, New Zealand, Norway, Sweden, and the UK using a common core protocol. Enrolled in the study have been 2,765 individuals with gliomas, 2,425 with meningiomas, 1,121 with acoustic neuromas, 109 with malignant parotid gland tumors and 7,658 controls. In addition to assessing brain cancer risk, particular attention has been paid to estimating the amount and direction of potential recall and participation biases and their impact upon study results. Results have been presented for countries individually with consistently no statistically-significant within-country association identified between phone use and brain cancer identified, as in Germany [160], [161], France [162], Sweden [163], and Japan [164]. One exception was in Israel, where the odds ratios (OR) for benign and malignant parotid gland tumors in the highest category of cumulative number of calls and call time without use of hand-free devices were 1.58 (95% confidence interval: 1.11, 2.24) and 1.49 (1.05, 2.13), respectively [165].

When INTERPHONE data from multiple countries has been compiled, there has been a significantly increased risk of glioma (OR = 1.40; 95% CI 1.03-1.89), but only among those in the highest 10% of recalled cumulative call time (more than 1640 h). Any increased risk was not statistically significant for meningiomas (OR = 1.15; 0.81-1.62) [166]. One issue raised by the investigators was that there were implausible values of reported use in the highest user group. Odds ratios for glioma did tend to be greater in the temporal lobe than in other lobes of the brain, but the CIs around the lobe-specific estimates were wide. The ORs for glioma also tended to be greater in subjects who reported usual phone use on the same side of the head as their tumor than on the opposite side. In terms of actual exposure, represented by total cumulative specific energy (TCSE; J/kg), when 553 glioma and 676 meningioma cases of brain tumor from the Australian, Canadian, French, Israeli and New Zealand components of the Interphone Study, whose tumors were localised by neuroradiologists, were compared with controls matched for age, sex and region, and compared against 1762 and 1911 controls, respectively, ORs for glioma were below 1.0 within the first four quintiles of TCSE, but above 1.0 in the highest quintile, 1.35, approaching but not quite achieving statistical significance (95% CI 0.96 to 1.90) [167]. In a complementary analysis in which 44 glioma and 135 meningioma cases in the most exposed area of the brain were compared against gliomas and meningiomas located elsewhere, increased ORs were noted for tumors in the most exposed part of the brain in those with 10 or more years of mobile phone use (OR 2.80, 95% CI 1.13 to 6.94 for glioma). And, in pooled analysis across the four Nordic countries and the UK, increased risk of a tumor on the same side of the head as reported phone use that has persisted for ≥ 10 years was noted (OR = 1.8, 95% CI: 1.1-3.1) [168].

No increased risk of acoustic neuroma was identified in any study [169]. Overall, the INTERPHONE investigators concluded that there were no conclusive data linking cell-phone use and risk of brain malignancies, except after prolonged and exorbitant use. Criticisms have been made of the INTERPHONE studies, however, relating, among other issues, to recall and misclassification biases potentially exacerbated by low response rates [170]- [172].

In a meta-analysis drawing from both sets of studies (Hardell et al and INTERPHONE), Hardell et al found that the odds ratio for glioma (1.0; 95% CI, 0.9-1.1) increased to 1.3 (1.1-1.6) after a 10-year latency period, with the highest risk identified for ipsilateral exposure (OR=1.9; 1.4-2.4) versus OR=1.2 (0.9-1.7) with contralateral exposure [173]. The odds of acoustic neuroma (OR=1.0; 0.8-1.1) also increased after a 10-year latency period, but just failed to achieve statistical significance (OR=1.3; 0.97-1.9), except when ipsilateral exposure was considered alone (OR=1.6; 1.1-2.4). No consistent pattern of increased risk was uncovered for meningiomas. In terms of age, the highest risk of brain cancer was identified among those who were under 20 years of age at the time they first started using wireless phones.

Outside these two sources of multiple studies, another source of data stems from the previously-mentioned SEER database in the U.S., drawing from which Little et al compared epidemiological data from 12 registries (Atlanta, Detroit, Los Angeles, San Francisco, San Jose-Monterey, Seattle, rural Georgia, Connecticut, Hawaii, Iowa, New Mexico, and Utah) against incidence trends reported by the INTERPHONE Study Group and Hardell's group in Sweden [174]. U.S. population-based data was evaluated for glioma incidence from 1992 to 2008, a period of time during which mobile phone use increased dramatically from virtually 0% to almost 100% of the U.S. population. During these years, 24,813 non-Hispanic Caucasians 18 years or older were diagnosed with glioma. Age-specific incidence rates of glioma remained generally stable from 1992 to 2008 (-0.02% change per year, 95% confidence interval -0.28% to 0.25%), despite the exponential increase in cell-phone use. The authors concluded that the decline in brain cancer rates they observed was inconsistent with the association between brain cancer and mobile phone use conjectured by Hardell's group, since rates should have been at least 40% higher than observed. On the other hand, they felt that the SEER data could be consistent with the glioma rates predicted based upon the small proportion of highly-exposed individuals reported in the INTERPHONE study.

Overall, results on the association between mobile phone use and brain cancer certainly might be considered suggestive, particularly in terms of long-term risk after years of exposure to cell phones, especially when used extensively. However, in two just-published reviews, Swerdlow et al [155] and Repacholi et al [11] both noted the inconclusiveness of current data, and on the limitations imposed by the absence of data both on exposures beyond 10 to 15 years, and on childhood cancers. Echoing Carpenter's concerns about EMF exposures in general [10], what is potentially alarming is the potential for further increases in brain cancer risk after latencies beyond ten years, especially given the now almost-universal use of cell phones and other hand-held electronic devices by adolescents and children.

7.3. Diet (maternal diet during pregnancy/childhood diet)

Many of the same methodological issues and sources of potential bias (e.g., recall and ascertainment bias) pertain to maternal and childhood diet as to electromagnetic field exposure, rendering research to address the association between diet and childhood brain cancer difficult. For that reason, the research into this issue is, again, inconclusive. The most consistently positive association between diet and childhood brain cancer risk has been for cured meats, like hot dogs. In Denver, Colorado, cured and broiled meat consumption by mothers during pregnancy and by children themselves was assessed in 234 childhood cancer cases (including 45 brain tumor patients) and 206 controls selected by random digit dialing [175]. Five meat groups (ham, bacon, or sausage; hot dogs; hamburgers; bologna, pastrami, corned beef, salami, or lunch meat; charcoal-broiled foods) were assessed. Exposures among U.S. standard metropolitan statistical areas were compared, with adjustments made for confounders. Maternal hot dog consumption once or more weekly was statistically associated with childhood brain tumors (OR = 2.3, 95%CI, 1.0-5.4). Meanwhile, among children, eating hamburgers once or more times per week was associated with a non-statistically increased risk of ALL (OR = 2.0, CI = 0.9-4.6), as was eating hot dogs once or more times weekly with brain tumors (2.1; 0.7-6.1). However, among children, the combination of no vitamins and eating cured meats was associated more strongly with both ALL and brain cancer than either no vitamins or meat consumption alone, producing ORs between 2 and 7, suggesting possible adverse effects of dietary nitrites and nitrosamines.

Bunin et al and the Children's Cancer Group conducted a case-control study specifically assessing the effects of maternal diet during pregnancy on the risk of childhood astrocytoma in 155 cases and 155 matched controls, all under age six, the controls selected by random-digit dialing [176]. A trend again was observed for consumption of cured meats (adjusted odds ratio [OR] for the highest versus lowest intake quartile = 1.7, p = 0.10). Iron supplements were associated with a significant decrease in astrocytoma risk (OR = 0.5, 95%CI, 0.3-0.8). No significant trends were observed for nitrosamine (OR = 0.8, p = 0.60); nitrites (1.3, p = 0.54); nitrates (0.7, p = 0.43); vitamin C (0.7, p = 0.37); or vitamin E (0.7, p = 0.48). Unfortunately, income level was a potential confounder.

In yet another high-profile case-control study, Bunin et al examined maternal diet relative to the risk of primitive neuroectodermal tumors (PNET) of the brain in offspring, with all 166 cases again under the age of six years at diagnosis [177]. As in the previously-mentioned study, controls were selected by random-digit dialing and matched for age and race. Telephone interviews with mothers included questions on the frequency of consumption of alcohol, vitamin and mineral supplements, and 53 specific foods during pregnancy. Significant protective trends were observed for vegetables (OR for the highest versus lowest quartile group for intake, 0.37; p = 0.005), fruits and fruit juices (OR = 0.28; p = 0.003), vitamin A (0.59; p = 0.03), vitamin C (0.42; p = 0.009), nitrate (0.44; p = 0.002), and folate (0.38; p = 0.005). Taking iron (0.43; p = 0.004), calcium (0.42; p = 0.05), and vitamin C (0.35; p = 0.04) supplements at any time during pregnancy and multivitamins over the first six weeks (0.56; p = 0.02) all were associated with decreased risk. On multivariate analyses, folate, early multivitamin use, and iron supplements remained protective [177]. A non-significant trend of increasing risk was observed for nitrosamine consumption (1.65; p = 0.15).

Concerns over the consumption of nitrates, nitrites and nitroamines have been expressed by others, given the susceptibility of rats to develop brain tumors in response to N-nitroso urea exposure, the morphological similarity between these tumors and those observed in humans, and the presence of nitrate salts in many fertilizers [178]. Consistent with this potential risk, one meta-analysis of brain cancer risk in U.S. farmers yielded a relative risk of 1.30 (95% CI, 1.09, 1.56) [179], though pesticides, to which farmers also often are exposed, are another potential explanatory factor. In yet another case-control study, an increased risk of childhood astrocytomas was detected in association with *in utero* exposure to nitrites via a residential water source [180].

7.4. Environmental neurocarcinogens and parental occupation

As confusing and diverse the literature on EMF and diet is, it is even more so with respect to environmental and occupational exposures, due to the difficulties ascertaining and quantifying levels of exposure, especially when that exposure is second-hand to a child.

Pesticide exposure, both first-hand and second-hand, has been shown to be associated with increased brain cancer risk in children in a number of studies; but effects have tended to be modest and sometimes conflicting. Daniels et al [181] reviewed the results of 31 studies published between 1970 and 1996 and noted methodological issues in most of them, including small sample sizes, inadequate measurement of actual exposure, and potential biases related to the selection of controls. A further inconsistency was the lack of an effect of direct exposure to the child in studies in which an effect of parental occupational exposure was identified, a clearly counter-intuitive discovery [181]. Risks also varied with the type of pesticide and type and level of exposure. For example, Shim et al compared 526 brain cancer cases diagnosed before age 10 years and identified from statewide cancer registries of four U.S. Atlantic Coast states versus one-to-one-matched controls selected via random digit dialing [182]. Exposure risk was assessed through computer-assisted telephone interviews with mothers. Using information on residential pesticide use and jobs held by fathers over the 2-year period prior to the child's birth, potential exposures to insecticides, herbicides, and fungicides were estimated. For each occupation, two raters independently classified the probability and intensity of exposure. A significantly increased risk of astrocytoma was associated with exposures to herbicides from residential use (OR = 1.9; 95% CI, 1.2-3.0). Combining parental exposures to herbicides from both residential and occupational sources, the elevated risk remained significant (1.8; 1.1-3.1). Little association was observed with primitive neuroectodermal tumors (PNET) for any of the pesticide classes or exposure sources considered. In another study, the risk of childhood brain cancer was again assessed relative to parental exposure to different classes of pesticide in 154 children diagnosed with astrocytoma and 158 children diagnosed with primitive neuroectodermal tumors (PNET) in the United States and Canada between 1986 and 1989 [183]. Controls again were selected by random digit dialing and were individually matched to cases by race, age, and geographic area. Each job in the fathers' work history and the usual occupation of mothers were assigned a probability, intensity, and frequency of exposure to insecticides, herbicides, and agricultural and non-agricultural fungicides. Elevated risks of astrocytoma were identified for paternal exposure (ever vs. never) to all four classes of pesticides (odds ratios (OR) = 1.4-1.6), while an increased risk of PNET was observed only for herbicides (OR = 1.5). For mothers, odds ratios for astrocytoma were elevated for insecticides, herbicides, and non-agricultural fungicides (OR = 1.3-1.6) but not agricultural fungicides (OR = 1.0). Concerns have been raised about the accuracy of the levels of probability, intensity, and frequency of exposure assigned to mothers and fathers. Interestingly, both studies that assessed the use of no-pest strips within the home identified increased childhood brain cancer risk [184], [185]. In the study by Leiss et al, this effect was dose dependent, with the odds ratio of brain tumors equal to 1.5 (95%CI, 0.9-2.4) when exposure was limited to just the last three months of pregnancy, versus 1.8 (1.2-2.9) when exposure was for the full two years prior to and throughout pregnancy [185]. One potential mechanism for direct pesticide-induced cancer risk is their conversion via nitrites in the stomach into potentially-carcinogenic N-nitroso compounds [186]; though how this might affect an unborn child is unclear.

Hair dyes are another environmental and occupational neurocarcinogen that has been shown to significantly increase brain cancer risk. In a population-based case-control study involving 112 white women in Nebraska newly diagnosed with glioma between July 1988 and June 1993, versus 215 controls, a 1.7-fold increased risk of glioma was observed among those who had ever used hair coloring products (95%CI = 1.0-2.9) [187]. This risk increased to 2.4 among those who had used permanent hair coloring products (95%CI, 1.3-4.5), and the risk of glioblastoma increased with duration of exposure, to 4.9 (95% CI, 1.6-15.7) after 21 or more years of permanent hair color use. Higher risks also were observed with earlier age at first use. In another study, the risk of brain cancer among children born on or after 1980 to women who had personally used hair dyes over the five years prior to pregnancy was increased 11-fold, though the confidence limits were broad (95%CI, 1.2-90) [188]. Childhood brain cancers also were associated with non-work-related maternal exposure to any beauty products (OR = 2.6, 95%CI, 1.2-5.9) and to hair sprays (3.4; 1.0-11).

Choi et al identified a significant risk of childhood brain cancer before age 5 in women living within one mile of a facility releasing toxic release inventory (TRI) chemicals while pregnant [189]. In 2008, Clapp, Jacobs and Loechler published a detailed review of environmental and occupational causes of cancer, a 40-page manuscript with extensive tables that list all chemicals and other environmental exposures associated with a variety of cancers. For brain cancers, evidence of an association is considered strong only for ionizing radiation [180].

Occupational exposures have been assessed both for the mother and father, but especially the latter, in terms of child cancer risk [4]. Besides farming/agriculture, associations have been reported for the aircraft, electronics, petroleum, and pulp and paper industries, as well as for any industries associated with increased exposures to paints, solvents, other chemicals, pesticides, ionizing radiation, and electromagnetic fields [4], [190]. Albeit now more than 20 years old, Savitz and Chen wrote a very thorough paper summarizing all studies performed to date assessing the risk of childhood brain cancers, hematopoietic malignancies, and other malignancies relative to both paternal and maternal occupations [191]. Occupations were subdivided into motor vehicle related occupations, machinist and factory workers, occupations with paint exposure, occupations with chemical exposure, the petroleum industry, occupations with exposure to aggregated hydrocarbons, electronics, occupations associated with ionizing radiation, occupations with metal exposure, agriculture, construction, pulp and paper, aerospace and aircraft industries, and other occupations (printing workers, graphic arts workers, and glass, clay and stone industry). For virtually every occupational category, there was at least one study identifying a statistically increased odds ratio for childhood nervous system cancer. Table 2 summarizes that list, noting the number of studies in each job category, the number of studies with an odds ratio for childhood brain cancer > 1.0, the number of studies with an odds ratio statistically greater than 1.0, and the range of odds ratios within that job category.

Note that, in no category for which there was more than a single study, was every odds ratio for childhood brain cancer statistically greater than one. Note also that the industries in which all odds ratios were > 1.0, even if not statistically significant, were the petroleum industry, electrical work, metal work, and pulp and paper. Note also that some industries, like health care, were not mentioned. Among mothers, the odds ratios for childhood brain cancer were 3.3 for occupations with chemicals on the skin, 3.0 for occupations involving inhaled chemicals of fumes, 1.6 for bakers, and 4.0 for occupations requiring protective clothing or equipment [191]; only the last OR was statistically greater than 1.0.

In a later and also quite thorough review of the literature, published in 1998, Colt and Blair reviewed 48 papers published between 1974 and 1987, encompassing relative risk estimates for over 1000 specific cancer/occupation and cancer/exposure combinations [192]. Of these papers, 23 contained data assessing the relationship between paternal occupations and childhood nervous system cancers other than neuroblastoma; maternal occupations only were evaluated in terms of childhood leukemia risk. In table form, these authors listed studies by exposure, categorizing into electromagnetic fields; paints and pigments; hydrocarbons; metals; and motor vehicle-related occupations. These results are summarized in Table 3.

As in the review by Savitz and Chen, the results were conflicting, the authors themselves concluding that the evidence was strongest in support of an association between paternal exposure to paints and pigments [192]. Results on maternal occupations were scant and yielded no statistically significant associations.

More recently published studies yield much the same diffuse and inconsistent results [193]-[196], including one recently published study (2008) in Taiwan in which no associations among

http://dx.doi.org/10.5772/52427

Occupation/Main Exposure	Number of studies	Number of OR "/> 1.0	# OR statistically "/> 1.0	Range of OR
Motor vehicles	7	3	1	0.6 - 2.8
Machinist & factory workers	5	3	1	0.7 - 4.4
Paint	4	3	1	1.0 - 7.0
Chemicals	6	5	3	0.8 - 10.0
Petroleum	3	3	0	1.3 - 3.1
Aggregated hydrocarbons	6	4	1	0.5 - 3.2
Electrical	4	4	2	1.6 - 11.8
Ionizing radiation	6	5	2	1.0 - 2.2
Metals	3	3	1	1.6 - 2.7
Agriculture	4	2	n/a	0.6 - 2.0
Construction	4	3	2	0.9 - 2.3
Pulp & paper	3	3	1	1.6 - 4.0
Aerospace & aircraft	3	2	1	1.0 - ∞*
Printing workers	1	1	1	4.5
Graphic arts	1	1	1	21.9
Glass, clay, stone	1	1	0	1.5
Total	61	46	18	0.5 - ∞*

Savitz and Chen, 1990 [1][9][1]

* ∞ = infinity

Table 2. Paternal Occupation and Childhood Nervous System Cancer Risk

202 young brain cancer cases, ages 0 to 29 years, were identified across a wide variety of occupations [197].

Finally, in one novel study, Rosso et al examined whether or not there was an association between a father's hobbies and brain cancer risk in their child, specifically looking at medulloblastomas and other PNET in 318 children under age 6 versus 318 randomly selected population controls [198]. On multivariate analyses, the only significant association was for lawn care with pesticides [during pregnancy: odds ratio (OR) = 1.6, 95% confidence interval (CI): 1.0, 2.5; after birth: OR = 1.8, 95% CI: 1.2, 2.8].

7.5. Other potential risk factors

Numerous other risk factors for childhood brain cancer have been reported, albeit mostly in single studies. Neonatal head circumference was found to be associated with an increased risk

Main Exposures	# RR estimates	Number of RR "/> 1.0	# RR statistically "/> 1.0	Range of RR
Electromagnetic fields	55	45	9	0.3 - 73.3
Paints & pigments	14	13	4	1.0 - ∞
Hydrocarbons	28	12	2	0.4 - 4.0
Metals	17	15	4	0.8 - 5.3
Motor vehicles, etc.	32	12	2	0.1 -5.9
Total	146	97	21	0.1 - ∞

Colt and Blair, 1998 [192]

* ∞ = infinity

Table 3. Paternal Occupation and Childhood Nervous System Cancer Risk

of brain cancer by Samuelson et al, who analysed 1,010,366 individuals with 12,378,172 person-years of follow-up, from which 453 individuals ages 0 to 15 years were diagnosed with brain cancer [199]. In this population, the relative risk of brain cancer was 1.27 (95%CI 1.16-1.38) for every 1 cm increase in head circumference, after adjusting for birth-weight, gestational age, and gender. In another study of 746 invasive CNS cancers in children less than 4 years old, after adjusting for parental education, elevated birth-weight was associated with an odds ratio of 1.71 for astrocytoma (95%CI, 1.01-2.90); but birth weight was not associated with an increased risk of PNET [42].

Prior malignancy has been associated with a variety of malignancies in the literature, including brain cancer. Some of this increased risk almost certainly is secondary to radiation therapy to the head and neck [129]. Yet even when head irradiation is not utilized, brain cancer risk may be increased. Maule et al identified a total of 133 second malignant neoplasms in 16,540 patients with hematopoietic malignancies (12,731 leukemias, 1246 Hodgkin's lymphomas, and 2563 non-Hodgkin's lymphomas) after an average follow-up of 6.5 years [200]. The most frequent second malignancies after leukemia were brain cancer (standardized incidence ratio [SIR] = 8.52; 95% CI = 5.13 to 13.3), non-Hodgkin's lymphoma (SIR = 9.41; 4.30 to 17.9), and thyroid cancer (SIR = 18.8; 8.60 to 35.7). The most frequent after non-Hodgkin's lymphoma were thyroid cancer (SIR = 40.4; 14.8 to 88.0) and brain cancer (SIR = 6.97; 1.90 to 17.9). There was no increased incidence of brain cancer following Hodgkin's lymphoma.

In Rio de Janeiro, in a hospital-based case-control study involving 231 adults with primary brain tumors and 261 controls matched for gender and age among in-patients hospitalized for various conditions unrelated to brain cancer, past head injury was found to be significantly more frequent among cases (46%) than controls (36%) (OR(adjusted) = 1.49; 95%CI = 1.03-2.15) [201]. Moreover, a dose-response effect was observed related to the number of head injuries, and a statistically-borderline association was observed specifically for meningioma (OR(adj) = 1.63; 0.96-2.75). These results have not yet been replicated and, to date, no such association has been identified for childhood brain cancer.

In a nationwide Danish study on the occurrence of cancer among 8,093 Danish individuals born with an oral cleft deformity between 1936 and 1998 and followed in the Danish Cancer Registry from 1968 through 1998, a total of 175,863 person-years, the possible association between cancer and oral clefts was assessed [202]. The expected overall number of all cancers was 131, but 140 incident cancers were found, corresponding to a standardized incidence ratio of 1.07 (95%CI, 0.90-1.26). Analyses of the 52 sites for all oral cleft cases and analyses stratified into three cleft subgroups and two sexes revealed only a few significant associations, one of which was the increased incidence of primary brain cancer among females, but not males, born with a cleft palate (SIR = 3.11; 1.14, 6.78).

Finally, medications are often listed as a potential risk factor for brain cancer [203], but there are almost no data scientifically supporting such a claim. In one case-control study of 163 matched pairs, patients under 15 years of age when diagnosed with astrocytoma between 1980 and 1986 were identified through the tumor registries of eight hospitals in Pennsylvania, New Jersey, and Delaware [204]. Controls were selected by random digit dialing, and matched to cases for age, race, and telephone area code and exchange. In this population, maternal anti-nausea medications significantly increased the risk of childhood astrocytoma [OR = 2.0, p = 0.04], while gestational exposure to marijuana was of borderline significance (OR = 2.8, p = 0.07). Gestational exposures to neurally-active medications, alcohol, and tobacco did not increase brain cancer risk, consistent with other studies [203]. The association between anti-emetics and increased brain cancer risk was not identified in another, Swedish study in which this was assessed [205]. In the Swedish study, no significant changes in risk were noted after exposure to iron supplementation, anti-emetics, analgesics, antibiotics or any other drug, with the exception that 10 children with a brain tumor had been exposed to some beta-blocking agent *in utero* versus just two children without brain tumor (adjusted OR 5.3, 95%CI 1.2-24.8). In addition, a tendency towards a protective effect was observed for prenatal exposure to folic acid (adjusted OR 0.6; 0.3-1.1). Finally, case-control data from M. D. Anderson Cancer Center and the University of California, San Francisco were pooled to conduct an analysis stratified by histological subtype of glioma to identify any potentiating effects of inflammation-related variables and antihistamine use [206]. An association was discovered between long-term antihistamine use and the increased risk of anaplastic gliomas, especially when the length of use was considered in conjunction with a history of asthma or allergy: anaplastic cases with no history of asthma or allergy were 2.94 times more likely than controls to report antihistamine use lasting 10 years or more; while anaplastic cases with a history of asthma or allergy were 2.34 times more likely. Conversely, anti-inflammatory medication use was protective against glioblastoma (OR = 0.80; 95%CI: 0.65, 0.99), especially among individuals with no history of asthma or allergies. No statistically-significant effects of anti-inflammatory drugs or antihistamines were evident for other histological subtypes of glioma.

8. Summary, clinical applications, and directions for future research

Brain cancer is one of the most fear-provoking and lethal of all illnesses, two reasons that concerns about the potential for increased rates from the use of hand-held electronic devices have been raised. To date, however, there is no evidence that brain cancer incidence rates have increased at all over the same time period that the use of these devices has escalated exponentially. In the U.S. and U.K., where data are available, brain cancer incidence rates appear to be stable or declining. Mortality rates also are declining. That being said, there are virtually no readily-accessible data outside the U.S. and the U.K., and there is some research evidence that any effects of such devices on brain cancer risk only become significantly and clinically manifest after years, if not decades of their use. Consequently, it may be too soon to have detected adverse effects and, if present, to determine the magnitude of such effects on brain cancer numbers.

Known risk factors for brain cancer are male gender, younger age among pediatric populations, and Caucasian race. A family or personal history of cancer, and in particular brain cancer appears to increase risk as well, as do radiation treatments to the head and neck area. In addition, a small percentage of brain cancer cases, likely 5 percent or less, occur within the context of a familial syndrome, the most common of which are neurofibromatosis and tuberous sclerosis. In such patients, the risk is high for a variety of intracranial and extra-cranial malignancies, so that continuous vigilance by qualified health care practitioners is paramount.

Unfortunately, research into a variety of suspected brain cancer risk factors has been fraught with difficulties, given problems accurately evaluating levels of exposure, controlling for numerous other potentially carcinogenic exposures, and issues like recall and ascertainment bias. As stated earlier, understanding about the true risk of hand-held devices like cell phones may not come until they have been in widespread use for several more years, at which point it may be too late to prevent whatever initial rise in cases results. The same is true for electromagnetic fields from the increasing number of household appliances, especially home computers that are entering our homes, though the trend has been towards negative-result studies as methodologies have advanced over the years. As for dietary factors, other than promoting good diet and moderation in the consumption of cured meats, little more can be said at this time. And all patients should be advised to exercise caution when partaking in any occupation, hobby or other activity that places one in regular close contact with chemicals or ionizing radiation.

Further research clearly is needed to clarify the huge number of yet-unanswered questions, but this must start with close and international monitoring of brain cancer rates, both overall and cancer-type specific. In the U.S., the SEER database is a huge advantage; but investigators need to utilize this database more and publish these results within the medical literature. The number and completeness of similar databases in other countries this author cannot say; but again, such databases need to be used for research purposes and resultant findings published on a regular basis, if changing trends in brain cancer incidence are to be detected early. As for establishing the magnitude of risk from devices like cell phones, if such risk actually exists, what are needed are large, prospective, longitudinal studies assessing dose-dependent effects, since it makes sense that the highest-volume users will be the ones most likely to present earliest with problems, a contention that already-published results support. Moreover, using prospective studies will largely counter the problems with recall and ascertainment bias that has plagued the numerous case-control studies published to date though, admittedly, such studies invariably must be larger and, hence costlier. This being said, it is important to recall those databases already in existence, like the SEER database and State and provincial cancer registries. Linking prospectively-acquired, multicenter exposure data with some database like these would provide a powerful research tool in the fight against brain cancer.

Author details

Adrianna Ranger

University of Western Ontario, London, Ontario, Canada

References

[1] Centers for Disease Control and Prevention (CDC)Trends in childhood cancer mortality--United States, (1990). MMWR Morb Mortal Wkly Rep 2007; , 56(48), 1257-1261.

[2] Linet, M. S, Ries, L. A, Smith, M. A, Tarone, R. E, & Devesa, S. S. Cancer surveillance series: recent trends in childhood cancer incidence and mortality in the United States. J Natl Cancer Inst (1999). , 91(12), 1051-1058.

[3] Bunin, G. R, Feuer, E. J, Witman, P. A, & Meadows, A. T. Increasing incidence of childhood cancer: report of 20 years experience from the greater Delaware Valley Pediatric Tumor Registry. Paediatr Perinat Epidemiol (1996). , 10(3), 319-338.

[4] Gurney, J. G, Smith, M. A, & Bunin, G. R. CNS and miscellaneous intra-cranial and intraspinal neoplasms. SEER Pediatric Monograph, National Cancer Institute, (2001). Ref Type: Serial (Book,Monograph), 51-63.

[5] National Cancer InstituteA Snapshot of Pediatric Cancers: Incidence on Mortality Rate Trends. (2011). Ref Type: Report

[6] Ellison, L. F. De P, Mery LS, Grundy PE, Canadian Cancer Society's Steering Committee for Canadian Cancer Statistics. Canadian cancer statistics at a glance: cancer in children. CMAJ (2009). Feb 17;, 180(4), 422-4.

[7] Rendón-macías, M. E, Ramos-becerril, C, Bernardez-zapata, I, & Iglesias-leboreiro, J. Cancer epidemiology in children and adolescents at private health care ((1995). Article in Spanish]. Rev Med Inst Mex Seguro Soc 2008; , 46(4), 353-360.

[8] Brain Tumor FactsAmerican Brain Tumor Association. (2012). Ref Type: Electronic Citation

[9] Chatenoud, L, Bertuccio, P, Bosetti, C, Levi, F, & Negri, E. La Vecchia C. Childhood cancer mortality in America, Asia, and Oceania, 1970 through 2007. Cancer (2010). , 116(21), 5063-5074.

[10] Carpenter, D. O. Electromagnetic fields and cancer: the cost of doing nothing. Rev Environ Health (2010). , 25(1), 75-80.

[11] Repacholi, M. H, Lerchl, A, Roosli, M, et al. Systematic review of wireless phone use and brain cancer and other head tumors. Bioelectromagnetics (2012). , 33(3), 187-206.

[12] Vrijheid, M, Deltour, I, Krewski, D, Sanchez, M, & Cardis, E. The effects of recall errors and of selection bias in epidemiologic studies of mobile phone use and cancer risk. J Expo Sci Environ Epidemiol (2006). , 16(4), 371-384.

[13] Deorah, S, Lynch, C. F, Sibenaller, Z. A, & Ryken, T. C. Trends in brain cancer incidence and survival in the United States: Surveillance, Epidemiology, and End Results Program, 1973 to 2001. Neurosurg Focus (2006). E1.

[14] Vutuc, C, Waldoer, T, & Haidinger, G. Cancer mortality in Austria: Wien Klin Wochenschr (2004). , 1970-2002.

[15] Fang, Z, Kulldorff, M, & Gregorio, D. I. Brain cancer mortality in the United States, 1986 to 1995: a geographic analysis. Neuro Oncol (2004). , 6(3), 179-187.

[16] Monteiro, G. T, & Koifman, S. Brain tumors mortality in Brazil, 1980-1998]. [Article in Portuguese]. Cad Saude Publica (2003). , 19(4), 1139-1151.

[17] Johannesen, T. B, Angell-andersen, E, Tretli, S, Langmark, F, & Lote, K. Trends in incidence of brain and central nervous system tumors in Norway, 1970-1999. Neuroepidemiology (2004). , 23(3), 101-119.

[18] De Vocht, F, Burstyn, I, & Cherrie, J. W. Time trends (1998-2007) in brain cancer incidence rates in relation to mobile phone use in England. Bioelectromagnetics (2011). , 32(5), 334-349.

[19] Yeole, B. B. Trends in the brain cancer incidence in India. Asian Pac J Cancer Prev (2008). , 9(2), 267-270.

[20] Smith, M. A, Freidlin, B, Ries, L. A, & Simon, S. L. Trends in reported incidence of primary malignant brain tumors in children in the United States. J Natl Cancer Inst (1998). , 90(17), 1269-1277.

[21] Mcnally, R. J, Kelsey, A. M, Cairns, D. P, Taylor, G. M, Eden, O. B, & Birch, J. M. Temporal increases in the incidence of childhood solid tumors seen in Northwest England (1954-1998) are likely to be real. Cancer 92 [7], (2001). Ref Type: Electronic Citation, 1967-1976.

[22] The SEER databaseNational Cancer Institute. (2012). Ref Type: Electronic Citation

[23] Brain Cancer Fact Sheet: The SEER databaseNational Cancer Institute. (2012). Ref Type: Electronic Citation

[24] Age-adjusted SEER Incidence Rates by YearRace and Sex- Cancer of the Brain and Other Nervous System (Invasive). National Cancer Institute. (2012). Ref Type: Electronic Citation

[25] Age-adjusted Incidence and Mortality Rates: The SEER databaseNational Cancer Institute. (2012). Ref Type: Electronic Citation

[26] Mao, Y, Desmeules, M, Semenciw, R. M, Hill, G, Gaudette, L, & Wigle, D. T. Increasing brain cancer rates in Canada. CMAJ (1991)., 145(12), 1583-1591.

[27] Preston-martin, S, Lewis, S, Winkelmann, R, Borman, B, Auld, J, & Pearce, N. Descriptive epidemiology of primary cancer of the brain, cranial nerves, and cranial meninges in New Zealand, Cancer Causes Control 4 [6], 529-538. (1993). Ref Type: Electronic Citation, 1948-88.

[28] Legler, J. M, Ries, L. A, Smith, M. A, et al. Cancer surveillance series [corrected]: brain and other central nervous system cancers: recent trends in incidence and mortality. J Natl Cancer Inst (1999)., 91(16), 1382-1390.

[29] Grovas, A, Fremgen, A, Rauck, A, et al. The National Cancer Data Base report on patterns of childhood cancers in the United States. Cancer (1997)., 80(12), 2321-2332.

[30] Khatua, S, Sadighi, Z. S, Pearlman, M. L, Bochare, S, & Vats, T. S. Brain Tumors in Children- Current Therapies and Newer Directions. Indian J Pediatr (2012). Feb 1 [Epub ahead of print] 2012.

[31] Khalatbari, M. R, Hamidi, M, & Moharamzad, Y. Glioblastoma multiforme with very rapid growth and long-term survival in children: report of two cases and review of the literature. Childs Nerv Syst (2011)., 27(8), 1347-1352.

[32] MacDonadl TJAguilera D, Kramm CM. Treatment of high-grade glioma in children and adolescents. Neuro Oncol (2011)., 13(10), 1049-1058.

[33] Sievert, A. J, & Fisher, M. J. Pediatric low-grade gliomas. J Child Neurol (2009)., 24(11), 1397-1408.

[34] Qaddoumi, I, Sultan, I, & Gajjar, A. Outcome and prognostic features in pediatric gliomas: a review of 6212 cases from the Surveillance, Epidemiology, and End Results database. Cancer (2009)., 115(24), 5761-5770.

[35] Taylor, M. D, Sanford, R. A, & Boop, F. A. Cerebellar pilocytic astrocytomas. In: Albright AL, Pollack IF, Adelson PD, editors. Principles and Practice of Pediatric Neurosurgery. New York: Thieme Medical pUBLISHERS, iNC.; , 655-667.

[36] Epstein, F, & Mccleary, E. L. Intrinsic brain-stem tumors of childhood: surgical indications. J Neurosurg (1986)., 64(1), 11-15.

[37] Khatua, S, Moore, K. R, Vats, T. S, & Kestle, J. R. Diffuse intrinsic pontine glioma-current status and future strategies. Childs Nerv Syst (2011). , 27(9), 1391-1397.

[38] Farmer, J-P, Mcneely, P. D, & Freeman, C. R. Brainstem Gliomas. In: Albright AL, Pollack IF, Adelson PD, editors. Principles and Practice of Pediatric Neurosurgery. New York: Thieme Medical Publishers, Inc.; , 640-654.

[39] Diller, L, Chow, E. J, Gurney, J. G, et al. Chronic disease in the Childhood Cancer Survivor Study cohort: a review of published findings. J Clin Oncol (2009). , 27(14), 2339-2355.

[40] Davis, D. L, Ahlbom, A, Hoel, D, & Percy, C. Is brain cancer mortality increasing in industrial countries? Am J Ind Med (1991). , 19(4), 421-431.

[41] Tseng, J. H, & Tseng, M. Y. Survival analysis of children with primary malignant brain tumors in England and Wales: a population-based study. Pediatr Neurosurg. 42 [2], (2006). Ref Type: Electronic Citation, 67-73.

[42] Von Behren, J, & Reynolds, P. Birth characteristics and brain cancers in young children. Int J Epidemiol. 32 [2], (2003). Ref Type: Electronic Citation, 248-256.

[43] Gajjar, A, Sanford, R. A, Heideman, R, et al. Low-grade astrocytoma: a decade of experience at St. Jude Children's Research Hospital. J Clin Oncol. 15 [8], (1997). ef Type: Electronic Citation, 2792-2799.

[44] Pollack, I. F, Gerszten, P. C, Martinez, A. J, et al. Intracranial ependymomas of childhood: long-term outcome and prognostic factors. Neurosurgery 37 [4], (1995). Ref Type: Electronic Citation, 655-666.

[45] Darefsky, A. S, & Dubrow, R. International variation in the incidence of adult primary malignant neoplasms of the brain and central nervous system. Cancer Causes Control (2009). , 20(9), 1593-1604.

[46] Bunin, G. Racial patterns of childhood brain cancer by histologic type. J Natl Cancer Inst (1987). , 78(5), 875-880.

[47] Farwell, J, & Flannery, J. T. Cancer in relatives of children with central-nervous-system neoplasms. N Engl J Med. 311 [12], (1984). Ref Type: Electronic Citation, 749-753.

[48] Hemminki, K, Li, X, & Collins, V. P. Parental cancer as a risk factor for brain tumors (Sweden). Cancer Causes Control 12 [3], (2001). Ref Type: Electronic Citation, 195-199.

[49] Hill, D. A, Inskip, P. D, Shapiro, W. R, et al. Cancer in first-degree relatives and risk of glioma in adults. Cancer Epidemiol Biomarkers Prev (2003). , 12(12), 1443-1448.

[50] Hill, D. A, Linet, M. S, Black, P. M, et al. Meningioma and schwannoma risk in adults in relation to family history of cancer. Neuro Oncol.2004 Oct;(2004). Ref Type: Electronic Citation, 6(4), 274-80.

[51] Blumenthal, D. T, & Cannon-albright, L. A. Familiality in brain tumors. Neurology (2008). , 71(13), 1015-1020.

[52] Ostrom, Q. T, Mcculloh, C, Chen, Y, et al. Family history of cancer in benign brain tumor subtypes versus gliomas. Front Oncol.2012;2:19.Epub 2012 Feb 28. (2012). Ref Type: Electronic Citation

[53] Kuitjen, R. R, & Bunin, G. R. Risk factors for childhood brain tumors. Cancer Epidemiol Biomarkers Prev. 2 [3], (1993). Ref Type: Electronic Citation, 277-288.

[54] Kuitjen, R. R, Strom, S. S, Rorke, L. B, et al. Family history of cancer and seizures in young children with brain tumors: a report from the Childrens Cancer Group (United States and Canada). Cancer Causes Control. 4 [5], (1993). Ref Type: Electronic Citation, 455-464.

[55] Wrensch, M, Lee, M, Miike, R, et al. Familial and personal medical history of cancer and nervous system conditions among adults with glioma and controls. Am J Epidemiol. 145 [7], (1997). Ref Type: Electronic Citation, 581-593.

[56] Korf, B. R. The phakomatoses. Clin Dermatol (2005). , 23(1), 78-84.

[57] Van Der Hoeve, J. Eye symptoms in tuberous sclerosis of the brain. Trans Ophthalmol Soc UK (1920). , 40, 329-334.

[58] Alaraj, A. M, Valyi-nagy, T, & Roitberg, B. Double phakomatosis; neurofibromatosis type-1 and tuberous sclerosis. Acta Neurochir (Wien) (2007). , 149(5), 505-509.

[59] Ferner, R. E. Neurofibromatosis 1 and neurofibromatosis 2: a twenty first century perspective. Lancet Neurol (2007). , 6(4), 340-351.

[60] Crump, T. Translation of case reports in Ueber die multiplen Fibrome der Haut und ihre Beziehung zu den multiplen Neuromen by F. v. Recklinghausen. Adv Neurol (1981). , 29, 259-275.

[61] Pearce JMSHistorical Note: Neurofibromatosis. J Neurol Neurosurg Psychiatry (2003).

[62] Lu-emerson, C, & Plotkin, S. R. The Neurofibromatoses. Part 1: NF1. Rev Neurol Dis (2009). EE53., 47.

[63] Lu-emerson, C, & Plotkin, S. R. The neurofibromatoses. Part 2: NF2 and schwannomatosis. Rev Neurol Dis (2009). EE86., 81.

[64] Evans, D. G, Howard, E, Giblin, C, et al. Birth incidence and prevalence of tumour prone syndromes: estimates from a UK genetic family register service. Am J Med Genet (2010). A:, 327-332.

[65] Ferner, R. E, Huson, S. M, Thomas, N, et al. Guidelines for the diagnosis and management of individuals with neurofibromatosis 1. J Med Genet (2007). , 44(2), 81-8.

[66] Legendre, C. M, Charpentier-cote, C, Drouin, R, & Bouffard, C. Neurofibromatosis type 1 and the "elephant man's" disease: the confusion persists: an ethnographic study. PLoS One (2011). e16409.

[67] Ferner, R. E. The neurofibromatoses. Pract Neurol (2010)., 10(2), 82-93.

[68] Hersh, J. H. American Academy of Pediatrics Committee on Genetics. Health supervision for children with neurofibromatosis. Pediatrics (2008)., 121(3), 633-642.

[69] Dodge, H. W, Lowe, J. G, Craig, W. M, et al. Gliomas of the optic nerves. Arch Neurol Psychiatr (1958)., 79, 607-621.

[70] Hottinger, A. F, & Khakoo, Y. Neuro-oncology of Neurofibromatosis Type 1. Curr Treat Options Neurol (2009)., 11(4), 306-314.

[71] Leonard, J. R, Perry, A, Rubin, J. B, et al. The role of surgical biopsy in the diagnosis of glioma in individuals with neurofibromatosis-1. Neurology (2006)., 67(8), 1509-1512.

[72] Evans, D. G. Neurofibromatosis type 2: genetic and clinical features. Ear Nose Throat J (1999)., 78(2), 97-100.

[73] Fontaine, B, Sanson, M, Delattre, O, et al. Parental origin of chromosome 22 loss in sporadic and NF2 neuromas. Genomics (1991)., 10(1), 280-283.

[74] Fontaine, B, Hanson, M. P, Vonsattel, J. P, et al. Loss of chromosome 22 alleles in human sporadic spinal schwannomas. Ann Neurol (1991)., 29(2), 183-186.

[75] Jacoby, L. B. MacCollin M, Parry DM, et al. Allelic expression of the NF2 gene in neurofibromatosis 2 and schwannomatosis. Neurogenetics (1999)., 2(2), 101-108.

[76] Neurofibromatosis Conference StatementNational Institutes of Health. Consensus Development Conference. Arch Neurol (1988)., 45(5), 575-578.

[77] Gutmann, D. H, Aylsworth, A, Carey, J. C, et al. The diagnostic evaluation and multidisciplinary management of neurofibromatosis 1 and neurofibromatosis 2. JAMA (1997)., 278(1), 51-57.

[78] Osborne, J. P, Fryer, A, & Webb, D. Epidemiology of tuberous sclerosis. Ann NY Acad Sci (1991)., 615, 125-127.

[79] Hong, C. H, Darling, T. N, & Lee, C. H. Prevalence of tuberous sclerosis complex in Taiwan: a national population-based study. Neuroepidemiology (2009)., 33(4), 335-341.

[80] Morrison, P. J. Tuberous sclerosis: epidemiology, genetics and progress towards treatment. Neuroepidemiology (2009).

[81] Orlova, K. A, & Crino, P. B. The tuberous sclerosis complex. Ann N Y Acad Sci (2010). Jan):, 87-105.

[82] Grajkowska, W, Kotulska, K, Jurkiewicz, E, & Matyja, E. Brain lesions in tuberous sclerosis complex. Review. Folia Neuropathol (2010). , 48(3), 139-149.

[83] Goh, S, Butler, W, & Thiele, E. A. Subependymal giant cell tumors in tuberous sclerosis complex. Neurology (2004). , 63(8), 1457-1461.

[84] Hottinger, A. F, & Khakoo, Y. Neurooncology of familial cancer syndromes. J Child Neurol (2009). , 24(12), 1526-1535.

[85] Seizinger, B. R, Rouleau, G. A, Ozelius, L. J, et al. Von Hippel-Lindau disease maps to the region of chromosome 3 associated with renal cell carcinoma. Nature (1988). , 332(6161), 268-269.

[86] Glasker, S. Central nervous system manifestations in VHL: genetics, pathology and clinical phenotypic features. Fam Cancer (2005). , 4(1), 37-42.

[87] Hassard, A. D, Boudreau, S. F, & Cron, C. C. Adenoma of the endolymphatic sac. J Otolaryngol (1984). , 13, 213-216.

[88] Butman, J. A, Linehan, W. M, & Lonser, R. R. Neurologic manifestations of von Hippel-Lindau disease. JAMA (2008). , 300(11), 1334-1342.

[89] Richard, S, Campello, C, Taillandier, L, Parker, F, & Resche, F. Haemangioblastoma of the central nervous system in von Hippel-Lindau disease. French VHL Study Group. J Intern Med (1998). , 243(6), 547-553.

[90] Wanebo, J. E, Lonser, R. R, Glenn, G. M, & Oldfield, E. H. The natural history of hemangioblastomas of the central nervous system in patients with von Hippel-Lindau disease. J Neurosurg (2003). , 98(1), 82-94.

[91] Thayer, S. P. di Magliano MP, Heiser PWeal. Hedgehog is an early and late mediator of pancreatic cancer tumorigenesis. Nature (2003). , 425(6960), 851-856.

[92] Shanley, S, Ratcliffe, J, Hockey, A, et al. Nevoid basal cell carcinoma syndrome: review of 118 affected individuals. Am J MedGenet (1994). , 50(3), 282-290.

[93] Kleihues, P, & Schauble, B. zur Hausen A, Esteve J, Ohgaki H. Tumors associated with germline mutations: a synopsis of 91 families. Am J Pathol (1997). , 53.

[94] Li, F. P. Fraumeni JFJ, Mulvihill JJ, et al. A cancer family syndrome in twenty-four kindreds. Cancer Res (1988). , 48(18), 5358-5362.

[95] Birch, J. M. Li-Fraumeni syndrome. Eur J Cancer (1994). A(13):1935-1941.

[96] Evans, D. G, Wu, C. L, & Birch, J. M. BRCA2: a cause of Li-Fraumeni-like syndrome. J Med Genet (2008). , 45, 62-63.

[97] Taylor, M. D, Mainprize, T. G, & Rutka, J. T. Molecular insight into medulloblastoma and central nervous system primitive neuroectodermal tumor biology from hereditary syndromes: a review. Neurosurgery (2000). , 47(4), 888-901.

[98] Foulkes, W. D. A tale of four syndromes: familial adenomatous polyposis, Gardner syndrome, attenuated APC and Turcot syndrome. QJM (1995). , 88(12), 853-863.

[99] Hamilton, S. R, Liu, B, Parsons, R. E, et al. The molecular basis of Turcot's syndrome. N Engl J Med (1995). , 332(13), 839-847.

[100] Paraf, F, Jothy, S, & Van Meir, E. G. Brain tumor-polyposis syndrome: two genetic diseases? J Clin Oncol (1997). , 15(7), 2744-2758.

[101] Mclaughlin, M. R, Gollin, S. M, Lese, C. M, & Albright, A. L. Medulloblastoma and glioblastoma multiforme in a patient with Turcot syndrome: a case report. Surg Neurol (1998). , 49(3), 295-301.

[102] Jamjoom, Z. A, Sadiq, S, Mofti, A. B, Al-mofleh, I, & Ajarim, D. Turcot syndrome: report of a case and review of the literature. Int Surg (1989). , 74(1), 45-50.

[103] Schroder, S, Moehrs, D, Von Weltzien, J, Winkler, R, & Otto, H. F. The Turcot syndrome. Report of an additional case and review of the literature. Dis Colon Rectum (1983). , 26(8), 533-538.

[104] Taylor, M. D, Mainprize, T. G, Rutka, J. T, Becker, L, Bayani, J, & Drake, J. M. Medulloblastoma in a child with Rubenstein-Taybi Syndrome: case report and review of the literature. Pediatr Neurosurg (2001). , 35(5), 235-238.

[105] Burton, B. J, Kumar, V. G, & Bradford, R. Granular cell tumour of the spinal cord in a patient with Rubenstein-Taybi syndrome. Br J Neurosurg (1997). , 11(3), 257-259.

[106] Enchondromatosis: In The Free Dictionary by Farlex at http://medical-dictionarythe-freedictionary.com/enchondromatosis. (2008).

[107] Baumgart, R, Bürklein, D, Hinterwimmer, S, Thaller, P, & Mutschler, W. The management of leg-length discrepancy in Ollier's disease with a fully implantable lengthening nail. J Bone Joint Surg Br (2005). , 87(7), 1000-1004.

[108] Shapiro, F. Ollier's Disease. An assessment of angular deformity, shortening, and pathological fracture in twenty-one patients. J Bone Joint Surg Am 1982 Jan;(1982). , 64(1), 95-103.

[109] Ranger, A, Szymczak, A, Hammond, R, & Zelcer, S. Pediatric thalamic glioblastoma associated with Ollier's disease (multiple enchondromatosis): a rare case of concurrence. J Neurosurg Pediatr (2009). , 4(4), 363-367.

[110] Schwartz, H. S, Zimmerman, N. B, Simon, M. A, Wroble, R. R, Millar, E. A, & Bonfiglio, M. The malignant potential of enchondromatosis. J Bone Joint Surg Am (1987). , 69(2), 269-274.

[111] Balcer, L. J, Galetta, S. L, Cornblath, W. T, & Liu, G. T. Neuro-ophthalmologic manifestations of Maffucci's syndrome and Ollier's disease. J Neuroophthalmol (1999). , 19(1), 62-66.

[112] Silve, C, & Jüppner, H. Ollier disease. Orphanet J Rare Dis (2006). Sep 22;1:37 2006; 1:37.

[113] Boinet, E. Enchondrose rachitiforme. Arch Gen de Med (1904). , 194, 2689-2717.

[114] Ranger, A, Szymczak, A, Hammond, R, & Zelcer, S. Do intracranial neoplasms differ in Ollier's disease and Maffucci's syndrome?- An in-depth analysis of the literature. [in press]. Neurosurgery (2009).

[115] Ranger, A, & Szymczak, A. The association between intracranial tumours and multiple dyschondroplasia (Ollier's disease or Maffucci's syndrome): do children and adults differ? J Neurooncol (2009). , 95(2), 165-173.

[116] Altay, M, Bayrakci, K, Yildiz, Y, Erekul, S, & Saglik, Y. Secondary chondrosarcoma in cartilage bone tumors: report of 32 patients. J Orthop Sci (2007). , 12(5), 415-423.

[117] Ozisik, Y, Meloni, A. M, Spanier, S. S, Bush, C. H, Kingsley, K. L, & Sandberg, A. A. Deletion 1p in a low-grade chondrosarcoma in a patient with Ollier disease. Canc Genet Cytogen (1998). , 105(2), 128-133.

[118] Bovee JVMGGraadt van Roggen JF, Cleton-Jansen AM, Taminiau AHM, Woude HJ, van der Hogendoorn PCW. Malignant progression in multiple enchondromatosis (Ollier"s disease): An autopsy-based molecular genetic study. Human Pathol (2000). , 31(10), 1299-1303.

[119] Chang, S, & Prados, M. D. Identical twins with Ollier's disease and intracranial gliomas: case report. Neurosurg (1994). , 34(5), 903-906.

[120] Robinson, D, Tieder, M, Halperin, N, Burshtein, D, & Nevo, Z. Maffucci's syndrome--the result of neural abnormalities? Evidence of mitogenic neurotransmitters present in enchondromas and soft tissue hemangiomas. Cancer (1994). , 74(3), 949-957.

[121] Mann, I, Yates, P. C, & Ainslie, J. P. Unusual case of double primary orbital tumour. Br J Ophthalmol. 37 [12], (1953). Ref Type: Electronic Citation, 758-762.

[122] Giles, D, Hewitt, D, Stewart, A, & Webb, J. Malignant disease in childhood and diagnostic irradiation in utero. Lancet 271 [6940], 447. (1956). Ref Type: Electronic Citation

[123] Stewart, A, Webb, J, & Hewitt, D. A survey of childhood malignancies. Br Med J. 1 [5086], (1958). Ref Type: Electronic Citation, 1495-1508.

[124] MacMahon BPrenatal x-ray exposure and childhood cancer. J Natl Cancer Inst. 28 [5], (1962). Ref Type: Electronic Citation, 1173-1191.

[125] Chowdhary, A, Spence, M. A, Sales, L, Rostomily, R. C, Rockhill, J. K, & Silbergeld, D. L. Radiation associated tumors following therapeutic cranial radiation. Surg Neurol Int.2012;3:48.Epub 2012 May 14. (2012). Ref Type: Electronic Citation

[126] Ron, E, Modan, B, et al. Tumors of the brain and nervous system after radiotherapy in childhood. N Engl J Med. 319 [16], (2012). Ref Type: Electronic Citation, 1033-1039.

[127] Ron, E, & Modan, B. Boice JDJr. Mortality after radiotherapy for ringworm of the scalp. Am J Epidemiol. 127 [4], (1988). Ref Type: Electronic Citation, 713-725.

[128] Shore, R. E, Albert, R. E, & Pasternack, B. S. Follow-up study of patients treated by X-ray epilation for Tinea capitis; resurvey of post-treatment illness and mortality experience. Arch Environ Health 31 [1], (1976). Ref Type: Electronic Citation, 21-28.

[129] Hardell, L, Mild, K. H, Pahlson, A, & Hallquist, A. Ionizing radiation, cellular telephones and the risk for brain tumours. Eur J Cancer Prev. 10 [6], (2001). Ref Type: Electronic Citation, 523-529.

[130] Thierry-chef, I, Simon, S. L, & Miller, D. L. Radiation dose and cancer risk among pediatric patients undergoing interventional neuroradiology procedures. Pediatr Radiol (2006). Suppl 2):159-162.

[131] Mezei, G, Gadallah, M, & Kheifets, L. Residential magnetic field exposure and childhood brain cancer: a meta-analysis. Epidemiology (2008). , 19(3), 424-430.

[132] Gurney, J. G, & Van Wijngaarden, E. Extremely low frequency electromagnetic fields (EMF) and brain cancer in adults and children: review and comment. Neuro Oncol (1999). , 1(3), 212-220.

[133] Kheifets, L, Sussman, S. S, & Preston-martin, S. Childhood brain tumors and residential electromagnetic fields (EMF). Rev Environ Contam Toxicol (1999). , 159, 111-129.

[134] Kheifets, L. Electric and magnetic field exposure and brain cancer: a review. Bioelectromagnetics (2001). Suppl 5):S5131., 120.

[135] Neutra, R. R. Panel exploring pro and con arguments as to whether EMFs cause childhood brain cancer. Bioelectromagnetics (2001). Suppl 5):S5149., 144.

[136] Savitz, D. A, Wachtel, H, Barnes, F. A, John, E. M, & Tvrdik, J. G. Case-control study of childhood cancer and exposure to 60-Hz magnetic fields. Am J Epidemiol (1988). , 128(1), 21-38.

[137] Savitz, D. A, John, E. M, & Kleckner, R. C. Magnetic field exposure from electric appliances and childhood cancer. Am J Epidemiol (1990). , 131(5), 763-773.

[138] Savitz, D. A, & Kaune, W. T. Childhood cancer in relation to a modified residential wire code. Environ Health Perspect (1993). , 101(1), 76-80.

[139] Kheifets, L, Ahlbom, A, Crespi, C. M, et al. A pooled analysis of extremely low-frequency magnetic fields and childhood brain tumors. Am J Epidemiol. 172 [7], (2010). Ref Type: Electronic Citation, 752-761.

[140] Wertheimer, N, & Leeper, E. Electrical wiring configurations and childhood cancer. Am J Epidemiol. 109 [3], (1979). Ref Type: Electronic Citation, 273-284.

[141] Tomenius, L. Hz electromagnetic environment and the incidence of childhood tumors in Stockholm County. Bioelectromagnetics 7 [2], 191-207. (1986). Ref Type: Electronic Citation, 50.

[142] Preston-martin, S, Gurney, J. G, Pogoda, J. M, Holly, E. A, & Mueller, B. A. Brain tumor risk in children in relation to use of electric blankets and water bed heaters. Results from the United States West Coast Childhood Brain Tumor Study. Am J Epidemiol (1996)., 143(11), 1116-1122.

[143] Feychting, M, & Ahlbom, A. Magnetic fields and cancer in children residing near Swedish high-voltage power lines. Am J Epidemiol. 138 [7], (1993). Ref Type: Electronic Citation, 467-481.

[144] Habash, R. W, Elwood, J. M, Krewski, D, Lotz, W. G, Mcnamee, J. P, & Prato, F. S. Recent advances in research on radiofrequency fields and health: J Toxicol Environ Health B Crit Rev. 12 [4], 250-288. (2009). Ref Type: Electronic Citation, 2004-2007.

[145] Miller, A. B, & Green, L. M. Electric and magnetic fields at power frequencies. Miller AB, Green LM. Chronic Dis Can (2010). Suppl 1):69-83.

[146] Wood, A. W. Computer screens and brain cancer. Australas Phys Eng Sci Med (1995)., 18(4), 167-176.

[147] Mutnick, A, & Muscat, J. E. Primary brain cancer in adults and the use of common household appliances: a case-control study. Rev Environ Health. 12 [1], (1997). Ref Type: Electronic Citation, 59-62.

[148] Tworoger, S. S, Davis, S, Schwartz, S. M, & Mirick, D. K. Stability of Wertheimer-Leeper wire codes as a measure of exposure to residential magnetic fields over a to 11-year interval. J Expo Anal Environ Epidemiol. 12 [6], 448-454. (2002). Ref Type: Electronic Citation, 9.

[149] Armstrong, B. G, Deadman, J, & Mcbride, M. L. The determinants of Canadian children's personal exposures to magnetic fields. Bioelectromagnetics 22 [3], (2001). Ref Type: Electronic Citation, 161-169.

[150] Wertheimer, N, & Leeper, E. Re: "Risk of premenopausal breast cancer and use of electric blankets" and "Use of electric blankets and risk of postmenopausal breast cancer". Am J Epidemiol. 142 [12], (1995). Ref Type: Electronic Citation, 1344-1345.

[151] Wertheimer, N, & Leeper, E. Bias in studies of electromagnetic fields. J Clin Epidemiol. 47 [9], (1994). Ref Type: Electronic Citation, 1081-1083.

[152] Jensen, J. K, Olsen, J. H, & Folkersen, E. Assessment of exposure to EMF in a Danish case-control study of childhood cancer. Rev Environ Health 10 [(3-4)], (1994). Ref Type: Electronic Citation, 187-195.

[153] Kaune, W. T, & Zaffanella, L. E. Assessing historical exposures of children to power-frequency magnetic fields. J Expo Anal Environ Epidemiol. 4 [2], (1994). Ref Type: Electronic Citation, 149-170.

[154] Kheifets, L, Bowman, J. D, Checkoway, H, et al. Future needs of occupational epidemiology of extremely low frequency electric and magnetic fields: review and recommendations. Occup Environ Med. 66 [2], (2009). Ref Type: Electronic Citation, 72-80.

[155] Swerdlow, A. J, Feychting, M, & Green, A. C. Leeka Kheifits LK, Savitz DA, International Commission for Non-Ionizing Radiation Protection Standing Committee on Epidemiology. Mobile phones, brain tumors, and the interphone study: where are we now? Environ Health Perspect. 119 [11], (2011). Ref Type: Electronic Citation, 1534-1538.

[156] Hardell, L, Nasman, A, Pahlson, A, & Hallquist, A. Hansson Mild K. Use of cellular telephones and the risk for brain tumours: A case-control study. Int J Oncol. 15 [1], (1999). Ref Type: Electronic Citation, 113-116.

[157] Hardell, L, & Carlberg, M. Hansson Mild K. Pooled analysis of case-control studies on malignant brain tumours and the use of mobile and cordless phones including living and deceased subjects. Int J Oncol. 38 [5], (2011). Ref Type: Electronic Citation, 1465-1474.

[158] Hardell, L, & Carlberg, M. Hansson Mild K. Mobile phone use and the risk for malignant brain tumors: a case-control study on deceased cases and controls. Neuroepidemiology 35 [2], (2010). Ref Type: Electronic Citation, 109-114.

[159] Cardis, E, Richardson, L, Deltour, I, et al. The INTERPHONE study: design, epidemiological methods, and description of the study population. Eur J Epidemiol. 22 [9], (2007). Ref Type: Electronic Citation, 647-664.

[160] Schuz, J, Bohler, E, Berg, G, et al. Cellular phones, cordless phones, and the risks of glioma and meningioma (Interphone Study Group, Germany). Am J Epidemiol. 163 [6], (2006). Ref Type: Electronic Citation, 512-520.

[161] Blettner, M, Schlehofer, B, Samkange-zeeb, F, Berg, G, Schlaefer, K, & Schuz, J. Medical exposure to ionising radiation and the risk of brain tumours: Interphone study group, Germany. Eur J Cancer 43 [13], (2007). Ref Type: Electronic Citation, 1990-1998.

[162] Hours, M, Bernard, M, Montestrucq, L, et al. Cell Phones and Risk of brain and acoustic nerve tumours: the French INTERPHONE case-control study]. [Article in French]. Rev Epidemiol Sante Publique. 55 [5], (2012). Ref Type: Electronic Citation, 321-332.

[163] Lonn, S, Ahlbom, A, Hall, P, & Feychting, M. Swedish Interphone Study Group. Long-term mobile phone use and brain tumor risk. Am J Epidemiol. 161 [6], (2005). Ref Type: Electronic Citation, 526-535.

[164] Takebayashi, T, Akiba, S, Kikuchi, Y, et al. Mobile phone use and acoustic neuroma risk in Japan. Occup Environ Med. 63 [12], (2006). Ref Type: Electronic Citation, 802-807.

[165] Sadetzki, S, Chetrit, A, Jarus-hakak, A, et al. Cellular phone use and risk of benign and malignant parotid gland tumors--a nationwide case-control study. Am J Epidemiol. 167 [4], (2008). Ref Type: Electronic Citation, 457-467.

[166] Cardis, E, Deltour, I, Vrijheid, M, et al. Brain tumour risk in relation to mobile telephone use: results of the INTERPHONE international case-control study. INTERPHONE Study Group. Int J Epidemiol. 39 [3], (2010). Ref Type: Electronic Citation, 675-694.

[167] Cardis, E, Armstrong, B. K, Bowman, J. D, et al. Risk of brain tumours in relation to estimated RF dose from mobile phones: results from five Interphone countries. Occup Environ Med. 68 [9], (2011). Ref Type: Electronic Citation, 631-640.

[168] Schoemaker, M. J, Swerdlow, A. J, Ahlbom, A, et al. Mobile phone use and risk of acoustic neuroma: results of the Interphone case-control study in five North European countries. Br J Cancer 93 [7], (2005). Ref Type: Electronic Citation, 842-848.

[169] Cardis, E, Deltour, I, Vrijheid, M, et al. Acoustic neuroma risk in relation to mobile telephone use: results of the INTERPHONE international case-control study. INTERPHONE Study Group. Cancer Epidemiol. 35 [5], (2011). Ref Type: Electronic Citation, 453-464.

[170] Kundi, M. Mobile phone use and brain cancer: is the association biased? Neuroepidemiology (2010). , 35(2), 115-116.

[171] Olsen, J. The interphone study: brain cancer and beyond. Bioelectromagnetics (2011). , 32(2), 164-167.

[172] Hardell, L. Hansson Mild K. Mobile phone use and risk of acoustic neuroma: results of the interphone case-control study in five North European countries. Br J Cancer 94 [9], (2006). Ref Type: Electronic Citation, 1348-1349.

[173] Hardell, L, & Carlberg, M. Hansson Mild K. Epidemiological evidence for an association between use of wireless phones and tumor diseases. Pathophysiology 16 [(2-3)], (2009). Ref Type: Electronic Citation, 113-122.

[174] Little, M. P, Rajaraman, P, Curtis, R. E, et al. Mobile phone use and glioma risk: comparison of epidemiological study results with incidence trends in the United States. BMJ.2012 Mar 8;344:e1147.doi:bmj.e1147. (2012). Ref Type: Electronic Citation

[175] Sarasua, S, & Savitz, D. A. Cured and broiled meat consumption in relation to childhood cancer: Denver, Colorado (United States). Cancer Causes Control (1994). , 5(2), 141-148.

[176] Bunin, G. R, Kuitjen, R. R, Boesel, C. P, Buckley, J. D, & Meadows, A. T. Maternal diet and risk of astrocytic glioma in children: a report from the Childrens Cancer Group (United States and Canada). Cancer Causes Control 5 [2], (1994). Ref Type: Electronic Citation, 177-187.

[177] Bunin, G. R, Kuitjen, R. R, Buckley, J. D, Rorke, L. B, & Meadows, A. T. Relation between maternal diet and subsequent primitive neuroectodermal brain tumors in young children. N Engl J Med. 329 [8], (1993). Ref Type: Electronic Citation, 536-541.

[178] Forman, D. Commentary: Nitrites, nitrates and nitrosation as causes of brain cancer in children: epidemiological challenges. Int J Epidemiol (2004). , 33(6), 1216-1218.

[179] Khuder, S. A, Mutgi, A. B, & Schaub, E. A. Meta-analyses of brain cancer and farming. Am J Ind Med (1998). , 34(3), 252-260.

[180] Clapp, R. W, Jacobs, M. M, & Loechler, E. L. Environmental and occupational causes of cancer: new evidence 2005-2007. Rev Environ Health (2008). , 23(1), 1-37.

[181] Daniels, J. L, Olshan, A. F, & Savitz, D. A. Pesticides and childhood cancers. Environ Health Perspect (1997). , 105(10), 1068-1077.

[182] Shim, Y. K, Mlynarek, S. P, & Wijngaarden, E. Parental exposure to pesticides and childhood brain cancer: U.S. Atlantic coast childhood brain cancer study. Environ Health Perspect (2009). , 117(6), 1002-1006.

[183] Van Wijngaarden, E, Stewart, P. A, Olshan, A. F, Savitz, D. A, & Bunin, G. R. Parental occupational exposure to pesticides and childhood brain cancer. Am J Epidemiol (2003). , 157(11), 989-997.

[184] Davis, J. R, Brownson, R. C, Garcia, R, Bentz, B. J, & Turner, A. Family pesticide use and childhood brain cancer. Arch Environ Contam Toxicol (1993). , 24(1), 87-92.

[185] Leiss, J. K, & Savitz, D. A. Home pesticide use and childhood cancer: a case-control study. Am J Public Health 85 [2], (1995). Ref Type: Electronic Citation, 249-252.

[186] Inskip, P. D, Linet, M. S, & Heineman, E. F. Etiology of brain tumors in adults. Epidemiol Rev. 17 [2], (1995). Ref Type: Electronic Citation, 382-414.

[187] Heineman, E. F, Ward, M. H, Mccomb, R. D, Weisenburger, D. D, & Zahm, S. H. Hair dyes and risk of glioma among Nebraska women. Cancer Causes Control (2005). , 16(7), 857-864.

[188] Efird, J. T, Holly, E. A, Cordier, S, et al. Beauty product-related exposures and childhood brain tumors in seven countries: results from the SEARCH International Brain Tumor Study. J Neurooncol. 72 [2], (2005). Ref Type: Electronic Citation, 133-147.

[189] Choi, H. S, Shim, Y. K, Kaye, W. E, & Ryan, P. B. Potential residential exposure to toxics release inventory chemicals during pregnancy and childhood brain cancer. Environ Health Perspect (2006). , 114(7), 1113-1118.

[190] Mckean-cowden, R, Preston-martin, S, Pogoda, J. M, Holly, E. A, Mueller, B. A, & Davis, R. L. Parental occupation and childhood brain tumors: astroglial and primitive neuroectodermal tumors. J Occup Environ Med. 40 [4], (1998). Ref Type: Electronic Citation, 332-340.

[191] Savitz, D. A, & Chen, J. H. Parental occupation and childhood cancer: review of epidemiologic studies. Environ Health Perspect (1990).

[192] Colt, J. S, & Blair, A. Parental occupational exposures and risk of childhood cancer. Environ Health Perspect. 106 [Suppl 3], (1998). Ref Type: Electronic Citation, 909-925.

[193] Ali, R, Yu, C. L, Wu, M. T, et al. A case-control study of parental occupation, leukemia, and brain tumors in an industrial city in Taiwan. J Occup Environ Med. 46 [9], (2004). Ref Type: Electronic Citation, 985-992.

[194] Mutanen, P, & Hemminki, K. Childhood cancer and parental occupation in the Swedish Family-Cancer Database. J Occup Environ Med. 43 [11], (2001). Ref Type: Electronic Citation, 952-958.

[195] Cordier, S, Mandereau, L, Preston-martin, S, et al. Parental occupations and childhood brain tumors: results of an international case-control study. Cancer Causes Control 12 [9], (2001). Ref Type: Electronic Citation, 865-874.

[196] Cordier, S, Lefeuvre, B, Filippini, G, et al. Parental occupation, occupational exposure to solvents and polycyclic aromatic hydrocarbons and risk of childhood brain tumors (Italy, France, Spain). Cancer Causes Control 8 [5], (1997). Ref Type: Electronic Citation, 688-697.

[197] Mazumdar, M, Liu, C. Y, Wang, S. F, et al. No association between parental or subject occupation and brain tumor risk. Cancer Epidemiol Biomarkers Prev. 17 [7], (2008). Ref Type: Electronic Citation, 1835-1837.

[198] Rosso, A. L, Hovinga, M. E, Rorke-adams, L. B, Spector, L. G, & Bunin, G. R. Children's Oncology Group. A case-control study of childhood brain tumors and fathers' hobbies: a Children's Oncology Group study. Cancer Causes Control 19 [10], (2008). Ref Type: Electronic Citation, 1201-1207.

[199] Samuelson, S. O, Bakketeig, L. S, Tretli, S, Johannesen, T. B, & Magnus, P. Head circumference at birth and risk of brain cancer in childhood: a population-based study. Lancet Oncol (2006). , 7(1), 39-42.

[200] Maule, M, Scelo, G, Pastore, G, et al. Risk of second malignant neoplasms after childhood leukemia and lymphoma: an international study. J Natl Cancer Inst (2007). , 99(10), 790-800.

[201] Monteiro, G. T, Pereira, R. A, Koifman, R. J, & Koifman, S. Head injury and brain tumours in adults: A case-control study in Rio de Janeiro, Brazil. Eur J Cancer (2006). , 42(7), 917-921.

[202] Bille, C, Winther, J. F, Bautz, A, Murray, J. C, Olsen, J, & Christensen, K. Cancer risk in persons with oral cleft--a population-based study of 8,093 cases. Am J Epidemiol (2005). , 161(11), 1047-1055.

[203] Mcbride, M. L. Childhood cancer and environmental contaminants. [Article in English, French]. Can J Public Health 89 [Suppl 1], SS62. (1998). Ref Type: Electronic Citation, 53.

[204] Kuitjen, R. R, Bunin, G, Nass, C. C, & Meadows, A. T. Gestational and familial risk factors for childhood astrocytoma: results of a case-control study. Cancer Res. 50 [9], (1990). Ref Type: Electronic Citation, 2608-2612.

[205] Stalberg, K, Haglund, B, Stromberg, B, & Kieler, H. Prenatal exposure to medicines and the risk of childhood brain tumor. Cancer Epidemiol. 34 [4], (2010). Ref Type: Electronic Citation, 400-404.

[206] Scheurer, M. E, Amirian, E. S, Davlin, S. L, Rice, T, Wrensch, M, & Bondy, M. L. Effects of antihistamine and anti-inflammatory medication use on risk of specific glioma histologies. Int J Cancer 129 [9], (2011). Ref Type: Electronic Citation, 2290-2296.